Clinical Cardiology in the Elderly

Second Edition

Edited by

Elliot Chesler, M.D.

**Futura Publishing
Company, Inc.**
Armonk, NY
1999

Library of Congress Cataloging-in-Publication Data

Clinical cardiology in the elderly / edited by Elliot Chesler. — 2nd ed.
    p. cm.
    Includes bibliographical references and index.
    ISBN 0-87993-421-2
    1. Geriatric cardiology. I. Chesler, Elliot.
    [DNLM: 1. Heart Diseases—in old age. 2. Heart Dis-
eases—therapy.   WG 200C6415 1999]
    RC682.C566 1999
    618.97′612—dc21
    DNLM/DLC
    for Library of Congress   98-42493
                                        CIP

Copyright 1999
Futura Publishing Company, Inc.

Published by
Futura Publishing Company, Inc.
135 Bedford Road
Armonk, New York 10504-0418

LC #: 98-42493
ISBN #: 0-87993-421-2

Printed in the United States of America.

This book is printed on acid-free paper.

Contents

Part 2. Diseases of the Heart and Pulmonary Vasculature

Part 5. Noncardiac Surgery

Part 6. Ethics

Contributors

Inderjit Anand, M.D. Director, Heart Failure Clinic, Cardiovascular Section, VA Medical Center, Minneapolis, Professor of Medicine, University of Minnesota

Stephen L. Archer, M.D. Professor and Head, Division of Cardiology Walter C. Mackenzie, Health Science Center University of Alberta Edmonton, Alberta Canada

Howard B. Burchell, M.D. Professor Emeritus and Chief of Cardiology, University of Minnesota. Consultant in Medicine Emeritus, Mayo Clinic, Rochester, Minnesota

Christine K. Cassel, M.D. Professor and Chairman, The Henry L. Schwartz Department of Geriatrics & Adult Development, Mt. Sinai Medical Center, New York, New York

Elliot Chesler, M.D. Chief, Cardiovascular Section, VA Medical Center, Minneapolis and Professor of Medicine, University of Minnesota

Andrew Clark, L.M.A., M.D., M.R.C.P. Senior Registrar in Cardiology, Western Infrimary Glasgow UK

Leighton E. Cluff, M.D. Former President, The Robert Wood Johnson Foundation, VA Medical Center, Minneapolis

Andrew J.S. Coats, D.M., M.R.C.P. Professor of Cardiology, Royal Brompton National Heart and Lung Institute London UK.

Jenifer Daley, M.D. Division of General Medicine and Primary Care, Department of Medicine, Beth Israel Deaconess Medical Center, Harvard Medical School.

Jesse E. Edwards, M.D. Senior Consultant, Registry of Cardiovascular Disease, United Hospitals, St. Paul, Minnesota and Professor of Pathology, University of Minnesota

Emily J. Erbelding, M.D. Assistant Professor of Medicine, Division of Infectious Diseases, John's Hopkins Medical School, Baltimore, Maryland

Steven Fannin, M.D. Instructor, Department of Medicine, Divisions of Cardiology and Geriatrics, University Hospital, Case Western Reserve University School of Medicine, Cleveland, Ohio

Arthur H.L, From, M.D. Director, Electrocardiography Laboratory, Cardiovascular Section, VA Medical Center, Minneapolis, and Professor of Medicine, University of Minnesota

Julius M. Gardin, M.D. Professor of Medicine, Department of Medicine/ Cardiology, University of California, Irvine, California. President Emeritus Council of Geriatric Cardiology

Dale Gerding, M.D. Professor and Associate Chairman, Department of Medicine, Northwestern University, Chief Medical Service, Lakeside VA Medical Center, Chicago, Illinois

Bernard J. Gersh, M.B., Ch.B., D. Phil W. Proctor Harvey Professor of Medicine, Chief Division of Cardiology, Georgetown University Medical Center, Washington, DC

Charles C. Gornick, M.D. Director, Electrophysiology Laboratory, Cardiovascular Section, VA Medical Center, Minneapolis, and Assistant Professor, University of Minnesota

Diederick E. Grobbee, M.D., Ph.D. Department of Epidemiology and Biostatics, Erasmus University Medical School, Rotterdam, The Netherlands

Eugene A. Grossi, M.D. Division of Cardiothoracic Surgery, Department of Surgery, New York University Medical Center, New York

Jordan L. Holtzman, M.D. Chief, Therapeutics Section, VA Medical Center, Minneapolis, and Professor of Medicine, University of Minnesota.

Richard A. Josephson, M.D. Director of Cardiology Research and Education Summa Health System, Professor of Cardiology, Northeast Ohio Universities College of Medicine,Associate Professor of Biomedical Engineering, University of Akron, Ohio

Frank Lederle, M.D. General Internal Medicine Section, VA Medical Center, Minneapolis and Associate Professor of Medicine, University of Minnesota

Edward O. McFalls, M.D. Consultant Cardiovascular Section, VA Medical Center, Minneapolis, and Assistant Professor of Medicine, University of Minnesota

Henry D. McIntosh, M.D. Cardiologist, The Watson Clinic, Lakeland, Florida, and Clinical Professor of Medicine, University of Florida College of Medicine, Gainesville, Florida

Mary Ann Mclaughlin, M.D., M.P.H. Assistant Professor, The Henry L. Schwartz Department of Geriatrics and Adult Development, Department of Medicine, Division of Cardiology, The Mount Sinai Medical Center, New York, New York

Celia Oakley, M.D. Consultant Cardiologist, Hammersmith Hospital and the Royal Postgraduate Medical School, London.

Philip Podrid, M.D. Director Arrythmia Service University Hospital, Boston, and Associate Professor of Medicine, Boston University School of Medicine Boston, MA

Gordon L. Pierpont, M.D. Director, CCU, Cardiovascular Section, VA Medical Center, Minneapolis and Associate Professor of Medicine, University of Minnesota

Alfredo Rego, M.D., Ph.D. Department of Surgery University of Minnesota, Minneapolis, Minnesota

Joseph Rinaldi, M.D. Internist Summa Health System, Cleveland, Ohio

Hanna Rubins, M.D. Department of Medicine, VA Medical Center, Minneapolis and Associate Professor of Medicine, University of Minnesota

Luis F. Santamarina Department of Cardiothoracic Surgery VA Medical Center, University of Minnesota, Minneapolis, Minnesota

Norman Shumway, M.D. Department of Cardiothoracic Surgery, University of Minnesota, Minneapolis, MN; Department of Cardiovascular Surgery, Stanford University Medical Center, Stanford, CA

Sara Shumway, M.D.   Department of Cardiothoracic Surgery, University of Minnesota, Minneapolis, MN; Department of Cardiovascular Surgery, Stanford University Medical Center, Stanford, CA

Geza Simon, M.D.   Director, Hypertension Clinic, VA Medical Center, and Associate Professor of Medicine, University of Minnesota, Minneapolis, Minnesota

George, E. Thibault, M.D.   Chief Medical Officer Brigham and Women's Hospital Associate Professor of Medicine, Harvard Medical School.

Randall C. Thompson, M.D.   Consultant, Division of Cardiovascular Diseases, Mayo Clinic Jacksonville, Florida, and Assistant Professor of Medicine, Mayo Medical School; Rochester, Minnesota

Jack L. Titus, M.D.   Director, Registry of Cardiovascular Disease, United Hospitals, St. Paul, Minnesota and Professor of Pathology, University of Minnesota

Tom Treasure, M.D., M.S., F.R.C.S.   Consultant Cardiothoracic Surgeon, St. Georges Hospital, London, UK. Jonathan Unsworth-White, BSsc, FRCS(CTh) Consultant Cardiothoracic Surgeon St. Georges Hospital, London, UK

Herbert Ward, M.D.   Chief, Cardiovascular Surgery, VA Medical Center, Minneapolis and Thoracic Surgery Staff, University of Minnesota

E. Kenneth Weir, M.D.   Director, Cardiac Catheterization Laboratory, Cardiovascular Section, VA Medical Center, Minneapolis and Professor of Medicine, University of Minnesota

Timothy Wilt, M.D.   General Internal Medicine Section, VA Medical Center, Minneapolis and Associate Professor of Medicine, University of Minnesota

Steven Wright Ph.D.   Health Research Scientist, Health Services Research and Development West Roxbury, VA Medical Center, Boston Massachusetts

Preface

There is no dearth of textbooks dealing with the many facets of cardiology. Why yet another? Most cardiologists, including the contributors to this book, are not geriatricians, but because of demographic changes in western countries, they treat more and more elderly patients. Our earlier experience in adult and even pediatric cardiology permitted quick, accurate bedside diagnosis and appropriate, often curative treatment. In the elderly, however, valued tools such as cardiac auscultation and electrocardiography are improved by more precise noninvasive techniques such as echocardiography. Treatment is also more complicated because decisions have to be carefully weighed against a background of multiple chronic diseases and the expectations of patients and their families about duration and quality of life.

The goal in compiling this book has not been to encapsulate information about geriatric cardiology that might be found in various sections of well-known textbooks. The contributors are qualified to provide perspective into problems as diverse as cardiac defibrillators, cardiopulmonary resuscitation, clinical trials, the doctrine of informed consent, and euthanasia. The second edition is completely revised and there are new contributions dealing with issues such as peripheral vascular disease, abdominal aortic aneurysms, heart muscle disease and quality of life following cardiac surgery, etc. Hopefully, their knowledge will help us better manage elderly patients in an era when expenditures perspective into problems as diverse as cardiac defibrillators, cardiopulmonary resuscitation, clinical trials, the doctrine of informed consent, and euthanasia. The second edition is completely revised and there are new contributions dealing with issues such as peripheral vascular disease, abdominal aortic aneurysms, heart muscle disease and quality of life following cardiac surgery, etc. Hopefully, their knowledge will help us better manage elderly patients in an era when expenditures on health care costs are at the forefront of political and ethical thinking.

Elliot Chesler, M. D.

Guest Introduction

"If wrinkles must be written upon our brows, let them not be written upon the heart. The spirit should not grow old."

James A. Garfield

Since the end of World War II, most industrialized societies have experienced a revolution in longevity. There are now more than 30 million Americans—12% of the population—older than 65 years, constituting a greater proportion of the population than those under 25 years old. It is predicted that by the year 2000, the proportion above age 80 years will have doubled because of declining mortality rates, and that by the year 2030 more than half of all Americans now alive will have survived until at least their 85th birthday.[1,2]

Clearly, a large growing share of the American health care dollar will be spent on the elderly in general, and on the "oldest-old" in particular. Currently, health care for people over age 65 years is responsible for almost 40% of American's health care expenditure.[3] For every nine dollars spent on health care for the elderly, only one dollar is spent on health care for children. In this era of cost containment, it is important for a wide array of physicians—including geriatricians, cardiologists, family care physicians, internists, surgeons, and other subspecialists—to be aware of the most current information regarding the evaluation and treatment of cardiovascular problems in the elderly.

It is because of these consideration that a book focusing on clinical geriatric cardiology is of such importance. The second edition of *Clinical Cardiology in the Elderly*, edited by Dr. Elliot Chesler, and with contributions from 40 other experts, however, is not merely another book in the field. Rather, it is a superb compilation of chapters dealing with every aspect of geriatric cardiology ranging from the anatomy and pathophysiology of aging, presentation and treatment of common cardiac diseases, peculiarities of drug action and disposition, and cardiac and noncardiac surgery to socioeconomic and ethical considerations in the care of the elderly. I would like to share with you briefly my personal thoughts on the contributions presented in the various chapters of this book. Although these reflections cannot do justice to the scope of the work presented, I hope they will provide a helpful overview and introduction.

McLaughlin and Cassel provide important perspectives in a new chapter (Chapter 1) on "Demography and Epidemiology of Cardiovascular Disease in Old Age." It is well know that the risk of death due to congenital heart disease (CHD) is delayed, on average, by 10 years in women compared to men. Of interest, CHD death rates are 34% higher for black women than white women, and 5% higher for black men than white men. Although the relative importance of CHD risk factors (e.g., hypertension, hyperlipidemia, diabetes, and smoking) decreases somewhat with age, these factors continue to impart substantial risk in the elderly due to the high incidence and prevalence of coronary disease in this population. Stroke, the third leading cause of death in the U.S., is also believed to be the leading cause of disability. Although the mortality from stroke has been declining (e.g., by 20% from 1984 to 1994), it still has a prevalence of approximately 5% and 2% in 65–69 year old men and women, respectively, and 10% in men 80–84 years of age. Importantly, African-American men and women are 2.5 more time likely to die of stroke than are Caucasians. Although the decline in CHD mortality over the past 20 years has been multifactorial, it appears that treatment of patients with CHD, e.g., by an increase in use of revascularization procedures, has contributed more to the decline of CHD mortality than have primary prevention measures.

In Chapter 2, Drs. Titus and Edwards present a very cogent discussion of the pathological changes that are characteristic of the aging heart that involve the valves, myocardium, conduction system, aorta, and pericardium. Aortic sclerosis and calcification of the mitral annulus, senile atrophy, and amyloid infiltration of the myocardium and sigmoid (ventricular) septum are just a few of the conditions discussed in detail.

In the third chapter, "Physiology of the Aging Heart," Drs. Josephson and Fannin present the important concept that the primary age-related changes in cardiovascular physiology are similar to those accompanying systemic hypertension, namely, decreased arterial distensibility related to loss of elastic tissue, deposition of calcium, and increased amount and altered composition of collagen in the arterial wall. This primary decrease in arterial compliance results in increased left ventricular wall thickness and abnormal left ventricular early diastolic relaxation and filling. Other accompaniments of the aging process include a blunting of the cardiovascular response to catecholamine stimulation and impaired calcium release by the sarcoplasmic reticulum.

In a new Chapter (Chapter 5), deBruyne and colleagues describe the "Prevalence and Prognosis of Electrocardiographic Findings in the Elderly." Because of the relatively high prevalence of ECG abnormalities combined with the relatively high incidence of cardiac disease in the elderly, the ECG may prove valuable as a screening tool for older individuals at risk for future coronary heart disease. For example, the authors note that the prevalence of silent myocardial infarction (detected by ECG) in the Rotterdam Study was in the range of 4%, with the prognosis of these ECG findings being similar to that of clinical myocardial infarction. Furthermore, the prognosis of left ventricular hypertrophy by ECG was reported to be similar to that of silent myocardial infarction in the Framingham Heart Study. In asymptomatic men and women, non-specific ST-T wave abnormalities have been associated with a two-fold risk for future cardiovascular events. Atrial fibrillation on ECG is a well-known indicator of future risk, having been associated with such outcomes as thrombotic stroke, cardiovascular and all — cause mortality and dementia.

In Chapter 6, Drs. Erbelding, Gerding, and Chesler point out that over the past few decades, infective endocarditis has become a disease with a predilection for the elderly, and frequently exhibits an ambiguous clinical presentation (e.g., the absence of the so-called "classic" findings of fever, splinter hemorrhages, and changing murmur). Unlike earlier decades, when infective endocarditis disproportionately occurred on rheumatic valves in younger individuals, clinicians are increasingly seeing elderly individuals with nosocomial and prosthetic valve endocarditis. The fatality rate for infective endocarditis in the elderly is reported to be in the range of 45%! It is obvious that the clinician must have a high index of suspicion for infective endocarditis in the elderly, or the diagnosis may be missed, as it reportedly is initially in up to 60% of cases.

Drs. Archer and Weir discuss, in Chapter 7, pulmonary hypertension as it presents in the elderly. Paul Wood's classification of pulmonary hypertension is still quite useful, namely passive (i.e., secondary to LV failure); hyperkinetic (i.e., secondary to increased blood flow), obstructive/obliterative; and vasoconstrictive ("reactive"). The most common cause for pulmonary hypertension in the elderly appears to be passive, i.e., secondary to LV failure, with possibly superimposed pulmonary arterial remodeling and vasoconstriction. This chapter discusses in detail the diagnosis and therapy for primary and secondary pulmonary hypertension. In Chapter 8, Drs. Archer and Chesler highlight some of the difficulties involved in the diagnosis of valve disease in the elderly. For example, they point out that it is not uncommon for subacute bacterial endocarditis (SBE) to present in the elderly as clinical heart failure without a murmur, since 40% of SBE cases involve normal valves. Furthermore, mitral annular calcification has been shown, in the Framingham Heart Study (FHS), to be an independent risk factor for stroke, while embolization of thoracic aortic atherosclerotic debris is a common cause of intraoperative stroke.

Chapter 9 discusses the presentation and evaluation of ischemic heart disease. Dr. McIntosh points out that classic ischemic pain is not as frequent a presenting symptom in the elderly as it is in younger individuals, suggesting a possibly higher pain threshold in the elderly. In particular, in patients over 85 years of age, dyspnea is a more common presenting symptom of ischemia. In addition, silent ischemia is not uncommon in the elderly. Dr. Pierpont continues the discussion of ischemic heart disease in chapter 10, emphasizing a therapeutic approach that takes into account the severity of symptoms, myocardial damage, "at-risk" myocardium, and salvageable myocardium.

In new Chapter 11, Wright and colleagues tackle the interesting problem of "Cardiac Procedure Use and Outcomes of Elderly Patients with Acute Myocardial Infarction." These researchers analyzed a large database of VA hospitalizations (n = 72,276) between 1988 and 1997 for the principal diagnosis of acute myocardial infarction and compared these data to data available for patients with acute myocardial infarction admitted to both non-federal Medicare hospital and Canadian hospitals. When rates of coronary angiography, coronary angioplasty, and coronary bypass surgery for 1992 were compared, Medicare and VA patients had similar rates of coronary angiography (33%–-35%), but Medicare patients experienced nearly twice the rates of coronary angioplasty (11.7% versus 5.4%) and coronary bypass surgery (10.6% versus 4.8%). Procedure rates in Canada were substantially lower, being under 2% for coronary angioplasty and bypass surgery. Despite these differences, there was no significant difference among the three systems in unadjusted 1-year mortality rate (approximately 33%) in elderly acute myocardiac infarction patients. However, clinical trials such as SAVE and GUSTO have suggested that functional status and quality of life may be improved by the higher procedure rate prevalent to US versus Canada.

In Chapter 12, Dr. Pierpont presents a consideration of factors that may complicate therapy of angina in the elderly. These include resting bradycardia, atrioventricular conduction delay and susceptibility to heart block, orthostatic and postprandial hypotension, unexplained syncope of near-syncope, and multiple drug therapy. The discussion suggests that factors of potential importance in the decision of when to treat silent ischemia in the elderly include amount of myocardium at risk, status of left ventricular function, presence of related disorders, e.g., hypertension, and presence of life-threatening arrhythmias or hypotension.

In Chapter 13, Drs. Thompson and Gersh emphasize the increased mortality in the "oldest-old," i.e., those above 75 years of age, that accompanies both coronary artery bypass surgery and percutaneous transluminal coronary angioplasty (PTCA). Despite the fact that over 40% of coronary revascularization procedures in the United States and performed in patients above the age of 65 years, no direct randomized trial has been performed comparing medical therapy, PTCA, and coronary artery bypass surgery in the elderly. Although coronary artery bypass surgery provides good relief of angina and improved survival in "young-old" (ages 65 to 75 years) patients with left main or triple-vessel disease, there is an increased rate of stroke compared with that in individuals under age 65. Predictors of poor outcome post-PTCA include female gender, triple-vessel or diffuse coronary artery disease, and left ventricular ejection fraction less than 40%.

In a new chapter (Chapter 14), Dr. Rubins presents a comprehensive analysis of "Management of Lipid Disorders" in the elderly. Hypercholesterolemia is highly prevalent among the elderly: 46% of nearly 5,000 community-living persons over age 65 in the Cardiovascular Health Study had an LDL cholesterol >160 mg/dl. The relation between cholesterol level and coronary heart disease (CHD) in the elderly has been controversial. In 1992, an analysis of Manolio et al of 22 observational epidemiologic studies of 15,000 women and 49,000 men over age 65 concluded that the relative risk for CHD death in those with total cholesterol >240 mg/dl compared with cholesterol <200 mg/dl was 1.32 in men and 1.12 in women (both comparisons statistically significant). Although the increased relative risks related to higher cholesterol in the elderly appear relatively modest, especially compared with similar comparisons in younger-aged individuals, Rubins notes that because CHD is so much more prevalent among the elderly, a small increase in relative risk results in an important increase in excess (or attributable) risk. The chapter summarizes data from the 4S and CARE secondary prevention trials suggesting that cholesterol-lowering therapy with statin safely reduces the 5-year risk of CHD morbidity and mortality in elderly patients up to age 70–75, with a documented history of CHD and LDL-cholesterol >125 mg/dl. Dr. Rubins also provides a useful algorithm, based on the Framingham Multivariate Risk Function, for deciding who to screen and treat for hyperlipidemia among elderly persons without CHD.

In Chapter 15, Drs. Gornick and From present a comprehensive discussion of arrhythmias. Alterations in the normal conduction system with age may result in conduction delays that facilitate the development of reentrant arrhythmias. As in younger adults, elderly patients with the poorest ventricular function are at the highest risk for recurrence of significant ventricular tachyarrhythmias and sudden death. However, identifying tolerable antiarrhythmic drug therapy may be difficult in the elderly because of concomitant diseases (including pulmonary, hepatic, and renal), poor ventricular function, and acid-base or electrolyte disturbances. Automatic implantable cardiac defibrillators have proved quite successful, but in elderly patients who are not candidates for this therapy, e.g., those with intractable CHF, multisystem disease, etc., amiodarone may probe to be useful.

In Dr. Gornick's presentation on evaluation and treatment of the elderly patient with syncope (Chapter 16), the prevalence of syncope in a free-living population above the age of 75 years (FHS) is reported as 5.6% in men, compared to 0.7% in men in the 35- to 44-year age group. Etiologies for syncope include cardiac (e.g., aortic stenosis); "neurally mediated" ("vasovagal"), which is associated with hypotension and/or bradycardia, and can often be diagnosed by autonomic maneuvers such as head-up tilt testing; and neurological/psychiatric, e.g., seizures, sleep disorders, etc. There is an extensive discussion of orthostatic hypotension, which is reportedly present in up to 30% of medical outpatients above the age of 75 years. This condition confers an increased risk for subsequent falls and syncope and, almost paradoxically, appears to be more prevalent in patients with supine hypertension. A related problem, postprandial hypotension, is reportedly present in 15% of institutionalized elderly individuals. The chapter includes a useful discussion of the relative cost-effectiveness of electrophysiological studies (most useful in those with structural heart disease) and provocative autonomic studies, e.g., carotid sinus massage and head-up tilt testing (most useful in patients without structural heart disease).

In Chapter 17, "Hypertension in the Elderly," Dr. Simon points out that systolic hypertension was discovered in the FHS to be more predictive of future cardiovascular complications than was diastolic hypertension.[4] The prevalence of isolated systolic hypertension increased from 6% in the 60- to 69-year age decade to 18% in those over 80 years of age in the Systolic Hypertension in the Elderly Program (SHEP) study.[5] A number of studies, including SHEP, have demonstrated a decrease in stroke attributable to treatment of systolic hypertension in the elderly. This chapter presents a reasoned discussion of the advantages and side effects of various proposed antihypertensive therapies in the elderly.

Dr. Celia Oakley, an expert on cardiomyopathies, provides a new Chapter (Chapter 18) entitled "Heart Muscle Disease.". Although primary cardiomyopathy accounts for only a small proportion of (elderly) patients with heart failure—myocardial infarction and hypertension being much more important—the hypertrophic, dilated, and restrictive forms of cardiomyopathy present an interesting spectrum. The reader should find fascinating the discussion of the confusion involved in differentiating *hypertensive hypertrophic* from *senile pseudo-hypertrophic* from *genetic hypertrophic cardiomyopathy*, as well as the discussion of the pathophysiology of cardiac amyloidosis—amyloid being the major cause of severe restrictive cardiomyopathy in the elderly.

Dr. Anand presents a new in-depth review of "Pathophysiology of Chronic Heart Failure" in Chapter 19. He emphasizes the concept that age-related changes in cardiovascular structure and function act to reduce the capacity of older individuals to respond normally to both physiological stress and disease states, greatly increasing the risk of developing congestive heart failure in the elderly. For example, approximately 35% of total cardiac myocytes may be lost with aging due to a process known as *apoptosis* —programmed cell death. Since adult cardiac myocytes are terminally-differentiated and cannot divide, the apoptotic myocytes are replaced by hypertrophy of the remaining myocytes and increased interstitial connective tissue. These and other physiological alterations with aging result in increased myocardial and aortic stiffness, as well as impaired LV relaxation, result in impaired left ventricular diastolic filling. These changes help account for the fact LV diastolic dysfunction accounts for heart failure syndrome in a substantial portion of elderly patients, especially women. In addition, the contractile response to B_1-adrenergic receptor stimulation is attenuated with aging. Dr. Anand points out that the important adaptive mechanisms in response to left ventricular dysfunction include activation of neurohormones, the Frank-Starling mechanism, and myocardial hypertrophy. He emphasizes the important and complex role of neurohormonal activation, including the vasoconstrictor hormones—e.g., norepinephrine, the renin-angiotensin-aldosterone system and arginine vasopressin; vasodilator hormones—e.g., atrial and brain natriuretic peptides, prostaglandins, and the kallikrein-kinin system. Although neurohormonal activation initially helps to maintain circulatory homeostasis, prolonged neurohormonal activation, associated with congestive heart failure, ultimately becomes deleterious.

In Chapter 20, "Management of Congestive Heart Failure," congestive heart failure (CHF) is defined as decreased functional capacity due to inability of the heart to circulate blood adequately to meet physiological demands. In addition to brief discussions of high output failure and primary right heart failure, Dr. Pierpont presents an extensive discussion of left heart failure, including the importance of diastolic dysfunction in the elderly. It has been estimated that LV diastolic dysfunction in the presence of normal systolic function may account for more than one third of cases of heart failure in the elderly.[6] Patients with decreases in both LV diastolic compliance and peripheral arterial compliance have left ventricles that operate on the steeper portion of the LV pressure-volume curve. These elderly patients are, therefore, more sensitive to changes in intravascular volume and can more easily develop symptomatic heart failure. Practical guidance is provided regarding appropriate treatment for acute decompensation as well as chronic CHF, including the appropriate role for diuretics, inotropics, digoxin, vasodilators, antiarrhythmic agents, and nasal oxygen.

Clark and Coats present considerations related to "Physical Exercise and Training in Congestive Heart Failure" in a new chapter (Chapter 21). The authors note that many of the changes seen in the periphery in patients with chronic heart failure are similar to those seen in deconditioned normal subjects—mainly, activation of the renin-angiotensin system, loss of skeletal muscle, and depletion of oxidative enzymes. Reports in the literature suggest that exercise training can produce an improvement of approximately 20% in exercise capacity. Of interest, exercise training apparently produces little change in central hemodynamics, but measurable improvements primarily in skeletal muscle structure and metabolism. Training programs as short as 4 weeks have resulted in improvements in exercise capacity, with training effects reaching a plateau in 4 to 6 months. Furthermore, programs featuring training at 50% of maximal exercise capacity have been associated with measurable improvement in exercise capacity and quality of life—at less risk than higher-intensity exercise programs.

In a new contribution (Chapter 22), Rego and associates summarize the experience with "Cardiac Transplantation" in older patients, defined as over age 55. There have been very few heart transplant recipients older than 70 years. Of interest, survival rates among the "elderly" have been found in several clinical series to be comparable to younger patients undergoing heart transplantation. The elderly are not as likely to reject a transplanted heart, but appear to be at increased risk to develop infection, malignancy, osteoporosis, and steroid-induced diabetes following transplantation. Although immunosuppression should be scaled down in the elderly, including initiating a more rapid tapering of steroids, the authors conclude that age alone is not a significant criterion for exclusion from heart transplantation.

Drs. Ward and Santamarina offer important insights regarding cardiac surgery in Chapter 23. They reiterate that in elderly patients, coronary artery bypass surgery relieves angina as frequently as it does in younger patients. However, data from multiple centers suggest that in addition to age above 75 years, important risk factors for poor postoperative outcome include urgency of surgery (elective: 4%, urgent: 11%, and emergency: 26% mortality in their series); pump time, need for intraoperative balloon pump; and reoperation. The higher incidence of perioperative stroke in the elderly may be due to factors such as hypotension, hypoperfusion during cardiopulmonary bypass, heparin-induced intracerebral bleed, or atheromatous emboli from the aorta. With regard to valve surgery, the mortality from a combined multicenter series was reportedly 10.6%, with no difference in perioperative mortality between aortic and mitral valve replacement. Risk factors for valve surgery in the elderly include multiple valve surgery, isolated aortic regurgitation, emergency operation, previous cardiac surgery, and concomitant coronary artery disease.

In Chapter 24, Grossi et al. review the literature and summarize their results at New York University related to "Mitral Valve Repair" in the elderly. Because of improvements in the techniques of cardiopulmonary bypass and cardiac anesthesia, the risk of surgery in the elderly, including octogenarians, has been reduced dramatically. Operative mortality for isolated mitral valve repair was 5.7% in patients ≥70 years, compared to 1.4% in those <70 years of age. However, the addition of an operation for concomitant coronary artery disease, more common in the elderly, increases the operative mortality in the >70 age group to 16%, compared to 7.4% for combined mitral valve repair and CABG in the <70 year old group. The authors make the important point that elderly patients who were referred for mitral valvuloplasty early in their disease process, i.e., when asymptomatic with well-preserved ventricular function, had a low operative risk—not significantly different from that of younger patients. In addition, the authors point out that the presence of mitral annular calcification in elderly patients does not preclude successful mitral valvuloplasty.

In new Chapter 25, Unsworth-White and Treasure provide some important insights regarding "Quality of Life after Cardiac Surgery in Patients Older Than Seventy Years." The authors point out that after indicated cardiac surgery, elderly patients appear to perceive just as much gain in their quality of life as their younger counterparts, albeit they may register lower scores on specific health measurements reflecting physical role and social functions, etc., and have had to accept greater risks of surgery and post-operative complications. In particular, the incidence of post-operative stroke (approximately in 6.5%) and cognitive impairment is higher in the elderly. The authors cite interesting work from the Middlesex Hospital which is the use of a 40-micron filter on the arterial side of the cardiopulmonary bypass circuit resulted in a decreased embolic load (as detected by transcranial Doppler signals), accompanied by a reduced post-operative incidence of neuropsychological deficits and depression.

In a new chapter (Chapter 26), Lederle summarizes the literature and his experience with "Abdominal Aortic Aneurysms." Aortic aneurysms constitute the tenth leading cause of death in older men, their principal victims. Multiple factors contribute to aneurysm formation, including atherosclerosis, genetic factors, and smoking. Smokers have more than five times the risk of developing abdominal aortic aneurysms compared with non-smokers. There is some controversy regarding the appropriate use of resources in the detection and management of abdominal aneurysms. If ultrasound screening is undertaken (in addition to abdominal palpation), the author suggests that it would be most cost-effective to focus on men over age 60, particularly smokers and former smokers. Also, there is general agreement that large aneurysms ($\geq$ 6.0 cm) in patients with low surgical risk should be repaired.

"Diagnosis and Management of Peripheral Arterial Disease," a new chapter (Chapter 27) by Wilt, provides important insights about an entity which afflicts one million individuals in the U.S. annually. Of interest, approximately one-half of the patients with peripheral arterial disease remain symptomatically stable or show some improvement 5 years after the onset of systems. Major risk factors for peripheral arterial disease are similar to those for CHD, including cigarette smoking, diabetes, hypertension and hypercholesterolemia. With regard to physical diagnosis, the lack of a posterior tibial pulse may be the single best clinical predictor of peripheral arterial disease. Among diagnostic tests, a ratio of the ankle-to-arm systolic blood pressure (ankle:brachial index ABI) of <0.9 has a sensitivity of 95% in detecting angiographically-positive disease, while an ABI $\geq$ 0.9 is virtually 100% specific for identifying patients without clinical disease. The proper diagnostic roles for plethysmography, Doppler velocity and color Doppler ultrasound studies, and transcutaneous oxygen tension measurements, as well as exercise testing and reactive hyperemia studies, are outlined. Most patients with peripheral arterial disease can be treated with non-interventional therapy—i.e., risk factor modification, exercise rehabilitation, and, in some cases, pharmacotherapy. This chapter emphasizes the importance of smoking cessation and the fact that a model walking program can achieve improvement in claudication which is comparable to that produced by vascular bypass surgery or percutaneous transluminal angioplasty.

In Chapter 28, "Preoperative Assessment of the Elderly Patient for Noncardiac Surgery," Dr. McFalls summarizes some of the clinical variables previously reported to be associated with increased operative risk, including age greater than 70 years, myocardial infarction within the previous six months, CHF, significant aortic stenosis, significant arrhythmias, poor general medical condition, poor functional class, prior cerebrovascular accident, and abnormal electrocardiogram. The authors point out that thallium stress testing may be useful in further stratifying the group felt to be at *intermediate* risk, i.e., those having one or two of the above-mentioned clinical risk variables, as to their risk for noncardiac surgery. The advantages and disadvantages of prophylactic coronary artery revascularization (either surgery or PTCA) are discussed, as is the appropriate preoperative medical management of high-risk patients not amenable to preoperative revascularization.

In Chapter 29, Dr. McIntosh presents a historically-based discussion on attaining and maintaining autonomy in the elderly. This chapter also has an excellent discussion of advanced directives, including Informed Consent, Living Will, and Durable Power of Attorney. These doctrines have emanated from the Nuremberg Codes post—World Ward II, and represent a shift from the public's acceptance of the physician's role based on Beneficence and Paternalism to an insistence on the Patient's Right of Self-Determination.

Dr. Podrid discusses cardiopulmonary resuscitation (CPR) in the elderly in Chapter 30. In the largest series (503 patients) of CPR in the elderly, Murphy and associates reported that CPR was initially effective in 22%, but only 3.8% were discharged from the hospital, and only 1.8% were able to return home and regain normal function.[7] Prognosis for survival approached zero if the cardiac arrest was out-of-hospital and unwitnessed; if no vital signs could be detected or the rhythm was asystole or electromechanical association at the time of discovery; or if CPR duration was greater than 5 minutes.

An important discussion of socioeconomic circumstances and the elderly is presented in Chapter 31 by Dr. Cluff. Health care for residents in the United States older than 65 years is responsible for almost 40% of the nation's health care expenditures. Nursing home care represents an important contributor to these expenses, since 22% of people older than 85 years live in long-term care facilities. Of additional importance is the limited access to health care, especially in nursing home; one-fifth of the elderly are poor or near-poor, three-fourths of the poor elderly are women, one-third are black, and one-fourth are Hispanic.

The concluding chapter by Dr. Burchell, "Reflections on Bioethics in the Elderly Cardiac," presents an important discussion of issues that include "conflict of interest" with respect to marketing, billing, etc.; the Living Will; "Do Not Resuscitate" orders; hospice care; and dismal success rate of CPR in patients over 80 years old; ethical and cost-benefit considerations of surgery in the elderly; euthanasia and assisted suicide; rotating of health care; and clinical trials in the elderly.

Although my previous clinical and research endeavors have included a heavy emphasis on geriatric cardiology, my knowledge and understanding of the problems and opportunities involved in the cardiovascular care of the elderly have been greatly enriched by reading this volume. I am confident that others who read this work will benefit significantly.

Julius M. Gardin, M.D.
Professor of Medicine
Department of Medicine
Division of Cardiology
University of California, Irvine Orange, California

Part 1

Cardiovascular Aging

Chapter 1

Demography and Epidemiology of Cardiovascular Disease in Old Age

Mary Ann McLaughlin, Christine K. Cassel

Demography

Over the last century, we have witnessed a dramatic and unprecedented change in our population. Increased longevity has led to increasing numbers and increasing proportion of older people in the United States and in other developed countries. Rapid declines in death rates have occurred throughout the age structure. Reductions in infant mortality and adult mortality have resulted in a considerable increase in the proportion of each birth cohort surviving beyond age 65.

Within populations, certain age groups may grow at different rates. In many countries, the oldest-old (those over age 80 years) are the fastest growing portion of the elderly population. According to the U.S. Census, the oldest-old constituted 16% of the world's elderly in 1992, 22% in developed countries and 12% in developing countries. In the United States, however, the oldest-old comprised 22% of the elderly population in 1990, and this is expected to increase until the year 2025.[1] The growth in this group of oldest-old presents an important public health challenge, because this group will consume disproportionate amounts of health care and long-term care.

Although an overall reduction in the death rate due to cardiovascu-

From *Clinical Cardiology in the Elderly. Second Edition,* edited by Elliot Chesler. © 1999, Futura Publishing Company, Armonk, NY.

lar disease in the United States has occurred over the last several decades, cardiovascular diseases, particularly coronary heart disease (CHD) and stroke, remain the leading cause of death of both men and women. Yet today, heart disease strikes later than was the case 20 years ago. Importantly, during the 1980s and 1990s, the death rates from CHD declined more rapidly in men than in women.

Data from the National Center for Health Statistics reveals that the death rate from acute coronary disease declined more rapidly than the death rate from chronic coronary disease.[2] Thus, although absolute mortality rates declined, absolute prevalence rates of coronary disease increased, especially in the elderly. In fact, the age-adjusted death rates from cardiovascular disease may start to rise as increasing numbers of patients with heart disease remain at risk for death from CHD.[3] The increase in prevalence of CHD will have significant medical, social, and economic implications.

Life Expectancy

Life expectancy is a summary measure of the expected duration of life, calculated from observed death rates for a population. *Lifespan* may be defined as the theoretical length of life for an individual under "ideal" living conditions; *average lifespan* is the average individual life span in a population.

As individuals in a cohort pass through childhood, middle age, and older ages, the observed probabilities of death take on a characteristic shape (Figure 1). There is high mortality at birth, a rapid decline in the risk of death to its lowest point at sexual maturity, and an exponential rise in the death rate until very old ages (>85 years), after which the rate of increase in the death rate decelerates. Senescence may be considered the passage of biological time, while aging may be considered the passage of chronological time.[4] While individuals in a cohort age at the same rate, the random nature of damage that accumulates in cells and tissues, combined with genetic variability in inherited mortality risk, leads to different rates of senescence and varying mortality risks among individuals in a population.

Specific mortality can be demonstrated in a survival curve. Figure 2 demonstrates survival curves for Americans from 1840 to 1980. At the beginning of the century, a large initial decline in death rates occurred secondary to improvements in infant mortality. In the late 1800s, more than half of the population died before middle age. In 1900, life expectancy was 45 to 50 years; in 1980, it increased to 74 years. Today, age-adjusted mortality rates are decreasing throughout the entire population, with the greatest declines occurring in the population over 80 years of age.[3]

Demographic Transitions and Cardiovascular Disease

Periods in history where dramatic changes in mortality rates occur are know as demographic transitions. The usual consequence of a tran-

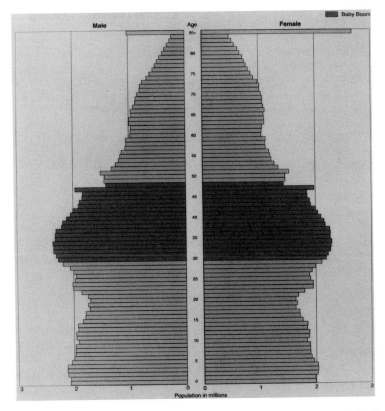

Figure 1: *Population by age and sex: July 1, 1994. (U.S. Bureau of the Census. Current Population Reports, Special Studies, P23–190, 65+ in the United States. U.S. Government Printing Office, Washington, DC, 1996.)*

sition is a redistribution of deaths from the young to the old.[5] The age distribution of the population during most of human history resembles the shape of a pyramid. The epidemiological transition theory originally described three phases of transition.

Phase I of the transition, which lasted until about 1850, is typically described as the age of pestilence and famine. It is characterized by the fluctuation of birth and death rates between peaks and troughs, largely in response to the periodic effects of infectious and parasitic disease. During this phase, cardiovascular disease consisted of rheumatic heart disease, as well as infectious and deficiency induced cardiomyopathies, and accounted for 5%–10% of deaths (Table 1).[6]

During the 19th century, Phase II of the transition was marked by the age of receding pandemics (1850–1920), largely due to improvements in sanitation, water supply, and developments in public health and medicine. As a result of these advances, the risk of death at younger

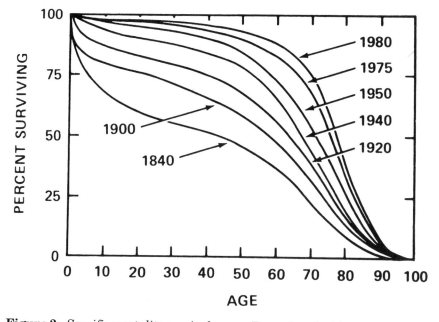

Figure 2: *Specific mortality survival curve. (Reproduced with permission from Cassel CK, Brody JA. Demography, epidemiology, and aging. In: Cassel CK, Riesenberg DE, Sorensen LB, Walsh JR (eds): Geriatric Medicine. Second Edition. New York: Springer-Verlag; 1990, p. 17.)*

ages, particularly among infants and women of childbearing ages, declined rapidly. Cardiovascular diseases began to include hypertensive disease and hemorrhagic stroke, in addition to rheumatic heart disease and cardiomyopathies, and accounted for 10%–35% of deaths.

The eventual transformation of birth rates and death rates to a lower level of equilibrium at approximately 10 per thousand occurred in most of today's developed nations. Phase III, or the age of degenerative and man-made disease, set the stage for population aging. During this phase, atherosclerosis from high fat diets, sedentary lifestyles, and smoking contributed to an increased incidence of ischemic heart disease and stroke, accounting for 35%–50% of deaths.

Olshansky and Ault[7] added the concept of a fourth phase of demographic transition, known as the "age of delayed degenerative diseases." During this recent mortality transition (end of 20th century), the majority of the gain in life expectancy at birth has been attributable to declines in death rates among the middle and older segments of the population (age >50 years). This period is marked by improved education and reduction of cardiovascular risk factors, with postponement of death from ischemic heart disease and stroke until older age.

Table 1
Circulatory System Disease at Various Stages of the
Epidemiologic Transition

Phase of Epidemiological Transition*	% of Deaths Due to Circulatory Disease	Nature of Circulatory Problems	Nature of Risk Factors
1. Age of pestilence and famine	5%–10%	Rheumatic heart disease; infectious & deficiency-induced cardiomyopathies.	Uncontrolled infection; deficiency conditions.
2. Age of receding pandemics	10%–35%	The above plus hypertensive heart disease and hemorrhagic stroke.	High-salt diets leading to hypertension; increased smoking.
3. Age of degenerative and man-made diseases	35%–55%	All forms of stroke; ischemic heart disease.	Atherosclerosis from fatty diets; sedentary lifestyles; smoking.
4. Age of delayed degenerative diseases	Probably under 50%	Stroke and ischemic heart diseases at older ages and as a smaller proportion of deaths.	Educated behavior leading to lower levels of risk factors.

* Omraon (1971) introduced the concept of epidemiological transition with discussion of phases 1, 2, and 3; Olshansky and Ault (1986) added the concept of a fourth phase.

Epidemiology

Epidemiology is the study of patterns of disease in populations. Both morbidity and mortality measuares are used. This science (1) provides the basic descriptors of cardiovascular disease frequency and trends, (2) measures the average levels and distribution of risk factors in the population, and their change over time, and (3) establishes relationships between population risk characteristics and population rates of disease.[8]

The development of disease is often an irregularly evolving process, and the point at which a person should be labeled, "diseased" rather than "not diseased" is often arbitrary. Chronic diseases, which may last years or decades, have a natural history. By natural history, we refer to the course of the disease over time, unaffected by treatment. Chronic disease often progresses through a series of stages, and it is apparent that factors favoring the development of chronic disease often are present early in life, antedating the appearance of clinical disease by many years. The age of occurrence of certain cardiac diseases has been delayed, which may be related, in part, to primary prevention—reduction in smoking and improved diet and exercise.

Cardiovascular Morbidity and Mortality

Ischemic Heart Disease

In 1993, CHD claimed the lives of 239,701 women (48.9% of all CHD deaths) and 250,360 men (51.1% of all CHD deaths).[9] The risk of death due to CHD occurs 10 years later in women than men (Figure 3). Therefore, although women have a marked advantage in age-specific risk of CHD death, their greater likelihood to survive to advanced ages produces nearly equal numbers of actual deaths due to CHD in men and women. In fact, the Cardiovascular Health Study reported a prevalence of myocardial infarction of 9.7% for women aged 65–69 years, but 17.9% for women over the age of 85.[10]

Declines in CHD death rates also show ethnic variations. CHD death rates are 34% higher for African-American women than white women and 5% higher for African-American men than white men. Although death rates for CHD and cardiovascular disease in general have been reported to be markedly lower for Mexican-American men compared with white men, this advantage has not held true for Mexican-American women.[11] Recent data from the Corpus Christi Heart Project

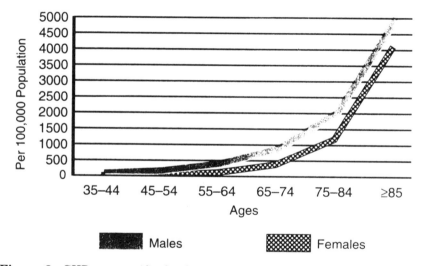

Figure 3: *CHD age-specific death rates by age and sex, United States: 1993 mortality, final data. (Reproduced with permission from 1997 Heart and Stroke Statistical Update. Dallas, TX, American Heart Association, 1996.)*

also demonstrated higher hospitalization rates for myocardial infarctions and incident myocardial infarctions in Mexican-American compared with non-Hispanic whites for both men and women. In addition, this study found a higher case-fatality rate after myocardial infarction in Mexican-Americans and women compared with non-Hispanic whites and men, respectively.[12]

Risk Factors for CHD in the Elderly

There is strong evidence that risk factors for CHD are the same in elderly patients as in younger populations. Hypertension, hyperlipidemia, diabetes, smoking, and obesity are prevalent among elderly patients. Although their relative importance decreases somewhat with age, they continue to impart substantial risk due to the high incidence and prevalence of coronary disease in this population.

Hyperlipidemia. The association of serum lipids with CHD in subjects 60 years of age or older was evaluated in the Systolic Hypertension in the Elderly Program (SHEP). Total cholesterol concentration, low-density lipoprotein (LDL) cholesterol, and the ratios of total to high-density lipoprotein (HDL) cholesterol, and LDL to HDL were found to be predictive of CHD events. The Adult Treatment Panel of the National Cholesterol Education Program (NCEP) recommends that all adults with total blood cholesterol level be evaluated and that those with elevated LDL cholesterol levels be treated. Based on NCEP guidelines, approximately one-third of elderly men and one-half of elderly women have cholesterol levels that warrant intervention. In fact, the estimated percentage of Americans with blood cholesterol 200 mg/dL or higher are even more striking (Figure 4). Recommendations of lipid

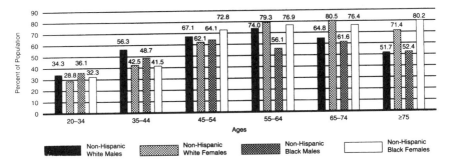

Figure 4: *Estimated percentage of Americans with blood cholesterol of 200 mg/dL or more by age, race and sex. Source: Centers for Disease Control and Prevention/National Center for Health Statistics: Unpublished data from Phase I, National Health and Nutrition Examination Survey III (NHANES III), 1988–1991. (Reproduced with permission from 1997 Heart and Stroke Statistical Update. Dallas, TX: American Heart Association, 1996.)*

lowering in the elderly are predominantly based on extrapolation of data from younger populations. The Scandinavian Simvastatin Survival Study (4S), however, with participants aged 50–70 years (at baseline) followed for 5 years, found treatment beneficial regardless of age.[13] The role of triglycerides in CHD risk remains controversial, but observational studies suggest they may be particularly important in predicting risk in women and the elderly.[14]

There are no conclusive data regarding the benefit of lipid modification for primary prevention of CHD in those over age 65. A diet restricted in saturated fat and cholesterol and high in vegetables, fruits, and grains is recommended for the older adult.

Hypertension. Hypertension occurs in over half of the United States population over age 65. Although systolic blood pressure increases as one enters the eighth and ninth decades, diastolic pressure levels off at age 50–60. Therefore, isolated systolic hypertension is prominent in geriatric populations.[15,16] Epidemiological studies document a strong association between high levels of both systolic and diastolic blood pressure and risk of CHD. In addition, hypertension contributes to the development of stroke, renal failure, heart failure and aortic aneurysm rupture. Control of hypertension decreases the risk of complications. In SHEP, antihypertensive therapy resulted in a 25% reduction in CHD and a 36% reduction in stroke.[17] Pharmacological studies have shown that cardiovascular morbidity and mortality is reduced in patients with treated hypertension, as well as isolated systolic hypertension.[18,19]

Diabetes. The prevalence of diabetes mellitus increases with age and is a common risk factor for CHD in the elderly.[20] In addition, asymptomatic hyperglycemia is associated with an atherogenic profile. Patients with diabetes have higher levels of very-low-density lipoprotein and triglyceride levels and lower HDL cholesterol levels. Although diabetes is a significant risk factor for coronary disease and mortality in the elderly, there is a lack of data regarding the effect of serum glucose control on reduction of risk.

Smoking. Cigarette smoking is associated with an increased risk of sudden cardiac death and reinfarction. Smoking cessation decreases cardiovascular risk, independent of the age at smoking cessation.[21] The Coronary Artery Surgery Study (CASS) revealed that smoking cessation decreased the risk of mortality and myocardial infarction in older men and women with angiographically proven coronary artery disease.[22]

Physical Activity. Physical activity has a protective effect on coronary disease in the elderly; conversely, lack of physical activity has been established as a risk factor for coronary disease in the elderly. Regular endurance exercise maintains muscle mass and increases fat loss in patients on weight-loss therapy. Older patients also improve submaximal endurance capacity in response to aerobic conditioning. It is possible that improvements in aerobic capacity may mitigate the stiffening of the arterial tree that accompanies aging.[23]

Stroke

Stroke is the third leading cause of death in the United States. It is also the leading cause of disability, with an estimated cost of $30 billion per year.[24] Strokes account for half of acute neurological hospitalizations. Survivors of stroke are at greater risk of dementia and disability than men and women without a history of stroke.[25]

The prevalence of stroke is higher in men than in women, but increases with age in both groups (Figure 5). Among older adults, gender differences disappear after adjustment for age.[26] The Cardiovascular Health Study reported the prevalence of stroke in older American men was 5.3% for ages 65–69 and 9.8% for ages 80–84. For older women, stroke prevalence was 2.2% for those aged 65–69 and 7.8% for those over 85 years. African-American men and women are 2.5 times more likely to die of stroke. The 1993 death rates for stroke were 26.8 for

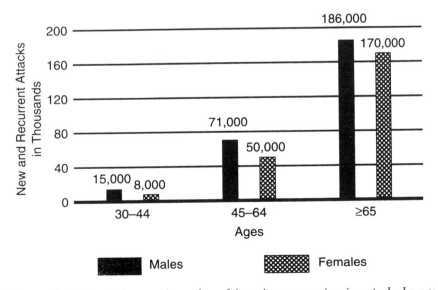

Figure 5: *Estimated annual number of Americans experiencing stroke by age and sex. Source: Framingham Heart Study, 24-year follow-up. (Reproduced with permission from 1997 Heart and Stroke Statistical Update. Dallas, TX: American Heart Association, 1996.)*

white males and 52.0 for black males, 22.7 for white females and 39.9 for black females. Although the lifetime risk of stroke is higher in men, women are more likely to die of stroke, probably due to their older age at stroke occurrence and longer life expectancy. Importantly, mortality from stroke has been declining for both men and women during the last decade. Between 1984 and 1994, the death rate from stroke declined by 19.8%.[9]

Age and ethnicity are important predictors of survival after a stroke. The National Longitudinal Mortality Study[27] reported 5-year cumulative mortality rates from stroke among whites, African-Americans, and Hispanics, according to age of occurrence. Among all ethnic groups, mortality rates from stroke increased with increasing age, but the greatest rate of change occurred in the non-Hispanic white women (0.12%). By age 75 and older, stroke mortality had increased to 3.92% in non-Hispanic white women, 4.07% in African-American women, and 1.85% in Hispanic women.

Congestive Heart Failure

Congestive heart failure (CHF) is the most frequent hospital discharge diagnosis for patients older than 65 years of age. A majority of the 2.5 million patients diagnosed with heart failure are elderly. The American Heart Association, with the National Health and Nutrition Examination Survey III, estimate that 11.1% of people older than age 80 have CHF (Figure 6). The increase in prevalence of CHF in the elderly may be attributed to (1) age-related changes in cardiac structure and function, (2) increased prevalence of systolic hypertension with age, and (3) increased prevalence of coronary artery disease with age.[28]

A profound development in recent years has been the recognition of the clinical significance of left ventricular diastolic dysfunction. Abnormalities in cardiac and coronary vascular structure, as well as loading conditions, result in impairment of left ventricular relaxation and decreased compliance. Echocardiography has substantially improved the recognition of heart failure in elderly patients and helped to differentiate between predominantly systolic versus diastolic dysfunction. Coronary atherosclerotic heart disease, hypertensive cardiovascular disease, and valvular aortic stenosis are the most prevalent causes of heart failure. Diastolic dysfunction may be present in as many as half of all elderly patients with clinical manifestations of heart failure. Several studies have reported that 40% of elderly patients hospitalized for heart failure have intact systolic function.[29,30]

Population-based cohort studies indicate one-year mortality rates of 20%.[31] Taffet et al[32] reported a 1-year mortality rate of 30%, and a 5-year mortality rate of 50% in elderly men (mean age 82 years). Patients with CHF and normal systolic function are reported to have better survival than those with reduced ejection fractions.

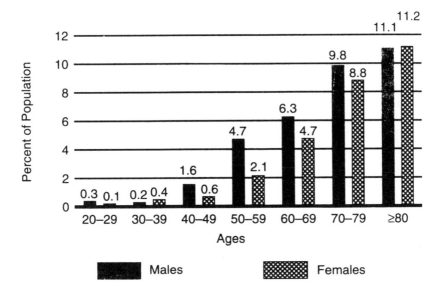

Figure 6: *Estimated prevalence of congestive heart failure by age and sex. Source: Phase I, National Health and Nutrition Examination Survey III (NHANES III), 19881991, and the American Heart Association. (Reproduced with permission from 1997 Heart and Stroke Statistical Update. Dallas, TX: American Heart Association, 1996.)*

Improvements in Cardiovascular Mortality

The recent increases in life expectancy at birth and at older ages has resulted from a decline in death rates due to major degenerative diseases, most notably, cardiovascular disease.[33] Explanations for decline in mortality attributable to CHD are likely multifactorial:

(1) *The effect of risk factor reductions (primary prevention).* The percentage decline in CHD mortality owing to primary prevention has been difficult to determine. The Minnesota Heart Study demonstrated that cholesterol levels, prevalence of smoking and systolic blood pressure declined from 1985 to 1992. In addition, an increase in the use of aspirin occurred during this time period. Investigators from this study reported an annual decline in the rate of first myocardial infarction of 1% from 1980 to 1990.[34]

(2) *The effect of treatment of myocardial infarction.* The number of elderly patients experiencing acute myocardial infarction is growing rapidly. Although hospital mortality remains high, mortality after acute myocardial infarction declined in the 1990s with

the introduction of new therapeutic models, such as thrombolytic therapy.

(3) *Increase in revascularization procedures.* Recent analysis by Hunink et al[3] supports data from the Framingham Heart Study and the Australian national survey, that between 1980 and 1990, the management of patients with CHD contributed more to the decline in CHD mortality than primary prevention measures. The Task Force on Research in Epidemiology and Prevention of Cardiovascular diseases concluded that, "The remarkable coalescence on the causes and prevention of cardiovascular disease resulted in major changes in health policy and practice and in modified attitudes and lifestyles among large numbers of Americans. Nevertheless, the epidemic continues."[35]

References

1. Bureau of the Census, International Population Reports P95/92–3, An Aging World II. US Government Printing Office, Washington, DC, 1992.
2. National Center for Health Statistics: Vital Statistics of the United States 1990, Vol II: Mortality, Part A. Hyattsville, MD; US Dept. of Health and Human Services, Public Health Service, Centers for Disease Control and Prevention, 1994.
3. Hunink MG, Goldman L, Tosteson AN, et al. The recent decline in mortality from coronary heart disease, 1980–1990. *JAMA* 177:535–542, 1997.
4. Carnes BA, Olshansky SJ: Evolutionary perspectives on human senescence. *Popul Dev Rev* 19:793–806, 1993.
5. Omraon AR: The epidemiologic transition: A theory of the epidemiology of population change. *Milbank Q* 49:508–538, 1971.
6. See Pearson TA, Jamison DT, Trejo-Gutierrez J: Health Sector Priorities Review. Cardiovascular Disease. Population, Health and Nutrition Division, Population and Human Resources Department, The World Bank, Washington, D.C., November, 1990.
7. Olshansky SJ, Ault B: The fourth stage of the epidemiologic transition: The age of delayed degenerative diseases. *Milbank Q* 64:355–391, 1986.
8. Blackburn H: Contributions of epidemiology to cardiovascular health. *Am J Cardiol* 78:1267–1272, 1996.
9. *1997 Heart and Stroke Statistical Update*: Dallas, TX: American Heart Association, 1996.
10. Mittlemark MB, Psaty BM, Rautaharju PM, et al: Prevalence of cardiovascular disease among older adults: The Cardiovascular Health Study. *Am J Epidemiol* 137:311–317, 1993.
11. Mitchell BD, Hazuda HP, Haffner SM, et al: Myocardial infarction in Mexican Americans and non-Hispanic whites: The San Antonio Heart Study. *Circulation* 83:45–51, 1991.
12. Goff DC Jr, Ramsey DJ, Labarthe DR, et al: Greater case-fatality after myocardial infarction among Mexican Americans and women than among non-Hispanic whites and men. The Corpus Christi Heart Project. *Am J Epidemiol* 139:474–483, 1994.

13. Randomised trial of cholesterol lowering in 4444 patients with coronary heart disease: The Scandinavian Simvastatin Survival Study (4S). *Lancet* 344:1383–1389, 1994.
14. LaRosa JC: Triglycerides and coronary risk in women and the elderly. *Arch Intern Med* 157:961–968, 1997.
15. National High Blood Pressure Education Program Working Group: National High Blood Pressure Education Program Working Group report on hypertension in the elderly. *Hypertension* 23:275–285, 1994.
16. Staessen J, Amery A, Fagard R: Isolated systolic hypertension in the elderly. *J Hypertens* 8:393–405, 1990.
17. SHEP Cooperative Research Group: Prevention of stroke by antihypertensive drug treatment in older persons with isolated systolic hypertension. *JAMA* 265:3255–3264, 1991.
18. Collins R, Peto R, MacMahon S, et al: Blood pressure, stroke, and coronary heart disease, Part 2. Short term reductions in blood pressure: overview of randomised drug trials in their epidemiological context. *Lancet* 335: 827–838, 1990.
19. MacMahon S, Peto R, Cutler J, et al: Blood pressure, stroke, and coronary heart disease. Part 1: Prolonged differences in blood pressure: Prospective observational studies corrected for the regression dilution bias. *Lancet* 335: 765–774, 1990.
20. Wilson PWF, Anderson KM, Kannel WB: Epidemiology of diabetes mellitus in the elderly. The Framingham Study. *Am J Med* 80:3–8, 1986.
21. Jajich CL, Ostfeld AM, Freeman DH Jr: Smoking and coronary heart disease mortality in the elderly. *JAMA* 252:2831–2834, 1984.
22. Hermanson B, Omenn GS, Kronmal RA, et al: Beneficial six-year outcome of smoking cessation in older men and women with coronary artery disease. Results from the CASS Registry. *N Engl J Med* 319:1365–1369, 1988.
23. Vaitkevicius PV, Fleg JL, Engel JH, et al: Effects of age and aerobic capacity on arterial stiffness in healthy adults. *Circulation* 88:1456–1462, 1993.
24. Heros RC: Stroke: Early pathophysiology and treatment. Summary of the fifth annual decade of the brain symposium. *Stroke* 25:1877–1881, 1994.
25. Prencipe M, Ferretti C, Casini AR, et al: Stroke, disability and dementia. Results of a population survey. *Stroke* 28:531–536, 1997.
26. Manikui TA, Kronmal RA, Burke GL, et al: Short-term predictors of incident stroke in older adults. The Cardiovascular Health Study. *Stroke* 27: 1479–1486, 1996.
27. Howard G, Anderson R, Sorlie P, et al: Differences in stroke mortality between non-Hispanic whites, Hispanic whites, and blacks. The National Longitudinal Mortality Study. *Stroke* 25:2120–2125, 1994.
28. M, Redfield MM: Congestive heart failure in the elderly. *Mayo Clin Proc* 72:453–460, 1997.
29. Vasan RS, Benjamin EJ, Levy D: Prevalence, clinical features and prognosis of diastolic heart failure: An epidemiologic perspective. *J Am Coll Cardiol* 26:1565–1574, 1995.
30. Vasan RS, Benjamin EJ, Evans JC, et al: Prognosis of diastolic heart failure: Framingham heart study. *Circulation* 92(Suppl 1):I-665, 1995.
31. Rodeheffer RJ, Jacobsen SJ, Gersh BJ, et al: The incidence and prevalence of congestive heart failure in Rochester Minnesota. *Mayo Clin Proc* 69: 1143–1150, 1993.
32. Taffet GE, Teasdale TA, Bleyer AJ, et al: Survival of elderly men with congestive heart failure. *Age Ageing* 21:49–55, 1992.

33. Cassel CK, Brody JA: Demography, epidemiology, and aging. In: Cassel CK, Riesenberg DE, sorensen LB, Walsh JR, (eds): *Geriatric Medicine.* Second Edition. New York: Springer-Verlag; 1990, p. 17
34. McGovern PG, Pankow JS, Shahar E, et al: Recent trends in acute coronary heart disease; Mortality, morbidity, medical care and risk factors. *N Engl J Med* 334:884–890, 1996.
35. Report of a Task Force on Research in Epidemiology and Prevention of Cardiovascular Diseases. U.S. Dept. of Health Services, National Institutes of Health, 1994.

Chapter 2

Pathology of the Aging Heart

Jack L. Titus, Jesse E. Edwards

The name of this chapter, which deals with the heart in the aged, has been deliberately chosen to be, as given, the aging heart. Titles such as senile heart disease, the heart in geriatric subjects, and the aged heart have been discarded by the authors. Also, we have chosen not to introduce a so-called iron curtain or specific age between the young and the old for the following reasons.

There are certain conditions in the heart that take years to develop. In some individuals, such a process may be present in a "younger" person, while a number of substantially older persons may not have that particular condition. For the conditions presented as part of the aging heart, there is no hard and fast age limit under which such conditions do not occur. For conditions to be part of the aging heart, there is a positive but not absolute correlation between age and the occurrence of that condition.

Changes observed in the aging heart are frequently a composition of various pathological states. Against a background of alterations specifically related to normal aging, there may be superimposed another active process such as infective endocarditis, or the residual of other conditions such as the congenital bicuspid aortic valve or systemic hypertension. Unlike the young, among whom the clinical picture is commonly a result of one process and therefore straightforward, in older patients it is frequently complex.

The conditions covered are of two general types, one age-specific, the other conditions nonage-specific, but may be observed in the aged.

From *Clinical Cardiology in the Elderly. Second Edition,* edited by Elliot Chesler. © 1999, Futura Publishing Company, Armonk, NY.

Age-Specific Lesions

The Valves

Aging changes may cause nonspecific fibrous thickening (sclerosis) related to sites of valve closure. Two common specific valvular lesions are associated with aging change. These are calcification of the mitral ring and calcification of aortic cusps. An uncommon condition is that of amyloid infiltration of the valves to the exclusion of amyloid infiltration of the other layers of the heart.

Valvular Sclerosis

In the aged, it is not uncommon to find that there is thickening at the line of closure of leaflets or cusps. Histologically, this thickening is caused principally by collagen and elastic tissue. The underlying spongiosa commonly is thickened, as well. The process may be termed sclerosis of valvular tissue. It is primarily a reaction to "wear and tear." The process may be detected in echocardiograms.[1]

While sclerosis of valves may be considered as a minor and unimportant phenomenon, it may have more serious import. At sites of sclerosis, it is probable that there is recurrent endothelial desquamation. Such a process may underlie the occurrence of infective endocarditis. It may be significant that in the aged, infective endocarditis is common upon "normal" valves.[2] The process of sclerosis may be fundamental in explaining this phenomenon.

Calcification of the Mitral Ring

Calcification of the mitral ring or annulus appears to start as a fatty alteration of annular tissue related to the basal insertion of the posterior mitral leaflet (Figures 1 and 2).[3,4] In some instances organized fibrinous mural thrombi at this site may contribute. The altered tissue invites calcium, and ultimately calcification of annular connective tissue occurs. As the process progresses, it bulges from its annular location toward or into the left ventricular cavity beneath the posterior leaflet. The larger extensions may adhere to the posterior mitral leaflet, making the base of this leaflet immobile. The lesion starting in the annular area also may extend for varying distances into the left ventricular myocardium. Uncommonly the major portion of the lesion may be liquid resembling a myocardial abscess (Figure 1, lower). Calcification of the mitral ring tends to be confined to the base of the posterior leaflet and is essentially "C" shaped. Uncommonly, calcification of the mitral ring may be associated with independent calcification of the anterior mitral

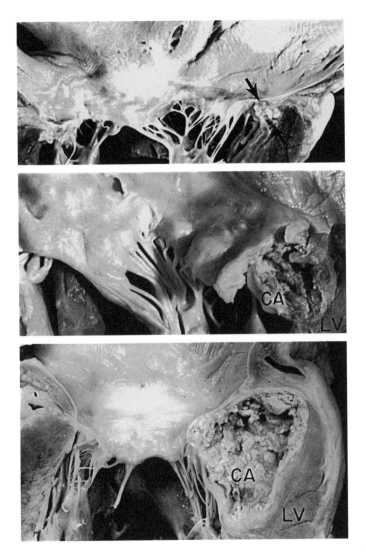

Figure 1: Upper: *Left atrium mitral valve, and a portion of left ventricle from a 77-year-old man. At the junction of the left atrium and posterior mitral leaflet and left ventricle is white lesion (between arrows) representing calcification of the mitral ring.* **Center:** *From a 79-year-old man. One portion of the mitral valve and adjacent structures shown. Beneath the posterior mitral leaflet is a calcified mass (CA), which pushes the leaflet upward. The mass also invades the left ventricle (LV).* **Lower:** *A portion of the left atrium and left ventricle, as well as mitral valve, in a 72-year-old woman. there is a major liquefaction of a lesion representing calcification of the mitral ring (CA). Major extension into the left ventricular myocardium (LV) is evident. Note that in illustration at* **center,** *the lesion causes upward deviation of the posterior mitral leaflet, so-called "jutting angulation."*

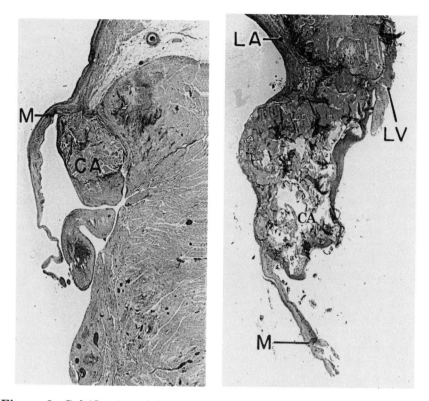

Figure 2: *Calcification of the mitral ring.* **Left:** *Low-power photomicrograph of posterior mitral leaflet (M) and adjacent portions of left atrium and left ventricle from a 57-year-old woman. In the angle between the leaflet and the left atrial and left ventricular walls is a mass (CA) representing calcification of the mitral ring that has protruded from the annulus into the left ventricular cavity. Elastic tissue stain × 5.* **Right:** *From an 84-year-old woman. Photomicrograph of the left atrium (LA), posterior mitral leaflet (M), and a small portion of the left ventricular wall (LV) showing calcification of the mitral ring (CA), which has extended into the left ventricular cavity and has become attached to the basilar portion of the posterior mitral leaflet. Elastic tissue stain × 5.*

leaflet. This may result in a configuration of a circle of "O" in roentgenograms.[5]

Histologically, the lesion is characterized by amorphous, calcified accumulations (Figure 2). These accumulations are surrounded by nonspecific connective tissue, usually of loose, relatively avascular nature. The interstitial tissue may be infiltrated by leukocytes, in limited number, usually lymphocytes and macrophages. Polymorphonuclear leukocytes also may be observed.[6] Uncommonly, the condition is characterized by white or tan, often grumous, fluid which, after escaping during dissection, may lead to an incorrect diagnosis of an annular myocardial abscess (Figure 2, lower).

Calcification of the mitral ring is seen only in adults. Its incidence increases with age. It is noteworthy that the condition is significantly more common in the female than in the male. Pomerance[7] found that in subjects over 50 years of age calcification of the mitral ring was present in 8.5% of cases, being twice as common in females (11.5%) as compared with males (4.6%). In males under 70 years, the incidence was 1.4%, and in females 3.2%. In subjects over 90 years of age, the incidence in males was 17% and in females 43.5%. Somewhat comparable figures were found by Lie and Hammond.[8]

The functional effect of calcification of the mitral ring is usually of no particular significance. It has been pointed out that among subjects with mitral annular calcification, murmurs are common. It is probable that this sign is coincidental to the mitral calcification. Nevertheless, some examples of mitral regurgitation caused by annular calcification do occur but these are probably uncommon.

Simon and Liu[9] explained the occurrence of mitral insufficiency due to annular calcification, and concurred with Korn and associates,[10] as follows. The mitral orifice is normally made smaller during systole by contraction of the left ventricular myocardium. With extensive calcification in the mitral ring, left ventricular contraction could be prevented from reducing the circumference of the mitral orifice, thereby contributing an element that permits mitral regurgitation.

Korn and associates[10] also pointed out that either adhesion of the calcific mass to mitral chordae or pressure by the mass on the chordae could be another basis for mitral regurgitation. These authors also agreed that adhesion of the mass to the ventricular aspect of the posterior mitral leaflet could immobilize all or part of this leaflet.

Korn and associates[10] expressed the view that in rare cases with massive calcification, the mitral orifice might be materially reduced and mitral stenosis might occur. Nevertheless, a presystolic murmur in mitral annular calcification is probably not indicative of mitral stenosis according to Simon and Liu.[9] These authors explained a presystolic murmur originated by the blood flowing over the "jutting angulation" of the mitral valve caused by the annular calcification (Figure 1, center and lower).[11]

In 1946, Rytand and Lipsitch[12] found that complete heart block was common in subjects with calcification of the mitral ring. Nevertheless, the ventricular septum was not commonly involved by the calcific process. The authors were of the view that complete heart block was coincidentally present.

Friction of the posterior mitral leaflet against the mass that presents into the left ventricle may be the basis for infection that uncommonly develops on the mitral valve in subjects with annular calcification.[13]

Among complications of mitral annular calcification is systemic embolism.[14] The latter may originate from vegetative material connected with complicating infective endocarditis, or from the constituents of the basic lesion resulting from fragmentation, or from small mural thrombi on the calcified mass or the valve.

Aortic Stenosis

The specific relationship between age and aortic valvular disease is that of calcification occurring in previously normally developed tricuspid aortic valves (Figure 3). Classically, there is no commissural fusion. This lesion commonly is called the senile or degenerative type of aortic valvular stenosis. The characteristic change is that of fatty alteration of the valvular collagen after which calcification occurs at tissue so altered.[13] The abnormality begins in and primarily involves the base of the cusps.

Multifocal masses of calcification may grow and coalesce. These masses tend to bulge more from the non-contact than from the contact surfaces (Figures 3 and 4).

Ultimately, the rigidity imparted to the cusps may be responsible for various degrees of aortic valvular stenosis. The histological appearance is essentially like that in calcification of the mitral annulus (Figure 5). The free aspects of the cusps are usually spared.

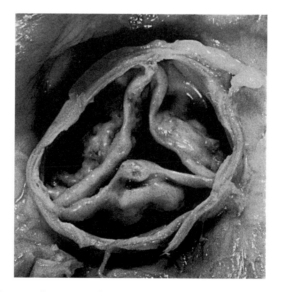

Figure 3: *Unopened aortic valve viewed from above in an autopsy specimen from an 83-year-old woman. Classic example of the senile or degenerative type of calcific aortic stenosis. Each of the three commissures is not fused. Numerous masses of calcium protrude principally from the sinus aspects of each cusp.*

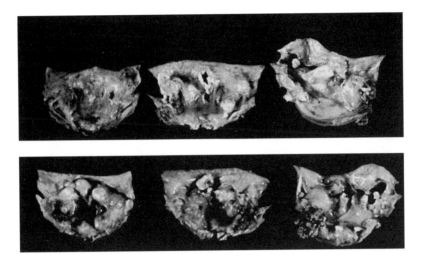

Figure 4: *Surgically removed aortic cusps from a 56-year-old man with the senile type of calcific aortic stenosis.* **Upper:** *The irregularities of the contact surfaces are caused by masses of calcium. Defects are artifactual.* **Lower:** *The sinus portions of the cusps show in greater relief the masses of calcium that protrude from the cusps toward the sinuses.*

Among patients having aortic valves replaced for aortic stenosis, the so-called senile type of aortic stenosis more commonly is represented by women than men. In the study of Peterson and associates[15] concerning this type of aortic stenosis, the ratio of female to male was 18:13. This is in contrast to the gender distribution in the other types of stenotic aortic valves in which males outnumber females. In the study of Peterson and associates[15] concerning stenotic aortic valves removed surgically, the senile type of aortic valvular stenosis was the second most common type of stenotic aortic valve. The most common type was the calcified, congenitally bicuspid valve, representing 48.6% of cases, while the senile type accounted for 27.6% of the cases.

Amyloid Infiltration of Valves

Amyloid infiltration of valves is a rare condition and is to be contrasted with amyloid infiltration of the myocardium (Figures 6 and 7). Among the few cases of amyloid involving only or principally the valves, the ages ranged from 74 to 84 years.[16] The process is more pronounced in the right-sided than the left-sided valves. Although valvular amyloid is an interesting condition, it does not cause recognized valvular malfunction.

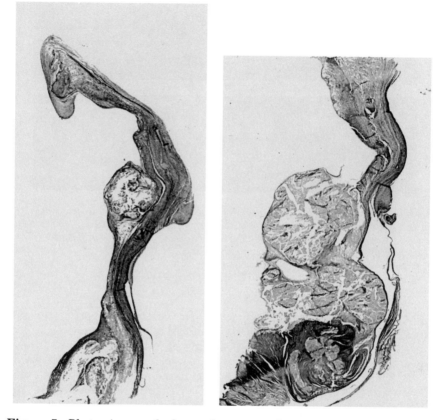

Figure 5: *Photomicrographs from valves removed surgically showing the characteristic histological picture in the senile type of calcific aortic stenosis.* **Left:** *From a 73-year-old man. Low-power view shows two accumulations, one at the center and one in the lower portion of the illustration of amorphous masses that protrude primarily toward the sinus aspects. Over the mass involving the center of the cusp, the contact surface (right side of illustration) shows localized fibrous thickening. Elastic tissue stain × 5.* **Right:** *From a 58-year-old man. Illustration taken through the center of the cusp showing a huge mass of amorphous, calcific material bulging toward the sinus (left side of illustration). Over the mass of calcium, the cuspid tissue has become markedly attenuated. Elastic tissue stain × 10.*

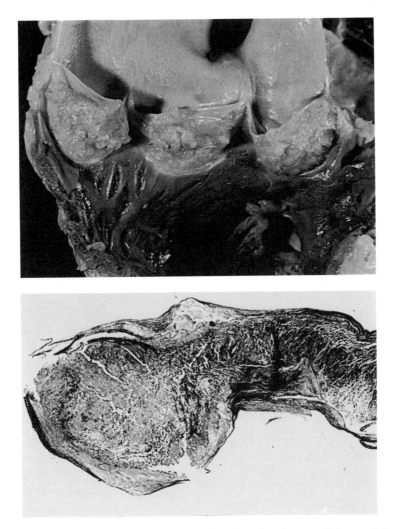

Figure 6: *Pulmonary valve with amyloid infiltration from an 84-year-old man.* **Upper:** *Gross specimen shows major nodularity of the valve cusps.* **Lower:** *The nodularity is explained by the clear area representing major amyloid infiltration. Elastic tissue stain × 40. (Reproduced with permission from Yomtovian RA, Walley VM, Bollinger DJ, et al: Isolated valvular amyloid. Am J Cardiovasc Pathol 2:365, 1989.)*

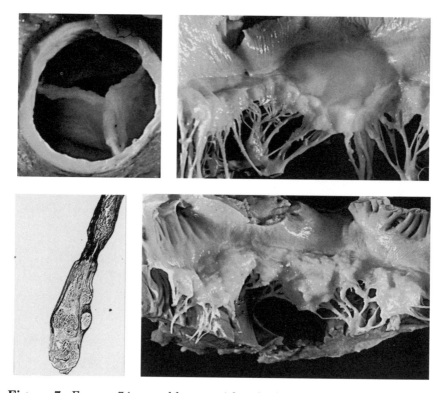

Figure 7: *From a 74-year-old man with valvular amyloidosis.* **Left upper:** *Unopened aortic valve from above. Nodularity of the cusp caused by amyloid infiltration similar to that shown in the pulmonary valve in Figure 6.* **Right upper:** *Opened mitral valve. The process of nodularity of the leaflets and chordae is evident but not as striking as in the tricuspid valve (right lower).* **Left lower:** *A cord of the mitral valve. In the lowermost part of the illustration there is bulbous thickening. This represents amyloid infiltration of the cord. Elastic tissue stain ×10.* **Right lower:** *Tricuspid valve opened. Nodularity of the cusps and chordae represents amyloid infiltration. (Reproduced with permission from Yomtovian RA, Walley VM, Bollinger DJ, et al: Isolated valvular amyloid. Am J Cardiovasc Pathol 2:365, 1989.)*

The Myocardium

Senile Atrophy

Classically, the effect of aging on the myocardium is that of atrophy, so-called brown atrophy or senile atrophy. The myocardium is relatively atrophic, based on measurement of fibers and weight of the organ. Within the myocardial fibers, the paranuclear lipofuscin pigment becomes increased.[17] This, along with atrophy of the fibers, causes the myocardium to have a more brown shade than the myocardium in younger persons.

Myocardial atrophy may be a contributing factor to the tortuosity of the coronary arteries that occurs with age, because the arteries do not atrophy. Interstitial fibrosis, especially in the posterior wall of the left ventricle, has been reported in the aging myocardium.[18,19] This condition was represented by an increase in thickening of the basement membranes related to the myocardial fibers and to be distinguished from myocardial scarring. In the study of Burns and associates,[18] hypertrophy of myocardial fibers was found in the posterior wall but not in other sites.

Amyloid Infiltration

Amyloid infiltration confined to the heart, or nearly so, is a relatively common state among the aged. The condition has been called senile amyloidosis of the heart, or amyloidosis localized to the heart.[20,21] Not only is the myocardium involved, but it is common to find infiltrate in the mural endocardium of the atria (Figure 8, left).

Amyloid infiltration of the myocardium occurs under certain other circumstances beside aging. These include the secondary type complicating chronic inflammation, the primary systemic type, and that associated with multiple myeloma. Smith and associates[22] compared the clinicopathological features of senile cardiac amyloidosis with the cardiac involvement in primary systemic amyloidosis or the amyloid infiltration of multiple myeloma, these two latter forms being grouped as one entity (called primary amyloidosis). In that study, men were more commonly represented than women in both groups. The male to female ratio in the primary systemic group was 1.6:1. The male dominance was greater with the senile group, the ratio being 5.5:1. Patients with the senile type were older, the age range being 70 to 89 years (mean age 83 years). In the primary type at the time of diagnosis the age range was 35 to 85 years. Only 4 of 21 patients in the primary group were older than 70 years.

In a study by Lie and Hammond[8] on cardiac findings at autopsy in subjects 90 years or older, cardiac amyloid was found in 66% of the male and 65% of the female subjects. These authors referred to the myocardial infiltrates as being of one of two types, namely the nodular (Figure 8, right) and the perifiber pattern. They graded the amount of myocardial infiltration in four grades of severity. The perifiber type of infiltrate was more common than the nodular in the higher degrees of infiltrate and with the primary systemic type of disease.

In the study by Lie and Hammond,[8] symptoms of cardiac origin were observed among the systemic type but in none of the cases of the senile type of amyloid infiltration. In some of the latter, it was difficult to differentiate cardiac symptoms due to amyloid infiltration from those resulting from other coincidental cardiac disease, and to establish the

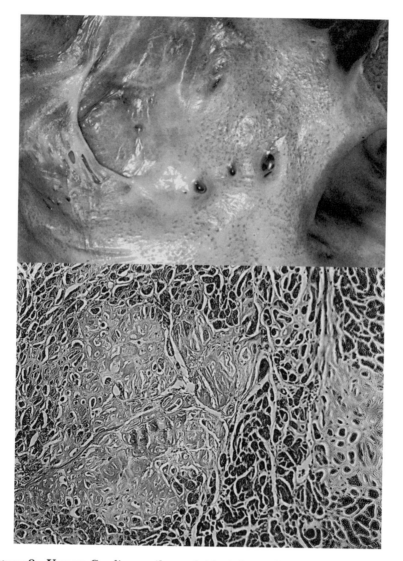

Figure 8: Upper: *Cardiac senile amyloidosis in an 82-year-old man. The septal wall of the right atrium shows numerous dot-like elevations representing foci of amyloid involving the mural endocardium.* **Lower:** *From a 79-year-old man. Nodular type of amyloid infiltration of myocardium in a case of senile amyloidosis. The lesion is characterized by replacement of myocardial fibers in a nodular distribution. H & E × 100.*

relative part each played in causing symptoms. This report, restricted to individuals 90 years of age or older, concluded that cardiac amyloid was the primary cause of death in 9% of the men and in 10% of the women.

Involvement of the atrial mural endocardium by amyloid is common. In subjects 90 years of age and older, Lie and Hammond[8] found cardiac amyloid was confined to the atrial mural endocardium in about two-thirds of the patients.

Infiltration of valves, epicardium, and the walls of intramyocardial blood vessels occurred in both groups but less commonly in the senile type. Involvement of extracardiac organs may occur in each group but is significantly more common in the primary type. Nevertheless, it is of importance to note that among the 26 cases of senile cardiac amyloidosis in the study of Smith and associates[22] there were 2 instances in which involvement was identified in the kidneys, spleen, lungs, and adrenal gland and 1 instance each of involvement of the colon and the liver.

Lipomatous Hypertrophy of the Atrial Septum

Lipomatous hypertrophy of the atrial septum or lipomatosis of the atria, is to be distinguished from localized lipoma. In lipomatosis of the atrial septum, there is an increase in the normal fat within the atrial septum. McAllister[23] indicated that among 32 patients with lipomatous hypertrophy of the atrial septum, the majority of the patients were over 60 years of age but observed that this condition may occur at younger ages. The youngest in McAllister's series was 22 years of age.

The lesion causes thickening of the atrial septum with prominence of the landmarks that present particularly from the right atrial side (Figure 9). This is often expressed as a prominence of the edges of the foramen ovale with increased height of the fossa ovalis.

The process is composed of cells containing neutral fat. Some are typical adult adipose cells, while others are spindle in shape and have a granular cytoplasm. The latter stains positive for neutral fat and resembles fetal fat. The process may interdigitate with myocardium, rarely including conduction tissue.

It is still unclear as to whether or not lipomatous hypertrophy has an influence on the circulation. The opinions in the literature are divided on this point.[24]

The Conduction System

Normal anatomic features, and pathological processes of the cardiac conduction system in adults, have been recorded in many studies and reviews, such as the monographs by Lev,[25] Davies,[26] and Davies et al.[27]

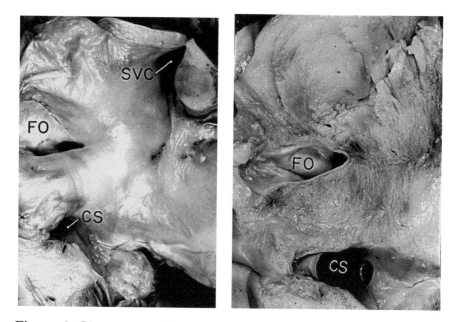

Figure 9: *Lipomatous infiltration of the atrial septum in an 81-year-old woman. **Left:** The septal wall of the right atrium occupies the major portion of the illustration. In the left lowermost portion of the illustration is the ostium of the coronary sinus (CS). Above this is the fossa ovalis (FO). the entrance of the superior vena cava (SCV) is shown in the upper right portion of the illustration. Thickness of the atrial septal wall is shared by the anterior wall near the entrance of the superior vena cava. **Right:** A section has been made through the atrial septum parallel to its surface. A probe lies in the coronary sinus (CS). The wall of the fossa ovalis (FO) is above. The area is in about the central portion of the illustration. The major thickening of the atrial septum is caused by fatty infiltration.*

Age-related, morphological changes in the sinus (sinoatrial) node, the atrioventricular node, the His bundle and the bundle branches occur. Many, but not all, such changes progress with increasing age from neonatal to adult to older adult life, and are not associated with electrocardiographic abnormalities of rhythm or conduction. For this reason, such changes may be regarded, in a sense, as maturational events. In some older patients, with defined atrial or ventricular abnormalities of conduction, apparent exaggeration of these normal, age-related changes may be responsible for electrocardiographically identified dysfunction.

Sinus Node

Well-defined histopathological changes in the structure of the sinus node occur with aging but without changes in the electrocardiogram. The most obvious of these is a progressive increase in fibrous tissue (mainly collagen with some elastic fibers) in the node, with a decrease in the volume of nodal myocardial fibers.[28] The mass of the specialized myocardium of the sinus node relative to the mass of atrial myocardium is large in the fetus and infant, but small in adults of all ages. In individuals older than 70 years of age with normal sinus node function, only about 10% to 40% of the sinus node is muscle. Other morphological changes that occur with age are decrease in the number of ordinary atrial fibers in the immediate perinodal regions (approaches to the sinus node), and some increase in normal fat cells in the atrial myocardium contiguous to the sinus node. As in other parts of the heart, amyloid deposits often (about 10%) may be found in the atrial myocardium in individuals older than 70 years, and in some instances may be close to the sinus node, but not have associated electrocardiographic abnormalities.

With aging, exaggeration of normal, maturational-type changes in the sinus node artery may occur without evident dysfunction of the sinus node. These changes are nonatherosclerotic, intimal, fibroelastic thickening with luminal narrowing, and medial fibrosis with decrease in medial smooth muscle mass.

In general, pathological abnormalities of the sinus node that might account for various atrial arrhythmias, especially sinus node disorders, such as sinus bradycardia or sinus node arrest (sick sinus syndromes), have not been established in most cases. Davies and colleagues[27] stated that 4 morphological patterns may be found in patients with chronic sinus node disease. These are amyloid deposition in the node (uncommon in our experience), marked loss of nodal cells (greater than anticipated for age) of unknown cause, apparent atrophy or hypoplasia—possibly a congenital anomaly,[29] and no morphological abnormality.

Atrioventricular Node

Apparent age-related changes in the atrioventricular (AV) node are less obvious than those in other components of the cardiac conduction system. Increase in the quantity of fat in atrial muscle adjacent to the node occurs, but rarely encroaches on the node. A slight increase in relatively fine collagen fibers in the deeper portions of the node (ie, contiguous to the central fibrous body) may be found in the hearts of older individuals with normal electrocardiograms. Frequently, the AV node partially extends into the central fibrous body; this finding may reflect time-dependent "molding" of the AV node, and exaggeration of the process has been implemented as a possible mechanism of fatal AV nodal dysfunction in young individuals. Nonatherosclerotic changes in the AV nodal artery, as described in the sinus node artery, often occur with aging; sometimes, the artery may be nearly occluded.

His Bundle and Bundle Branches

Because of the normal anatomic relationships of the origins of the bundle branches from the His (main AV conduction) bundle, and the similarities of age-related histological changes,[30] these components are discussed together.

Slight increases in fibrous tissue may be present in the His bundle of older individuals with normal electrocardiograms. More marked fibrotic changes develop in the bundle branches at or near their origins from the His bundle. Fibrosis, often relatively loose collagen occasionally with adipose tissue, may obliterate the origins of some fibers of the left bundle branch from the His bundle. Often, microfoci of calcification are associated with the fibrosis. The same process may be found in the more distal portions of both left and right bundle branches on or in the ventricular septum. These changes are common by the seventh or eighth decades of life, and often are associated with nonspecific increases in endocardial, subendocardial, and intramyocardial connective tissues (collagen and elastica) that are recognized to be age-related conditions. Although these changes may be marked, continuity of some myocardial conduction fibers can be identified if the electrocardiogram did not demonstrate some type of His bundle or bundle branch block.

Heart Block

Morphological abnormalities that are correlated with electrocardiographic abnormalities are best known in instances of complete (third degree), permanent heart block.[31-34] No specific correlations of pathological abnormalities of the AV conduction system can be made with first- or second-degree heart block except Mobitz type II second degree block in whom, rarely, significant abnormalities may be identified.

The majority of patients studied have been in the seventh and eighth decades of life, and the recognized abnormalities of the conduction system might be regarded as exaggeration of normal aging changes. It should be noted that, uncommonly, identical abnormalities causing permanent complete heart block may be found in younger adult patients.

With permanent complete heart block, serial histological sections demonstrate complete interruption of some part of the AV conduction system. The anatomic locations of the interruptive lesions are most commonly the left and right bundle branches, being found in about one-half of cases.[34,35] The bifurcating His bundle and left bundle branch or the penetrating His bundle are sites of involvement, each occurring in about one-fifth of cases. AV nodal and nodal-bundle regions account for the remainder. The pathological bases for the interruptive lesions are, in order of frequency; idiopathic bilateral bundle branch fibrosis (approximately 40%); coronary heart disease (<20%); calcific (usually related to calcification of aortic or mitral valves and annuli) lesions (about 10%); and a heterogenous group including dilated cardiomyopathy in the remainder.

The Ascending Aorta

Senile Dilatation

With increasing age, the caliber of the thoracic aorta widens.[36] This is most evident in the ascending portion. The process leads to the potential for aortic insufficiency, although this state appears to be uncommon compared to the common state of dilatation of the ascending aorta with age. The mechanism for the aortic insufficiency of this cause is stretching of the aortic cusps in a manner similar to the cause of aortic insufficiency in other types of dilatation of the ascending aorta.

A rare complication of senile dilatation of the aorta is through-and-through rupture that results in hemopericardium. This uncommon process is not associated with classic aortic dissection. It may be related to excessive degrees of age-related medial degenerative changes that are characterized by loss of medial smooth muscle cells and elastic fibers, accompanied by increased amounts of acid mucopolysaccharide (glycosamino-glycans) ground substance.

Calcification of Sinotubular Ridge

The ascending aorta consists of the sinus and tubular portions. The former is dilated relative to the latter. At the junction of the two segments, at the superior margin of the valvular cusps, is a ridge, the sinotubular ridge. In this area, there is a tendency for a calcific lesion to develop. This has the basic histological appearance like that in calcified mitral ring and in the senile type of calcified aortic valves. While atheromatous lesions of the aorta may also occur in this area, the histological appearance of calcification of the sinotubular ridge is different from that in atherosclerosis. Additionally, the lesions involve not only the intima but also the media of the aorta. Once formed at the sinotubular ridge, the process may extend into the lumen of the aorta as a spur that may override the ostium of a coronary artery, more frequently the right ostium than the left. The lesion may extend in the opposite direction to invade the aortic wall and the ostium of a coronary artery (Figures 10 and 11, upper left and upper right).

In 37 specimens with this lesion, Tveter and Edwards[37] found emboli in the coronary arteries in 10 cases (Figure 11, lower left and lower right). In 5 of these specimens, calcific lesions with potential for embolism were found at the aortic sinotubular ridges in four cases and of the aortic sinuses in one. Healed myocardial infarction commonly was

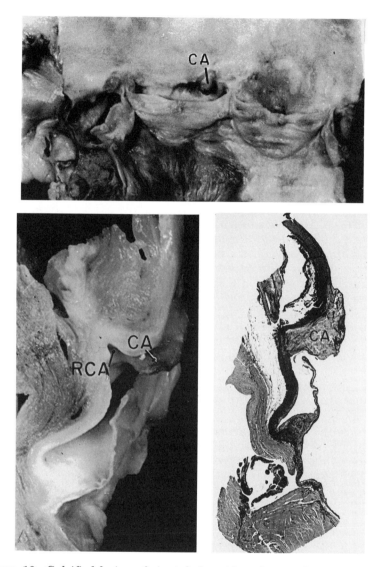

Figure 10: *Calcified lesion of sinotubular ridge of aorta from a 77-year-old woman.* **Upper:** *The opened aortic valve. A mass of calcified material (CA) is at the sinotubular ridge.* **Lower Left:** *Longitudinal section through the right aortic sinus and related portions of the ascending aorta revealing the ostium of the right coronary artery (RCA). At the ridge, near the ostium of the artery, is the calcified (CA) mass shown in the upper illustration.* **Lower right:** *Low power photomicrograph through the ostium of the right coronary artery, the right coronary cusp, and related structures. The mass of calcium seen in the other illustrations is illustrated (CA). Elastic tissue stain × 4.*

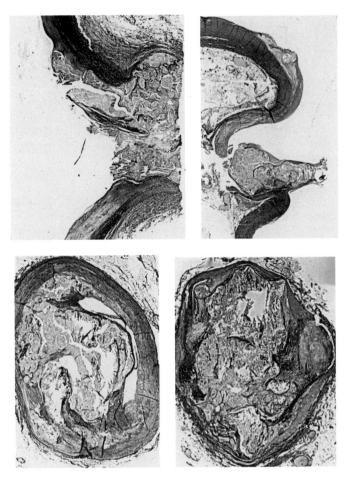

Figure 11: *Calcific lesion of sinotubular ridge of aorta.* **Left upper:** *From a 65-year-old man. Ostium of right coronary artery and longitudinal section of adjacent portion of aorta. The ostium of the artery is occluded by a collection of amorphous, calcified masses. There is involvement of the aortic wall as well. In the lower portion of the illustration is an atheromatous lesion of aorta, additionally. Elastic tissue stain × 5.* **Right upper:** *From a second patient, ostium of right coronary artery and longitudinal section of the aorta. A mass of calcified, amorphous material obstructs the ostium of the coronary artery. An atheromatous lesion of aorta lies above the artery. Elastic tissue stain × 5.* **Lower:** *Right coronary artery (left), left circumflex coronary artery (right), each from the patient whose ostium of the right coronary artery is illustrated in* **right upper**. *In each of the coronary arteries, there is some atheromatous disease, but the major obstruction is formed by amorphous masses of calcified material considered to be embolic from the sinotubular lesion seen in the* **right upper** *illustration.* **Right upper, left lower** *and* **right lower** *from a 49-year-old man.*

present in the cases with emboli but atherosclerotic coronary lesions were frequently associated. In the series of Tveter and Edwards,[37] the ages of the 37 patients studied ranged from 49 to 88 years (men: mean 68.3 years, women: mean 75.2 years; the male to female ratio was 1:3:1).

Left Ventricular Cavity

Sigmoid Septum of the Left Ventricle

Along with the aging change, the outflow tract of the left ventricle tends to assume a shape different from that in the young. In the latter, the direction of the outflow tract of the left is more or less straight. In contrast is the so-called "sigmoid septum." This is characterized by a sigmoid course as the blood flows from the left ventricular apex to the ascending aorta (Figure 12). This is accomplished in part by subaortic prominence of the ventricular septum toward the left ventricular cavity, in addition to apparent deviation toward the right of the wide aortic origin. Goor and associates[38] studied 50 cardiac specimens. They graded the degree of "sigmoidity" and compared this with cardiac

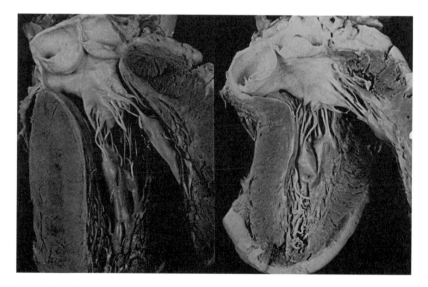

Figure 12: *Frontal sections of the ventricular septum revealed adjacent portions of the left ventricle and the aortic valve.* **Left:** *The ventricular septum is straight.* **Right:** *The ventricular septum shows a major deformity characteristic of the sigmoid septum. Reproduced with permission from The American Roentgen Ray Society.*[38]

weight and age. These investigators found that there was, in general, an inverse relationship between age and heart weight and degree of "sigmoidity." These observations underpin the conclusion that the "sigmoid septum" phenomenon is part of the aging heart. The deformity does not appear to have an influence on the circulation, although the shape of the left ventricular outflow tract resembles that in hypertrophic muscular subaortic stenosis.

Pericardium

The pericardial tissues do not show changes in the aged that are materially different from those in the young. The fat of the epicardium reflects changes in body nutrition. Cachexia, regardless of the cause, is associated with atrophy of epicardial adipose tissue. This process is associated with loss of yellow color grossly and with loss of cytoplasmic fat histologically. As the process progresses, the adipose cells may become fusiform and take on a stainable substance. The interstitial tissue of the fatty tissue may become mucoid in appearance leading to the term, serous atrophy of fat.

Tuberculous pericarditis has become uncommon. Nevertheless, of the cases described, an inordinate number occurs in aged persons.

Nonspecific, not significant clinically or pathologically, foci of slight fibrosis ("soldier's patch") may be more common with aging.

Nonage-Specific Conditions

Valves

Infective Endocarditis

The aged are not immune to infective endocarditis. The probability is that the calcified aortic valve is susceptible to infective endocarditis. The particular situation, by force of circumstance, is more common in the aged than in the young. In general, infective endocarditis in the aged may be masked by the fact that in general, fever is less common in the aged with infective endocarditis than in younger persons. This may act as a negative factor in the clinical suspicion of this condition. Because of the factor of age, cerebral complications of endocarditis tend to be regarded as part of the aging process, as it affects the brain, and so lead away from the true diagnosis (Figure 13).

In Chapter 6, Gerding and Chesler[2] review 100 autopsied cases of infective endocarditis in subjects older than 60 years. The background conditions and relative incidence were as follows. Normal valves were observed in about one-third of the cases. Myxomatous mitral valves were next in frequency, followed by prosthetic valves and aortic valvu-

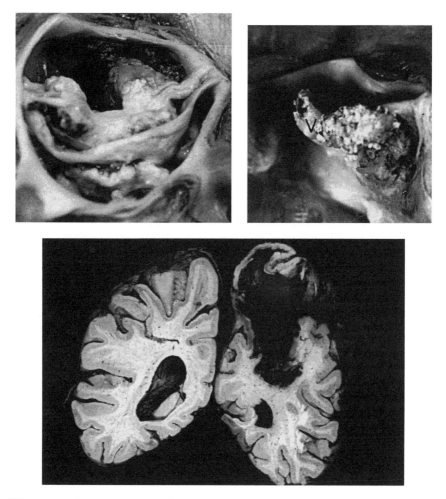

Figure 13: *From a 70-year-old female patient in a nursing home. She developed an illness thought to be a primary stroke. The autopsy showed a congenital bicuspid aortic valve with bacterial endocarditis and a hemorrhagic cerebral infarct of the brain secondary to embolism from the aortic valve.* **Left upper:** *Aortic valve. Congenital bicuspid state with calcific stenosis. Vegetations of infective endocarditis are also evident.* **Right upper:** *Opened aortic valve revealing the calcified state and vegetation (V) of infective endocarditis.* **Lower:** *Brain. Hemorrhagic infarct secondary to embolism from the infected aortic valve.*

lar disease. The latter were either calcified of various background types, or noncalcified congenital bicuspid or unicuspid valves. Rheumatic mitral valvular disease was observed but was uncommon. A rare case of infection of a tricuspid valve with amyloid infiltration was noted. No cases of infective endocarditis in calcification of the mitral ring was noted in that study.

The Myxomatous Mitral Valve

Although the myxomatous mitral valve has been considered a condition of the young to mid-life adult, it is a condition that may be seen at all ages.[39] In some aged, the condition is not materially different from that in younger persons (Figures 14 and 15, upper). Nevertheless, one sees examples of scarred valves that tend to be called rheumatic, when they are probably part of the myxomatous valve syndrome including the effects of healed infectious endocarditis (Figure 15, lower). The mural endocardium of the left ventricle in relation to chordae inserting into the posterior leaflets shows linear or patch-like, fibrous thickening. Such lesions are consistent with the friction lesions of the left ventricular mural endocardium seen in the floppy or myxomatous mitral valve.[40] Coexistence of the changes of myxomatous valve with calcification of the mitral ring may occur.

The histological appearance of the mitral valve leaflets are consistent with those of the floppy mitral valve or mitral valve prolapse, including invasion of fibrosa by spongiosa elements, fibrosis of the atrialis and fibrous deposits upon the ventricular surface of the leaflets. Aging of the fibrous deposits on both sides of the leaflets causes not only thickening of the leaflets and chordae, but contracture and distortion.

Myxomatous valvular disease is to be distinguished from histologically similar changes involving mainly the free edges only of the valves. Commonly, nodule aranti of the aortic valve have myxomatous appearance in older hearts.

Congenital Heart Disease

The finding of congenital heart disease in the aged is uncommon. Yet there are instances that are hemodynamically of consequence either through the primary effects of the anomaly or through secondary changes resulting from it.

The most common situation relates to the congenital bicuspid aortic valve. This condition uncommonly remains essentially normal into the aged class. The bicuspid aortic valve has a strong tendency to develop significant problems. Among these is infective endocarditis. The most common tendency is for the congenital bicuspid valve to become calcified and stenotic, and it is the most common condition causing

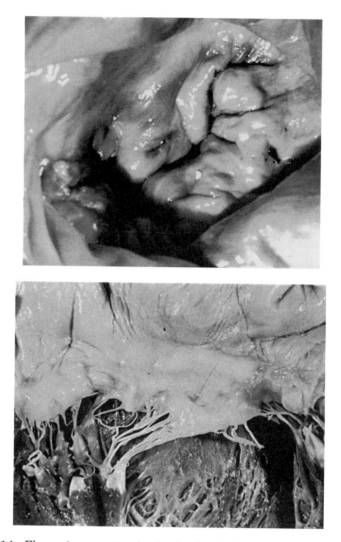

Figure 14: *Floppy (myxomatous) mitral valve in the aged.* **Upper:** *Unopened mitral valve from above in an 84-year-old woman. Numerous upward protrusions involve principally the posterior leaflet, as well as the lateral aspect of the anterior leaflet.* **Lower:** *From a woman, 100 years of age. The opened mitral valve shows minor degrees of hooding of mitral valve tissue toward the atrium.*

aortic stenosis in the older adult. Although this state is usually reached in young adulthood or mid-life, there are cases of stenotic calcific aortic stenosis in the congenital bicuspid aortic valve that do occur in advancing age (Figure 16).

Congenital bicuspid aortic valve occurs in at least 50% of cases of

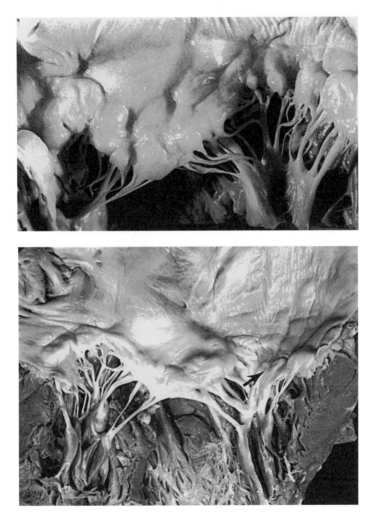

Figure 15: *Floppy (myxomatous) mitral valve in the aged.* **Upper:** *From an 86-year-old woman. The opened mitral valve shows numerous sites of interchordal hooding, including considerable involvement of the anterior leaflet (center of illustration).* **Lower:** *From an 89-year-old man. The opened mitral valve shows numerous sites of prolapse. The commissures are not fused. There is some adhesion (point of arrow) of the posterior mitral leaflet and chordae to a mural thickening involving the underlying left ventricular mural endocardium. The illustration may be not only of a myxomatous mitral valve but also of healed endocarditis involving the posterior leaflet. The endocardial thickening of the ventricular septum (lower portion of center of illustration) may represent healed mural endocarditis secondary to an antecedent active bacterial endocarditis.*

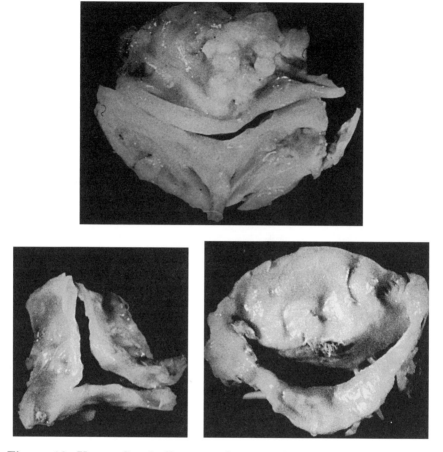

Figure 16: *Upper:* *Surgically removed aortic valve in a 73-year-old woman showing a congenitally bicuspid state with calcific stenosis. The conjoined cusp is at the lower portion of the illustration. A congenital raphe leads onto the aortic surface of this cusp. The free edge of the conjoined cusp is relatively smooth.* **Lower:** *From an 80-year-old woman. Surgically removed valves.* **Left:** *The aortic valve. The conjoined cusp lies in the lower part of the illustration. In contrast to the relatively smooth surface of the conjoined cusp of congenital bicuspid aortic valve (see above), there is a V-shaped defect that is considered to be part of an acquired fusion between two adjacent cusps.* **Right:** *The surgically excised mitral valve viewed from above shows major thickening of the cusps without commissural fusion. The probability is that this is an example of rheumatic mitral regurgitation.*

aortic coarctation. It is to be recognized, therefore, that among patients with aortic coarctation in whom the aortic condition either has or has not been cured surgically, there is the potential for the development of calcific aortic stenosis.

Among aged subjects, there are not only sequelae of congenital heart disease but also of acquired disease. For example, Figure 16, lower, shows the aortic and mitral valves removed at operation from an 80-year-old woman. The aortic valve shows an acquired, bicuspid state with secondary calcific stenosis, and the mitral valve shows the fibrous type of mitral regurgitation. The condition appears to be consequences of rheumatic valve disease.

Congenital heart disease of the common types but untreated is uncommon in the aged. The most consistent types are forms of low pressure shunts. In the study by Lie and Hammond[8] there was a 91-year-old man with atrial septal defect. The defects described in the aged are the fossa ovalis ("secundum" type) and interatrial ostium primum associated with cleft mitral valve (so-called partial type of common atrioventricular canal) (Figure 17).[41]

Isolated cases of partial anomalous pulmonary venous connection are occasionally observed in older patients. In instances of anomalous pulmonary venous connection among the aged, the strong tendency is for the process to be partial, involving only one lobe or, at most, one lung. The most common site of termination for partial anomalous venous connection from the left lung is the left innominate vein.

Partial anomalous pulmonary venous connection from the right lung may either be a self-contained condition or part of a syndrome. As a self-contained condition, part or all of the venous drainage of the right lung is to the superior vena cava or the azygos vein.

When partial anomalous pulmonary venous connection of the right lung occurs as part of a syndrome, one or three types is usually present. The first is that in which veins of all or the upper part of the right lung join either the superior vena cava or the right atrium near a sinus venosus type of atrial septal defect. The second type is part of the so-called scimitar syndrome. In this condition, a right lower pulmonary vein descends to the area of the diaphragm, where either above or below the diaphragm the vessel joins the inferior vena cava. While most cases have been reported in children, adults with this condition have been observed. Frequently, some degree of hypoplasia of the right lung is present. Symptoms vary in part, with the particular anomalies associated. In a review of 67 patients by Kiely and associates,[42] there were 7 without symptoms. Intracardiac anomalies and bronchial anomalies may also occur. In the third type of partial anomalous pulmonary venous connection from the right lung, the veins terminated in the right atrium. This is part of the polysplenia syndrome of which the members do not reach advanced age.

Without an exhaustive study, the authors have observed the following congenital conditions in the relatively old: persistent truncus arteriosus, age 53 years; anomalous origin of the left coronary artery from

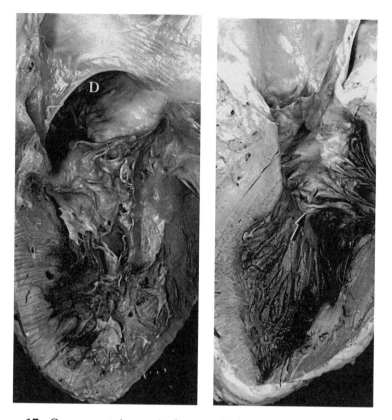

Figure 17: *Common atrioventricular canal of the partial type including the presence of interatrial ostium primum in a 78-year-old man.* **Left:** *Right atrium, right ventricle. There is a defect (D) of the ostium primum type immediately above the tricuspid valve.* **Right:** *Left ventricle and aorta. The anterior mitral leaflet shows a cleft, the upper extremity of which is at the point of arrow. (Reproduced with permission from the American Heart Association.[41])*

the pulmonary trunk, age 59 years, and Ebstein anomaly of the tricuspid valve, age 95 years.

Considering that modern surgery for congenital heart disease is less than 40 years old, there awaits for the profession a series of aging patients who, having been born with congenital heart disease and adequately treated, will be among aged patients with "cured" congenital heart disease. Among these, one would anticipate relatively few with significant residual changes, because inadequacies in achieving cure would, in general, prevent survival to the aging category. Nevertheless, one may look to the future with interest on the subject of congenital heart disease in the aged in whom surgical or other treatment had been done in earlier years.

The Coronary Arteries

In the aging, coronary atherosclerosis is commonly present. However, in some, the process may be less severe than average, reflecting the point that the degree of coronary atherosclerosis need not progress with age. In some arteries, the lumen is wide, while there is segmental atherosclerosis causing little obstruction. In many such segments in the aged there is calcification of the lipid accumulations. The picture suggests that individuals who live into the aged category have experienced the process of atherogenesis many years earlier and some or all lesions have failed to progress.

In an individual in the aged category, one may find signs of nonfatal events that may have occurred earlier. Thus, in the coronary arteries, processes that have occurred over time may be reflected by the finding of complex coronary arterial lesions. These may be related to organized thrombosis with recanalization of varying degrees. Signs of organized intimal hemorrhage may be observed, as well as the multilayering of atheromatous progression.

Tortuousity of the epicardial coronary arteries increases with age. In the absence of stenosing atherosclerotic lesions, no functional abnormality results.

In the aged, the coronary arteries may manifest nonatherosclerotic calcification in or near the internal elastic membrane constituting Mönckeberg sclerosis. No functional abnormality results. Recognition of this possibility is important in evaluation of coronary arterial calcifications that may be seen radiographically.[43]

Myocardium

In the aging, there may be observed changes in the myocardium that relate to events that have occurred months or years earlier.

It is not uncommon that in the aged there are features of chronic obstructive pulmonary disease associated with right ventricular hypertrophy alone, or right ventricular hypertrophy and dilatation as manifestation of right ventricular failure.

Left ventricular concentric hypertrophy is fairly common, reflecting the presence of systemic hypertension. It is noteworthy that left ventricular hypertrophy as a consequence of systemic hypertension tends to be of lesser degree in the female than in the male for corresponding levels of hypertension over time.

Healed myocardial infarction is commonly observed. The most common type of healed myocardial infarction in the aged is subendocardial in type, involving the basilar part of the inferior wall of the left ventricle. In many such cases, the acute infarct or the scar of the healed stage may have escaped identification even in electrocardiograms. In some such cases, mitral insufficiency may have been present as a consequence of the infarction in relation to the papillary muscles of the mitral valve.

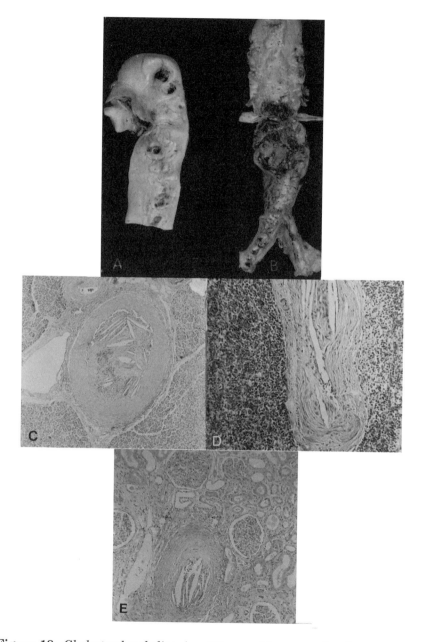

Figure 18: *Cholesterol embolism in a 77-year-old woman showing severe atherosclerosis of descending thoracic aorta (A), abdominal aorta (B). Emboli are present in pancreatic (C), splenic (D), and renal arteries (E).*

In the aged, acute transmural myocardial infarction causing death has a strong tendency to be observed in the female, the mechanism of death being left ventricular rupture with resulting acute hemopericardium.

Aorta

Atherosclerosis and Cholesterol Embolism

The prevalence of aortic atherosclerosis increases with age. When the ascending aorta is involved, aortotomy for insertion of saphenous vein bypass grafts may result in stroke and intraoperative tranesophageal echocardiography has been used to avoid such lesions. Atherosclerosis of the aortic arch is an important cause of postoperative stroke.

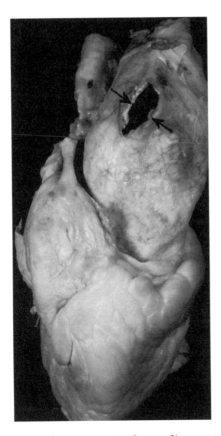

Figure 19: *Ruptured saccular aneurysm of ascending aorta as a result of medionecrosis.*

Severe atherosclerosis with ulcerating plaques may result in spontaneous discharge of cholesterol emboli to various organs resulting in a clinical picture of fever, eosinophilia and elevated erythrocyte sedimentation rate simulating polyarteritis nodosa or infective endocarditis (Figure 18). Cholesterol embolism is an important cause of morbidity and mortality after aortic or coronary angiography and may result in mesenteric infarction shortly after the procedure.

Aortic Aneurysm

Among the aged, aneurysms of the ascending aorta are usually a result of cystic medial degeneration. Enlargement is usually confined to the ascending aorta and there is a strong tendency for rupture and dissection of varying portions of the aorta (Figure 19).

Aneurysms associated with atherosclerosis most frequently in-

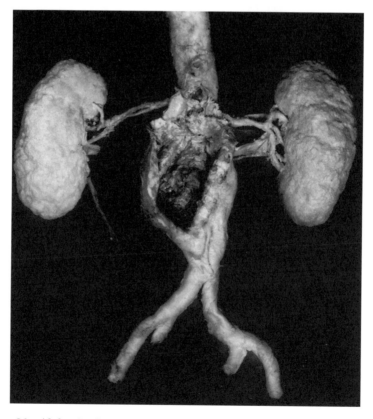

Figure 20: *Abdominal aortic aneurysm in typical position below renal arteries.*

volve the thoraco-abdominal or abdominal segments. Abdominal aortic aneurysms are almost invariably infrarenal but chacteristically spare the renal arteries (Figure 20). Rupture of these aneurysms is a leading, preventable cause of death among the elderly (see Chapter 28).

References

1. Sahasakul Y, Edward WD, Naessens JM, et al: Age-related changes in aortic and mitral valve thickness: Implications for two-dimensional echocardiography based on an autopsy study of 200 normal human hearts. *Am J Cardiol* 62:424, 1988.
2. Gerding DN, Chesler E: Infective endocarditis. Unpublished data.
3. Sell S, Scully RE: Aging changes in the aortic and mitral valves. Histologic and histochemical studies, with observations on the pathogenesis of calcific aortic stenosis and calcification of the mitral annulus. *Am J Pathol* 46: 345,1965.
4. Kim KM, Valigorsky JM, Mergner WJ, et al: Ageing changes in the human aortic valve in relation to dystrophic calcification. *Hum Pathol* 7:47, 1976.
5. Roberts WC, Waller BF: Mitral valve "annular" calcium forming a complete circle or "O" configuration: Clinical and necropsy observations. *Am Heart J* 101:619, 1981.
6. Pomerance A: Pathological and clinical study of calcification of the mitral ring. *Br J Clin Pathol* 23:354, 1970.
7. Pomerance A: Cardiac pathology and systolic murmurs in the elderly. *Br Heart J* 30:687, 1968.
8. Lie JT, Hammond PI: Pathology of the senescent heart: Anatomic observations on 237 autopsy studies of patients 90–105 years old. *Mayo Clin Proc* 63:552, 1988.
9. Simon MA, Liu SF: Calcification of the mitral valve annulus and its relation to functional valvular disturbance. *Am Heart J* 48:497, 1954.
10. Korn D, DeSanctis RW, Sell S: Massive calcification of the mitral annulus. A clinicopathologic study of fourteen cases. *N Engl J Med* 267:900, 1962.
11. Edwards JE: *An Atlas of Acquired Diseases of the Heart and Great Vessels. Vol I, Diseases of the Valves and Pericardium.* Philadelphia: WB Saunders; 1961, p. 385.
12. Rytand DA, Lipsitch LS: Clinical aspects of calcification of the mitral annulus fibrosus. *Arch Intern Med* 78:544, 1946.
13. Burnside JW, DeSanctis RW: Bacterial endocarditis on calcification of the mitral anulus fibrosus. *Ann Intern Med* 76:615, 1972.
14. Lin C-S, Schwartz IS, Chapman I: Calcification of the mitral annulus fibrosus with systemic embolization. *Arch Pathol Lab Med* 111:411, 1987.
15. Peterson MD, Roach RM, Edwards JE: Types of aortic stenosis in surgically removed valves. *Arch Pathol Lab Med* 109:829, 1985.
16. Yomtovian RA, Walley VM, Bollinger DJ, et al: Isolated valvular amyloid. *Am J Cardiovasc Pathol* 2:365, 1989.
17. Strehler BL, Mark DD, Milidvan SA, et al: Rate and magnitude of age pigment accumulation in the human myocardium. *J Gerontol* 14:430, 1959.
18. Burns TR, Klima M, Teasdale TA, et al: Morphometry of the aging heart. *Mod Pathol* 3:336, 1990.
19. Klima M, Burns TR, Chopra A: Myocardial fibrosis in the elderly. *Arch Pathol Lab Med* 114:938, 1990.

20. Josselson AJ, Pruitt RD, Edwards JE: Amyloid disease of the heart. *Med Clin North Am* 34:1137, 1950.
21. Pomerance A: The pathology of senile cardiac amyloidosis. *Br J Pathol Bacteriol* 91:357, 1966.
22. Smith TJ, Kyle RA, Lie JT: Clinical significance of histopathologic patterns of cardiac amyloidosis. *Mayo Clin Proc* 59:547, 1984.
23. McAllister HA Jr: Primary tumors and cysts of the heart and pericardium. *Curr Prob Cardiol* 4:1, 1979.
24. Erhardt LR: Abnormal atrial activity in lipomatous hypertrophy of the interatrial septum. *Am Heart J* 87:571, 1974.
25. Lev M: The conduction system. In: Gould SE (ed): *Pathology of the Heart and Blood Vessels.* Edition 3. Springfield, IL: Charles C Thomas Publisher; 1968, p. 180.
26. Davies MJ: *Pathology of Conducting Tissue of the Heart.* London: Butterworths, 1971.
27. Davies MJ, Anderson RH, Becker AE: *The Conduction System of the Heart.* London: Butterworths, 1983.
28. Lev M: Aging changes in the human sinoatrial node. *J Gerontol* 9:1, 1954.
29. Evans R, Shaw DB: Pathological studies in sino-atrial disorder (sick sinus syndrome). *Br Heart J* 29:778, 1977.
30. Erickson EE, Lev M: Aging changes in the human atrioventricular node, bundle, and bundle branches. *J Gerontol* 7:1, 1952.
31. Lenègre J: Etiology and pathology of bilateral bundle branch block in relation to complete heart block. *Prog Cardiovasc Dis* 6:409, 1964.
32. Lev M: The pathology of complete atrio-ventricular block. *Prog Cardiovasc Dis* 6:317, 1964.
33. Lev M: Anatomic basis for atrioventricular block. *Am J Med* 37:740, 1964.
34. Davies MJ, Harris A: Pathologic basis of primary heart block. *Br Heart J* 31:219, 1969.
35. Edwards JE, Titus JL: Pathology of complete heart block in adults. Unpublished data.
36. Wellman WE, Edwards JE: Thickness of the media of the thoracic aorta in relation to age. *Arch Pathol* 50:183, 1959.
37. Tveter KJ, Edwards JE: Calcified aortic sinotubular ridge: A source of coronary ostial stenosis or embolism. *J Am Coll Cardiol* 12:1510, 1988.
38. Goor D, Lillehei CW, Edwards JE: The "sigmoid septum." Variation in the contour of the left ventricular outlet. *Am J Roentgenol* 107:366, 1969.
39. Lucas RV Jr, Edwards JE: The floppy mitral valve. *Curr Prob Cardiol* 7: 1, 1982.
40. Salazar AE, Edwards JE: Friction lesions of ventricular endocardium. Relation to chordae tendinae of mitral valve. *Arch Pathol Lab Med* 90:364, 1970.
41. Tandon R, Moller JH, Edwards JE: Unusual longevity in persistent common atrioventricular canal. *Circulation* 50:619, 1974.
42. Kiely B, Filler J, Stone S, et al: Syndrome of anomalous venous drainage of the right lung to the inferior vena cava: A review of 67 reported cases and three new cases in children. *Am J Cardiol* 20:102, 1967.
43. Titus JL, Kim H-S: Blood vessels and lymphatics. In: Kissane JM (ed): *Anderson's Pathology.* Edition 9). St. Louis, MO: CV Mosby, 1990.

Chapter 3

Physiology of the Aging Heart

Richard A. Josephson, Steven Fannin, Joseph Rinaldi

The cardiovascular system undergoes significant alterations in structure and physiological function with age. These alterations result from a complex interaction between the effects of aging, disease, and lifestyle. Interest in the effects of aging on the cardiovascular system has increased due to the growth in the elderly population and the discovery that age-related changes can significantly modify disease states and make the medical care in the elderly unique from younger patients. The study of these changes has been difficult because the effects of aging are subtle and difficult to separate from the effects of disease and lifestyle.

Because approximately 85% of the people over the age of 65 have 1 or more chronic conditions, it has been difficult to study disease-free elderly populations.[1] Early studies on aging screened participants by history and physical examination to exclude those individuals with overt disease; however, until special techniques were developed to stress or alter basal physiological function, occult disease usually remained undetected. When techniques were developed to noninvasively detect occult coronary artery disease (CAD), it was found that asymptomatic CAD had increasing prevalence with age and could significantly affect cardiac performance during stress even though symptoms were absent at rest.[2] Early aging studies using participants unscreened for CAD found a general decline in myocardial performance with age.[3] This work suggested that there was a large deterioration in cardiac performance with increasing age. In these earlier studies the difference in cardiac output (CO) between healthy young and putatively healthy

From *Clinical Cardiology in the Elderly. Second Edition,* edited by Elliot Chesler. © 1999, Futura Publishing Company, Armonk, NY.

elderly people was similar in magnitude to the difference in cardiac output between healthy young and young people with documented severe cardiovascular pathology. Subsequent work in this area, utilizing highly-screened individuals suggested that the deterioration in cardiovascular performance with advancing age was modest. There was a decline in Vo_2max with advancing age, but a significant portion of this decline could be accounted for by changes in body composition.[4] In these select populations, there did not appear to be a change in cardiac output across the age spectrum. More recent work in this area, utilizing a large number of patients, of more diverse background, and varying physical fitness suggests indeed that there is a diminution in cardiac output with advancing age. This decrease is moderate in magnitude, and the measured differences in cardiac output between individuals of varying ages is similar in magnitude to the variations in cardiac output in different individuals of the same age.[5-7] Therefore, to study age-related changes in cardiovascular function in isolation from disease states, participants must be vigorously screened for conditions that significantly affect cardiovascular performance.

Lifestyle variables can also modify the age-related changes in cardiovascular function, but their interaction has been poorly investigated. Two of the more frequently studied variables, physical conditioning and dietary habits, are known to alter age- related change. Physical conditioning has a major influence on the cardiovascular system and has been found to delay or partially regress age-related changes in cardiovascular function. Studies of physically fit elderly have found that their cardiac physiology is similar to younger individuals.[8-10] Changes thought strictly due to aging may be partially secondary to deconditioning effects.[8,11] Similarly, dietary habits have also been found to effect age-related change indirectly. In a study of 2 Chinese populations, the effects of regional differences in salt intake on age-related arterial stiffness were compared.[12] The urban population, which had greater salt intake, was found to have a premature increase in arterial stiffness that subsequently led to a higher prevalence of hypertension with age (Figure 1). Thus, lifestyle variables can influence the effects of aging on the cardiovascular system in positive or negative ways.

Research methods may also confound the results of aging studies. Cross-sectional studies, frequently used in geriatric research, are greatly influenced by the high disease prevalence and lifestyle variability in aging populations. In addition, survival bias becomes important because the process of aging selects for individuals who may be more genetically fit to live longer. Prospective longitudinal studies, such as the Framingham Study and the Baltimore Longitudinal Study on Aging, are more accurate for detecting age-related change and make it easier to control confounding variables and biases. However, these studies are time consuming and more difficult to perform. Despite these limitations, prospective longitudinal studies have significantly contributed to our understanding of aging physiology. Animal models have

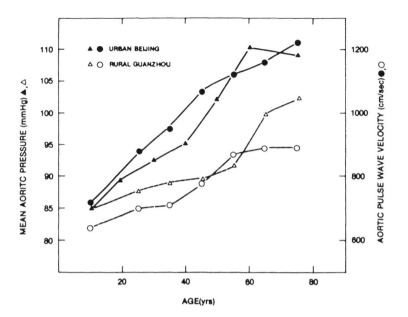

Figure 1: *Arterial stiffness as measured indirectly by pulse wave velocity (the distance that the pulse wave travels through an arterial segment per unit time) and blood pressure as a function of age in an urban (high-salt intake) and rural (low-salt intake) Chinese population. Reproduced by permission of the American Heart Association from Avolio AP, Fa-Quan D, Wei-Qiang L, et al: Effects of aging on arterial distensibility in populations with high and low prevalence of hypertension: Comparison between urban and rural communities in China. Circulation 71:202–210, 1985.*

also been useful in defining biochemical and physiological changes associated with aging, but the direct application to human populations is often difficult.

Cardiovascular Changes and Normal Human Aging

Factors that may modulate or obfuscate age-related change in the cardiovascular system and hinder age-related study were discussed earlier. In the following sections, specific physiological changes in the cardiovascular system that occur with normal aging are described. This description is with the acknowledgment that the study of each physiological parameter in isolation from the rest has been virtually impossible. However, by taking account of many of these covariables, individual parameters may be understood in context with their physiological milieu.

The framework for discussion separates cardiac function according to 3 common and fundamental physiological parameters: afterload, preload, and contractility, and describes what is presently known about the age-related changes that affect these parameters. Within this framework, aging changes in electrophysiology and autonomic control, are also described. Initially, the discussion focuses on changes that occur during the resting state and exercise is discussed separately. Changes in cardiac structure are only discussed as they relate to function.

Afterload

Afterload is the resistance to the ejection of blood faced by the contracting heart and is primarily determined by the blood flow characteristics within the vascular system. Structural changes occur in arterial walls as they age that reduce their distensibility and cause a gradual increase in afterload. These structural changes result from the loss and destruction of the elastic tissue within the vascular media, the deposition of calcium in the vessel wall, and a change in the amount and composition of vessel wall collagen.[13,14] The endothelial cells of the vessel lining also change with age, becoming more heterogeneous in size, shape, and orientation, inhibiting laminar flow and increasing lipid deposition.[15,16] These structural changes and the resulting increase in afterload are theorized to act as the primary stimulus for other age-related structural and physiological changes that occur in the heart. Evidence to support this theory has been seen in study models of experimentally-induced hypertension where changes in cardiac physiology were found to be similar to age-related change. Table 1 lists some of the similar effects of aging and hypertension.[17]

Measurements of afterload have tried to determine how structural changes in the arterial system influence afterload. These measurements have found that afterload has both a steady-state (static) and a pulsatile (dynamic) component. The steady-state component, termed peripheral vascular resistance (PVR), is the resistance to mean blood flow and is measured from the mean cardiac output and pressure via Ohm's law. The pulsatile component, termed characteristic vascular impedance (CVI), is the resistance to pulsatile blood flow and is measured as the time variation in pressure/flow through the aorta. The age-related change in CVI and PVR has been measured by impedance spectral patterns.[18] CVI was found to be inversely proportional to arterial compliance (distensibility of the arterial wall) and PVR was found to be inversely proportional to the cross-sectional area of the peripheral vascular beds. CVI increased by 137% and PVR increased 37% from ages 20 to 60 (Figure 2). These impedance spectral patterns infer that there is a progressive decline in arterial compliance and a loss af peripheral vascular beds with age. The study concluded that the decline in arterial compliance contributes more significantly to the age-related

Table 1
Similar Effects of Aging and Hypertension

A. Qualitative similarities in cardiovascular structure and function in hypertensive
   patients and healthy (normotensive) elderly subjects
   Increased arterial stiffness
   Increased arterial pressure
   Increased left ventricular mass
   Increased peripheral resistance[A]
   Increased characteristic aortic impedance at rest
   Decreased left ventricular early diastolic filling rate at rest
   Decreased left ventricular early diastolic filling volume at rest
   Increased left atrial dimension at rest
   Decreased cardiovascular response to catecholamines
B. Myocardial changes in hearts of younger animals with experimental pressure
   overload and in healthy animals of advanced age
   Increased left ventricular mass
   Decreased protein synthesis and degradation rates
   Decreased myocardial catecholamine content
   Increased myocardial collagen content
   Altered viscoelastic properties
   Altered excitation-contraction coupling mechanisms
      Prolonged contraction duration
      Prolonged action potential duration
      Prolonged myoplasmic free Ca^{++} transient duration
      Altered myosin isoenzyme composition
      Diminished myosin ATPase activity
   Diminished response to catecholamines

[A] Not observed in all elderly populations studied.

increase in afterload than the loss of peripheral vascular beds. Another measurement technique, pulse wave velocity (PWV), measures the propagation speed of pressure waves traveling from proximal to distal arterial segments and has been used clinically as an indirect index of afterload. PWV has been found to increase as arteries become less compliant and is related to the degeneration of the vascular media independent of atherosclerosis. PWV has also been shown to increase with age and supports the evidence that the decline in arterial compliance is the major factor in the age-related increase in afterload.[19]

The major clinical manifestation of increased afterload is blood pressure elevation. Epidemiological studies have shown that there is an age-related increase in pulse pressure and systolic blood pressure.[20] The rise in systolic blood pressure with aging has been found to be approximately 1 mm Hg per year in both men and women up to age 70, then the rise in women increases 1.2 mm Hg per year after age 70.[21] Diastolic blood pressure slightly increases until the sixth decade, then slightly declines over the next 20 years (Figure 3).[21]

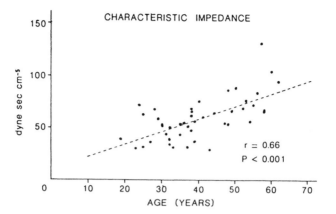

Figure 2A: *Change in the characteristic vascular impedance (CVl) with age. Reproduced by permission from Nichols WW, O'Rourke MF, Avolio AP, et al: Effects of age on ventricular-vascular coupling.* Am J Cardiol 55:1179–1184, 1985.

The mechanism that causes blood pressure to increase with age involves a progressive impedance mismatch between the energy of ventricular ejection and the energy of aortic flow. As aortic compliance deteriorates, the transfer of kinetic energy from the blood ejected during systole to potential energy stored in the elasticity of the aortic wall is reduced. As a result, the return of this potential energy within the aortic wall back to the kinetic energy of blood flow during diastole is

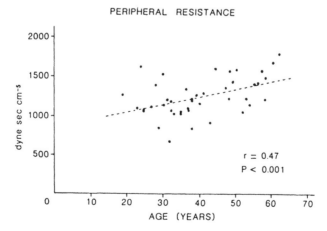

Figure 2B: *Changes in peripheral vascular resistance (PVR) with age. Reproduced with permission from Nichols WW, O'Rourke MF, Avolio AP, et al: Effects of age on ventricular-vascular coupling.* Am J Cardiol 55:1179–1184, 1985.

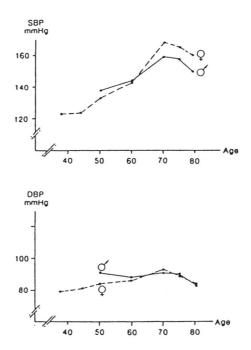

Figure 3: *The change in systolic and diastolic blood pressure with age in subjects without antihypertensive treatment. Reproduced with permission from Landahl S, Bengtsson C, Sigurdsson JA, et al: Age-related change in blood pressure.* Hypertension *8:1044–1049, 1986.*

also reduced. To maintain adequate cardiac output, the ventricle must empty its stroke volume into a less compliant aorta with greater force and pressure. Additionally, the increased PWV enhances the return of reflected waves from distal arterial segments back to the aorta, causing the pressure in the aortic root to continue to increase and peak later in systole, thus contributing to the elevated systolic pressure and widened pulse pressure. This increased late systolic peak resulting from the early reflected fluid wave can be quantified using applanation tonometry and is termed the arterial pressure pulse augmentation index (Figure 4).[22] The arterial pressure pulse augmentation index and late systolic peak are important determinants of the extent to which the left ventricular (LV) reactively hypertrophies.

Neurohumoral factors may also play a role in the age-related increase in afterload. Circulating levels of catecholamines are found to increase with age. However, -adrenergic vasoconstriction has been shown not to change and contributes little to the afterload changes seen with aging.[23] In contrast, β-adrenergic vasodilation of vascular smooth muscle declines with aging.[24] This has been confirmed with isoproterenol-induced vasodilation in the human forearm.[25] The mechanism of

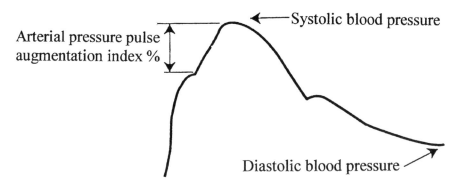

Figure 4: *Schematic of arterial pulse pressure augmentation index % determined from the arterial pressure waveform.*

this decline includes reduced β-adrenoceptor number and impaired actation of adenylate cyclase. The impaired vasodilatory response to β-adrenergic stimulation is found to be most important during exercise. Other humoral factors, such as histamine, renin, and angiotensin have not been found to produce consistent age-related changes in vascular tone.[26] Serotonin has some enhanced vasoconstricting effects with age in animal models, but its significance in humans is unknown.[26] Age-related baroreceptor insensitivity has also been proposed as a mechanism for increased blood pressure in the elderly, but definitive evidence for this is lacking.

The deterioration in arterial compliance and the resulting elevation in systolic blood pressure is translated to the myocardium as increased LV wall stress. Systolic blood pressure (BP), ventricular radius, and myocardial wall thickness are determinants of myocardial wall stress and are related via Laplace's law (LV wall stress = systolic BP × ventricular radius/2 × wall thickness). To compensate for the age-associated increase in blood pressure, the myocardium reactively hypertrophies, which results in a normalization of wall stress. Although the wall thickness increases, LV cavity size remains normal. From age 25 to 90, heart weight increases 1 to 1.5 g/year and ventricular wall thickness increases 30%.[27,28] However, the ventricular wall thickness never exceeds the upper limits of normal without the presence of concomitant disease (e.g., hypertension, aortic stenosis). Echocardiographic measurement of LV posterior wall thickness in healthy normotensive men aged 25 to 80 is shown in (Fig. 5).[29] As mentioned above, the arterial pressure pulse augmentation index and late systolic peak are important stimuli for this reactive hypertrophy. Kobayashi et al.[30] studied the effects of early and late systolic loading on LV mass in rats through proximal and distal aortic banding. While both types of banding caused similar increases in total systemic resistance, only the distal banding was associated with a late systolic peak, attributed to the fluid wave reflection, and a greater amount of concentric hypertrophy. Human studies suggest that females have a more prominent late systolic peak than men starting in the 4th decade and a greater arterial pressure pulse augmentation index after the first decade of life.[31] This gender difference may relate to differences in stature. Because intensity of wave reflection depends on the distance to the reflecting sites, gender differences in height come into play. The study authors also suggest the gender differences in arterial pressure pulse augmentation index and late systolic peak could account for the increased age-related left ventricular hypertrophy (LVH) in women than in men. Furthermore, others have shown that while increased characteristic impedance and early reflected fluid waves can promote the formation of LVH, pharmacological agents that can attenuate these factors may halt or even reverse the hypertrophy process.[32] While both hydralazine and zofenopril equally decrease mean arterial pressure, zofenopril was associated with a decrease in characteristic impedance, less wave reflection, and a regression in the LV weight-to-body weight ratio. Therefore the efficacy of the pharmacological agent is determined not only by its effect on blood pressure, but also by its effect on pulsatile vascular afterload.

The pervading dogma has been that this age-related hypertrophy of the ventricular wall occurs through cellular hypertrophy and fibrotic change rather than hyperplasia. Studies have shown that the aging process is accompanied by a gradual loss of ventricular myocytes with

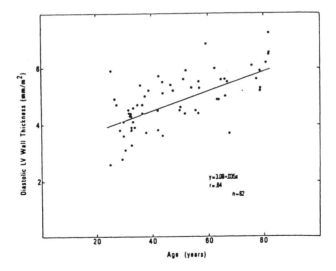

Figure 5: *Linear regression plot of the relationship between age and diastolic left ventricular (LV) wall thickness. Reproduced by permission of the American Heart Association from Gerstenblith G, Fredericksen J, Yin F, et al: Echocardiographic assessment of a normal adult aging population.* Circulation 56: 273–278, 1977.

reactive hypertrophy of the remaining cells and proliferation of connective tissue.[33] A recent report in humans has shown that myocytes may retain the ability to hypertrophy *and* proliferate in the aging heart.[34] These provocative data suggests that the age related alterations in structure are due to both hypertrophy and hyperplasia, with a net loss of myocytes coupled with reactive hypertrophy of the remaining myocytes and proliferation of the connective tissue to maintain wall thickness.[15] The cellular hypertrophy occurs mainly due to the addition of morphologically similar sarcomeres.[35] In an interesting study of 53 men and 53 women screened for cardiovascular disease, diabetes, malignancies and considered to represent normal aging, Olivetti et al[36] found no change in the size, shape or proportion of mononucleated or binucleated myocardial cells in women with age. Furthermore, they found no loss of myocytes or decrease in weight of the female hearts with increasing age, and found there was myocyte loss and weight loss of approximately 1% and 1 g per year, respectively, in the male hearts with aging. In males, the remaining myocytes were found to undergo reactive hypertrophy.[36] Additional studies are needed to see if this qualitative gender difference in myocyte behavior with advancing age is a universal phenomenon and to understand its cellular genetic basis.

Preload

Preload is the physiological concept that relates the extent of ventricular filling to myocardial contractile performance. As the ventricle progressively fills, the force of contraction is augmented by an increased sensitivity of the contractile proteins to calcium as the sarcomere is stretched. This is the basis of the ventricular function curves as described by the Frank-Starling mechanism in which stroke volume is related to LV end-diastolic volume. Preload is determined by the mechanical properties of the ventricle during diastolic filling, as well as many external factors that influence blood return to the heart.

Radionuclide ventriculography and echocardiography have shown that ventricular volumes at rest are not significantly different between healthy elderly and younger individuals, which infers that resting preload does not change with age.[29,37] Although resting preload is unchanged, the physiology of diastolic filling has been found to be altered with aging. As the myocardium undergoes structural and biochemical changes with age, the stiffness of the ventricular wall gradually increases. This results in changes in the mechanical properties of the ventricle that reduces its compliance and limits early diastolic filling. Studies have shown that ventricular filling during early diastole declines 50% from age 20 to 80, potentially impairing the maintenance of adequate preload in the elderly.[29,38,39]

The rate at which the myocardium actively relaxes after contraction and passively fills while relaxed determines the degree of early diastolic filling. Active relaxation occurs during the isovolumic phase of diastole and is an energy-requiring process that causes disengagement of the contractile proteins, actin and myosin. During this phase, the sarcoplasmic reticulum sequesters calcium fueled by the hydrolysis of adenosine triphosphate (ATP) and thereby reduces the myoplasmic calcium concentration. As the myoplasmic calcium concentration falls, calcium is detached from troponin and the interaction between actin and myosin is inhibited, resulting in ventricular relaxation. In studies of senescent animals, alterations in the excitation-contraction coupling mechanism occur that are associated with impaired release and reuptake of calcium by the sarcoplasmic reticulum.[40,41] This impairment is thought to be caused by a decreased rate of calcium pumping by the sarcoplasmic reticulum. As a result, the flux of calcium into and out of the myoplasm, termed the myoplasmic calcium transient, is prolonged in senescent animals that both extends the duration of the myofilament-calcium interaction and increases the time course of cardiac muscle relaxation (Figure 6).

Passive ventricular filling occurs during the rapid filling and diastasis phases of early diastole. It denotes the filling properties of the ventricle that are dependent on the mechanical properties of the relaxed myocardium and not on excitation properties. It is controversial whether the mechanical properties of the left ventricle, which determine passive filling, contribute to the reduced filling in early diastole. Animal data have shown that passive ventricular filling is decreased in senescent animals due to multiple factors, including changes in the

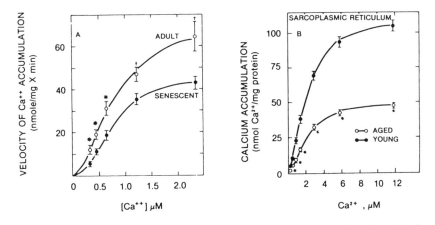

Figure 6: *A: The velocity of calcium accumulation in sarcoplasmic reticulum isolated from adult and senescent Wistar rat hearts.* ***B:*** *Effects of varying calcium concentrations on adenosine triphospate (ATP)-supported calcium accumulation by cardiac SR from young and aged Fisher rat hearts. Reprinted by permission of the American Heart Association from Gerstenblith G, Fredericksen J, Yin F, et al: I Echocardiographic assessment of a normal adult aging population.* Circulation 56:273–278, 1977.

intrinsic viscoelastic properties of the myocardium, the configuration and thickness of the left ventricle, and the external constraints to filling.[42] Human studies have not consistently confirmed an age-related decrease in passive ventricular filling. There is some evidence in humans that passive ventricular filling may be impaired from an increase in ventricular wall thickness, changes in the amount and characteristics of collagen, in particular the replacement of lost myocytes mentioned above with less distensible fibrous tissue, and possibly from the accumulation of senile amyloid.[14,15] To compensate for these age-related factors that limit early diastolic filling, atrial contraction becomes more vigorous to increase late diastolic filling, which acts as an adaptive mechanism to maintain preload. It has been determined that by age 80, up to 46% of the stroke volume may be dependent on atrial contraction.[38] Consequently, the atrial "kick" may be an important mechanism to overcome the reduced ventricular compliance with age.

The altered physiology of diastolic filling in the elderly has been investigated by transmitral blood flow patterns as measured by pulsed-Doppler echocardiography. It has been demonstrated by this technique that there is an increased maximal late diastolic flow across the mitral valve during left atrial contraction (A) in response to reduced early diastolic flow (E).[43] Furthermore the ratio of early diastolic flow to late diastolic flow (E:A ratio) has been found to decrease linearly with age (Figure 7), reflecting the decreased compliance of the left ventricle with

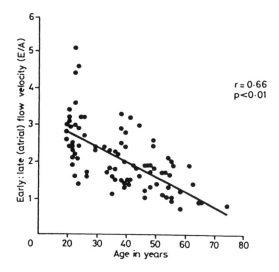

Figure 7: *Linear regression plot of the relationship between age and the ratio of maximal early diastolic to late diastolic flow velocities (E:A) Reprinted with permission from Spirito P, Maron BJ: Influence of aging on doppler echocardiographic indices of left ventricular diastolic function.* Br Heart J 59:672–679, 1988.

age. Although the E:A ratio may be influenced by many other factors, it has been found to be a reasonable index of ventricular compliance during diastole. Associated with the decreased E:A ratio is an age-related increase in left atrial size that is thought to result form increased wall stress from elevated intraatrial pressure to counteract the effects of reduced ventricular compliance with age.[37]

It is known that diastolic filling is altered with advancing age. Whether this is secondary to age associated changes in activity/fitness, or is a true aging phenomenon was unclear. Recent studies of elderly men have shown that the institution of regular aerobic exercise could improve diastolic filling, in particular the early diastolic filling phase.[8,44] However further observations of older endurance male athletes show impairment of early diastolic LV filling similar to that of their sedentary peers.[45] This data suggests that impaired early diastolic filling truly is a "normal" aging phenomenon and not due strictly to deconditioning.

Contractility

The intrinsic ability of the heart to generate force does not change appreciably with age. Echocardiography in humans has shown no age-associated deterioration in ejection fraction index and circumferential fiber shortening in healthy subjects.[29] A similar study using radionuclide multigated cardiac blood-pool scans (MUGA) has also shown that resting stroke volume and cardiac index are only modestly decreased with age.[5-7,46] Although these studies have been useful to evaluate cardiac performance with age, they have been limited by the use of indirect measures of contractility and the inability to experimentally control preload and afterload in humans. Studies in senescent animals using isolated heart and cardiac muscle preparations under controlled conditions have yielded the greatest knowledge of age-associated changes in contractile function. These animal studies have demonstrated that there is no deterioration in myocardial tension-generating ability with age, although alterations in contractile physiology have been discovered between young and senescent animals (Fig. 8).[35,41,42,47]

The most significant age-related alteration in myocardial contractile physiology is the prolongation of the duration of contraction and relaxation,[35,47] which can increase as much as 15% to 20% in senescent as compared to younger animals (Figure 9).[42]

Noninvasive measurements of LV ejection time have demonstrated that this occurs in aging humans as well.[48] The prolongation of the duration of contraction in senescent animals is associated with an increase in muscle stiffness and a prolongation of the action potential duration (Figure 10). These age-related alterations in contractile physiology are linked to cellular changes in the excitation-contraction coupling mechanism and may be an adaptive mechanism to preserve contractile performance in response to an age-associated increase in

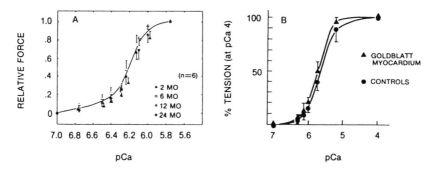

Figure 8: *Relative force as a function of pCa in thin papillary muscles from Wistar rates of varying age. Reprinted with permission from Lakatta EG: Do hypertension and aging have similar effects on the myocardium?* Circulation *75(suppl I):169-I77, 1987.*

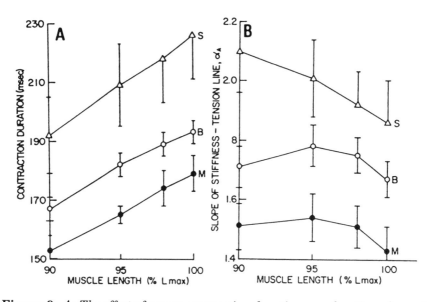

Figure 9: *A: The effect of age on contraction duration as a function of muscle lengths in trabecular muscles of rats isolated from adults, 10 months (M); senescent, 24 months (S); and adult animals in which aorta was banded to induce cardiac hypertrophy. B: The effect of age on slope of stiffness-tension relationship in the same animals. Reprinted with permission from Lakatta EG, Yin FCP: Myocardial aging: Functional alterations and related cellular mechanisms. Am J Physiol 242:H927-H941, 1982.*

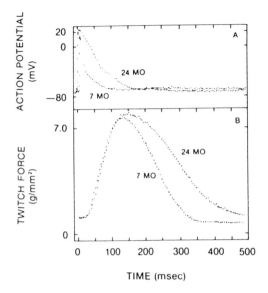

Figure 10: *Simultaneously measured transmembrane potential (**A**) and isometric contraction (**B**) in adult (7 months) and senescent (24 months) right ventricular rat muscle. Reprinted with permission from Lakatta EG: Do hypertension and aging have similar effects on the myocardium?* Circulation 75(suppl I):I69-I77, 1987.

afterload. Animal studies have shown that the force development in trabeculae carneas from senescent hearts is not compromised by changing calcium perfusate, which suggests that the calcium-dependent cell functions are unchanged by aging. However, other contractile parameters have been found to be altered by aging. These parameters include the time to peak tension and time to peak shortening, which increase with age, and the velocity of shortening, which decreases with age. These alterations reflect a reduction in the rate of myofilament shortening during early systole, which is primarily determined by the rate of myofilament hydrolysis of ATP. The rate of ATP hydrolysis in senescent myocardium is reduced compared to younger animals because of a gradual shift in myosin adenosine triphosphatase (ATPase) isoenzymes to slower forms during aging.[42] The V1 isoenzyme of myosin, which has the most rapid ATP hydrolytic rate, progressively declines with age. The V3 isoenzyme, which has the slowest ATP hydrolytic rate, increases and becomes more than 80% of the myosin isoenzyme content in senescent myocytes. This change in genetic expression of the myosin isoenzyme system has been associated with a decrease in muscle shortening velocity and an increase in time to peak force. The myoplasmic calcium transient is prolonged in senescent myocytes due to the deterioration in calcium pumping ability of the sarcoplasmic reticulum. The prolonged myoplasmic calcium transient has little effect on the rate of myofilament shortening in early systole, but plays a more important role during late systole and early diastole by determining the duration of myofilament interaction and, as a result, the duration of relaxation (previously discussed in the physiology of preload). In addition to these changes, the action potential duration lengthens in association with the prolongation in the duration of contraction and is hypothesized to be an important factor in maintaining the timing of contraction. The lengthening of the action potential duration may compensate for the reduced rates of ATP hydrolysis and calcium pumping by the aging myocyte by primarily prolonging contraction to maintain the maximum tension-generating ability of the sarcomere with aging.

Contractile physiology in senescent animals is also affected by the blunted response to inotropic stimulation by catecholamines and cardiac glycosides. There is an age-related decrement in the maximal rate of force development to both of these inotropic agents.[42] The decreased inotropic response to catecholamines is not due to a decrease in receptor affinity or number but is probably due to a biochemical alteration distal to the receptor.[42] Because the myofilament response to calcium release is probably unchanged with aging, the difference is likely caused by a decline in catecholamine-mediated augmentation of calcium release by the sarcoplasmic reticulum. The mechanism for decreased inotropic response to cardiac glycosides is not well known, but may involve the sodium-potassium ATPase receptor.[42]

These age-associated changes in excitation-contraction coupling mechanisms are thought to be adaptive responses to the alteration in myocardial loading characteristics with age (ie, afterload). It has been frequently hypothesized that myocardial hypertrophy, induced by increased ventricular load, is causally related to changes in excitation-contraction coupling. Studies of experimentally-induced cardiac hypertrophy in young rats have supported this hypothesis since the cellular changes in these animals are similar to senescent animals.[17] Other experimental evidence in rats have contradicted this causal relationship and have suggested a dissociation between myocardial hypertrophy and age-associated cellular changes in excitation-contraction coupling.[17,49] This evidence comes from 3 experimental observations. First, physical conditioning in senescent rats can reverse the age-associated cellular changes in excitation-contraction coupling independent of changes in cardiac mass (Figure 11). Secondly, there is less prolongation of the duration of contraction and relaxation and shift of the V1 to V3 myosin ATPase isoenzyme in young rats with experimentally-induced cardiac hypertrophy even though they have greater degrees of hypertrophy than senescent rats. Thirdly, similar cellular changes occur in nonhypertrophied senescent right ventricular papillary muscles. It can be concluded from these studies that changes in excitation-contraction coupling is not causally related to ventricular hypertrophy in all circumstances. There is evidence to suggest that aging may act as a stimulus for changes in excitation-contraction coupling that is independent of cardiac hypertrophy. Furthermore, other stimuli, such as physical conditioning, are able to modulate changes in the excitation-

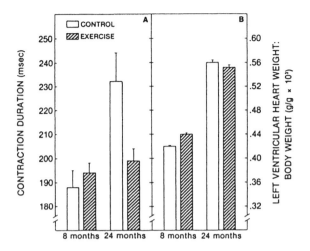

Figure 11: *A. The effect on long-term exercise on contraction duration and B. Relative heart mass in aduit (8 months) and senescent (24 months) rats. Reprinted with permission from Lakatta EG: Do hypertension and aging have similar effects on the myocardium?* Circulation 75(suppl I):I69-I77, 1987.

contraction coupling mechanism in senescent myocardium. These observations have made it clear that there are many complex and interrelated influences on excitation-contraction coupling making the influence of aging difficult to determine.

Age-Related Cardiovascular Response to Exercise and Stress

It has been difficult to evaluate the cardiovascular response to exercise as a function of age. Because exercise challenges cardiac reserve, it can amplify the effects of conditions that are not apparent at rest. CAD is one condition that can be asymptomatic at low levels of activity but can significantly impair cardiac performance during exercise. Additionally, deconditioning due to a sedentary lifestyle can also degrade exercise response. This is especially applicable to the elderly in whom levels of physical fitness vary widely. Other factors, such as smoking and body weight, must be taken into account in any evaluation of exercise response. Because of these factors, the data on exercise performance in the elderly are conflicting.

Maximum aerobic capacity, as measured by the maximum oxygen uptake (VO_2max), has been used to evaluate cardiovascular performance during exercise. Many studies have found that VO_2max declines with age after the 3rd decade, falling 5% to 10% per decade between the ages of 25 and 75 years.[50] Because VO_2max is calculated to be equal to the maximal cardiac output multiplied by the A-VO$_2$ difference, studies have extrapolated the decline in VO$_2$max to an age-related decline in maximal cardiac output.[51,52] Many of these studies were done in unselected populations. More recent studies in better screened populations suggest that while resting CO decreases modestly with advancing age, both max CO and A-VO$_2$ difference decline more substantially with age.[5-7] In other words, there is a diminution with age in the cardiac reserve to aerobic stress. Maximal CO decreases through both a decrease in max HR and a decreased stroke volume (SV) with aging. The A-VO$_2$ difference decline is determined by numerous peripheral factors. For example, when VO$_2$max is normalized for muscle mass, which decreases approximately 10% from middle age to senescence, the age-related decline of VO$_2$max is reduced.[53] Other peripheral factors which may contribute to age-related decline in VO$_2$max, include a reduced ability to shunt blood to active muscles, a decrease in capillary density, and a deterioration of muscle oxidative capacity.[52,53] The decline of VO$_2$max is highly variable between individuals and is significantly dependent of the level of physical conditioning. Physical conditioning has been found to blunt the age-related decline in VO$_2$max, as in elderly master athletes in whom the decline of VO$_2$max is one half that of sedentary persons.[6,9] In a recent study of highly trained older men, it was shown that the higher aerobic capacity attainable through regular exercise was achieved through both central and peripheral mechanisms, each of similar magnitude. These elder athletes were able to increase peak CO (through increased SV and EF with lower SVR) and A-VO$_2$ difference, much like their younger athlete counterparts.[53] Because VO$_2$max does not exclusively reflect central circulation performance, maximal cardiac output may be a better measure of cardiac performance during exercise.

As in the resting state, there are many age-related alterations in cardiac physiology that occur during exercise. An early study by the Baltimore Longitudinal Study on Aging (BLSA) evaluated the exercise response in 61 individuals previously screened with maximal exercise thallium scans to exclude CAD.[46] It was found that the maximal heart rate response to exercise declined significantly with age and exercise stroke volume was augmented to help maintain cardiac output. The augmentation of stroke volume resulted primarily from an increase in end-diastolic volume (preload) by use of the Frank-Starling mechanism. This was in contrast to the response in the non-elderly, in which stroke volume only modestly increased by a decrease in end-systolic volume and a slight increase in end-diastolic volume, and the heart rate response was mainly responsible for exercise cardiac output (CO). This seminal work produced results that were at variance with later investigators,[5-7] who detected a significant age associated decrease in resting CO and in exercise associated increases in CO. Some of the differences in these findings may have been methodological in nature (eg, treadmill vs. bicycle stress, technique of measuring CO). The limitations inherent in subgroup analysis of studies with small numbers of subjects, as well as baseline fitness levels of study subjects likely contributed to the apparently contradictory findings.

More recent studies, involving larger numbers of subjects, with careful adjustments for baseline fitness level, method of producing stress, and gender have helped to better elucidate the complex alterations in cardiovascular function with increasing age and its variation with gender and fitness/training level, etc. A recent study in another 200 individuals in the BLSA has helped determine the age-related alterations in cardiac physiology that occur during exercise between men and women.[5] These patients were screened with maximal exercise thallium scans to exclude CAD. It was found that both men and women showed a parallel decrease in peak work rate with age. Men, however, maintained a higher exercise capacity across the age spectrum. As in the previous study, older men, unlike their female counterparts, had

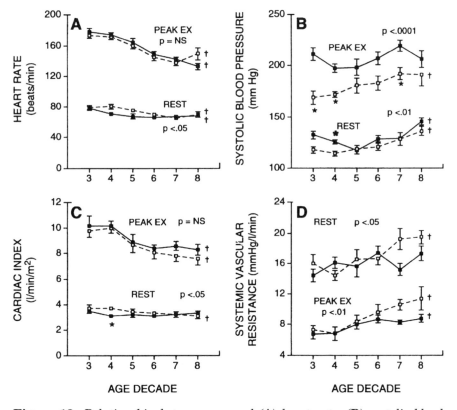

Figure 12: *Relationship between age and (**A**) heart rate, (**B**) systolic blood pressure, (**C**) cardiac index, and (**D**) systemic vascular resistance in males (■) and females (□). Reproduced with permission from Fleg JL, O'Connor F, Gerstenblith G, et al: Impact of age on the cardiovascular response to dynamic upright exercise in healthy men and women.* J Appl Physiol 78(3):890–900, 1995.

age-related increases in cardiac volumes and thus increased utilization of the Frank-Starling mechanism both at rest and with exercise. It was also found that indices of peak pump performance (EF, CI, SBP/ESVl) all showed similar declines in both men and women with age, except for SVI at exhaustion, which was not found to be age related.

Cardiovascular reserve, or "the ability to augment cardiovascular performance from resting levels"[5] was shown to decline at similar rates in both sexes, except HR reserve, which declined at a more rapid rate in men. Lastly, it did not appear that exogenous estrogens affected hemodynamics. Figures 12 and 13 graphically demonstrate these and other age-related changes in exercise physiology.

These differences in physiological response to exercise between nonelderly and elderly are thought to be mediated in part by changes in the sensitivity to β-adrenergic stimulation.[54] In the nonelderly, β-

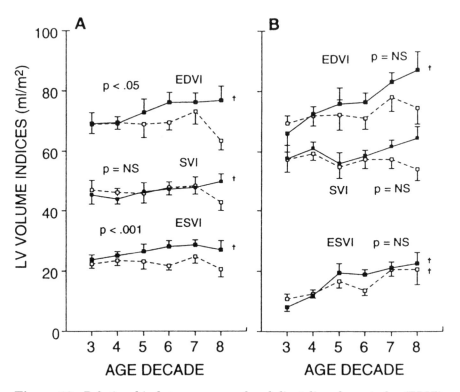

Figure 13: *Relationship between age and end diastolic volume index (EDVl), stroke volume index (SVl), end systolic volume index (ESVl), in males (■) and females (□) at rest (**A**) and at peak exercise (**B**). Reproduced with permission from Fleg JL, O'Connor F, Gerstenblith G, et al: Impact of age on the cardiovascular response to dynamic upright exercise in healthy men and women. J Appl Physiol 78(3):890–900, 1995.*

adrenergic stimulation results in significant heart rate elevation and modest stroke volume augmentation through diminished end-systolic volume, reflecting enhanced chronotropy, inotropy, and vasodilation. These same responses have been found to be blunted in the elderly even though catecholamine levels are greater in the elderly during exercise compared to the nonelderly.[55,56] This suggests that catecholamine response with aging is impaired by a receptor or postreceptor defect in catecholamine stimulation.[56] To overcome the impaired catecholamine response with exercise, the elderly, particularly men, rely on an enhanced end-diastolic volume that helps maintain exercise cardiac output by the Frank-Starling mechanism.

Clinical Implications of the Aging Heart

Age-related changes in cardiovascular physiology have many clinical implications. First, it is important not to attribute abnormalities or symptoms in elderly patients to "normal" aging. The definitions of "normal" in elderly populations are continually being refined and many changes once thought secondary to aging are now known to be false. For example, a common belief that was widely accepted for many years was that cardiac performance declined with age. It is now known that if individuals are thoroughly screened for CAD, there is minimal to no age-related decline in many important measures of cardiac performance.[46] Another misconception in the past was that the age-associated increase in systolic blood pressure had been considered "normal" regardless of the degree of elevation. The Framingham Study found that elevation of systolic blood pressure was associated with increased cardiovascular morbidity and mortality.[57] The Systolic Hypertension in the Elderly Program (SHEP) demonstrated that treatment of systolic blood pressure above 160 mm Hg can reduce the incidence of stroke by 36% and reduce the incidence of nonfatal myocardial infarction and coronary deaths by 27%.[58] In addition, the LV hypertrophy induced by systolic blood pressure elevation had also been considered a normal finding with age, but is now known to be associated with increased risk of myocardial ischemia, infarction, and sudden death.[59]

Second, a thorough knowledge of the age-related changes in cardiovascular physiology is also necessary to understand cardiac dysfunction that may occur during times of stress. Reduced compliance of the myocardium and diminished cardiac and vascular responsiveness to beta-adrenergic stimulation make the elderly particularly dependent on the Frank-Starling mechanism to augment cardiac output. Consequently, volume changes are not well-tolerated in the elderly. Reduced intravascular volume, impediment of venous return, or sudden vasodilation by disease states or drugs decrease LV preload and may dramatically reduce cardiac output and increase the risk of hypotension. Hospitalized elderly may be at significant cardiovascular risk when placed "nil per mouth" for prolonged periods of time or given vasodilatory anesthetic agents during surgery. Conversely, the elderly may not be able to tolerate sudden increases in intravascular volume as well. Reduced LV compliance with age can potentially impair diastolic filling and cause marked increases in LV end-diastolic pressure with small increases in LV volume. Consequently, intravascular volume expansion may increase LV filling pressure to such an extent that pulmonary congestion develops even though systolic function is normal. Furthermore, the loss of atrial contraction (atrial kick) may also contribute to diastolic dysfunction since atrial contraction can contribute up to 50% of the ventricular filling in poorly compliant ventricles. The development of atrial fibrillation may cause deterioration in cardiac output and lead to pulmonary congestion because of the loss of the atrial contribution to ventricular filling and reduced diastolic filling time with high ventricular rates. For this reason, elderly patients should be considered for cardioversion if no contraindications exist because of the hemodynamic benefits and the reduced incidence of stroke with sinus rhythm. If cardioversion cannot be accomplished, the ventricular response needs to be aggressively controlled so as to allow adequate time for diastolic filling, reduce ventricular filling pressures, and maximize stroke volume.

Third, age-related changes in cardiovascular physiology may affect the choice of medication prescribed for hypertension in the elderly. Elderly hypertensives have been characterized as having a contracted intravascular volume, low plasma renin activity, and increased peripheral vascular resistance.[60] Antihypertensive agents that cause vasodilation, enhanced diastolic filling, and avoid volume depletion may be better tolerated in the elderly. Calcium channel blocking agents have these properties and may be excellent antihypertensive agents in elderly patients who do not have systolic dysfunction or fluid overload. They have also been shown in at least one study to reverse the impairment in early diastolic filling in elderly subjects.[61] Diuretics, although efficacious and well tolerated in elderly patients, may theoretically cause adverse reactions through their effects on preload. One study has found significant orthostatic blood pressure change during tilt-table testing in elderly patients after a modest diuretic-induced sodium depletion.[62] Preload reduction in the elderly can result in a significant blood pressure decline with upright posture secondary to the impaired heart rate response and the reduced compliance characteristics of the aging ventricle.

Finally, physical conditioning may play an important role in modifying age-related changes in cardiovascular physiology. Animal studies have shown that the age-related changes in the excitation-contraction coupling mechanism, which prolong contraction and reduce diastolic relaxation, can be modified with chronic physical conditioning.[49] In humans, long-term exercise in the elderly has been associated with a 30% increase in VO_2max.[10,54] Although this point is still controversial,[9] at least 1 study has shown that the age-associated impairment in LV diastolic function may be ameliorated by physical conditioning.[8] This study of LV filling dynamics in young adults, sedentary old, and old master athletes found that old master athletes had filling dynamics similar to young adults. Therefore, physical conditioning has the potential to enhance diastolic filling, increase aerobic capacity, and reduce risk factors for cardiovascular morbidity and mortality. For these reasons and others, elderly individuals should be encouraged to participate in physical activity as tolerated.

Age-related changes in cardiovascular function make homeostatic balance very precarious in the elderly. Although these changes are initially adaptive in nature, they can become maladaptive and contribute to pathological derangements. This may predispose the elderly to increased morbidity and mortality from stresses easily tolerated in younger individuals. This emphasizes the need for all physians to be knowledgeable in the age-related changes of the cardiovascular system.

Summary

The physiological and hemodynamic changes associated with aging are outlined as follows:

- It is important to differentiate the effects of aging with those from alterations in lifestyle or occult diseases.
- The ability of the heart to generate force does not decline with age; however, the duration of myocardial contraction and relaxation are prolonged.
- Afterload increases modestly with age, and is related to a decrease in arterial compliance. This results in the tendency for the systolic blood pressure and pulse pressure to increase with age. Diastolic blood pressure may also increase with age, but to a lesser extent than the systolic blood pressure.
- The left ventricle reactively hypertrophies to reduce the wall stress imposed by the age-related increase in afterload. Early diastolic filling declines with age secondary to decreased ventricular compliance and impaired diastolic relaxation. The atrial contribution to LV filling increases during late diastole, which helps maintain stroke volume.
- Circulating levels of catecholamines increase with age; however, the response to β-adrenergic stimulation is muted. Therefore, the heart rate response is diminished and the vasodilatory capacity is reduced. α-Aadrenergic vasoconstriction remains intact.
- VO_2max declines with age due to a reduction in both peripheral oxygen utilization and a modest decline in maximal cardiac output.
- During exercise, the maximal heart rate response declines with age and exercise stroke volume is augmented to help maintain cardiac output by the Frank-Starling mechanism.
- The aging heart is particularly dependent on preload for maintenance of cardiac output because of the reduction in ventricular compliance and relaxation. There is greater reliance on atrial contraction and the Frank-Starling mechanism to augment stroke volume.

Overall cardiac performance does not necessarily deteriorate markedly with age. However, the homeostatic balance may be easily upset in the elderly during times of stress.

References

1. Kovar MG: Health of the elderly and use of health services. *Public Health Res* 92:9–19, 1979.
2. Gerstenblith G, Fleg JL, Vantosh A, et al: Stress testing redefines the prevalence of coronary artery disease in epidemiologic studies. *Circulation* 62:111–308, 1980.
3. Brandforbrener M, Landowne M, Shock NW: Changes in cardiac output with age. *Circulation* 12:557–566, 1955.
4. Tzankoff SP, Norris HH: Effects of muscle mass decrease on age-related BMR changes. *J Appl Physiol* 43:1001–1006, 1977.
5. Fleg JL, O'Connor F, Gerstenblith G, et al: Impact of age on the cardiovascular response to dynamic upright exercise in healthy men and women. *J Appl Physiol* 78(3):890–900, 1995.
6. Ogawa T, Spina RJ, Martin WH III, et al: Effects of aging, sex, and physical training on cardiovascular responses to exercise. *Circulation* 86:494–503, 1992.
7. Stratton JR, Levy WC, Cerqueira MD, et al: Cardiovascular responses to exercise: Effects of aging and exercise training in healthy men. *Circulation* 89:1648–1655, 1994.
8. Forman DE, Manning WJ, Hauser R, et al: Enhanced left ventricular diastolic filling associated with long-term endurance training. *J Gerontol* 47: M56-M58, 1992.
9. Heath GW, Hagberg JM, Ehsani AA, et al: A physiologic comparison of young and older endurance athletes. *J Appl Physiol* 51:634–640, 1981.
10. Seals DR, Hagberg JM, Hurley BF, et al: Endurance training in older men and women. I. Cardiovascular response to exercise. *J Appl Physiol* 57: 1024–1029, 1984.
11. Spurgeon HA, Steinbach MF, Lakatta EG: Chronic exercise prevents characteristic age-related changes in rat cardiac contraction. *Am J Physiol* 244: H513-H518, 1983.
12. Avolio AP, Fa-Quan D, Wei-Qiang L, et al: Effects of aging on arterial distensibility in populations with high and low prevalence of hypertension: Comparison between urban and rural communities in China. *Circulation* 71:202–210, 1985.
13. Learoyd B, Taylor M: Alterations with age in the viscoelastic properties of human arterial walls. *Circ Res* 18:278–292, 1966.
14. Fleg JL: Alterations in cardiovascular structure and function with advancing age. *Am J Cardiol* 57:33c-44c, 1986.
15. Forman DE, Wei JY: Age-related cardiovascular changes. Cardiovasc Rev Rep 47–51, 1994.
16. Yin FCP: The aging vasculature and its effects on the heart. *Aging Heart* 12:137–213, 1980.
17. Lakatta EG: Do hypertension and aging have similar effects on the myocardium? *Circulation* 75(suppl I):I69-I77, 1987.
18. Nichols WW, O'Rouke MF, Avolio AP, et al: Effects of age on ventricular-vascular coupling. *Am J Cardiol* 55:1179–1184, 1985.

19. Avolio AP, Chen S, Wang R, et al: Effects of aging on changing arterial compliance and left ventricular load in a northern Chinese urban community. *Circulation* 68:50–58, 1983.
20. Schoenberger J: Epidemiology of systolic and diastolic BP elevation in the elderly. *Am J Cardiol* 37:45c-51c, 1986.
21. Landahl S, Bengtsson C, Sigurdsson JA, et al: Age-related change in blood pressure. *Hypertension* 8:1044–1049, 1986.
22. Vaitkevicius PV, Fleg, JL, Engel, et al: Effects of age and aerobic capacity on arterial stiffness in healthy adults. *Circulation* 88:1456–1462, 1993.
23. Buhler F, Kowski W, Van Brumeler P: Plasma catecholamines and cardiac, renal and peripheral vascular adrenoceptor mediated response in different age groups in normal and hypertensive subjects. *Clin Exp Hypertens* 2: 409–426, 1980.
24. Pan HY, Hoffman BB, Pershe RA, et al: Decline in beta-adrenergic receptor-mediated vascular relaxation with aging in man. *J Pharmacol Exp Ther* 239:802–807, 1986.
25. van Brummelen P, Buhler FR, Kiowski WC: Age-related decrease in cardiac and peripheral vascular responsiveness to isoprenaline: Studies in normal subjects. *Clin Sci* 60:571–577, 1981.
26. Vanhoutte P: Aging and vascular responsiveness. *J Cardiovasc Pharmacol* 12:s11-s19, 1988.
27. Linzbach A, Akuamoa-Boateng E: dis Alernsuersanderungen des wenschlichen berzens. I. Das berzgenwieht in alter. *Klin Wochenschr* 51: 156–163, 1973.
28. Sjogen A: Left ventricular wall thickness in patients with circulatory overload of the left ventricle. *Ann Clin Res* 4:310–318, 1972.
29. Gerstenblith G, Fredericksen J, Yin F, et al: Echocardiographic assessment of a normal adult aging population. *Circulation* 56:273–278, 1977.
30. Kobayashi S, Yano M, Kohno M, et al: Influence of aortic impedance on the development of pressure-overload left ventricular hypertrophy in rats. *Circulation* 94:3362–3368, 1996.
31. Hayward CS, Kelly RP: Gender-related differences in the central arterial pressure waveform. *JACC* 30:1863–1871, 1997.
32. Mitchell GF, Pfeffer MA, Finn PV, et al: Equipotent antihypertensive agents variously affect pulsatile hemodynamics and regression of cardiac hypertrophy in spontaneously hypertensive rats. *Circulation* 94: 2923–2929, 1996.
33. Olivetti G, Melissari M, Capasso J, et al: Cardiomyopathy of the aging human heart: Myocyte loss and reactive cellular hypertrophy. *Circulation* 68:1560–1568, 1991.
34. Olivetti, G, Melissari M, Balbi T, et al: Myocyte nuclear and possible cellular hyperplasia contribute to ventricular remodeling in the hypertrophic senescent heart in humans. *JACC* 24:140–149, 1994.
35. Fraticelli A, Josephson R, Danziger R, et al: Morphological and contractile characteristics of rat cardiac myocytes from maturation to senescence. *Am J Physiol* 257:H259-H265, 1989.
36. Olivetti G, Giordano G, Corradi D, et al: Gender differences and aging: Effects on the human heart. *JACC* 26:1068–1079, 1995.
37. Gardin JM, Henry WL, Savage DD, et al: Echocardiographic measurements normal subjects: Evaluation of an adult population without clinically apparent heart disease. *J Clin Ultrasound* 7:437–447, 1977.
38. Bryg RJ, Williams GA, Labovitz AJ: Effect of aging on left ventricular diastolic filling in normal subjects. *Am J Cardiol* 59:971–974, 1987.

39. Iskandrian AS, Aakki A: Age related changes in left ventricular diastolic performance. *Am Heart J* 112:75–78, 1986.
40. Yin FCP, Spurgeon HA, Weisfeldt MI, et al: Mechanical properties of myocardium from hypertrophied rat hearts. *Circ Res* 46:292–300, 1980.
41. Wei JY, Spurgeon HA, Lakatta EG: Excitation-contraction in rat myocardium: Alterations with adult aging. *Am J Physiol* 246:H784-H791, 1984.
42. Lakatta EG, Yin FCP: Myocardial aging: Functional alterations and related cellular mechanisms. *Am J Physiol* 242:H927-H941, 1982.
43. Spirito P, Maron BJ: Influence of aging on doppler echocardiographic indices of left ventricular diastolic function. *Br Heart J* 59:672–679, 1988.
44. Levy W, Cerqueira MD, Abrass IB, et al: Endurance exercise training augments diastolic filling at rest and during exercise in healthy young and older men. *Circulation* 88:116–126, 1993.
45. Fleg JL, Shapiro EP, O'Connor F, et al: Left ventricular diastolic filling performance in older male athletes. *JAMA* 273:1371–1375, 1995.
46. Rodeheffer RJ, Gerstennblith G, Becker LC, et al: Exercise cardiac output is maintained with advancing age in healthy human subjects: Cardiac dilation and increased stroke volume compensate for a diminished heart rate. *Circulation* 69:203–213, 1984.
47. Capasso JM, Malhotra A, Remly RM: Effects of age on mechanical and electrical performance of rat myocardium. *Am J Physiol* 245:H72-H81, 1983.
48. Willens JL, Roelandt J, De Deest H, et al: The left ventricular ejection time in elderly subjects. *Circulation* 42:37–42, 1970.
49. Spurgeon HA, Steinbach MF, Lakatta EG: Chronic exercise prevents characteristic age-related changes in rat cardiac contraction. *Am J Physiol* 244:H513-H518, 1983.
50. Gerstenblith G, Lakatta E, Weisfeld M: Age change in myocardial function and exercise response. *Prog Cardiovasc Dis* 19:1–21,1976.
51. Conway J, Wheeler R, Samerstedt R: Sympathetic nervous activity during exercise in relationship to age. *Cardiovasc Res* 5:577–581, 1971.
52. Julius S, Avery A, Whitlock LS, et al: Influence of age on the hemodynamic response to exercise. *Circulation* 36:222–230, 1967.
53. Fleg JL, Schulman SP, O'Connor, et al: Cardiovascular responses to exhaustive upright cycle exercise in highly trained older men. *J Appl Physiol* 77(3):1500–1506, 1994
54. Lakatta EG: Age-related alterations in the cardiovascular response to adrenergic-mediated stress. *Fed Proc* 39:3173–3177, 1980.
55. Lakatta EG: Altered autonomic modulation of cardiovascular function with adult aging: Perspectives from studies ranging from man to cell. In HL Stone, WB Weglicki (eds): *Pathobiology of Cardiovascular Injury*. Boston, MA, Martinus Nijhoff, 1983, pp 441–460.
56. Fleg JL, Txankoff SP, Lakatta EG: Age-related augmentation of plasma catecholamines during dynamic exercise in healthy males. *J Appl Physiol* 59:1033–1039, 1985.
57. Kannel WB, Dawber TR, McGee DL: Perspectives on systolic hypertension: The Framingham study. *Circulation* 61:1179–1182, 1980.
58. SHEP Cooperative Research Group: Prevention of stroke by antihypertensive drig treatment in older persons with isolated systolic hypertension. *JAMA* 265:3255–3264, 1991.

59. Pearson AC, Pasierski T, Labovitz AJ: Left ventricular hypertrophy: Diagnosis, prognosis, and management. *Am Heart J* 121:148–157, 1991.

60. Lakatta EG: Mechanisms of hypertension in the elderly. *J Am Geriatr Soc* 37:780–790, 1989.

61. Manning WJ, Shannon RP, Santinga JA, et al: Reversal of changes in left ventricular diastolic filling associated with normal aging using diltiazem. *Am J Cardiol* 67:894–896, 1991.

62. Shannon RP, Wei JY, Rosa RM, et al: The effect of age and sodium depletion of cardiovascular response to orthostasis. *Hypertension* 8:438–443, 1986.

Chapter 4

The Effect of Age on the Action and Disposition of Drugs Used in the Treatment of Cardiovascular Disease

Jordan L. Holtzman

The current literature on studies in animal models and humans suggests that elderly individuals are at increased risk for adverse drug reactions. Although this increase may result from a greater sensitivity to a given level of drug, the primary cause is thought to be due to a reduced capacity of the elderly to clear drugs from the body. In view of the importance of this decreased clearance in the increased incidence of adverse events in the elderly, this chapter first describes the basic methodology used in human subjects and in animal models to evaluate changes in the clearance of drugs. This is followed by a short overview of the metabolic processes involved in the disposition of drugs and how these processes are affected by age. Finally, the individual cardiovascular drug classes and how age affects the patient's sensitivity to these agents and the disposition of the drugs is outlined.

The Effect of Age on the Absorption, Distribution, Metabolism, and Excretion of Drugs

The administration of medications or other foreign compounds to a patient leads to a multistep process in which the agent is first ab-

From *Clinical Cardiology in the Elderly. Second Edition,* edited by Elliot Chesler. © 1999, Futura Publishing Company, Armonk, NY.

sorbed from the intestinal tract, distributed in the body to the site of action, metabolized, and then excreted. In intact subjects these processes are most readily studied by determining the pharmacokinetics and pharmacodynamics of the drug. In pharmacokinetic studies the concentration of the drug is determined at various times after administration (Fig. 1). The data are usually analyzed by the determination of the clearance of the drug. This determination is fundamentally the same as the determination of the creatinine clearance and is given by the formula:

$$\text{Clearance} = \text{Dosage/AUC} \qquad (1)$$

where the clearance is the volume of blood from which the drug is totally removed per unit time and is usually given in liters per hour (L/h), the dosage is the amount of drug administered, and the AUC is the area under the time versus concentration curve. This procedure is exemplified in a study of the pharmacokinetics of lovastatin in a normal, male volunteer (Figure 1).

The AUC is calculated by multiplying the time interval between points, t, by the average height of the curve, h, between each pair of

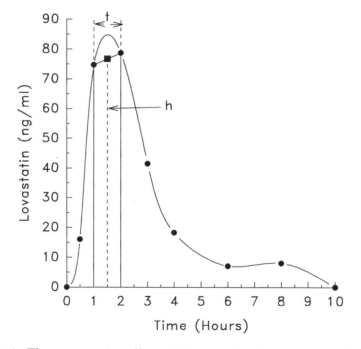

Figure 1: *The concentration of lovastatin versus time in a normal, male subject (age 40 years). The subject received 20 mg of lovastatin and blood samples were drawn at regular time intervals. The lovastatin concentration was determined by the inhibition of rat, hepatic, microsomal HMG-CoA reductase.*

points. In this example (Fig. 1), the area under the curve is 19.6 (ng/mL) × hours. With a dosage of 20 mg, this gives a clearance for lovastatin of 102 L/hr.

A major problem with this analysis is that for many drugs that are administered orally such as nifedipine or propranolol, only a small fraction of the drug actually reaches the systemic circulation. The remainder is metabolized by the liver before the drug leaves the portal blood. This phenomenon is referred to as the "first-pass effect." A high first-pass effect gives a "reduced bioavailability." The bioavailability of a drug can be estimated by dividing the AUC of the drug when it is given orally to that observed when it is given parentally. If a drug has a high first-pass effect and therefore only a low bioavailability, then the "dose" term used in equation 1 must be corrected for the reduced amount of drug reaching the systemic circulation.

The second set of parameters of interest are the half life, $t_{1/2}$ and the volume of distribution, V_d, of the drug in the body. The half-life is the time it takes half the drug to be metabolized or excreted from the body. This parameter is of importance because, as a rule of thumb, the dosing interval is usually taken as approximately 1 half-life. If the half-life lengthens with aging, then the dosing interval should be increased proportionately. In estimating this parameter, it is assumed that when the data are plotted as the log (concentration) versus time, the resulting curve is a straight line. This procedure is illustrated for the study shown in Figure 2 in which the same data are replotted as a log (concentration) versus time graph. The volume of distribution, V_d, is determined from the extrapolated concentration at t = 0 minutes, C_0, and is given as:

$$V_d = Dose/C_0 \qquad (2)$$

In a normal, human subject the total body water is about 650 mL/kg. Hence, if the drug has a V_d of 650 mL/kg, it is said to distribute evenly in the body water.

In the above example after receiving a 20-mg dose, the C_0 was 224 ng/mL, or 224 mg/L. This gives a V_d of 89 L. A 70-kg man has a body water of 46 L. Hence lovastatin would appear to distribute into a space that is equal to approximately twice the body water. There are 3 usual explanations for such a large volume of distribution. First, the drug may have a high first-pass effect so that only a small fraction of the drug actually reaches the systemic circulation. Such is the case with lovastatin. Hence in calculating V_d, it is necessary to correct the "Dose" in equation 2 for the reduced bioavailability.

$$Cl = F*Dose/AUC \qquad (3)$$

where F is the fraction of drug that is systemically bioavailable.

Second, the large V_d may indicate that the drug either binds to some tissue receptor, such as is seen with agents like digoxin, or that it dissolves in the body fat. This is seen with highly lipophilic drugs, such as amiodarone. Hence for drugs that either have a high bioavail-

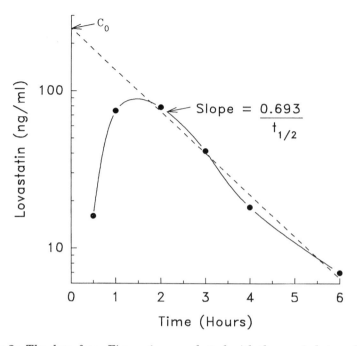

Figure 2: *The data from Figure 1 are replotted with the y-axis being changed to the log of the lovastatin concentration. The dashed line is the estimated slope of the disappearance of the lovastatin.*

ability, that is a low first-pass effect, or for which it is possible to correct the V_d for the first-pass effect, calculations of V_d can offer insights into the changes in drug distribution that are seen with aging or the differences that are observed in drug distribution between males and females. In both cases, an increased V_d would be expected to be due to the lower percentage of fat found in young, adult males as compared with the elderly of both sexes and adult females. Hence, with aging there is an increase in the fraction of body weight that is due to fat, even if there is no change in the total weight or body weight index. Similarly, young adult females have a higher percentage of body fat than young adult males. For highly lipophilic drugs, the elderly of both sexes and young females should have a greater V_d than young adult males. These differences in the pharmacokinetic parameters between males and females and the young adult and the elderly is one reason why the Food and Drug Administration (FDA) has recently required pharmaceutical companies to provide pharmacokinetic data in populations other than the usual young, male adult volunteer.

The half-life and V_d can be used to determine the peak concentration and the length of time which the drug will remain at either its therapeutic or toxic concentrations. Unfortunately, these parameters are much more difficult to estimate than clearances because the body is not a single, homogeneous pool of fluid in which the drug distributes and from which it is metabolized and excreted. Rather, pharmacokinetic studies indicate that it is divided into innumerable compartments, each of which has a characteristic V_d and half-life. As a result, the type of curve represented in Figure 2, is unusual. In most studies, the graph of the log (concentration) versus time data gives a curved instead of a straight line. It is generally accepted that this curvature represents a summation of the pharmacokinetic parameters due to each of the individual pools (Figure 3).

Because it is often not possible to determine a single half-life and volume of distribution for a drug in the whole subject, most pharmacokinetic studies are analyzed by determining the clearance of the drug. Hence, in many of the studies discussed below, the stated conclusions are based on clearance analyses of the data.

Another factor that can significantly affect the patient's response to a medication is the binding of the drug to serum proteins. When a drug binds to the serum proteins, it is not available to interact with the tissues, such as the heart. Yet, it is only the free, and not the bound, drug that can bind to the tissue receptors. There are 3 serum proteins that are involved in the major portion of the nonspecific binding of drugs: albumin, α_1-acid glycoprotein and serum lipoproteins.[1] Some

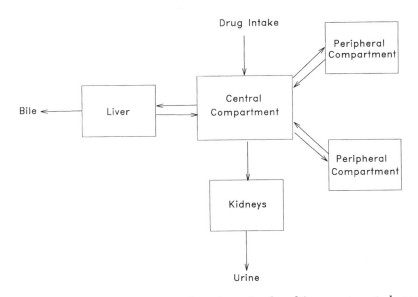

Figure 3: *A schematic representation of standard multicompartment pharmacokinetic model in which the drug enters the central compartment (vascular space) from the gastrointestinal tract, distributes into several peripheral compartments, is metabolized by the liver and is then excreted through the bile or the urine.*

drugs, such as digoxin, show little binding to serum proteins. Others, such as warfarin, are greater than 99% bound to serum albumin. Finally, drugs, such as lidocaine and quinidine, are 60%–70% bound to α_1-acid glycoprotein. Binding of drugs to serum proteins is a dynamic process and therefore is only important in determining the concentration of the drug which is available to bind to tissue receptors. Serum binding has little or no long term effect on clearance. For example, propranolol is about 90% bound to α_1-acid glycoprotein. This would suggest that only 10% of drug can be cleared from the blood with each passage through the liver; whereas in fact over 90% is cleared on each passage. This high clearance is probably due to the rapid release of the drug from the protein after the free drug is taken up by the hepatocytes, although it has been suggested that the binding protein, α_1-acid glycoprotein, may facilitate the uptake of the drug by the liver.

There are 2 caveats concerning the interpretation of data reporting to show changes in the effect of drugs in the elderly. The first is that the elderly have a high incidence of a variety of chronic diseases. It has been shown in animal models, where the effect of disease can be examined in isolation, that both acute and chronic disease can have a a major effect on both the response to and the clearance of drugs. In any study examining the effect of age on any physiological process, it is extremely important to determine whether the subjects are truly healthy.

A second major problem with many of the reports in the literature is that they have only examined the pharmacokinetics and pharmacodynamics in single-dose studies. Yet, medications are administered chronically. There can be marked differences in the results between single-dose and multi-dose studies. and the results of single-dose studies may have little meaning in the care of patients. This problem is well exemplified in studies on the pharmacokinetics of phenytoin in the elderly.[2,3] In the first study Hayes et al[2] found that in a single-dose study, phenytoin clearance was significantly greater in the elderly than in the young adult. This increased clearance correlated with a lower serum albumin concentration that they found in their elderly subjects. They postulated that because phenytoin binds to serum albumin, the lower levels of this protein would increase the free drug and give a higher clearance of the drug. This is only true in single-dose studies. After multiple doses, the body clears the extra drug and the clearance returns to normal. In fact, Bauer and Blouin[3] found that elderly epileptics (60–79 years) required 21% less phenytoin than young adults epileptics (20–39 years) in order to maintain the same serum levels of drug. Data such as these serve to indicate that reports in the literature on the effect of aging on drug metabolism may be accurate, but misleading. Hence, great care should be exercised in interpreting such data and using them in the treatment of patients. Hence, ideally for the clearances and half-lives to be of clinical significance, they should be determined for subjects who are in a steady state after receiving multiple doses of drug.

The Metabolism and Excretion of Drugs

The pharmacokinetic parameters in intact subjects are a reflection of the changes in the body composition and the metabolic processes that determine the metabolism and excretion of drugs. The primary routes of excretion of most foreign compounds are either through the urine or the bile. A few drugs, such as digoxin, are readily excreted unchanged in the urine. Yet most drugs must first be converted to more water-soluble metabolites before they can be excreted. As a result, the clearance of drugs is usually determined by their rate of metabolism to polar metabolites. The liver is the primary organ which metabolizes drugs, although there is also significant metabolism by the kidneys, the lungs, and the intestines. In animal studies, to be discussed below, the effect of aging on the drug metabolism has been directly investigated by examining the changes in the concentration and activity of these enzymes in aged animals.

There are 2 enzyme systems in these organs that metabolize drugs to polar compounds. The first are the cytochrome P-450 family of enzymes. These enzymes catalyze the insertion of a hydroxyl group on to a carbon atom in the drug molecule. This leads to the production of more water soluble compounds that are either directly excreted by the kidneys or the liver or may be further metabolized by the addition of another water soluble compound to the hydroxyl group to form an even more soluble product.

The cytochrome P-450 systems are found in a membranous, intracellular organelle, the endoplasmic reticulum. There are a number of isozymes of this cytochrome that have varying degrees of specificity. Some forms will insert a hydroxyl group onto only a certain functional group of the drug molecule, while others appear to be important in the metabolism of a wide range of compounds and functional groups. The concentration of a number of isozymes of cytochrome P-450 is increased by the administration of various inducing agents. Each of these agents appears to increase the concentration of only 1 or 2 isozymes of this cytochrome. Since the free-living human population is exposed to some or all of these agents, this induction can have profound effects on the interpretation of the changes in drug metabolism with age.

Probably the most ubiquitous group of inducing agents are the polycyclic aromatic hydrocarbons. These inducers are major toxic constituents of flue gases and cigarette tars. They are also thought to be the primary carcinogens found in cigarette smoke. These agents induce a specific family of cytochrome P-450, the IA isozymes. This induction has significant affects on the clearance of such agents as theophylline and diazepam and is the basis for the interaction of cigarette smoking with drug clearance.[4] Dioxin, the toxin found in Agent Orange and in flue gases, has a similar inductive effect. Several investigators have suggested that some of the decrease in drug clearance that is observed with age may be due to a failure of the liver of the elderly to respond to these agents.[5-9] Hence, the decreases in clearances seen in the elderly may be unrelated to the loss of constitutive enzymes. Instead it may be secondary to the inability of aged smokers to respond to the inducing agents found in cigarette smoke.

A second group of inducers are the barbiturates, of which phenobarbital has been the best studied. These agents induce the IIB family of isozymes of cytochrome P-450. Since today the barbiturates are primarily restricted to the treatment of convulsive disorders, their administration is a much less frequent source of drug interactions. Other anticonvulsants, such a phenytoin and carbamazepine, also appear to induce this family of isozymes. There are no studies on the effect of age on the induction of these isozymes.

The third important inducing agent is ethanol. This agent induces the IIE family of cytochromes P-450. As a result of this induction such agents as acetaminophen and the N-nitrosoamines are much more toxic in heavy drinkers than in abstainers. Again there is no literature on the effect of age on the induction of this isozyme.

Finally, a number of agents induce another important family of cytochromes P-450, called the IIIA isozymes. This group of isozymes were first purified from human liver because they catalyze the metabolism of nifedipine, and probably are important in the metabolism of similar antihypertensives. The common agents that induce the IIIA isozymes include erythromycin, rifampin, and dexamethasone. Erythromycin is also metabolized by the IIIA isozymes. Hence, it both markedly inhibits the metabolism of other drugs, which are substrates for this isozyme, as a well as increasing the content of this isozyme in the liver. As a result of these properties the introduction of agents, such as erythromycin, can profoundly alter the metabolism of other drugs. Initially, erythromycin blocks the metabolism of a drug like nifedipine, but with continued administration it induces the IIIA isozyme and will increase metabolism. Based on the metabolism of erythromycin, there is no decrease in the activity of this system in the elderly.[10] However, as noted above for the inductive effects of the polycyclic aromatic hydrocarbons on the cytochrome P-450 system, the elderly show less induction of these isozymes when they receive rifampin.[11] Again, many of the effects of age may be due to the decreased ability of the elderly to induce these isozymes.

A second major form of drug interaction is the inhibition of the cytochrome P-450 system by a variety of therapeutic agents. Of these the best studied and by far the most important is cimetidine.[12,13] A number of years ago we reported that this agent, which contains an imidazole ring, binds to some isoforms of cytochrome P-450 and blocks their activity.[13] The only other H2-blocker available at that time was ranitidine, which does not contain this moiety and did not inhibit the cytochrome P- 450 system. In light of the continued importance of cimetidine in the treatment of dyspesia, this interaction is of great clinical importance. The azole antifungal agents, such as ketoconazole, fluconazole and intraconazole, containing similar structures have also been reported to block the activity of this enzyme system and represent a potential hazardous interaction with agents such as warfarin.[14–16]

The other system that is important in the metabolism of drugs is the conjugative enzymes. The major conjugative enzymes catalyze the addition of a sugar acid, glucuronic acid, to the drug molecule to form the glucuronide. Glucuronides are very water soluble and are actively excreted by the renal tubules. Bilirubin is metabolized by this same system. A second conjugative system catalyzes the formation of sulfate esters, which are also very water soluble and are actively excreted by the renal tubules. There are a variety of other conjugating systems that metabolize some drugs, but are of much less importance than these 2.

In adults the conjugating systems have an extremely high capacity. Hence, there has to be almost an 80% loss of liver function before there is a loss of conjugation. The one situation where limitations on conjugations have proven to be of significance is in the newborn to whom chloramphenicol is given. The young infant is unable to conjugate this antibiotic. The accumulation of the chloramphenicol leads to the formation of methemoglobinemia, the so-called "gray baby syndrome."

The Effect of Aging on Drug Metabolism

Although a few studies have indicated that drug metabolism may not decline with age,[12] the majority of the literature suggests that the elderly metabolize many drugs more slowly than young, adults. This decline is due to many factors including changes in body composition, renal function and the activity of the drug metabolizing enzymes of the liver.[17–20] These observations in humans have been confirmed in a number of biochemical studies investigating the mechanism of the decline with age in rodents.[21–30]

A second interesting aspect of these studies on the effect of aging on drug disposition is that *in vitro* studies of human liver have suggested that the decrease in metabolism seen in the elderly may be due more to decreases in the size of the liver rather than to changes in the enzymatic activity per unit weight.[31–36] This decrease in the size of the liver is due, at least in part, to the infirmities associated with age, but appears to also occur in apparently elderly, healthy individuals.

Finally, a major, general observation from the studies of the effect of aging on drug metabolism is that the clearance of drugs that are metabolized by the conjugative enzymes appears to be far less affected by age than those drugs which are cleared by oxidative metabolism. Hence, the clearance and half-life of agents, such as the short acting benzodiazepenes[17,18,37,38] and acetaminophen,[39] which are cleared primarily through the formation of conjugative metabolites, are not affected by aging. As a result it is not necessary to alter either the dosage or the frequency of dosing of these drugs in the elderly.

Effect of Age on the Cardiovascular System: The Implications of the Changes on the Use of Cardiovascular Drugs

There is an extensive literature indicating that with age there are major changes in the autonomic nervous system, the heart, and the peripheral vasculature.[40-44] Many of these changes are due to a decrease in physical activity as individuals age.[45,46] Yet exercise alone cannot completely reverse the changes seen with aging. For example, Kasch et al.[45] found, in an 18-year longitudinal study of a small cohort of physically active men, that with age there were significant decreases in both the basal and maximum heart rates. But the maximum exercise capacity of these individuals, as measured by the VQO_2, did not change over the 18 years of follow-up. Furthermore, even after a myocardial insult, the deconditioning that occurs with a more sedentary life can be at least partially reversed in the elderly.[47] The decreases in both the basal and maximal heart rates are probably due to a combination of a loss of autonomic function, as discussed below, and the marked decreases in the cellularity of the conduction system within the heart.

Although deconditioning appears to be a major factor in the changes seen in the cardiovascular system with aging in the general population, in the usual patient with hypertensive or cardiovascular disease, there are other significant changes in the elderly. In particular, it has been found that there are increases in the total peripheral resistance and decreases in the cardiac output.[41] Similarly, although less dramatic, these same changes are seen in the normotensive elderly who have no evidence of cardiovascular disease.[48] These changes are due to decreases in the elderly in the diastolic filling that may be related to the increased amyloid and fibrotic deposits seen in the aged heart.[42,44] Similar changes are seen in the peripheral, arterial vasculature both in humans[44] and in otherwise healthy, old experimental animals.[49]

Effect of Age on the Action and Metabolism of Specific Classes of Cardiovascular Agents

β-Blockers

The use of β-adrenergic blockers for the treatment of cardiovascular disease in the elderly has been widely reviewed. On the basis of biochemical and short-term clinical studies on the action of these agents many authors have speculated on how they should be used in the elderly. They have particularly questioned whether these agents should be used to treat hypertension.

It is difficult to draw any general conclusions concerning the hazard of using these agents in the elderly since this a large family of drugs which have a wide range of chemical structures. All of these agents share only one chemical characteristic: they all contain the 3-N-isopropyl-propanediol side chain. As a result of these major differences in chemical structure, they show marked differences in their distribution, pathways of metabolism and mode of excretion. It is therefore not possible to draw broad conclusions concerning the effect of aging on their metabolism, adverse reactions and pattern of activity. Yet they obviously show the common property of blocking the action of β-adrenergic agonists. I shall discuss the basic biochemical and clinical studies which have led to the current concern about the use of β-adrenergic blocking agents in the elderly. Finally, the therapeutic trials which have investigated whether these concerns are warranted are summarized.

Studies by a number of investigators have suggested that, due to changes in the adrenergic autonomic system seen with aging, the β-blockers may not be as useful in the elderly as the young or middle aged adult in the treatment of a variety of cardiovascular conditions.[50–55] With aging there are significant changes in the functional activity of the autonomic nervous system which have been well studied for the β-adrenergic agonists. These changes can be seen in studies ranging from investigations in intact human subjects to the level of the fundamental biochemistry of the system. At the clinical level, for example, the changes seen in the basal and maximum exercise heart rates[45] are consistent with studies in intact humans[56,57] and experimental animals[49,58–60] that have indicated that in the elderly there are significant decreases in the activity of the β-adrenergic nervous system, particularly in the β_1-system.[59] These decreases in β-adrenergic activity present a major problem in the care of the elderly. As a result of this reduced capacity of the autonomic system to respond to normal activities of daily living, the elderly are more dependent on their fluid status to maintain adequate cardiovascular function.[61–63] In particular, any activity that causes a redistribution of the circulation, such as a large meal or certain medications, like nitrates, can lead to profound changes in blood pressure. When the elderly are compared to the young adult, they show a marked increase in the variability in cardiac output and blood pressure during normal, daily activities.[63]

The relative decrease in the responsiveness of the autonomic nervous system in the elderly presents a therapeutic problem since it is more difficult to adjust medication to achieve an optimal response without a significant increase in the incidence of serious side-effects. Furthermore, the decreased capacity of the autonomic nervous system, even in the absence of overt disease, leads to vasomotor instability that is associated with an increase in the incidence of falls and other disabilities that limit the functional capacity of the elderly.[63] It is of interest that food deprivation, a treatment which is known to decrease the rate of aging, reverses the decrease in β-response seen in the elderly.[64]

A large number of studies have utilized several *in vitro* systems to determine what is the primary defect which leads to the loss with age of the β-adrenergic response. These studies have incorporated recent information concerning the basic biochemical processes mediating the response to β-adrenergic agents (Figure 4). When a cell is stimulated by a β-adrenergic agent, there is an increase in the formation of a second messenger, cyclic-adenine monophosphate (cAMP).[65] This second messenger is formed from adenine triphosphate (ATP) through the action of the enzyme adenyl cyclase. The process begins with a β-agonist, such as epinephrine, binding to a receptor on the plasma membrane. This activates the receptor which in turn binds to and activates an intermediate protein termed the GTP-binding stimulatory protein (Gs). The G-proteins are a large family of regulatory proteins that require guanine triphosphate (GTP) in order to function. With the formation of this complex of the receptor with the Gs protein, the receptor is further activated so that it now has a higher affinity for β-adrenergic agents. The stimulated Gs-protein activates adenyl cyclase, which then catalyzes the conversion of ATP to cAMP. The cyclase is deactivated by an inhibitory G-protein, Gi. As discussed below, the inhibitory system is controlled by the α_2-adrenergic system. The β-stimulation is terminated by the endocytosis of the β-receptor into the interior of the cell. The intracellular pool of receptors is then recycled to the plasma membrane to form new β-adrenergic complexes.

The effect of aging on the β-response has been extensively studied with *in vitro* preparations. These studies have included the examina-

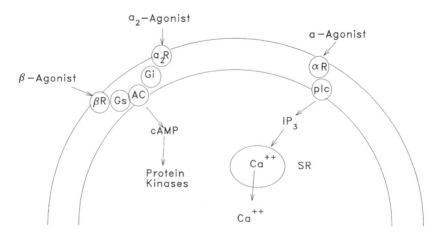

Figure 4: *A scheme of the α- and β-adrenergic receptors and their affecters in muscle cells. In this scheme aR and bR are the α- and β-receptors respectively; Gs and Gi are the stimulatory and inhibitory GTP-dependent proteins respectively; AC is adenyl cyclase; cAMP is cyclic adenosine monophosphate; plc is phosphatydilinositol specific phospholipase C; IP3 is inositol-1,4,5-triphosphate and SR is the sarcoplasmic reticulum.*

tion of such tissues as skeletal[66] and smooth muscle,[67-71] leukocytes,[72-74] lymphocytes,[76,77] cardiac muscle,[67,76,78-80] brain,[88,89] liver,[64]
and adipose tissue.[90] All of these studies have indicated that in tissues
taken from the elderly, when compared with the response of tissues
taken from young adults, there is a significant decrease in the rate of
formation of cAMP after treatment with a β-agonist. This decreased
response is probably not due to a decrease in the number of β-receptors,
because some studies have found a decrease,[91] while others have found
no change,[64,74,79] and still others have reported that there is a significant increase in the number of β-receptors.[69] Such inconsistency would
suggest that the decreased response is not due to changes in the number
of receptors, but rather to their functional capacity. Similarly, the decrease in response to β-agonists is not due to a decrease in the total
activity of the Gs protein or in activity of the adenyl cyclase that forms
the cAMP, because when the system is stimulated by drugs that act
directly on the G-proteins, without binding to the receptor, the rate of
formation of cAMP is the same in preparations from the elderly and
the young adult.[74] Taken together, these data would suggest that the
changes seen in the elderly are due to changes in the coupling between
the β-receptors and the Gs GTP-binding protein. However, more recent
studies have suggested that there is a shift in the ratio of the Gi/Gs
GTP-binding proteins in old rats.[75] This ratio was decreased in young
rats that had undergone cardiovascular conditioning, but not in the old.
Again there appears to be inconsistencies in the results in the numerous
studies. Yet, even though the studies on the mechanism have failed
to consistently identify the basis for the marked decrease in the β-
adrenonergic response with age, they have all shown this decline is a
consistent phenomenon.

Similar decreases in the responsiveness of the β-adrenergic nervous system in the elderly have been reported in clinical investigations.
Studies by Vestal et al[50] and others[51-53,55] have demonstrated that
there is a decrease in both the β-response to isoproterenol and the blockade of this response by propranolol. Colangelo et al[55] found that this
effect, although statistically significant, was very modest.

In spite of all of these observed differences in well controlled clinical
studies, there is little evidence to indicate that β-blockers are contraindicated in the treatment of either angina or hypertension in elderly
patients who are not otherwise at risk for heart failure.[43,62,92-95] In the
few studies which have been performed the β-blockers appear to be as
efficacious in the elderly as in the young. Similarly, the adverse effects
of β-blockers is the same in young and elderly asthmatics.[96] Hence even
though sophisticated clinical studies would indicate that there should
be an effect of age on the response to these agents, the sparse body
of clinical data do not support this concept. A partial reason for the
discrepancy between well-controlled, clinical studies and the observed
efficacy of these agents in the elderly is that, at least in the treatment
of hypertension, it is not clear how these agents act to reduce blood
pressure.[97] Hence many of the clinical studies on the effect of these

agents on the peripheral vasculature may not be relevant to the actual mode of action of these agents.

A further problem with the use of these agents in the treatment of hypertension is that, even though they have been clearly demonstrated to reduce blood pressure, in most long-term studies they have not been shown to be as effective as diuretics in reducing the incidence of either strokes or cardiovascular events.[98,99] As a result many of the current long-term trials that are examining the question of the outcome of the treatment of hypertension have elected to compare the newer classes of antihypertensive agents to diuretics.

Similarly, clearance studies comparing the disposition of several β-blockers have reported varying results. For example in single dose studies for the β-blockers epanolol,[100] celiprolol,[95] and R- and S-propranolol[54] the clearances were unaffected by age. Furthermore, Cockshott[100] reported that age had no effect on the clearance of epanolol in multidose studies. However, a number of workers have observed modest decreases with aging in the clearance of propranolol[101] and pindolol[102] in single-dose studies and multiple dose studies of pindolol and propranolol[102,103] or bopindolol.[105]

Of interest Hitzenberger et al[103] reported that there was no interaction between smoking and aging in the metabolism of propranolol. This is contrary to the observations of Vestal et al,[6] who found that propranolol clearance decreased with age more in smokers than nonsmokers. The difference in results between these 2 studies may be due to differences in patient selection. Yet, it would not be expected that smoking would have a major effect on the clearance of propranolol since this drug is primarily metabolized by glucuronidation, which is not affected by smoking. Furthermore, the increased clearance of propranolol in smokers could explain lack of efficacy observed for this agent in the prevention of strokes in the Medical Research Council (MRC) trial in the treatment of hypertension.[104]

One final phenomenon that has been associated with the β-adrenergic system is the up and down regulation seen after the administration of β-blockers and β-agonists. The administration of β-agonists decreases the activity of the β-adrenergic nervous system. It is generally thought that this is due to an increase in the endocytosis of the β-receptors with repeated stimulation. Yet, recent studies have suggested that both the downregulation and the upregulation discussed below are due to changes in the rate of synthesis of the receptor protein.[106] This increases the fraction of the receptors which are resident in cellular organelles rather than on the plasma membrane. The β-blockers apparently decrease this endocytosis and thereby leave more receptors within the β-complex on the plasma membrane. Even if there is a decline in the β-response with aging, the β-system still shows downregulation and upregulation after the administration of β-agonists and β-blockers, respectively.[67,73,80]

The observation that the elderly retain the ability to both upregulate and downregulate the β-adrenergic system is of clinical importance. Hence elderly patients, like middle-aged patients, who are on β-blocking agents actually have an increased sensitivity to β-agonists. As a result, when these agents are used in the treatment of angina in both elderly and middle aged adults, the sudden withdrawal of β-adrenergic blocking agents can lead to a marked increase in angina. Therefore, even long-acting agents, such as atenolol and nadolol, should probably be tapered over a 3- to 6-day period in the elderly as well as in the middle-aged patient.

Recently carvedilol, a combined α_1- and β-blocker has been introduced for the treatment of congestive heart failure.[81–85] This agent has been shown to improve cardiac performance and increase longevity in patients receiving the standard maximal therapy for their failure. This improvement in clinical status is associated with remodeling of the failing heart.[84] Carvedilol is rapidly metabolized by the liver so that hepatic failure would be expected to decrease clearance.[86,87] Age has no effect on either its clearance or efficacy.[86,87]

Angiotensin–Converting Enzyme Inhibitors and Angiotensin–Receptor Blockers

Over the past decade angiotensin-converting enzyme (ACE) inhibitors have become a major form of therapy for the treatment of congestive heart failure and hypertension. The use of these agents in the treatment of congestive heart failure represents a logical extension of our basic understanding of the pathophysiolgy of this condition in both the young and the elderly. As the heart fails, there is a concomitant increase in the production of angiotensin II. This is a normal regulatory response to the decreased perfusion pressure in the kidney. Similarly, the administration of diuretics also leads to an increase in renin production and a commensurate increase in the production of angiotensin II. These increases in angiotensin II cause an increase in the systemic vascular resistance. Yet the failing heart is unable to maintain adequate function with the added work load resulting from this increased system vascular resistance. Because blocking the formation of angiotensin II reduces the resistance, the use of ACE inhibitors acts to reduce the afterload and hence compensate for the reduced cardiac functional capacity. A number of clinical studies have demonstrated that the introduction of ACE inhibitors has been a major advance in the treatment of congestive heart failure in patients of all ages.[107]

Similarly, the ACE inhibitors have gained wide acceptance for the treatment of hypertension in the both the young and the elderly.[108–119] Yet a number of clinical investigations have suggested that these agents should not be efficacious in the treatment of hypertension in the elderly.[120–122] This conclusion is based on the observation that there is a progressive decrease in serum renin with age and that a much larger fraction of the elderly have low renin hypertension than do young adults.[120-124] Hence, hypertension in the elderly should be primarily dependent on fluid status rather than excess function of the renin-angiotensin system. As a result ACE inhibitors should have decreased efficacy in the elderly because there should be a less angiotensin I to convert to angiotensin II. Yet, the ACE inhibitors have been found to be efficacious in the treatment of hypertension in the elderly. This would suggest that the increased vascular resistance associated with hypertension in the elderly results from an increased sensitivity of the vascular system to angiotensin II. And indeed clinical studies have indicated that the elderly do show an increased sensitivity to angiotensin II.[123,125] Some studies have shown that they are more efficacious than the Ca^{2+} channel blockers[128] although others find that the Ca^{2+} channel blockers are more efficacious.[129] Hence, even though the elderly have a lower production of angiotensin II, their increased sensitivity to this hormone represents a logical explanation for their efficacy in the treatment of hypertension in all age groups.

Another mechanism that could also explain the high incidence of low renin hypertension in the elderly is that the vascular resistance associated with hypertension could be due to hyperplasia of the resistance vessels, such as medial hypertrophy. This would be analogous to the development of the left ventricular hypertrophy seen in chronic hypertension. Yet it is unclear whether this hypertrophy is a result of pressure overload or is a response to the trophic effects of hormones such as angiotensin II. In line with this latter hypothesis it is known that with long- term use, the ACE inhibitors do lead to remodeling of the hypertrophied heart.[130] Hence, much of the long-term effects of ACE inhibitors could result from a similar remodeling of the resistance vessels that is unrelated to the decrease in blood pressure seen with these agents.[131]

An alternative mechanism for hypertension in the elderly is that there could be an increase in the α-adrenergic activity with age. This does not appear to be the case because in the elderly, α-adrenergic activity is actually reduced. This point will be discussed in detail in the section on α-adrenergic blockers and agonists. Furthermore, clinical studies have shown that ACE inhibitors do not alter the function of the α-adrenergic nervous system.[132,133] Hence, it is unlikely that the effects of ACE inhibitors are mediated through a diminution in the activity of the α-adrenergic system.

Finally, an alternative mechanism for the increased vascular resistance seen in the elderly could be due to a loss of vasodilating activity of the arteries rather than to an increased response to angiotensin II. In particular, there would appear to be a loss of capacity of the endothelial to produce the critical relaxing factor, nitric oxide (NO). The interest in this area began with the seminal studies of Furchgott and Zawadski[134] who identified this important central element in not only hormone and neurotransmission, but also in the phagocytic action of macrophages. In their original studies they demonstrated that with acetylcholine stimulation the endothelium released a very labile relaxing factor. They termed this endothelial derived relaxing factor (EDRF). Other workers went on to demonstrate that EDRF was in fact NO.[135,136] Of some interest in the original description of the role of NO in the EDRF-like activity, Ignarro and coworkers[135] demonstrated that the action of nitrates and nitroprusside was due to the conversion of these compounds to NO. The NO activates an enzyme, guanyl cyclase, which converts guanosine triphosphate to cyclic guanosine 3':5'-monophosphate (cGMP).[135] This nucleotide in turn causes relaxation of the vascular smooth muscle. The endogenous NO is synthesized by 2 unrelated families of enzymes, NO-synthases.[137] One of these families has been purified from neuronal tissues and is not inducible.[137] The second is found in macrophages and is inducible by a variety of stimuli.[138] Both types of NO-synthase metabolize L-arginine to give L-citrulline and NO. The vasodilatory effects of several hormones, such as bradykinin is mediated by the stimulation of NO synthesis.

In animals it has been found that there is a decrease in endothelial NO production with age.[139,140] This would suggest that one component of the hypertension seen in the elderly could result from a decrease in NO synthesis and hence a decreased response to vasodilatory hormones such as bradykinin. As a result the vasoconstrictive action of angiotensin II would be relatively unopposed. If such is the case, then the low renin hypertension seen in the elderly could result from an imbalance between the vasoactivity of angiotensin II and the vasodilatory actions of such hormones as bradykinin.

Irrespective of the ultimate mechanism whereby the decreased production of angiotensin II leads to a clinical response, age appears to have little effect on the either the pharmacokinetics of the ACE inhibitors or their clinical efficacy.[115,141-145] The effects on the clearance of these agents that have been observed are primarily due to decreases in renal clearance of the drugs. Many of these agents, such as captopril, lisinopril, and fosinopril are administered as the active agent. While other members of this class of drugs, such as enalapril, benazepril, cilazapril, pentopril, ramipril, quinapril and spiropril are actually prodrugs, which must first be converted to the active agent through the removal of the ethyl esters. This conversion is catalyzed by nonspecific esterases. The activity of these enzymes does not appear to decrease with age. The active drugs are primarily excreted by the kidneys. Hence, there is a decreased clearance with decreasing renal function. This effect is of relatively little clinical importance because these agents are usually begun at a minimum dose and titrated until the patient either responds or the maximum recommended dose has been administered. With this approach there are rarely problems with accumulation of the active agents.[146] Finally, a major advantage of these agents is that, unlike the β-adrenergic blockers and the diuretics none of them have any effect on serum lipids or glucose metabolism.[147] As a result they have a significant theoretical advantage in the long-term prevention of cardiovascular disease.

One of the most common side effects of the ACE inhibit is the production of a dry cough. As a result of this side effect a number of agents have been developed that block the angiotensin II receptors rather than blocking the production of this hormone. These agents include losartan, valsartan and ibasartan. All of them appear to be as effective as the ACE inhibitors in reducing blood pressure and have unusually good side-effect profiles. Yet, because these agents are highly specific in their receptor blocking action and because differences in the activation of different angiotensin receptors may have different cellular effect, the angiotensin II receptor blockers may actually have some therapeutic advantages over the ACE inhibitors.

Various *in vitro* studies have shown that there are at least 2 major subtypes of angiotensin II receptors, AT1 and AT2.[148,149] All of the currently available angiotensin receptor blockers bind specifically to the AT1 receptor. This specificity may represent a significant advantage for the use of these agents as opposed to the use of the ACE inhibitors in the treatment of both hypertension and congestive heart failure. The reason for this is that AT1 and AT2 receptor blockers appear to have opposite effects on the heart and vasculature.[149,150] While the AT1 receptor stimulates the growth of myocytes and vasculature smooth muscle cells, the AT2 receptor is thought to have the opposite effect. Hence, a potential advantage of the specific AT1 receptor blockers could therefore be to enhance remodeling with a decrease in cardiac and vascular hypertrophy. Since the ACE inhibitors simply block the formation of angiotensin II, they would only enhance remodeling by preventing the growth stimulatory effects of the hormone. However, the AT1 blockers would permit the continued stimulation of the growth inhibitory effects of the AT2 receptor site. In line with the potential enhanced benefit of the AT1 blockers over ACE inhibitors it was found in the ELITE trial that elderly patients receiving losartan for the treatment of congestive heart failure had a better outcome, including a lower mortality and decreased hospital admissions, than those receiving captopril.[151] This was a small trial that is currently being repeated with both losartan and other AT1 blockers.

Studies would suggest that the use of the AT1 blockers is equally effective in the young and the elderly.[152] This is true even thought losartan has an active metabolite which appears to provide a significant fraction of the therapeutic efficacy. Apparently, with aging there is a balance between the formation and further metabolism of this active metabolite.

Calcium Channel Blockers

The Ca^{2+} channel blockers are a highly effective group of agents for the treatment of hypertension and angina. As a result of a large body of basic studies we now have a firm understanding of their mode of action. These studies have indicated that the contraction of the vascular and myocardial musculature is initiated by an increase in the cytosolic Ca^{2+} concentration. This increase results from both an increased influx of Ca^{2+} during membrane depolarization and the release of Ca^{2+} from the intracellular stores found in the sarcoplasmic reticulum. The increased influx occurs through the plasma membrane, voltage sensitive, slow channels. There are 3 classes of these channels: L, N, and T. The Ca^{2+} channel blockers prevent the opening of the L channels during membrane depolarization and thereby decrease the force of contraction of cardiac muscle. Similarly, they relax the vascular smooth muscle by reducing the peak cytosolic Ca^{2+} concentration.

There are 4 chemically and pharmacologically distinct classes of Ca^{2+} channel blockers currently used in the treatment of cardiovascular disease and hypertension: the phenylalkylamines, of which verapamil is the only agent available in the United States; the benzothiazepines, of which diltiazem is similarly the only available agent; the dihydropyridines of which there are 6 on the market for the treatment of cardiovascular disease: nifedipine, nicardipine, isradipine, felodipine, nisoldipine and amlodipine; and the tetranapthols of which the only agent available is mibefradil. This latter agent presumably inhibits both the L and T Ca^{2+}-channels. It has been withdrawn from the market because of serious toxicities. Since both the L and T channels are found primarily in the vascular smooth muscle and the myocardium, the Ca^{2+} channel blockers primarily cause vasodilatation of the arterial bed, including the coronary arteries, and thereby reduce vascular resistance. All 4 classes of Ca^{2+} channel blocking agents have similar effects on the vascular smooth muscle, but, at pharmacological concentrations, they have markedly different effects on cardiac muscle and the myocardial conduction system. At pharmacological concentrations verapamil and, to a lesser extent, diltiazem have significant negative inotropic and chronotropic effects. However, the agents found in the dihydropyridine tetranapthol groups have no direct effect on the heart at concentrations that are achieved during treatment. At much higher concentrations, all of the Ca^{2+} channel blockers have negative inotropic and chronotropic effects.

Verapamil is the oldest of the Ca^{2+} channel blockers. It was originally shown by Hass and Hartfelder[153] to be a coronary vasodilator. Fleckenstein et al[154] suggested that its effect on cardiac muscle was secondary to a decreased influx of Ca^{2+}. This is the only Ca^{2+} channel blocker that is used in the treatment of not only hypertension and angina, but also in the suppression of cardiac arrhythmias, such as supraventricular tachycardia. It has the most pronounced negative inotropic and chronotropic effect of all the Ca^{2+} channel blockers, but it is an effective and inexpensive agent for the treatment of angina, hypertension and a variety of arrhythmias. As a result it has remained relatively popular and is less expensive than the other Ca^{2+} channel blockers. A number of pharmaceutical firms have marketed extended release forms of the drug. A side effect of this agent is that about 20% of the patients will complain of significant constipation and a small percentage will have some pedal edema not related to congestive heart failure. Because of its significant negative inotropic effects, it can precipitate congestive heart failure in patients with borderline cardiac function. This clearly represents a significant consideration in the use of this agent in those elderly who might have mild failure. Yet in low doses this agent (80 mg tid) has been found to be quite safe.[155]

A major advantage of all of the Ca^{2+} channel blockers is that, unlike the β-adrenergic blockers and the diuretics, none of them have any effect on serum lipids or glucose metabolism. As a result they have a significant theoretical advantage in the long-term prevention of cardiovascular disease. Furthermore, studies have indicated that these agents are as efficacious in the elderly as in the young adult.[120–122,156]

A major advance in the use of these agents has been the introduction of sustained release preparations that meter out the drug over 12–27 hours. Until the introduction of isradipine, and more recently amlodipine, all of the available Ca^{2+} channel blockers had relatively short half-lives when administered in standard rapid-absorption preparations. Hence, the 3 agents that were initially marketed in the United States, verapamil, diltiazem and nifedipine, had to be given 3 to 4 times a day to achieve 24 hour control. Even with this dosing schedule, it was difficult to achieve constant serum concentrations of drug. The marked variation in the serum concentration led to a poor side-effect profile. In particular, this problem was a major concern in the use of these agents in patients with compromised ventricular function. For example, in light of our recent recognition of the value of vasodilator therapy in the treatment of congestive heart failure, we would assume that nifedipine should have been an excellent choice of agents in this condition. In fact, it was found that the standard preparation of nifedipine actually had a deleterious effect on survival in heart failure.[157] This effect was probably due to the significant decrease in blood pressure that compromised coronary perfusion of the heart during the peak effect of the drug. However, the newly introduced sustained release preparations appear to have a neutral effect when used in patients with congestive heart failure.

Furthermore, as noted below, in the PRAISE trial it was reported that amlodipine, an agent with a long half-life, was found to be possibly beneficial in the treatment of congestive heart failure secondary to non-ischemic cardiomyopathy.[158]

Both basic, *in vitro* studies and specialized physiological studies in humans have reported decreases and increases in the effects of the various Ca^{2+} channel blockers in the elderly. Binding studies have suggested that there is a small decrease in the density of Ca^{2+} channel sites with age in rat brain[161,162] and hamster heart.[163] In spite of these observations there appears to be an increased sensitivity to verapamil in the hearts from senescent rats compared with young, mature animals.[164,165] Wanstall and O'Donnell[166] observed a similar effect on rat aorta with felodipine and diltiazem in reversing the vasoconstrictor effects of norepinephrine. Barringer and Bunag[167] found a similar effect with verapamil. However, other workers have observed that even though the aorta from aged rats is more sensitive to norepinephrine, the response to nifedipine was unchanged.[168] Similarly, in human subjects Rosendorff et al[125] found that older subjects were more sensitive to the hypertensive effects of norepinephrine and angiotensin II. Furthermore, they found that nitrendipine had a greater effect in the angiotensin II induced increased blood pressure in the elderly but less of an effect on the norepinephrine effect. Yet in studies with the hemodynamic response to a tilt table, Shannon et al[169] found that diltiazem had a greater effect on changes in blood pressure in the elderly than in the young. Lund-Johansen[62] has reported a particularly elegant series of studies in which he has examined the effect of age on the changes seen in the cardiovascular system. He has found that the elderly have an increase in vascular resistance and a decrease in cardiac index. While the β-blockers only decreased cardiac output, the Ca^{2+} channel blockers primarily deceased the peripheral resistance. This would suggest that the latter agents are more desirable for use in the elderly population. Similarly, Abernethy et al[170] reported that in single-dose studies, verapamil showed increasing efficacy with increasing age. This increase in response was associated with a decrease in clearance of the drug. Similarly Manning et al[171] have suggested in a single-dose, echocardiographic study that diltiazem may improve the ventricular filling defect associated with aging in humans.

In summary the *in vitro* and detailed clinical studies would suggest that there is no consensus of whether the Ca^{2+} channel blockers are more effective in the elderly or the young. These seemingly confusing set of results would suggest that the various authors have reported only small changes that are highly dependent on the particular experimental conditions. Although some of the detailed studies on the action of the Ca^{2+} channel blockers have suggested that the young and the elderly may have differing responses to these agents, there is unanimity in the literature that these agents are highly effective in both populations.[140,156,172–182] In a more detailed study, Imai et al[183] have examined the effect of the Ca^{2+} channel blockers on the circadian rhythm in blood pressure. Generally, it has been found that the blood pressure reaches a peak on awakening and remains elevated until late afternoon at which time it begins to decrease until it reaches a nadir at about midnight. The pressure at 9 AM is about 10–15 mm Hg higher than at midnight. In hypertensive patients, the entire curve is shifted up to higher blood pressures by a constant amount. In the study by Imai et al[183] they found that there were some minor changes in the circadian pattern with age, but that 3 channel blockers, nifedipine, nitrendipine and nisoldipine, all caused a parallel decreased in both the peak and the trough blood pressures.

Furthermore, the Ca^{2+} channel blockers appear to be more effective in reducing the left ventricular hypertrophy seen in about 30%–40% of hypertensive patients than do the diuretics or the β-adrenergic blockers. This has been seen in both echocardiographic studies in humans[184,185] and animal studies.[186,187] This represents an important consideration in the treatment of hypertension, because left ventricular hypertrophy is the most significant predictor of future adverse cardiac events secondary to hypertension.[188] It is thought that lowering blood pressure alone does not fully protect against the adverse effects of hypertension. Hence, many investigators recommend the use of agents, such as the Ca^{2+} channel blockers, which may reverse the associated effects of hypertension. Arrighi et al[189] have reported that the short-term administration of verapamil can also improve diastolic dysfunction. If this borne out other studies, it might suggest an important role for these agents in the treatment of heart disease. In light of other studies on the neutral effect of these agents in the long term treatment of congestive heart failure, it is unlikely that they will become major therapeutic modalities in the pharmacotherapy of this entity.

Yet in spite of the excellent therapeutic effects of the Ca^{2+} channel blockers some care must be used in their use with other agents. This is particularly true of verapamil that can increase the serum digoxin concentration, very much like the effect seen with quinidine.[190-193] This is due to a decrease clearance of the digoxin.[193] The increase appears to be due to a decrease in the biliary secretion of digoxin.[194] As a result of this interaction, the digoxin levels in patients receiving both of these agents can be increased. Hence, the digoxin levels should be monitored. A similar interaction has not been observed between digitoxin and verapamil[195] nor between diltiazem[196] or isradipine[193] and digoxin.

This agent can also act synergistically with β-blockers to cause severe or even complete atrioventricular (AV) heart block. Even though this interaction has been most often seen with the intravenous administration of these drugs, verapamil, and possibly diltiazem, probably should not be used with β-blockers. An unusual interaction has been observed between the flavonoids found in grapefruit juice and the first pass metabolism of nifedipine and felodipine.[197] This suggests that an occasional patient may show a change in response to these agents with changes in diet.

All of the Ca^{2+} channel blockers are primarily cleared by hepatic metabolism. As a result there appears to be a reduced clearance with age for all of the agents.[198] These effects appear to be small and since all of these agents are titrated by effect, these decreases in clearance seen with age and hepatic failure do not usually present a significant problem in therapy. There have been several single-dose studies on the effect of aging on verapamil clearance.[170,199-206] These authors have found that there was a small, but statistically significant decrease in clearance with age. However, Hosie et al[207] and Ahmed et al[208] found that there was no significant difference in the pharmacokinetics after multiple dosing, suggesting that in the therapeutic setting, age has no effect on the clearance of this agent. Similarly, both single- and multiple-dose studies indicate that age has no effect on diltiazem clearance.[209-211]

Several groups have examined the effect of age on the metabolism of various dihydropyridine Ca^{2+} channel blockers.[212-217] These studies have indicated that in the elderly there is an increase in the terminal half-life and a decrease in the clearance for amlodipine in single dose[212,213,216] and multiple dose studies.[214–216] A more marked effect was reported for felodipine.[217] These data suggest that there is a small decrease in the clearance of these agents with age. Yet, the changes are small and should have no effect on the use of these agents in the elderly population.

A recent retrospective chart review by Psaty et al[219] has suggested that the use of Ca^{2+} channel blockers may lead to an increased mortality in the treatment of hypertension. In support of this evaluation they noted that in a prospective trial comparing isardipine to hydrochlorothiazide (the MIDAS study) that there was an increased mortality among those patients receiving the former agent.[220] Yet neither study is convincing because the former study examined only patients receiving the short- acting preparations. As noted above these have been supplanted by the long-acting formulations which have far better pharmacokinetic and pharmacodynamic profiles. The rapid release formulations may well have been dangerous in the long-term treatment of patients because of the hazard of decreasing the blood pressure during diastole. This would compromise cardiac perfusion and could lead to myocardial ischemia. The MIDAS study was too small to have sufficient power to definitively resolve the issue.

However, in the PRAISE trial examining the effect of amlodipine in the treatment of congestive heart failure, for patients with ischemic cardiomyopathy there was no statistical difference between the treatment and control groups in either all cause mortality or hospitalizations.[158] In contrast, among patients with nonischemic disease, amlodipine reduced the combined risk of fatal and nonfatal events by 31% (p = 0.04) and decreased the risk of death by 46% ($p < 0.001$). Current studies scheduled to be completed in the next few years should clarify the question of whether these agents are beneficial or harmful in primary prevention of cardiovascular disease.

α_1-Adrenergic Blockers

The α_1-adrenergic nervous system is the primary mediator of sympathetic vascular tone as well as the chronotropic and inotropic responses of the heart. The major agonist mediating the actions of this system is norepinephrine. In the past decade there has been a vast increase in our knowledge of the basic mechanism of action of this agonist. Firstly, the α_1-adrenergic receptors have been cloned and sequenced.[159,160] Three subtypes have been identified: α_{1a}, α_{1b}, and α_{1d}. A form α_{1c} was proposed, but the sequencing studies indicated that this was an error and that this form was actually α_{1a}. The response of the vascular system to the α_1-agonists is mediated primarily through α_{1b}. Although the new α_1-adrenergic blocker, tamsulosin, was thought to be specific for the prostate, the current evidence would suggest that this agent as well as all of the other currently available therapeutic agents, block all 3 classes of receptors.

A second major advance in our understanding of the action of α_1-adrenergic agents has been the elucidation of the biochemical pathway involved in the transduction of this response. It is currently thought that the stimulation of the noradrenergic system by norepinephrine is mediated through a second and a third messenger. In the first step, norepinephrine binds to a receptor on the plasma membrane and activates an enzyme termed phosphatydilinositol specific phospholipase C (Figure 4). This enzyme hydrolyzes a phospholipid, phosphatydilinositol-4,5-diphosphate, thereby releasing a phosphorylated sugar, inositol 1,4,5 triphosphate. The inositol 1,4,5 triphosphate migrates to the endoplasmic reticulum and stimulates the release of a third messenger, Ca^{2+}. The increased cytosolic Ca^{2+} activates a variety of cellular components leading to such activities as smooth muscle contraction.

There are conflicting studies in animals concerning the effect of aging on the α_1-adrenergic system. Some workers have found that there is an increase in response[168]; others a decrease in the activity of this system[89,166,218–227]; while others have reported that there is little or no change.[49,78,88,228–232] Studies on the density of receptors and distribution of the various classes of receptors have yielded similar mixed results.[233–238] In human subjects Lund-Johansen[62] and Shannon et al[169] have found that the elderly depend on fluid status and increased vascular resistance to maintain their blood pressure while the young adult relies on alterations in cardiac output. This would suggest that in the elderly there is an increase in the response to α_1-adrenergic agents. Yet Elliott et al,[239] Rosendorff et al[125] and Hogikyan and Supiano[126] have reported that the elderly show a decreased response to infused α_1-adrenergic agents. Nielsen et al[127] demonstrated *in vitro* a similar loss of responsiveness of human resistance. Rosendorff et al[125] went on further to show that the middle-aged and elderly adult showed a similar response to infused angiotensin II. Bunag and Teravainen[60] have observed similar results in aged rats. These data would suggest that the increased vascular resistance seen in the elderly may be more dependent on the renin- angiotensin system rather than the α_1-adrenergic system. One system that appears to show an increased response in man is the smooth muscle of the corpus cavernosum.[240] These authors have suggested that this increased response may be one of the reasons for the increased incidence of impotence in the older population because an erection depends on dilation of this body. This hypothesis is supported by the observation in the TOMES trial that the administration of doxazosin led to a nonsignificant decrease in sexual dysfunction while all of the other agents were associated with a reported increase.[241]

These data might suggest that α_1-blockers agents should not be efficacious for the treatment of hypertension in the elderly. Yet clinical studies have indicated that the elderly show a good response to α_1-adrenergic blockers.[239,242–244] However, irrespective of age, these agents are not effective as afterload reducers in the treatment of congestive heart failure, because tolerance quickly develops to their vasodilator effects.[245-250] The reason for this difference in the effects of these agents in hypertension and congestive heart failure has yet to be elucidated.

There does appear to be a significant decrease in the clearance of these agents with age.[243,251-253] These changes in clearance appear to have little effect on their use in the elderly. Although it may be more important to begin with low doses and carefully titrate the dosage on the basis of the observed response.

The α_1-adrenergic antagonist are a particularly attractive class of agents for the treatment of hypertension in the elderly. These agents not only decrease blood pressure, but also improve the lipid profile, decrease the left ventricular hypertrophy associated with hypertension and decrease the symptoms associated with benign prostatic hypertrophy.[243,244,254-258] Materson et al[259] have recently reported that prazosin has a moderately high incidence of central nervous system (CNS) effects, with about 13% of the patients showing increasing sleepiness. In our clinical experience with the longer acting α_1-adrenergic blockers, such as a sustained release form of prazosin and doxazosin and terazosin, we have found them to be relatively free of adverse CNS effects. As was noted above for the Ca^{2+} channel blockers, these observations with prazosin may be related to the marked variations in serum concentrations seen in this agent when administered in rapid release forms. In spite of these reports, we still feel that this is a class of agents which probably should be used more often in the clinical treatment of hypertension.

α_2-Adrenergic Agonists

The α_2-adrenergic agonists are currently used only in the treatment of hypertension. In the peripheral tissues these agents raise blood pressure, while centrally they depress it.[260] This may be the basis for the well-known rebound hypertension seen with the sudden withdrawal of clonidine where there is a more rapid loss of the central effects than the peripheral effects. This would leave the unopposed peripheral effect to increase the vascular resistance. The prominent central effects of these agents have made them less popular than other agents for the treatment of hypertension in all age groups. A study in monkeys has basically confirmed the deleterious effect of clonidine on memory.[261,262] In this study they found a triphasic effect in which the monkeys had improved memory performance at moderate doses, but decreases in performance at both low and high doses. Recent studies have shown that clonidine causes significant sleepiness in about 30% of the patients, which was 3 times the rate for any other agent.[259] In view of these effects, this is probably not an ideal class of agents to use in the elderly.

A number of investigators have examined the effect of age on the α_2-adrenergic system in animal preparations. All have observed that there is little change in the density of receptors for the α_2-adrenergic agonists with age, but there was reduced activity of this system.[78,89,224,263-266] A few investigators reported that there was no of change this system with age.[231,267] Docherty and O'Malley[221] and Klein et al[268] have found in that in intact humans there was little change or at best a modest decrease in the response of this system with age. Klein et al[268] reported that there appeared to be a balanced decrease in the activity of the β- and α-adrenergic systems so that there was no net effect.

Diuretics

The 2 major classes of diuretics used in the treatment of cardiovascular disease are the thiazide diuretics and the loop diuretics. These agents compete with Na^+ for re-uptake from the lumen of the proximal portion of the distal tubule. This can lead to a decrease in extracellular volume. These agents are not effective in the treatment of hypertension in anephric subjects, suggesting that this deceased volume may account for the antihypertensive action of these agents. However, during long-term therapy there is a tendency for the volume to be replenished with continued treatment and no loss of therapeutic response. This is an expected result because the administration of diuretics leads to a marked increase in the activity of the renin angiotensin system with retention of sodium. Furthermore, the low dosages currently used in the treatment of hypertension have little effect on the extracellular volume. Similarly, in spite of the wide range of half-lives all these agents are administered once a day, because the pharmacodynamic action appears to far exceed the serum half-life. In fact, it can take several weeks for the effect of these agents to disappear.[156] Finally, these agents do cause vasodilatation. The mechanism of this vasodilatation is unknown. It was thought that the diuretics may stimulate the renal production of vasodilating prostaglandins, but this hypothesis has fallen into disrepute.

There are number of the benzothiadiazides that have been used in the treatment of hypertension. Hydrochlorothiazide is by far the most commonly used agent in this family for the treatment of hypertension. These agents are effective in the elderly.[269-275] These observations are consistent with what we might think is the mode of action of these agents in the treatment of hypertension, because increased blood pressure in the elderly is highly dependent on their fluid status.[61-63] Yet, the thiazide diuretics do not appear to decrease blood pressure by deceasing vascular volume.

A major observation indicating that diuretics do not decrease blood pressure by merely decreasing vascular volume is that in recent years it has been observed that very low doses of hydrochlorothiazide or chlorthalidone (12.5 mg) is as effective as 100 mg.[276] Yet the lower dose has little effect on the patient's volume status. This observation has particularly important implications for the use of these agents in the elderly, because these low doses decrease the incidence of orthostatic changes in this population. This adverse reaction is very significant in the elderly because of their inability to compensate for decreases in intravascular volume by increasing their cardiac output and systemic vascular resistance.

These agents have been shown to decrease the incidence of stroke, but they do not appear to decrease left ventricular hypertrophy. Furthermore, in most studies, they either do not decrease the incidence of cardiovascular disease or show a decrease which is not commensurate with what would be predicted from the observed decrease in blood pressure.[272-274] One suggestion for this apparently poor response to diuretic therapy is that these agents may cause an increase in serum cholesterol which would partially offset the beneficial effects of reduced blood pressure. Yet studies, such as the European Working Party on High Blood Pressure in the Elderly, have found that the use of long-term low-dose diuretics does not affect the serum cholesterol.[277]

The loop diuretics, of which furosemide is still by far the most commonly used member of this class of drugs, remain the major diuretic agents used in the treatment of congestive heart failure. In studies in normal volunteers, there was a slight delay in onset of action of furosemide in the elderly but their overall water and sodium clearance was the same in the 2 populations.[278] Interestingly, the loop diuretics, even though they are much more potent in decreasing the extracellular volume than the thiazide diuretics, do not appear to be as effective in the treatment of hypertension as the thiazides, chlorthalidone and indapamide. This supports the concept that volume depletion is not the sole mechanism for the antihypertensive effect of the thiazide- like diuretics.

The major adverse effect of all diuretics is that they deplete K^+ and body Mg^{++}. The elderly do not appear to be more prone to develop these side effects than the young adult population. Of greater importance for the use of these agents in the elderly is that they can cause glucose intolerance. There are occasional patients whose glucose metabolism will markedly improve when these diuretics are discontinued, even if they are receiving only low dose therapy. In patients with poorly controlled noninsulin- dependent diabetes mellitus, it is worthwhile to discontinue the diuretic and determine whether glucose metabolism improves.

These agents are all primarily excreted by the kidneys. Hence, there is an increase in the half-life of furosemide[279-282] and hydrochlorothiazide[283-285] that is probably related to the decrease in renal function seen in the elderly. A similar problem is seen in patients of all ages who are in congestive heart failure, because they frequently have compromised renal function and therefore a decrease in renal clearance of drugs. These changes in the disposition of hydrochlorothiazide are of no clinical significance since these agents are well tolerated by patients of all age groups. Furthermore, as long as the clinician begins the administration of the diuretics at the lowest doses that are usually clinically effective and increases the dosage slowly, there are usually few problems. This is not true of amiloride since with standard dosing, both Sabanathan et al[284] and Ismail et al[285] found that elderly patients had higher steady- state concentrations of this agent. Similar results have been observed with spironolactone, although these data are not definitive because the elderly patients also had multiple medical conditions.[286] These increased serum levels could lead to an increased incidence of hyperkalemia when amiloride or spironolactone combinations are administered to the elderly.

Digitalis

Digitalis is the oldest of the agents currently used in the treatment of cardiovascular disease. It is most commonly prescribed as the purified glycoside, digoxin. The other digitalis glycosides are now only rarely used. Digoxin is used in 2 settings. First, it is the only agent used in clinical practice that enhances the inotropic action of the heart. It does so by increasing the cytosolic concentration of Ca^{2+} in the heart muscle. The increased Ca^{2+} concentration increases the force of contraction. This increased Ca^{2+} is a result of a decreased extrusion of Ca^{2+}. The Ca^{2+} concentration in the heart is regulated by a balance between the leakage of this ion into the cell through the Ca^{2+} channels in the plasma membrane and the removal of Ca^{2+} by the Na^+/Ca^{2+} antiporter (Figure 5). This antiporter system uses the high Na^+ gradient across the plasma membrane to force the Ca^{2+} out of the cell.

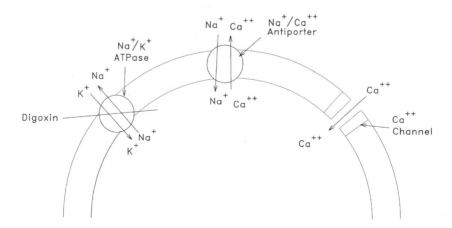

Figure 5: *Scheme outlining the mechanism for the ionotropic effect of digoxin.*

Digoxin acts by inhibiting the Na^+/K^+-ATPase of the myocardium, which pumps Na^+ out of the cell. This inhibition decreases the Na^+ extruded from the cell and leads to a decrease in the Na^+ gradient. The decreased gradient reduces the rate of removal of Ca^{2+} leaving a higher concentration of Ca^{2+} inside the cell than would normally be present. In spite of its use for over 200 years, its efficacy in congestive heart failure has only been recently demonstrated in a large clinical trial.[288] In this placebo-controlled trial, the investigators found that this agent did not decrease mortality, but it did decrease the rate of hospitalization.

Second, digoxin is used to block AV conduction to reduce the heart rate in patients with supraventricular tachycardias and atrial fibrillation.

Digoxin is primarily excreted by the kidney with 30% excreted by the intestines. Hence in anephric patients the half-life increases 3-fold and the required dosage decreases to a third.[287,289,290] In the elderly, there is a parallel increase in half-life with the decrease in renal function.[290] Animal studies would suggest that in the aged there is an increased sensitivity of the myocardium to digoxin,[291] although systolic time interval studies in humans have not confirmed this result.[292]

The digitalis glycosides have a very low therapeutic index. As a result in the elderly, or in any patient with impaired renal function, it is important to slowly titrate the dose of digoxin. In spite of the increased sensitivity of the elderly to this agent, the incidence of clinical significant toxicity is about 40% in all age groups.[293]

Furthermore, the clinical presentation is the same in the middle-aged and elderly adult.[293] Unfortunately, the serum levels of digoxin are of little value in adjusting the dosage of the drug.[294,295] It can be useful in confirming the presence of significant toxicity, but it should not be used to titrate the dosage.

The coadministration of digoxin and quinidine can lead to significant increases in the serum digoxin levels.[296–300] This effect has been attributed to both decreased renal and extrarenal clearance of digoxin[247,300–305] and displacement of digoxin from binding sites found in skeletal muscle.[301,306–308] This displacement leads to higher serum concentrations and an increased incidence of digoxin toxicity. Although dog studies suggest that the increased concentrations of digoxin do not lead to an increase in the inhibition of the cardiac Na^+/K^+ ATPase,[309] it is probably still prudent to closely monitor the digoxin concentrations when this agent is coadministered with quinidine. A similar interaction has been reported with verapamil[190,192,193,195] and amiodarone,[310] for digoxin but not with digitoxin.[311–314]

HMG–CoA Reductase Inhibitors

The introduction of the HMG-CoA reductase inhibitors has been one of the most important advances in the treatment and prevention of cardiovascular disease. Numerous primary and secondary prevention outcome trials have indicated that in middle aged and elderly individuals these agents significantly decrease the incidence of cardiovascular disease and prevent recurrent manifestations of the disease, irrespective of age, sex, or smoking status.[315-332] This effect appeared to be most significant in patients with low-density lipoprotein (LDL) cholesterol in excess of 160 mg/dL.[327,330,331] They have also been demonstrated to decrease the incidence of stroke.[333,334] Finally, they have been found to act synergistically with other classes of hypolipidemic agents to decrease the levels of LDL cholesterol and triglycerides in patients with severe hyperlipidemias and increase the concentrations of high-density lipoprotein (HDL) cholesterol.[335-339]

It is important to recognize that the improvement in cardiovascular outcome was discernible within 1 year after the initiation of therapy even in very elderly patients. These observations are surprising because many of the preventive measures which have become part of our recognized standard of care in both primary and secondary prevention are thought to be far less effective in the elderly. This assumption is based on the observation that there appears to be a natural aging process which compromises vascular function irrespective of the individual's blood pressure or serum lipid concentrations. Hence, on the basis of the published studies, it would appear to be reasonable to implement therapy for LDL cholesterols in excess of 160 mg/dL in the elderly as well as middle-aged patients. Furthermore, there is no published evidence to indicate that our therapeutic approach should be modified in treatment of the elderly.

Finally, one of the ironies of the introduction of this class of agents is that their development was predicated on the assumption that their primary effect would be to decrease the production of cholesterol by inhibiting an early step in its synthesis, yet a wide range of studies have suggested that they have multiple effects, the most important of which may be the induction of the synthesis of LDL receptors.[340] This increase leads to an increase in the rate of clearance of these lipoproteins rather than a decrease in synthesis.

Oral Anticoagulants

The oral anticoagulants, of which warfarin is the most commonly used, are probably the most dangerous drugs used for the treatment of non-neoplastic disease. Unlike even these latter agents, the effective use of anticoagulants requires that the patient's prothrombin time or international normalized ratio (INR) be maintained within a very narrow window. Yet, in spite of the absolute need for very careful monitoring of patients on these agents, there has been a recent increase in their usage. This increase has been a result of the recent demonstration of the value of anticoagulant therapy in the prevention of strokes in patients with chronic atrial fibrillation.

Warfarin blocks the reduction of vitamin K. Vitamin K is required for the synthesis of prothrombin through the δ-carboxylation of prepro-thrombin. During this conversion, vitamin K is oxidized. The oxidized vitamin is normally reduced by a specific enzyme in the liver which is inhibited by warfarin. This inhibition is readily overcome by the administration of therapeutic doses of vitamin K or by an increase in the consumption of green, leafy vegetables, the primary source of this vitamin in the diet. As a result of this balance in the action of vitamin K and the oral anticoagulants, the primary problem in utilizing these agents is that the patient must maintain a constant intake of the vitamin. This can be a problem in the elderly who frequently consume only modest quantities of these foods. Furthermore, changes in diet can lead to sudden changes in warfarin requirements. This is particularly a problem when patients become ill and stop eating.[341,342] Even though a decrease in the metabolism of warfarin with age has been noted, it does not appear to be specifically due to age, but rather is due to the increased incidence of serious disease in the elderly.[343-347]

Finally as noted above, one of the major problems is that great care must be exercised in the introduction of other therapeutic agents along with the warfarin. Cimetidine is the best studied of these agents.[13-16] But other agents, such as some of the antidepressants that inhibit warfarin metabolism and many of the anticonvulsants or erythromycin that induce its metabolism, can markedly affect the management of anticoagulation. This has become a particularly significant problem with the recent approval of cimetidine as an "over-the-counter" medication. Fortunately, there are many alternatively therapeutic agents that can be substituted for those agents that present a potential risk.

Antiarrhythmics

There have been few studies on the effect of age on the use of the class I antiarrhythmics. Studies in humans have indicated that in the elderly there is a decreased clearance of procainamide and N-acetylpro-cainamide,[348,349] disopyramide,[9] and lidocaine.[350] Roberts and Gold-berg[351] found in animal studies that the effects of quinidine decreased with age while the effect of lidocaine increased. Again in view of the standard practice of titrating the dose of these agents until there is a therapeutic response or significant changes in the electrocardiogram, none of these effects are probably of clinical significance.

One of the major areas in which antiarrhythmic agents have yet to show promise is in the long-term treatment of patients with severe myocardial disease. These patients have a very high incidence of sudden death due to ventricular arrhythmias. Unfortunately, as well documented in the CAST trials,[352] the classic antiarrhythmic agents not only fail to improve outcome, but actually increased long-term mortality. This effect was due to a well known proarrhythmic effect of these agents that was more pronounced in the elderly.[353] The only agent to show promise in this group of patients is amiodarone.[354–356] Unfortunately, this agent has an unusually high incidence of potentially serious side effects including both hyperthyroidism and hypothyroidism and pulmonary toxicity. It is hoped that more benign and yet efficacious agents will be able to supersede this agent.

Conclusions

It is clear that aging can alter the use of therapeutic agents in the treatment of cardiovascular disease. Yet, no single class of agents that is used in the young and middle-aged adult is contraindicated for use in the elderly. Rather, the use of all agents in all age groups should be initiated at the lowest dose that can give a response and then titrated to either the dose that gives the desired therapeutic response; the dose above which a response is unlikely; or the dose at which the patient has adverse reactions. Irrespective of the patient's age, this is the most judicious approach to initiation and maintenance of drug therapy.

References

1. Brinkschulte M, Breyer-Pfaff U: The contribution of alpha-1-acid glycoprotein, lipoproteins and albumin to the plasma binding of perazine, amitriptyline, and nortriptyline in healthy man. *N.S. Arch Pharmacol* 316: 61–66, 1980.
2. Hayes MJ, Langman MJ, Short AH: Changes in drug metabolism with increasing age: 2. Phenytoin clearance and protein binding. *Br J Clin Pharmacol* 2:73–79, 1975.
3. Bauer LA, Blouin RA: Age and phenytoin kinetics in adult epileptics. *Clin Pharmacol Ther* 31:301–304, 1982.
4. Jusko WJ: Role of tobacco smoking in pharmacokinetics. *J Pharmacokinet Biopharm* 6:7–39, 1978.
5. Vestal RE, Norris AH, Tobin JD, et al: Antipyrine metabolism in man: Influence of age, alcohol, caffeine and smoking. *Clin Pharmacol Ther* 18: 425–432, 1975
6. Vestal RE, Wood AJJ, Branch RA, et al: Effects of age and cigarette smoking on the disposition of propranolol in man. *Clin Pharmacol Ther* 26: 8–15, 1979.
7. Vestal RE, Wood AJJ: Influence of age and smoking on drug kinetics in man. *Clin. Pharmacokinet* 5:309–319, 1980.
8. Wood AJJ, Vestal RE, Wilkinson GR, et al: Effects of aging and cigarette smoking on antipyrine and indocyanine green elimination. *Clin Pharmacol Ther* 26:16–20, 1979.
9. Bonde J, Pedersen LE, Bidtker S, et al: The influence of age and smoking on the elimination of disopyramide. *Br J Clin Pharmacol* 20:453–458, 1985.
10. Hunt CM, Westerkam WR, Stave GM, et al: Hepatic cytochrome P-4503A (CYP3A) activity in the elderly. *Mech Ageing Dev* 64:189–199, 1992.
11. Smith DA, Chandler MH, Shedlofsky SI, et al: Age-dependent stereoselec-

tive increase in the oral clearance of hexobarbitone isomers caused by rifampicin. *Br J Clin Pharmacol* 32: 735–739, 1991.

12. Arora S, Kassarjian Z, Krasinski SD, et al: Effect of age on tests of intestinal and hepatic function in healthy humans. *Gastroenterology* 96: 1560–1565, 1989.

13. Knodell RG, Holtzman JL, Crankshaw DL, et al: Drug metabolism by rat and human hepatic microsomes in response to interaction with H2-receptor antagonists. *Gastroenterology* 8:82–84, 1982

14. Guengerich FP: Role of cytochrome P450 enzymes in drug-drug interactions. *Adv Pharmacol* 43:7–35, 1997.

15. Albengres E, Le Louet H, Tillement JP: Systemic antifungal agents. Drug interactions of clinical significance. *Drug Saf* 18:83–97, 1998.

16. Li AP, Jurima-Romet M: Overview: Pharmacokinetic drug-drug interactions. *Adv Pharmacol* 43:1–6, 1997.

17. Greenblatt DJ, Sellers EM, Shader RI. Drug disposition in old age. *N Engl J Med* 306:1061–1088, 1982.

18. Greenblatt DJ, Divoll M, Abernethy DR, et al: Physiologic changes in old age: Relation to altered drug disposition. *J Am Geriatrics Soc* 30:S6-S10, 1982.

19. Schmucker DL: Aging and drug disposition: An update. *Pharmacol Rev* 37:133–148, 1985.

20. Jackson SH, Johnston A, Woollard R, et al: The relationship between theophylline clearance and age in adult life. *Eur J Clin Pharmacol* 36: 29–34, 1989.

21. Kato R, Takanaka A: Metabolism of drugs in old rats (I). Activities of NADPH- linked electron transport and drug-metabolizing enzyme systems in liver microsomes of old rats. *Jpn J Pharmacol* 18:381–388, 1968.

22. Birnbaum LS: Altered hepatic drug metabolism in senescent mice. *Exp Gerontol* 15:259–267, 1980.

23. Schmucker DL, Wang RK: (1980) Age-related changes in liver enzymes. *Exp Gerontol* 15:321–329, 1980.

24. Schmucker DL, Wang RK: Age-dependent alterations in rat liver microsomal NADPH-cytochrome c (P-450) reductase: A qualitative and quantitative analysis. *Mech Ageing Dev* 21:137–136, 1983.

25. Schmucker DL, Wang RK: Age-dependent changes in rat liver microsomal NADPH-cytochrome c (P-450) reductase: A kinetic analysis. *Exp Gerontol* 15:313–321, 1983.

26. Rikans LE, Notley BA: Differential effects of aging on hepatic microsomal monooxygenase induction by phenobarbital and α-naphthoflavone. *Biochem Pharmacol* 31:2339–2343, 1982.

27. Sitar DS, Desai CD: Effect of aging on response to induction and metabolizing activity of the hepatic mixed-function oxidase system of male Sprague-Dawley rats. *Can J Physiol Pharmaco.* 61:89–94, 1983.

28. Kamataki T, Maeda K, Shimada M, et al: Age-related alteration in the activities of drug-metabolizing enzymes and contents of sex-specific forms of cytochrome P-450 in liver microsomes from male and female rats. *J Pharmacol Exp Ther* 233:222–228, 1985.

29. Sun J, Lau PP, Strobel HW: Aging modifies the expression of hepatic microsomal cytochromes P-450 after pretreatment of rats of with α-naphthoflavone or phenobarbital. *Exp Gerontol* 21:65–73, 1986.

30. Bandiera S, Ryan DE, Levin W, et al: Age- and sex-related expression of cytochromes P-450f and P-450g in rat liver. *Arch Biochem Biophys* 248: 658–676, 1986.

31. Woodhouse KW, Mutch E, Williams FM, et al: The effect of age on pathways of drug metabolism in human liver. *Age Ageing* 13:328–334, 1984.
32. Schnegg M, Lauterburg BH: Quantitative liver function in the elderly assessed by galactose elimination capacity, aminopyrine demethylation and caffeine clearance. *J Hepatol* 3:164–171, 1986.
33. Schmucker DL, Woodhouse KW, Wang RK, et al: Effects of age and gender on in vitro properties of human liver microsomal monooxygenases. *Clin Pharmacol Ther* 48:365–374, 1990.
34. Woodhouse KW, Wynne HA: Age-related changes in liver size and hepatic blood flow. The influence on drug metabolism in the elderly. *Clin Pharmacokinet* 15:287–294, 1988.
35. Wynne HA, Cope LH, James OF, et al: The effect of age and frailty upon acetanilide clearance in man. *Age Ageing* 18:415–418, 1989.
36. Woodhouse KW, James OF: Hepatic drug metabolism and ageing. *Br Med Bull* 46:22–35, 1990.
37. Ochs HR, Greenblatt DJ, Otten H: Disposition of oxazepam in relation to age, sex, and cigarette smoking. *Klin. Wochenschrift* 59:899–903, 1981.
38. Vozeh S: Pharmacokinetic of benzodiazepines in old age. *Schweiz Med Wochenschrift-J Suisse Med* 111:1789–1793, 1981.
39. Miners JO, Penhall R, Robson RA, et al: Comparison of paracetamol metabolism in young adult and elderly males. *Eur J Clin Pharmacol* 35:157–160, 1988.
40. Walsh RA: Cardiovascular effects of the aging process. *Am J Med* 82(suppl 1B):34–40, 1987.
41. Lund-Johansen P: The hemodynamics of the aging cardiovascular system. *J Cardiovasc Pharmacol* 12(suppl 8):S20-S30, 1988.
42. Morley JE, Reese SS: Clinical implications of the aging heart. *Am J Med* 86:77–86, 1989.
43. Collins KJ: Age related changes in autonomic control: The use of beta blockers in the treatment of hypertension. *Cardiovasc Drugs Ther* 4(suppl 6):1257–1262, 1991.
44. Wei JY: Age and the cardiovascular system. *N Engl J Med* 327:1735–1739, 1992.
45. Kasch FW, Wallace JP, Van Camp SP: Effects of 18 years of endurance exercise on the physical work capacity of older men. *J Cardiopulm Rehabil* 5:308–312, 1985.
46. Vaughan L, Zurlo F, Ravussin E: Aging and energy expenditure. *Am J Clin Nutr* 53:821–825, 1991.
47. Williams MA, Maresh CM, Esterbrooks DJ, et al: Early exercise training in patients older than age 65 years compared with that in younger patients after acute myocardial infarction or coronary artery bypass grafting. *Am J Cardiol* 55:263–266, 1985.
48. Downes TR, Nomeir A-M, Smith KM, et al: Mechanism of altered pattern of left ventricular filling with aging in subjects without cardiac disease. *Am J Cardiol* 64:523–527, 1989.
49. Frolkis VV, Bezrukov VV, Shevchuk VG: Hemodynamics and its regulation in old age. *Exp Gerontol* 10:251–271, 1975.
50. Vestal RE, Wood AJJ, Shand DG: Reduced beta-adrenoceptor sensitivity in the elderly. *Clin Pharmacol Ther* 26:181–185, 1979.
51. Bertel O, Buhler FR, Kiowski W, et al: Decreased beta-adrenoceptor responsiveness as related to age, blood pressure, and plasma catecholamines in patients with essential hypertension. *Hypertension* 2:130–138, 1980.

52. Klein C, Gerber JG, Gal J, et al: Beta-adrenergic receptors in the elderly are not less sensitive to timolol. *Clin Pharmacol Ther* 40:161–164, 1986.
53. Tenero DM, Bottorff MD, Burlew BS, et al: *J Cardiovasc Pharmacol* 16: 702–707, 1990.
54. Colangelo PM, Blouin RA, Steinmetz JE, et al: Age and propranolol stereoselective disposition in humans. *Clin Pharmacol Ther* 51:489–494, 1992.
55. Colangelo PM, Blouin RA, Steinmetz JE, et al: Age and β-adrenergic receptor sensitivity to S(-)- and R,S(+)-propranolol in humans. *Clin Pharmacol Ther* 51:549–545, 1992.
56. Lakatta EC: Age-related alterations in the cardiovascular response to adrenergic mediated stress. *Fed Proc* 39:3173, 1980.
57. Lakatta EC: Diminished beta-adrenergic modulation of cardiovascular function in advanced age. *Cardiol Clin* 4:185–200, 1986.
58. Rothbaum DA, Shaw DJ, Angell CS, et al: Age differences in the baroreceptor response of rats. *J Gerontol* 29:488–492, 1974.
59. Parfitt KD, Bickford-Wimer P: Age-related subsensitivity of cerebellar Purkinje neurons to locally applied beta$_1$-selective adrenergic agonist. *Neurobiol Aging* 11:591–596, 1990.
60. Bunag RD, Teravainen TL: Waning cardiovascular responses to adrenergic drugs in conscious ageing rats. *Mech Ageing Dev* 61:313–326, 1991.
61. Lipsitz LA, Marks ER, Koestner J, et al: Reduced susceptibility to syncope during postural tilt in old age. Is beta-blockade protective. *Arch Intern Med* 149:2709–2712, 1989.
62. Lund-Johansen P: Age hemodynamics and exercise in essential hypertension: Difference between β-blockers and dihydropyridine calcium antagonists. *J Cardiovasc Pharmacol* 14(suppl 10):S7-S13, 1989.
63. Jonsson PV, Lipsitz LA, Kelley M, et al: Hypotensive responses to common daily activities in institutionalized elderly. A potential risk for recurrent falls. *Arch Intern Med* 150:1518–1524, 1990.
64. Dax EM, Ingram DK, Partilla JS, et al: Food restriction prevents an age-associated increase in rat liver beta-adrenergic receptors. *J Gerontol* 44: B72-B76, 1989.
65. Heinsimer JA, Lefkowitz RJ: The impact of aging on adrenergic receptor function: Clinical and biochemical aspects. *J Am Geriatrics Soc* 33: 184–188, 1985.
66. Elfellah MS, Dalling R, Kantola IM, et al: Beta-adrenoceptors and human skeletal muscle characterization of receptor subtype and effect of age. *Br J Clin Pharmacol* 27:31–38, 1989.
67. Pitha J, Hughes BA, Kusiak JW, et al: Regeneration of β-adrenergic receptors in senescent rats: A study using an irreversible binding antagonist. *Proc Natl Acad Sci* 79:4424–4427, 1982.
68. Feldman RD, Limbird LE, Nadeau J, et al: Alterations in leukocyte β-receptor affinity with aging. A potential explanation for altered β-adrenergic sensitivity in the elderly. *N Engl J Med* 310:815–819, 1984.
69. Feldman RD: Physiological and molecular correlates of age-related changes in the human β-adrenergic receptor system. *Fed Proc* 45:48–50, 1986.
70. O'Donnell SR, Wanstall JC: Thyroxine treatment of aged or young rats demonstrates that vascular responses mediated by beta-adrenoceptor subtypes can be differentially regulated. *Br J Pharmacol* 88:41–49, 1986.
71. Mader SL: Influence of animal age on the beta-adrenergic system in cultured rat aortic and mesenteric artery smooth muscle cells. *J Gerontol* 47:B32-B36, 1992.

72. Zahniser NR, Parker DC, Bier-Laning CM, et al: Comparison between the effects of aging on antagonist and agonist interactions with beta-adrenergic receptors on human mononuclear and polymorphonuclear leukocyte membranes. *J Gerentol* 43:M151-M157, 1988.
73. Zahniser NR, Wiser A, Cass WA, et al: Terbutaline-induced desensitization of polymorphonuclear leukocyte β_2-adrenergic receptors in young and elderly subjects. *Clin Pharmacol Ther* 51:432–439, 1992.
74. Vanscheeuwijck P, Van de Velde E, Fraeyman N. Characterization of the beta- adrenergic transduction system in spleen mononuclear leukocyte membranes of young and senescent rats. *Biochem Pharmacol* 39: 2035–2040, 1990.
75. Roth DA, White CD, Podolin DA, et al: Alterations in myocardial signal transduction due to aging and chronic dynamic exercise. *J Appl Physiol* 84:177–184, 1998.
76. Scarpace PJ: Decreased β-adrenergic responsiveness during senescence. *Fed Proc* 45: 51–54, 1986.
77. Gietzen DW, Goodman TA, Weiler PG, et al: Beta receptor density in human lymphocyte membranes: Changing with aging? *J Gerontol* 46: B130-B134, 1991.
78. Goldberg PB, Kreider MS, McLean MR, et al: Effects of aging at the adrenergic cardiac neuroeffector junction. *Fed Proc* 45:45–47, 1986.
79. Matsumori Y, Ohyanagi M, Kawamoto H, et al: Intracellular distribution of cardiac beta-adrenoceptors in SHR and WKY. *Jpn Circ J* 53:113–120, 1989.
80. Tumer N, Houck WT, Roberts J: Effect of age on upregulation of the cardiac adrenergic beta receptors. *J Gerontol* 45:B48-B51, 1990.
81. Krum H, Sackner-Bernstein JD, Goldsmith, RL, et al: Double-blind, placebo- controlled study of the long-term efficacy of carvedilol in patients with severe chronic heart failure. *Circulation* 92:1499–1506, 1995.
82. Packer M, Bristow MR, Cohn JN, et al: The effect of carvedilol on morbidity and mortality in patients with chronic heart failure. U.S. Carvedilol Heart Failure Study Group. *N Engl J Med* 334:1349–1355, 1996
83. Cohn JN, Fowler MB, Bristow MR, et al: *J Cardiac Failure* 3:173–179, 1997.
84. Doughty RN, Whalley GA, Gamble G, et al: Left ventricular remodeling with carvedilol in patients with congestive heart failure due to ischemic heart disease. Australia-New Zealand Heart Failure Research Collaborative Group. *J Am Coll Cardiol* 29:1060–1066, 1997.
85. Anonymous: Randomised, placebo-controlled trial of carvedilol in patients with congestive heart failure due to ischaemic heart disease. Australia/ New Zealand Heart Failure Research Collaborative Group [see comments]. *Lancet* 349:375–380, 1997.
86. Morgan T, Anderson A, Cripps J, et al: Pharmacokinetics of carvedilol in older and younger patients. *J Hum Hypertens* 4:709–715, 1990.
87. Morgan T. Clinical pharmacokinetics and pharmacodynamics of carvedilol. *Clin Pharmacokinet* 26:335–346, 1994.
88. De Blasi A, Cotecchia S, Mennini T: Selective changes of receptor binding in brain regions of aged rats. *Life Sci* 31:335–340, 1982.
89. Greenberg LH: Regulation of brain adrenergic receptors during aging. *Fed Proc* 45:55–59, 1986.
90. Kobatake T, Watanabe Y, Matsuzawa Y, et al: Age-related changes in adrenergic α_1, α_2, and β receptors of rat white fat cell membranes: An

analysis using [3H]bunazosin as a novel ligand for the α_1 adrenoceptor. *J Lipid Res* 32:191–196, 1991.

91. Scarpace PJ, Mooradian AD, Morley JE: Age-associated decrease in beta-adrenergic receptors and adenylate cyclase activity in rat brown adipose tissue. *J Gerontol.* 43: B65-B70, 1988.

92. Wilkins MR, Kendall KJ: Beta-adrenoceptor blocking drugs and the elderly. *J R Coll Physicians* 18:42–45, 1984.

93. Fitzgerald JD: Age-related effects of β-blockers and hypertension. *J Cardiovasc Pharmacol* 12(suppl 8):S83-S92, 1988.

94. Man in 't Veld AJ, van den Meiracker AH, Schalekamp MA: Age dependency of blood pressure response to antihypertensive treatment: Some methodological considerations and observations on five β-adrenoceptor antagonists under different experimental conditions. *J Cardiovasc Pharmacol* 12(suppl 8):S93-S97, 1988.

95. Lamon KD: Evaluation of celiprolol, a new cardioselective beta1-adrenergic blocker with vasodilating properties in the treatment of mild to moderate hypertension in the elderly. *Cardiovasc Drugs Ther* 4(suppl 6): 1291–1295, 1991.

96. Tattersfield AD: Respiratory function in the elderly and the effects of beta blockade. *Cardiovasc Drugs Ther* 4(suppl 6):1229–1232, 1991.

97. Scriven AJ, Lewis PJ: Beta-adrenergic blocking drugs in the treatment of hypertension. *Pharmacol Ther* 20:95–131, 1983.

98. Dollery C, Brennan PJ: The Medical Research Council Hypertension Trial: The smoking patient. *Am Heart J* 115: 276–281, 1988

99. Kostis JB, Berge KG, Davis BR, et al: Effect of atenolol and reserpine on selected events in the systolic hypertension in the elderly program (SHEP). *Am J Hypertens* 8:1147–1153, 1995.

100. Cockshott ID: Pharmacokinetics of epanolol (ICI 141,292) in healthy young volunteers and comparative data in elderly patients with angina and subjects with renal or hepatic impairment. *Drugs* 38(suppl 2):10–17, 1989.

101. Bianchetti G, Brancaccio D, Forette F, et al: Pharmacokinetics of SL 75212 and propranolol in old age, uraemia and in healthy young adults. *Br J Clin Pharmacol* 9:299P, 1980.

102. Gretzer I, Alvan G, Duner H, et al: Beta-blocking effect and pharmacokinetics of pindolol in young and elderly hypertensive patients. *Eur J Clin Pharmacol* 31:415–418, 1986.

103. Hitzenberger G, Fitscha P, Beveridge T, et al: Influence of smoking and age on pharmacokinetics of β-receptor blockers. *Gerontology* 28(suppl 1): 93–100, 1982.

104. Anonymous: MRC trial of treatment of mild hypertension: Principal results. Medical Research Council Working Party. *Br Med J* 291:97–104, 1985.

105. Holmes D, Nuesch E, Houle JM, et al: Steady state pharmacokinetics of hydrolyzed bopindolol in young and elderly men. *Eur J Clin Pharmacol* 41:175–178, 1991.

106. Port JD, Huang LY, Malbon CC: β-Adrenergic agonists that down-regulate receptor messenger RNA up-regulate a Mr 35,000 protein(s) that selectively binds to β-adrenergic receptor messenger RNAs. *J Biol Chem* 267:24103–24108, 1992.

107. Tighe D, Brest AN: Congestive heart failure in the elderly. *Cardiovasc Clin* 22:127–138, 1992.

108. Cooper WD, Glover DR, Kimber GR: Influence of age on blood pressure response to enalapril. *Gerontology* 33(suppl 1):48–54, 1987.
109. Donohoe JF, Laher M, Doyle GD, et al: Influence of age on blood pressure response to enalapril. *Gerontology* 33(Suppl 1):36–42, 1987.
110. Schnaper HW, Stein G, Schoenberger JA, et al: Comparison of enalapril and thiazide diuretics in the elderly hypertensive patients. *Gerontololgy* 33(suppl 1):24–36,
111. Ball SG: Age-related effects of converting enzyme inhibitors: A commentary. *J. Cardiovasc Pharmacol* 12(suppl 8):S105–108, 1988.
112. Amery A, Van Hoof R, Bielen E, et al: Converting enzyme inhibitors in the treatment of elderly hypertensives. *Acta Cardiologica* 44:269–287, 1989.
113. Bursztyn M, Gavras I, Gavras H: Hypertension in the aging patient. Implications for the selection of drug therapy. *J Am Geriatrics Soc* 37:814–818, 1989.
114. Cummings DM, Amadio P Jr, Taylor EJ Jr, et al: The antihypertensive response to lisinopril: The effect of age in a predominantly black population. *J Clin Pharmacol* 29(1):25–32, 1989.
115. Kaiser G, Ackermann R, Dieterle W, et al: Pharmacokinetics and pharmacodynamics of the ace inhibitor benazepril hydrochloride in the elderly. *Eur J Clin Pharmacol* 38:379–385, 1990.
116. Saalbach R, Wochnik G, Mauersberger H, et al: Antihypertensive efficacy, tolerance, and safety of ramipril in young vs. old patients: A retrospective study. *J Cardiovasc Pharmacol* 18(Suppl 2):S134–136, 1991.
117. Smith WM, Gomez HJ: The use of benazepril in hypertensive patients age 55 and over. *Clin Cardiol* 14(8 suppl 4):IV79-IV90, 1991.
118. Frishman WH: Comparative pharmacokinetic and clinical profiles of angiotensin-converting enzyme inhibitors and calcium antagonists in systemic hypertension. *Am J Cardiol* 69:17C-25C, 1992.
119. Schnaper HW: Angiotensin-converting enzyme inhibitors for systemic hypertension in young and elderly patients. *Am J Cardiol* 69:54C-58C, 1992.
120. Buhler FR, Lutold BE: Renin and age as determinants of a predominantly betablocker-based antihypertensive drug program. *Adv Nephrol Necker Hosp* 6:303–317, 1976.
121. Buhler FR, Bolli P, Kiowski W, et al: Renin profiling to select antihypertensive baseline drugs. Renin inhibitors for high-renin and calcium entry blockers for low- renin patients. *Am J Med* 77(2A):36–42, 1984.
122. Breckenridge A: Age-related effects of angiotensin converting enzyme inhibitors. *J Cardiovasc Pharmacol* 12(suppl 8):S100–104, 1988.
123. Duggan J, Kilfeather S, O'Brien E, et al: Effects of aging and hypertension on plasma angiotensin II and platelet angiotensin II receptor density. *Am J Hypertens* 5:687–693, 1992.
124. Luft FC, Fineberg NS, Weinberger MH: The influence of age on renal function and renin and aldosterone responses to sodium-volume expansion and contraction in normotensive and mildly hypertensive humans. *Am J Hypertens* 5:520–528, 1992.
125. Rosendorff C, Kalliatakis B, Radford HM, et al: Age dependence of the pressor sensitivity to noradrenaline and angiotensin II during calcium channel blockade in hypertensive patients. *J Cardiovasc Pharmacol* 12(suppl 4):S69-S71, 1988.
126. Hogikyan RV, Supiano MA: Arterial alpha-adrenergic responsiveness is decreased and SNS activity is increased in older humans. *Am J Physiol* 266:E717–724, 1994.

127. Nielsen H, Hasenkam JM, Pilegaard HK, et al: Age-dependent changes in alpha- adrenoceptor-mediated contractility of isolated human resistance arteries. *Am J Physiol* 263:H1190-H1196, 1992.
128. Jensen HA: Efficacy and tolerability of lisinopril compared with extended release felodipine in patients with essential hypertension. *Clin Exp Hypertens* A14:1095–1110, 1992.
129. Bursztyn M, Ghanem J, Kobrin I, et al: Comparison of verapamil and captopril in elderly hypertensive subjects: Results of a randomized, double-blind, crossover study. *J Cardiovasc Pharmacol* 21:84–88, 1993.
130. Michel JB, Salzmann JL, Cerol ML, et al: Myocardial effect of converting enzyme inhibition in hypertensive and normotensive rats. *Am J Med* 84: 12–21, 1988.
131. Chillon JM, Capdeville-Atkinson C, Lartaud I, et al: Chronic antihypertensive treatment with captopril plus hydrochlorothiazide improves aortic distensibility in the spontaneously hypertensive rat. *Br J Pharmacol* 107: 710–714, 1992.
132. Ajayi AA, Reid JL: Renin-angiotensin modulation of sympathetic reflex function in essential hypertension and in the elderly. *Int J Clin Pharmacol Res* 8:327–333, 1988.
133. Bernasconi M, Marone C, Beretta-Piccoli C, et al: Cardiovascular pressor reactivity after chronic converting enzyme inhibition. *Am J Hypertension* 4:348–355, 1991.
134. Furchgott RF, Zawadzki JV: The obligatory role of endothelial cells in the relaxation of arterial smooth muscle by acetylcholine. *Nature* 288: 373–376, 1980.
135. Gruetter CA, Gruetter DY, Lyon JE, et al: Relationship between cyclic guanosine 3':5'-monophosphate formation and relaxation of coronary arterial smooth muscle by glyceryl trinitrate, nitroprusside, nitrite and nitric oxide: Effects of methylene blue and methemoglobin. *J Pharmacol Exp Ther* 219:181–186, 1981.
136. Palmer RM, Ferrige AG, Moncada S: Nitric oxide release accounts for the biological activity of endothelium-derived relaxing factor. *Nature* 327: 524–526, 1987.
137. Bredt DS, Snyder SH: Isolation of nitric oxide synthetase, a calmodulin-requiring enzyme. *Proc Natl Acad Sci USA* 87:682–685, 1990.
138. Stuehr DJ, Cho HJ, Kwon NS, et al: Purification and characterization of the cytokine-induced macrophage nitric oxide synthase: An FAD- and FMN-containing flavoprotein. *Proc Natl Acad Sci USA* 88:7773–7777, 1991.
139. Lang MG, Noll G, Luscher TF: Effect of aging and hypertension on contractility of resistance arteries: modulation by endothelial factors. *Am J Physiol* 269:H837–844, 1995.
140. Chou TC, Yen MH, Li C, et al: Alterations of nitric oxide synthase expression with aging and hypertension in rats. *Hypertension* 31:643–648, 1998.
141. Rakhit A, Kochak GM, Tipnis V, et al: Pharmacokinetics of pentopril in the elderly. *Br J Clin Pharmacol* 24(3):351–357, 1987.
142. Thomson AH, Whiting B. (1987) Population pharmacokinetics of lisninopril in hypertensive patients. *Gerontology* 33(suppl 1):17–24, 1987.
143. Williams PE, Brown AN, Rajaguru S, et al: A pharmacokinetic study of cilazapril in elderly and young volunteers. *Br J Clin Pharmacol* 27(suppl 2):211S-215S, 1989.
144. Laher MS, Mulkerrins E, Hosie J, et al: The effects of age and renal

impairment on the pharmacokinetics of co-administered lisinopril and hydrochlorothiazide. *J Hum Hypertens* 5(Suppl 2):77–84, 1991.

145. Weisser K, Schloos J, Jakob S, et al: The influence of hydrochlorothiazide on the pharmacokinetics of enalapril in elderly patients. *Eur J Clin Pharmacol* 43:173–177, 1992.

146. Cody RJ: Pharmacology of angiotensin-converting enzyme inhibitors as a guide to their use in congestive heart failure. *Am J Cardiol* 66:7D-13D, 1990.

147. Wada S, Nakayama M, Masaki K: Effects of diltiazem hydrochloride on serum lipids: Comparison with beta-blockers. *Clin Ther* 5:163–173, 1982.

148. Whitebread S, Mele M, Kamber B, et al: Preliminary biochemical characterization of two angiotensin II receptor subtypes. *Biochem Biophys Res Commun* 163:284–291, 1989.

149. Tufro-McReddie A, Johns DW, Geary KM, et al: Angiotensin II type 1 receptor: role in renal growth and gene expression during normal development. *Am J Physiol* 266: F911-F918, 1994.

150. Weber MA: Comparison of type 1 angiotensin II receptor blockers and angiotensin converting enzyme inhibitors in the treatment of hypertension. *J Hypertens* 15(suppl):S31-S36, 1997.

151. Pitt B, Segal R, Martinez FA, et al: Randomised trial of losartan versus captopril in patients over 65 with heart failure (Evaluation of Losartan in the Elderly Study, ELITE) *Lancet* 349:747–752, 1997.

152. Burrell LM, Johnston CI: Angiotensin II receptor antagonists. Potential in elderly patients with cardiovascular disease. *Drugs Aging* 10:421–434, 1997.

153. Hass VH, Hartfelder G: α-Isopropyl-α-[(N-methyl-N-homoveratryl)-γ-amino-propyl]-3,4-dimethoxyphenylacetonitril, eine Substanz mit coronargefasserweiternden Eigenschaften. *Arznmittel-Forschung* 12: 549–558, 1962.

154. Fleckenstein JA, Kammermeier H, Doring H, et al: ZumWirkungs-Mechanismus neuartiger Koronardilalatoren mit gleichzeitig Sauerstoff-einsparenden, myokard- Effekten. Prenylamin und Iproveratril. *Z Kreislaufforsch* 56:716–744, 839–853, 1967.

155. Ahmed JH, Elliott HL, Meredith PA, et al: Low-dose verapamil in middle-aged and elderly patients with angina pectoris: No evidence of increased susceptibility to the cardiac effects. *Cardiovasc Drugs Ther* 6:153–158, 1992.

156. Holtzman JL, Abrams A, Cutler R, et al: Multicenter comparison of once and twice daily isradipine to hydrochlorothiazide for the treatment of hypertension in the elderly. *Clin Pharmacol Ther* 48:590–597, 1990.

157. Elkayam U, Amin J, Mehra A, et al: A prospective, randomized, double-blind, crossover study to compare the efficacy and safety of chronic nifedipine therapy with that of isosorbide dinitrate and their combination in the treatment of chronic congestive heart failure. *Circulation* 82:1954–1961, 1990.

158. Packer M, O'Connor CM, Ghali JK, et al: Effect of amlodipine on morbidity and mortality in severe chronic heart failure. Prospective Randomized Amlodipine Survival Evaluation Study Group. *N Engl J Med* 335: 1107–1114, 1996.

159. Hieble JP, Bylund DB, Clarke DE, et al: International Union of Pharmacology. X. Recommendation for nomenclature of α_1-adrenoceptors: Consensus update. *Pharmacol Rev* 47:267–270, 1995.

160. Andersson KE, Lepor H, Wyllie MG: Prostatic alpha 1-adrenoceptors and uroselectivity. *Prostate* 30: 202–215, 1997.
161. Huguet F, Huchet AM, Gerard P, et al: Characterization of dihydropyridine binding sites in the rat brain: Hypertension and age-dependent modulation of [3H](+)-PN 200–110 binding. *Brain Res* 412:125–130, 1987.
162. Waki H, Kon K, Tanaka Y, et al: Age-related changes in the uptake of calcium channel blockers by brain capillary endothelial cells and synaptosomal fractions. *Neurosci Lett* 116:367–371, 1990.
163. Howlett SE, Nicholl PA: Density of 1,4-dihydropyridine receptors decreases in the hearts of aging hamsters. *J Mol Cell Cardiol* 24:885–894, 1992.
164. Schwartz JB: The effects of aging on responses to verapamil in isolated right atria. *J Gerontol* 44:M201-M205, 1989.
165. Schmidlin O, Garcia J, Schwartz JB: The effects of aging on the electrophysiologic responses to verapamil in isolated perfused rat hearts. *J Pharmacol Exp Ther* 258:130–135, 1989.
166. Wanstall JC, O'Donnell SR: Influence of age on calcium entry blocking drugs in rat aorta is spasmogen-dependent. *Eur J Pharmacol* 159: 241–246, 1989.
167. Barringer DL, Bunag RD: Differential age-dependent attenuation of reflex tachycardia by verapamil in rats. *Mech Ageing Dev* 58:111–125, 1991.
168. Olah ME, Rhwan RG: Age-related changes in responsiveness of the rat aorta to depolarizing and receptor-mediated contractile stimuli and to calcium antagonism. *Pharmacol.* 35:163–173, 1987.
169. Shannon RP, Maher KA, Santinga JT, et al: Comparison of differences in the hemodynamic response to passive postural stress in healthy subjects greater than 70 years and less than 30 years of age. *Am J Cardiol* 67: 1110–1116, 1991.
170. Abernethy DR, Schwartz JB, Todd EL, et al: Verapamil pharmacodynamics and disposition in young and elderly hypertensive patients. Altered electrocardiographic and hypotensive responses. *Ann Intern Med* 105: 329–336, 1986.
171. Manning WJ, Shannon RJ, Santinga JA, et al: Reversal of changes in left ventricular diastolic filling associated with normal aging using diltiazem. *Am J Cardiol* 67:894–896, 1991.
172. Buhler FR, Kiowski W: Age and antihypertensive response to calcium antagonists. *J Hypertens* 5(suppl 4):S111-S114, 1987.
173. Ram CV: Calcium antagonists as antihypertensive agents are effective in all age groups. *J Hypertens* 5(suppl 4):S115-S118, 1987.
174. Buhler FR: Age and pathophysiology-oriented antihypertensive response to calcium antagonists. *J Cardiovasc Pharmacol* 12(suppl 8):S156-S166, 1988.
175. Bohmer F, Barousch R, Reinfrank J: Treatment of isolated systolic hypertension in the elderly with verapamil slow-release 240 mg. *J Cardiovasc Pharmacol* 13(suppl 4):S45-S46, 1989.
176. Kaplan NM: Critical comments on recent literature. Age and the response to antihypertensive drugs. *Am J Hypertens* 2(suppl 3):213–215, 1989.
177. Elliott HL: Calcium antagonists in the treatment of hypertension and angina pectoris in the elderly. *J Cardiovasc Pharmacol* 13(suppl 4):S12-S16, 1989.
178. Wei JY: Use of calcium entry blockers in elderly patients. Special considerations. *Circulation* 80(suppl 6):IV171-IV177, 1989.

179. Djian J, Roy M, Forette B, et al: Efficacy and tolerance of sustained-release diltiazem 300 mg and a diuretic in the elderly. *J Cardiovasc Pharmacol* 16(suppl 1):S51-S55, 1990.
180. Larochelle P: Hypertension in the elderly. *Cardiovasc Drugs Ther* 4(suppl 5):947-950, 1990.
181. Elkik F, Claudel S, Carcone B, et al: Demographic factors and the antihypertensive effect of diltiazem. *J Cardiovasc Pharmacol* 17:685-691, 1991.
182. Zing W, Ferguson RK, Vlasses PH: Calcium antagonists in elderly and black hypertensive patients. Therapuetic controversies. *Arch Intern Med* 151:2154-2162, 1991.
183. Imai Y, Abe K, Sasaki S, et al: Influence of age on the nocturnal fall of blood pressure and its modulation by long-acting calcium antagonists. *Clin Exp Hypertens* 12:1077-1094, 1990.
184. Gerstenblith G: Special considerations in the elderly patient. *J Human Hypertens* 4(suppl 5):7-10, 1990.
185. Middlemost SJ, Sack M, Davis J, et al: Effects of long-acting nifedipine on casual office blood pressure measurements, 24-hour ambulatory blood pressure profiles, exercise parameters and left ventricular mass and function in black patients with mild to moderate systemic hypertension. *Am J Cardiol* 70:474-478, 1992.
186. Ohtsuka, M, Sakai, S, Miura, S, et al: Effects of nilvadipine, a new calcium entry blocker, on systemic blood pressure, cardiac hypertrophy and venous distensibility in spontaneously hypertensive rats. *Arch Int Pharmacodynamie Ther* 301:228-245, 1989.
187. Frohlich ED, Sasaki O, Chien Y, et al: Changes in cardiovascular mass, left ventricular pumping ability and aortic distensibility after calcium antagonists in Wistar-Kyoto and spontaneously hypertensive rats. *J Hypertens* 10:1369-1378, 1992.
188. Kannel WB: Prevalence and natural history of electrocardiographic left ventricular hypertrophy. *Am J Med* (Sept 26):4-11, 1983.
189. Arrighi JA, Dilsizian V, Perrone-Filardi P, et al: Improvement of the age-related impairment in left ventricular diastolic filling with verapamil in the normal human heart. *Circulation* 90:213-219, 1995.
190. Pedersen KE, Dorph-Pedersen A, Hvidt S, et al: Digoxin-verapamil interaction. *Clin Pharmacol. Ther* 30:311-316, 1981.
191. Belz GG, Doering W, Munkes R, et al: Interaction between digoxin and calcium antagonists and antiarrhythmic drugs. *Clin Pharmacol Ther* 33:410-417, 1983.
192. Doering W: Effect of coadministration of verapamil and quinidine on serum digoxin concentration. *Eur J Clin Pharmacol* 25:517-521, 1983.
193. Johnson BF, Wilson J, Marwaha R, et al: The comparative effects of verapamil and a new dihydropyridine calcium channel blocker on digoxin pharmacokinetics. *Clin Pharamcol Ther* 42:66-71, 1987
194. Hedman A, Angelin B, Arvidsson A, et al: Digoxin-verapamil interaction: Reduction of biliary but not renal digoxin clearance in humans. *Clin Pharmacol Ther* 49:256-262, 1991.
195. Kuhlmann J, Marcin S: Effects of verapamil on pharmacokinetics and pharmacodynamics of digitoxin in patients. *Am Heart J* 110:1245-1250, 1985.
196. Boden WE, More G, Sharma S, et al: No increase in serum digoxin concentration with high-dose diltiazem. *Am J Med* 81:425-428, 1986
197. Bailey DG, Spence JD, Munoz C, et al: Interaction of citrus juices with felodipine and nifedipine. *Lancet* 337:268-269, 1991.

198. Kates RE: Calcium antagonists. Pharmacokinetic properties. *Drugs* 25: 113–124, 1983.

199. Storstein L, Larsen A, Midtbo K, et al: Pharmacokinetics of calcium blockers in patients with renal insufficiency and in geriatric patients. *Acta Medica Scand* (Suppl 681):25–30, 1984.

200. Carosella L, Menichelli P, Alimenti M, et al: Verapamil disposition and cardiovascular effects in elderly patients after single intravenous and oral doses. *Cardiovasc Drugs Ther* 3:417–425, 1989.

201. Schwartz JB: Aging alters verapamil elimination and dynamics: Single dose and steady-state responses. *J Pharmacol Exp Ther* 255:364–373, 1990.

202. Schwartz JB, Troconiz IF, Verotta D, et al: Aging effects on stereoselective pharmacokinetics and pharmacodynamics of verapamil. *J Pharmacol Exp Ther* 265(2):690–698, 1993.

203. Abernethy DR, Wainer IW, Longstreth JA, et al: Stereoselective verapamil disposition and dynamics in aging during racemic verapamil administration. *J Pharmacol Exp Ther* 266:904–911, 1993.

204. Sasaki M, Tateishi T, Ebihara A: The effects of age and gender on the stereoselective pharmacokinetics of verapamil. *Clin Pharmacol Ther* 54: 278–285, 1993.

205. Schwartz JB, Capili H, Daugherty J: Aging of women alters S-verapamil pharmacokinetics and pharmacodynamics. *Clin Pharmacol Ther* 55: 509–517, 1994.

206. Schwartz JB, Capili H, Wainer IW: Verapamil stereoisomers during racemic verapamil administration: Effects of aging and comparisons to administration of individual stereoisomers. *Clin Pharmacol Ther* 56:368–376, 1994.

207. Hosie J, Hosie G, Meredith PA: The effects of age on the pharmacodynamics and pharmacokinetics of two formulations of verapamil. *J Cardiovasc Pharmacol* 13(suppl 4):S60-S62, 1989.

208. Ahmed JH, Meredith PA, Elliott HL: The influence of age on the pharmacokinetics of verapamil. *Pharmacol Res* 24:227–233, 1991.

209. Hermann P, Morselli PL: Pharmacokinetics of diltiazem and other calcium entry blockers. *Acta Pharmacol Toxicol* 57(suppl 2):10–20, 1985.

210. Montamat SC, Abernethy DR: N-monodesmethyldiltiazem is the predominant metabolite of diltiazem in the plasma of young and elderly hypertensives. *Br J Clin Pharmacol* 24:185–189, 1987.

211. Montamat SC, Abernethy DR: Calcium antagonists in geriatric patients: Diltiazem in elderly persons with hypertension. *Clin Pharmacol Ther* 45: 682–691, 1989.

212. Abernethy DR, Gutkowska J, Lambert MD: Amlodipine in elderly hypertensive patients: Pharmacokinetics and pharmacodynamics. *J Cardiovasc Pharmacol* 12(suppl 7):S67-S71, 1988.

213. Abernethy DR: The pharmacokinetic profile of amlodipine. *Am Heart J* 118:1100–1103, 1989.

214. Elliott HL, Green ST, Vincent J, et al: An assessment of the pharmacokinetics and pharmacodynamics of single doses of amlodipine in elderly normotensives. *Pharmacol Res* 26:33–39, 1992.

215. Elliott HL, Meredith PA, Reid JL, et al: A comparison of the disposition of single oral doses of amlodipine in young and elderly subjects. *J Cardiovasc Pharmacol* 12(suppl 7):S64-S66, 1988.

216. Abernethy DR, Gutkowska J, Winterbottom LM: Effects of amlodipine,

a long- acting dihydropyridine calcium antagonist in aging hypertension: Pharmacodynamics in relation to disposition. *Clin Pharmacol Ther* 48: 76–86, 1990.

217. Dequattro V: Efficacy and safety of felodipine, a new dihydropyridine calcium channel blocker, in elderly hypertensive patients. *Clin Exp Hypertens* 14:965–988, 1992.

218. Ito H, Hoopes MT, Roth GS, et al: Adrenergic and cholinergic mediated glucose oxidation by rat parotid gland acinar cells during aging. *Biochem Biophys Res Commun* 98:275–282, 1981.

219. Psaty BM, Smith NL, Siscovick DS, et al: Health outcomes associated with antihypertensive therapies used as first-line agents. A systematic review and meta- analysis. *JAMA* 277:739–745, 1997.

220. Borhani NO, Mercuri M, Borhani PA, et al: Final outcome results of the Multicenter Isradipine Diuretic Atherosclerosis Study (MIDAS). A randomized controlled trial. *JAMA* 276:785–791, 1996.

221. Docherty JR, O'Malley K: Ageing and alpha-adrenoceptors. *Clin Sci* 68(suppl 10):133s-136s, 1985.

222. Roth GS: Effects of aging on mechanisms of adrenergic and dopaminergic action. *Fed Proc* 45:60–64, 1986.

223. Handa RK, Duckles SP: Age-related changes in adrenergic vasoconstrictor responses of the rat hindlimb. *Am J Physiol* 253: H1566-H1572, 1987.

224. Docherty JR: The effects of ageing on vascular alpha-adrenoceptors in pithed rat and rat aorta. *Eur J Pharmacol* 146:1–5, 1988.

225. Burnett DM, Bowyer JF, Masserano JM, et al: Effect of aging on alpha-1 adrenergic stimulation of phosphoinositide hydrolysis in various regions of rat brain. *J Pharmacol Exp Ther* 255:1265–1270, 1990.

226. Vila E, Vivas NM, Tabernero A, et al: Alpha 1-adrenoceptor vasoconstriction in the tail artery during ageing. *Br J Pharmacol* 121:1017–1023, 1997.

227. Sawaki K, Baum BJ, Roth GS, et al: Decreased m3-muscarinic and alpha 1- adrenergic receptor stimulation of PIP2 hydrolysis in parotid gland membranes from aged rats: Defect in activation of G alpha q/11. *Arch Biochem Biophys* 322: 319–326, 1995.

228. Hamilton CA, Jones CR, Reid JL: α-Adrenoceptor regulation in vivo and in vitro in the rabbit. *Clin Sci* 68(suppl 10):125s-128s, 1985.

229. Schlicker E, Betz R, Gothert M: Investigation into the age-dependence of release of serotonin and noradrenaline in the rat brain cortex and of autoreceptor-mediated modulation of release. *Neuropharmacology* 28: 811–815, 1989.

230. Eikenburg DC: Age-related changes in vascular sympathetic neurotransmission in the rat kidney. *J Pharmacol Exp Ther* 259:176–181, 1991.

231. Yoshida M, Latifpour J, Nishimoto T, et al: Pharmacological characterization of alpha adrenergic receptors in the young and old female rabbit urethra. *J Pharmacol Exp Ther* 257:1100–1108, 1991.

232. Gurdal H, Friedman E, Johnson MD: Effects of dietary restriction on the change in aortic alpha 1-adrenoceptor mediated responses during aging in Fischer 344 rats. *J Gerontol A Biol Sci Med Sci* 50:B67-B71, 1995.

233. Villalobos-Molina R, Miyamoto A, Kowatch MA, et al: Alpha 1-adrenoceptors in parotid cells: Age does not alter the ratio of alpha 1A and alpha 1B subtypes. *Eur J Pharmacol* 226: 129–131, 1992.

234. Gascon S, Dierssen M, Marmol F, et al: Effects of age on alpha 1-adrenoceptor subtypes in the heart ventricular muscle of the rat. *J Pharm Pharmacol* 45:907–909, 1993.

235. Gurdal H, Cai G, Johnson MD: Alpha 1-adrenoceptor responsiveness in the aging aorta. *Eur J Pharmacol* 274:117–123, 1995.
236. Moriyama N, Kurimoto S, Inagaki O, et al: Renal aging change of alpha 1- adrenoceptor in Wistar rats. *Gen Pharmacol* 26:347–351, 1995.
237. Miller JW, Hu ZW, Okazaki M, et al: Expression of alpha 1 adrenergic receptor subtype mRNAs in the rat cardiovascular system with aging. *Mech Ageing Dev* 87:75- 89, 1996.
238. Xu KM, Tang F, Han C: Alterations of mRNA levels of alpha 1-adrenoceptor subtypes with maturation and ageing in different rat blood vessels. *Clin Exp Pharmacol Physiol* 24:415–417, 1997.
239. Elliott HL, Sumner DJ, McLean K, et al: Effect of age on the responsiveness of vascular alpha-adrenoceptors in man. *J Cardiovasc Pharmacol* 4: 388–392, 1982.
240. Christ GJ, Stone B, Melman A: Age-dependent alterations in the efficacy of phenylephrine-induced contractions in vascular smooth muscle isolated from the corpus cavernosum of impotent men. *Can J Physiol Pharmacol* 69:909–913, 1991.
241. Grimm RH Jr, Grandits GA, Prineas RJ, et al: Long-term effects on sexual function of five antihypertensive drugs and nutritional hygienic treatment in hypertensive men and women. Treatment of Mild Hypertension Study (TOMHS). *Hypertension* 29:8–14, 1997.
242. Elliott HL: Alpha 1-adrenoceptor responsiveness: The influence of age. *J Cardiovasc Pharmacol* 12(suppl 8):S116-S123, 1988.
243. Stokes GS: Age-related effects of antihypertensive therapy with alpha-blockers. *J Cardiovasc Pharmacol* 12(suppl 8): S109-S115, 1988.
244. Julius S: Clinical implications of pathophysiologic changes in the midlife hypertensive patient. *Am Heart J* 122:886–891, 1991.
245. Arnold SB, Williams RL, Ports TA, et al: Attenuation of prazosin effect on cardiac output in congestive heart failure. *Ann Intern Med* 91:345–349, 1979.
246. Desch CE, Magioren RD, Triffon DW, et al: Dvelopment of pharmacodynamic tolerance to prazosin in congestive heart failure. *Am J Cardiol* 44: 1178–1182, 1979.
247. Elkayam V, Lejemtel TH, Mathur M, et al: Marked early attenuation of hemodynamic effects of oral prazosin therapy in chronic congestive heart failure. *Am J Cardiol* 44:540–545, 1979.
248. Awan NA, Lee G, DeMaria AN, et al: Ambulatory prazosin treatment of chronic congestive heart failure development of late tolerance reversible by higher dosage and interrupted substitution therapy. *Am Heart J* 101: 541–547, 1981.
249. Packer M, Medina N, Yushak M: Role of the renin-angiotensin system in the development of tolerance to long-term prazosin therapy in patients with sever chronic heart failure. *J Am Coll Cardiol* 7:671–681, 1986.
250. Vincent J, Dachman W, Blaschke TF, et al: Pharmacological tolerance to α_1-adrenergic receptor antagonism mediated by terazosin in humans. *J Clin Invest* 90:1763–1768, 1992.
251. Elliott HL, Meredith PA, Vincent J, et al: Clinical pharmacological studies with doxazosin. *Br J Clin Pharmacol* 21(suppl 1):27S-31S, 1986.
252. McNeil JJ, Drummer OH, Conway EL, et al: Effect of age on pharmacokinetics of blood pressure responses to prazosin and terazosin. *J Cardiovasc Pharmacol* 10:168–175, 1987.
253. Charuel C, Comby P, Monro AM: Diurnal exposure profile in rats from

dietary administration of a chemical (doxazosin) with a short half-life: Interplay of age and diurnal feeding pattern. *J Appl Toxicol* 12:7–11, 1992.

254. Caine M: Medical management of prostatic hyperplasia. *Compr Ther* 12: 21–25, 1986.
255. Caine M: Alpha-adrenergic mechanims and dynamics of benign prostatic hypertrophy. *Urology* 32(suppl 6):16–20, 1988.
256. Dunzendorfer U: Clinical experience: Symptomatic management of BPH with terazosin. *Urology* 32(suppl 6):27–31, 1988.
257. Studer JA, Piepho RW: Antihypertensive therapy in the Geriatric Patient. 2. A review of the alpha$_1$-adrenergic blocking agents. *J Clin Pharmacol* 33:2–13, 1993.
258. Geller J: Benign prostatic hyperplasia: Pathogenesis and medical therapy. *J Am Geriatr Soc* 39:1208–1216, 1991.
259. Materson BJ, Reda DJ, Cushman WC, et al: Single drug therapy for hypertension in men: A comparison of six antihypertensive agents with placebo. *N Engl J Med* 328:914–921, 1993.
260. Martinotti E: α-Adrenergic receptor subtypes on vascular smooth musculature. *Pharmacol Res* 24:297–306, 1991.
261. Arnsten AF, Cai JX, Goldman-Rakic PS: The alpha-2 adrenergic agonist guanfacine improves memory in aged monkeys without sedative or hypotensive side effects: Evidence for alpha-2 receptor subtypes. *J Neurosci* 8:4287–4298, 1988.
262. Arnsten AF, Goldman-Rakic PS: Analysis of alpha-2 adrenergic agonist effects on the delayed nonmatch-to-sample performance of aged rhesus monkeys. *Neurobiol Aging* 11:583–590, 1990.
263. McAdams RP, Waterfall JF: The effect of age on the sensitivity of pre- and postsynaptic alpha-adrenoceptors to agonists and antagonists in the rat. *N-S Arch Pharmacol* 334:430–435, 1986.
264. Pellegrini A, Soldani P, Breschi MC, et al: Adrenergic innervation of the ductus deferences in young and aging rats: a morpho-functional investigation. *Acta Histochemica* 89:67–74, 1990.
265. Takayanagi I, Kawano K, Koike K: Effects of aging on alpha 2-adrenoceptor mechanisms in isolated guinea-pig tracheal preparations. *Eur J Pharmacol* 192:97–102, 1991.
266. Buchholz J, Tsai H, Friedman D, et al: Influence of age on control of norepinephrine release from the rat tail artery. *J Pharmacol Exp Ther* 260:722–727, 1992.
267. Periyasamy SM: Sodium regulation of alpha 2-adrenoceptor-agonist interactions in renal membranes of young and old Dahl rats. *Arch Int Pharmacodynamie Ther* 298:172–182, 1989.
268. Klein C, Hiatt WR, Gerber JG, et al: The balance between vascular alpha- and beta-adrenoceptors is not changed in the elderly. *Clin Pharmacol Ther* 42:260–264, 1987.
269. Amery A, Birkenhager W, Bulpitt C, et al: Mortality and morbidity results from the European Working Party on High Blood Pressure in the Elderly (EWPHE). *Lancet* 1:1349–1354, 1985.
270. Freis ED: Age and antihypertensive drugs (hydrochlorothiazide, bendroflumethiazide, nadolol and captopril). *Am J Cardiol* 61:117–121, 1988.
271. Materson BJ, Cushman WC, Goldstein G, et al: Treatment of hypertension in the elderly: I. Blood pressure and clinical changes. Results of a Department of Veterans Affairs Cooperative Study. *Hypertension* 15: 348–360, 1990.

272. SHEP Cooperative Research Group: Prevention of stroke by antihypertensive drug treatment in older persons with isolated systolic hypertension. *JAMA* 265:3255–3264, 1991.
273. Dahlof B, Lindholm LH, Hansson L, et al: Morbidity and mortality in the Swedish Trial in Old Patients with Hypertension (STOP-Hypertension). *Lancet* 338:1281–1285, 1991.
274. MRC Working Party: Medical Research Council trial of treatment of hypertension in older adults: Principal results. *Br Med J* 304:405–412, 1992.
275. Lund-Johansen P: Treatment of hypertension in the elderly—What have we learned from the recent trials? *Cardiovasc Drugs Ther* 6:571–573, 1992.
276. Beerman B, Groschinsky-Grind M: Antihypertensive effect of various doses of hydrochlorothiazide and its relation to the plasma level of the drug. *Eur J Clin Pharmacol* 13:195–201, 1978.
277. Amery A, Birkenhager W, Bulpitt C, et al: Influence of anti-hypertensive therapy on serum cholesterol in elderly hypertensive patiens. Results of trial by the European Working Party on High Blood Pressure in the Elderly. *Acta Cardiol* 37:235–244, 1982.
278. Chaudhry AY, Bing RF, Castleden CM, et al: The effect of ageing on the response to frusemide in normal subjects. *Eur J Clin Pharmacol* 27:303–306, 1984. 279. Luft FC, Fineberg NS, Miller JZ, et al: The effects of age, race and heredity on glomerular filtration rate following volume expansion and contraction in normal man. *Am J Med Sci* 279: 15–24, 1980.
280. Andreasen F, Hansen U, Husted SE, et al: The pharmacokinetics of furosemide are influenced by age. *Br J Clin Pharmacol* 16:391–397, 1983.
281. Kerremans AL, Tan Y, van Baars H, et al: Furosemide kinetics and dynamics in aged patients. *Clin Pharmacol Ther* 34:181–189, 1983.
282. Muhlberg W: Pharmacokinetics of diuretics in geriatric patients. *Arch Gerontol Geriatr* 9:283–290, 1989.
283. Williams RL, Thornhill MD, Upton RA, et al: Absorption and disposition of two combination formulations of hydrochlorothiazide and triamterene: Influence of age and renal function. *Clin Pharmacol Ther* 40:226–232, 1986.
284. Sabanathan K, Castleden CM, Adam HK, et al: A comparative study of the pharmacokinetics and pharmacodynamics of atenolol, hydrochlorothiazide and amiloride in normal young and elderly subjects and elderly hypertensive patients. *Eur J Clin Pharmacol* 32:53–60, 1987.
285. Ismail Z, Triggs EJ, Smithurst BA, et al: The pharmacokinetics of amiloride- hydrochlorothiazide combination in the young and elderly. *Eur J Clin Pharmacol* 37:167–171, 1989.
286. Platt D, Abshagen U, Muhlberg W, et al: The influence of age and multimorbidity on the pharmacokinetics and metabolism of spironolactone. *Arch Gerontol Geriatr* 3:147–159, 1984.
287. Doherty JE, Dalrymple GV, Murphy ML, et al: Pharmacokinetics of digoxin. *Fed Proc* 36:2242–2246, 1977.
288. The Digitalis Investigation Group: The effect of digoxin on mortality and morbidity in patients with heart failure. *N Engl J Med* 336:525–533, 1977.
289. Cusack B, Kelly J, O'Malley K, et al: Digoxin in the elderly: Pharmacokinetic consequences of old age. *Clin Pharmacol Ther* 25:772–776, 1979.
290. Algotsson A, Sanz E, Alvan G: Steady-state concentrations and dosage of digoxin in relation to kidney function in hospitalized patients over 70 years of age. *J Intern Med* 229:247–251, 1991.

291. Katano Y, Kennedy RH, Stemmer PM, et al: Aging and digitalis sensitivity of cardiac muscle in rats. *Eur J Pharmacol* 113:167–178, 1985.
292. Cokkinos DV, Tsartsalis GD, Heimonas ET, et al: Comparison of the inotropic action of digitalis and isoproterenol in younger and older individuals. *Am Heart J* 100:802–806, 1988.
293. Wofford JL, Hickey AR, Ettinger WH, et al: Lack of age-related differences in the clinical presentation of digoxin toxicity. *Arch Intern Med* 152: 2261–2264, 1992
294. Holtzman JL, Shafer RB, Erickson RR: Methodological causes of discrepancies in radioimmunoassay for digoxin in human serum. *Clin Chem* 20: 1194–1198, 1974.
295. Holtzman JL, Shafer RB: Discrepancies in the radioimmunoassay for digoxin. *JAMA* 233:817, 1975.
296. Ejvinsson G: Effect of quinidine on plasma concentrations of digoxin. *Br Med J* 1:278–280, 1978.
297. Leahey EB, Reiffel JA, Heissenbuttel RH, et al: Enhanced cardiac effect of digoxin during quinidine treatment. *Arch Intern Med* 139:519–521, 1979.
298. Leahey EB, Reiffel JA, Giardina E-GV, et al: The effect of quinidine and other oral antiarrhythmic drugs on serum digoxin. A prospective study. *Ann Intern Med* 92:605–608, 1980.
299. Doering W: Quinidine-digoxin interaction. Pharmacokinetics underlying mechanism and clinical implications. *N Engl J Med* 301:400–404, 1979.
300. Mungall DR, Robichaux RP, Perry W, et al: Effects of quinidine on serum digoxin concentration. *Ann Intern Med* 93:689–693, 1980.
301. Hager WD, Fenster P, Maversohn M, et al: Digoxin-quinidine interaction. Pharmacokinetic evaluation. *N Engl J Med* 300:1238–1241, 1979.
302. Leahey EB, Bigger JT, Butler VP, et al: Quinidine-digoxin interaction: Time course and pharmacokinetics. *Am J Cardiol* 48:1141–1146, 1981.
303. Ochs HR, Bodem G, Greenblatt DJ: Impairment of digoxin clearance by coadministration of quinidine. *J Clin Pharmacol* 21:386–400, 1981.
304. Doering W, Fichtl B, Herrmann M, et al: Quinidine-digoxin interaction: Evidence for involvement of an extrarenal mechanism. *Eur J Clin Pharmacol* 21:281–285, 1982.
305. Angelin B, Arvidsson A, Dahlqvist R, et al: Quinidine reduces biliary clearance of digoxin in man. *Eur J Clin Invest* 17:262–265, 1987.
306. Doherty JE, Straub KD, Murphy M., et al: Digoxin-quinidine interaction. Changes in cainine tissue concentration from steady state with quinidine. *Am J Cardiol* 45:1196–1200, 1980.
307. Schenck-Gustafsson K, Jogestrand T, Nordlander R, et al: Effect of quinidine on digoxin concentration in skeletal muscle and serum in patients with atrial fibrillation. Evidence for reduced binding of digoxin in muscle. *N Engl J Med* 305:209–211, 1981.
308. Jogestrand T, Schenck-Gustafsson K, Nordlander R, et al: Quinidine-induced changes in serum and skeletal muscle digoxin concentration; Evidence of saturable binding of digoxin to skeletal muscle. *Eur J Clin Pharmacol* 27:571–574, 1984.
309. Warner NJ, Leahey EB Jr, Hougen TJ, et al: Tissue digoxin concentrations during quinidine-digoxin interaction. *Am J Cardiol* 51:1717–1721, 1983.
310. Fenster PE, Powell JR, Graves PE, et al: Digitoxin-quinidine interaction: Pharmacokinetic evaluation. *Ann Intern Med* 93:698–701, 1980.

311. Fenster PE, White NW Jr, Hanson CD: Pharmacokinetic evaluation of the digoxin-amiodarone interaction. *J Am Coll Cardiol* 5:108–112, 1985.
312. Ochs HR, Pabst J, Greenblatt DJ, et al: Noninteraction of digitoxin and quinidine. *N Engl J Med* 303:672–674, 1980.
313. Garty M, Sood P, Rollins DE: Digitoxin elimination reduced during quinidine therapy. *Ann Intern Med* 94:35–37, 1981.
314. Kulhmann J, Dohrmann M, Marcin S: Effects of quinidine on pharmacokinetics and pharmacodynamics of digitoxin achieving steady-state conditions. *Clin Pharmacol Ther* 39:288–294, 1986.
315. Anonymous: Randomised trial of cholesterol lowering in 4444 patients with coronary: The Scandinavian Simvastatin Survival Study (4S). *Lancet* 344:1383–1389, 1994.
316. Shepherd J, Cobbe SM, Ford I, et al: Prevention of coronary heart disease with pravastatin in men with hypercholesterolemia. West of Scotland Coronary Prevention Study Group. *N Engl J Med* 333:1301–1307, 1995.
317. Anonymous: West of Scotland Coronary Prevention Study: Identification of high-risk groups and comparison with other cardiovascular intervention trials. *Lancet* 348:1339–1342, 1996.
318. Sacks FM, Pfeffer MA, Moye LA, et al: The effect of pravastatin on coronary events after myocardial infarction in patients with average cholesterol levels. Cholesterol and Recurrent Events Trial investigators. *N Engl J Med* 335:1001–1009, 1996.
319. Kroon AA, Aengevaeren WR, van der Werf T, et al: LDL-Apheresis Atherosclerosis Regression Study (LAARS). Effect of aggressive versus conventional lipid lowering treatment on coronary atherosclerosis. *Circulation* 93:1826–1835, 1996.
320. van Boven AJ, Jukema JW, Zwinderman AH, et al: Reduction of transient myocardial ischemia with pravastatin in addition to the conventional treatment in patients with angina pectoris. REGRESS Study Group. *Circulation* 94:1503–1505, 1996.
321. Kjekshus J, Pedersen TR: Reducing the risk of coronary events: Evidence from the Scandinavian Simvastatin Survival Study (4S). *Am J Cardiol* 76:64C-68C, 1995.
322. Byington RP, Jukema JW, Salonen JT, et al: Reduction in cardiovascular events during pravastatin therapy. Pooled analysis of clinical events of the Pravastatin Atherosclerosis Intervention Program. *Circulation* 92:2419–2425, 1995.
323. Waters D, Higginson L, Gladstone P, et al: Effects of cholesterol lowering on the progression of coronary atherosclerosis in women. A Canadian Coronary Atherosclerosis Intervention Trial (CCAIT) substudy. *Circulation* 92:2404–2410, 1995.
324. Furberg CD, Pitt B, Byington RP, et al: Reduction in coronary events during treatment with pravastatin. PLAC I and PLAC II Investigators. Pravastatin Limitation of Atherosclerosis in the Coronary Arteries. *Am J Cardiol* 76:60C-63C, 1995.
325. Tamura A, Mikuriya Y, Nasu M: Effect of pravastatin (10 mg/day) on progression of coronary atherosclerosis in patients with serum total cholesterol levels from 160 to 220 mg/dl and angiographically documented coronary artery disease. Coronary Artery Regression Study (CARS) Group. *Am J Cardiol* 79: 893–906, 1997.
326. Wenke K, Meiser B, Thiery J, et al: Simvastatin reduces graft vessel disease and mortality after heart transplantation: A four-year randomized trial. *Circulation* 96:1398–1402, 1997.

327. Anonymous: Baseline risk factors and their association with outcome in the West of Scotland Coronary Prevention Study. The West of Scotland Coronary Prevention Study Group. *Am J Cardiol* 79(6):756–762, 1997.
328. Miettinen TA, Pyorala K, Olsson AG, et al: Cholesterol-lowering therapy in women and elderly patients with myocardial infarction or angina pectoris: Findings from the Scandinavian Simvastatin Survival Study (4S). *Circulation* 96:4211–4218, 1997.
329. Boccuzzi SJ, Weintraub WS, Kosinski AS, et al: Aggressive lipid lowering in postcoronary angioplasty patients with elevated cholesterol (the Lovastatin Restenosis Trial). *Am J Cardiol* 81:632–636, 1998.
330. Herd JA, Ballantyne CM, Farmer JA, et al: Effects of fluvastatin on coronary atherosclerosis in patients with mild to moderate cholesterol elevations (Lipoprotein and Coronary Atherosclerosis Study [LCAS]). *Am J Cardiol* 80:278–286, 1997.
331. Pitt B, Mancini GB, Ellis SG, et al: Pravastatin limitation of atherosclerosis in the coronary arteries (PLAC I): Reduction in atherosclerosis progression and clinical events. PLAC I investigation. *J Am Coll Cardiol* 26: 1133–1139, 1995.
332. Pedersen TR, Kjekshus J, Pyorala K, et al: Effect of simvastatin on ischemic signs and symptoms in the Scandinavian simvastatin survival study (4S). *Am J Cardiol* 81:333–335, 1998.
333. Crouse JR 3rd, Byington RP, Hoen HM, et al: Reductase inhibitor monotherapy and stroke prevention. *Arch Intern Med* 157:1305–1310, 1997.
334. Bucher HC, Griffith LE, Guyatt GH: Effect of HMGcoA reductase inhibitors on stroke. A meta-analysis of randomized, controlled trials. *Ann Intern Med* 128:89–95, 1998.
335. Brown BG, Zambon A, Poulin D, et al: Use of niacin, statins, and resins in patients with combined hyperlipidemia. *Am J Cardiol* 81:52B-59B, 1998.
336. Wong PW, Dillard TA, Kroenke K: Multiple organ toxicity from addition of erythromycin to long-term lovastatin therapy. *S Med J* 91:202–205, 1998.
337. Pasternak RC, Brown LE, Stone PH, et al: Effect of combination therapy with lipid-reducing drugs in patients with coronary heart disease and "normal" cholesterol levels. A randomized, placebo-controlled trial. Harvard Atherosclerosis Reversibility Project (HARP) Study Group. *Ann Intern Med* 125:529–540, 1997.
338. Feher MD, Foxton J, Banks D, et al: Long-term safety of statin-fibrate combination treatment in the management of hypercholesterolaemia in patients with coronary artery disease. *Br Heart J* 74:14–17, 1995.
339. Vacek JL, Dittmeier G, Chiarelli T, et al: Comparison of lovastatin (20 mg) and nicotinic acid (1.2 g) with either drug alone for type II hyperlipoproteinemia. *Am J Cardiol* 76:182–184, 1995.
340. Witztum JL: Drugs used in the treatment of hyperlipoproteinemias. In: Hardman JG, Limbird LE, Molinoff PB, Ruddon RW, Gillman AG, eds. *The Pharmacological Basis of Therapeutics.* McGraw-Hill, New York, 1995, pp. 885–886.
341. O'Malley K, Stevenson IH, Ward CA, et al: Determinants of anticoagulant control in patients receiving warfarin. *Br J Clin Pharmacol* 4:309–314, 1977.
342. Forman WB, Cook CE, Zacharski LR, et al: Influence of age, performance status, body weight, and tumor type in individuals with cancer on the

disposition of warfarin and its enantiomers: Department of Veterans Affairs cooperative study number 75. *J Lab Clin Med* 119:280–284, 1992.

343. Shepherd AM, Hewick DS, Moreland TA, et al: Age as a determinant of sensitivity to warfarin. *Br J Clin Pharmacol* 4:315–320, 1977.

344. Hotraphinyo K, Triggs EJ, Maybloom B, et al: Warfarin sodium: Steady-state plasma levels and patient age. *Clin Exp Pharmacol Physiol* 5: 143–149, 1978.

345. Guggenheim R, Reidenberg MM: Serum digoxin concentration and age. *J Am Geriatr Soc* 28:553–555, 1980.

346. Gurwitz JH, Avorn J, Ross-Degnan D, et al: Aging and the anticoagulant response to warfarin therapy. *Ann Intern Med* 116:901–904, 1992.

347. Fihn SD, McDonell M, Martin D, et al: Risk factors for complications of chronic anticoagulation. A multicenter study. *Ann Intern Med* 118: 511–520, 1993.

348. Reidenberg MM, Camacho M, Kluger J, et al: Aging and renal clearance of procainamide and acetylprocainamide. *Clin Pharmacol Ther* 28:732–735, 1980.

349. Bauer LA, Black D, Gensler A, et al: Influence of age, renal function and heart failure on procainamide clearance and N-acetylprocainamide serum concentrations. *Int J Clin Pharmacol Ther Toxicol* 27:213–216, 1989.

350. Nation RL, Triggs EJ, Selig M: Lignocaine kinetics in cardiac patients and aged subjects. *Br J Clin Pharmacol* 4:439–448, 1977.

351. Roberts J, Goldberg PB: Changes in responsiveness of the heart to drugs during aging. *Fed Proc* 38:1927–1932, 1979.

352. Akiyama T, Pawitan Y, Greenberg H, et al: Increased risk of death and cardiac arrest from encainide and flecainide in patients after non-Q-wave acute myocardial infarction in the Cardiac Arrhythmia Suppression Trial. CAST Investigators. *Am J Cardiol* 68:1551–1555, 1991.

353. Akiyama T, Pawitan Y, Campbell WB, et al: Effects of advancing age on the efficacy and side effects of antiarrhythmic drugs in post-myocardial infarction patients with ventricular arrhythmias. The CAST Investigators. *J Am Geriatr Soc* 40:666–672, 1992.

354. Massie BM, Fisher SG, Radford M, et al: Effect of amiodarone on clinical status and left ventricular function in patients with congestive heart failure. CHF-STAT Investigators. *Circulation* 93:2128–2134, 1996.

355. Anonymous: Effect of prophylactic amiodarone on mortality after acute myocardial infarction and in congestive heart failure: Meta-analysis of individual data from 6500 patients in randomised trials. Amiodarone Trials Meta-Analysis Investigators. *Lancet* 350:1417–1424, 1997.

356. Sim I, McDonald KM, Lavori PW, et al: Quantitative overview of randomized trials of amiodarone to prevent sudden cardiac death. *Circulation* 96:2823–2829, 1997.

Chapter 5

Prevalence and Prognosis of Electrocardiographic Findings in the Elderly

Martine C. de Bruyne, Arno W. Hoes,
Diederick E. Grobbee

In most developed countries the proportion of elderly people in the population is expected to increase in the coming decades. Cardiovascular disease is a leading cause of death and disability in the elderly and it is predicted that the absolute incidence rates of cardiac disease in older adults will increase significantly in the years to come (see Chapter 29).

Since the invention of electrocardiography in 1902 by Willem Einthoven, the electrocardiogram (ECG) has gained an important position in clinical cardiology.[1] In the last decade, computer programs for ECG interpretation with good performance have become available,[2] improving the applicability of ECGs in medical practice and in epidemiological research. The ECG offers an inexpensive, noninvasive instrument to determine the presence of coronary heart disease as well as other cardiac abnormalities, such as ventricular hypertrophy and atrial fibrillation, known to be associated with the risk of future cardiovascular events. In addition, the ECG can be used to study subclinical cardiac disease processes, such as disturbances in autonomic balance or repolarization, which may infer a poor prognosis even in the absence of symptoms. Especially in the elderly, in whom medical histories may be

From *Clinical Cardiology in the Elderly. Second Edition,* edited by Elliot Chesler. © 1999, Futura Publishing Company, Armonk, NY.

troubled by concomitant diseases and are not always as reliable as one would desire, the ECG could serve as a useful diagnostic and prognostic instrument.

Since the 1950s, large epidemiological studies among young and middle-aged men and women have provided important information on the prevalence and prognosis of ECG abnormalities. Relatively few studies have been performed in the elderly. A comparison of individual studies is hampered because of differences in diagnostic criteria applied in the individual studies, although comparability has improved since the introduction in 1960 of the Minnesota Code as a standardized coding system for the ECG.[3] Recently, several studies reported that ECG indicators of autonomic balance, such as heart rate variability and QTc interval duration, may be strong predictors of cardiac and all-cause mortality, both in middle-aged and in older subjects.

In this chapter, the prevalence and prognosis of ECG abnormalities in the elderly is reviewed. The ECG abnormalities included are Minnesota Code items, myocardial infarction, left ventricular hypertrophy, ST-T wave changes, conduction defects, and atrial fibrillation. In addition, new developments concerning ECG parameters of autonomic balance and repolarization are discussed.

Methods

A thorough literature search using computerized literature databases and lateral literature references was performed. In addition, several recent reviews, concerning electrocardiography in epidemiology[4] and ECG findings in the elderly[5,6] were scrutinized.

The review of literature on the prevalence of ECG abnormalities was limited to studies that apply the Minnesota Code. In selecting studies reporting prevalence of Minnesota Code abnormalities, we only included studies that were performed in the general population aged 60 years or older, or studies in the general adult population that presented data in age strata. Studies limited to hospitalized patients or to men only were excluded. In total, 7 studies could be found in which prevalence of Minnesota Code items in the elderly population at large was reported.[7-13] In addition, we computed the prevalence of Minnesota Code items among men and women aged 60 years or older in the Rotterdam Study, a population-based study among men and women aged 55 years or older, living in the Rotterdam district of Ommoord.[14]

Prevalence of ECG Abnormalities According to the Minnesota Code

Selected characteristics of the 8 population-based cross-sectional studies are shown in Table 1. Tables 2, 3, and 4 summarize the major findings from these studies.

Table 1
Summary of Major Characteristics of Eight Population-Based Studies in the Elderly

	First Author (Reference)							
	Ostrander (9)	Kennedy (10)	Kitchin (11)	Campbell (7)	Östör (8)	Furberg (12)	Casiglia (13)	Rotterdam Study
Subjects (n)	663	400	487	2254	4118	5150	2254	5089
Men, %	46	48	44	39	49	43	36	40
Response rate (%)	>70	NR	NR	60	72	NR	73	70
Age range (y)	≥60	≥65	62–90	≥65	≥60	≥65	≥65	60–106
Mean age (y)	70	74	NR	71	68	73	NR	72
Men	70	74	NR	71	68	74	NR	70
Women	71	75	NR	71	67	73	NR	73

NR, not reported.

Table 2
Prevalence of Electrocardiographic Evidence of Myocardial Infarction (Q-QS abnormalities) in Eight Population-Based Studies in the Elderly

	First Author (Reference)							
	Ostrander (9)	Kennedy (10)	Kitchin (11)	Campbell (7)	Östör (8)	Furberg (12)	Casiglia (13)	Rotterdam Study
Q-Qs abnormalities, Code 1.1–1.3	6.8	9.5	7.7	6.3	4.5	NR	NR	15.7
Men	9.1		7.9	10.0	6.3			20.0
Women	4.7		7.4	4.0	2.7			12.9
Major Q-QS abnormalities Code 1.1–1.2	5.0	NR	5.4	4.7	3.1	5.2	2.3	8.7
Men	6.8		5.6	7.8	4.3	7.3	3.6	11.6
Women	3.6		5.2	2.4	2.0	3.6	1.4	6.8
Minor Q-QS abnormalities Code 1.3	1.8	NR	2.3	1.6	1.4	NR	NR	7.0
Men	2.3		2.3	2.2	2.0			8.3
Women	1.4		2.2	1.2	0.8			6.1

NR, not reported.

Table 3
Prevalence of Axis Deviation, Ventricular Hypertrophy, and ST-Segment and T-Wave Abnormalities in Eight Population-Based Studies in the Elderly

	First Author (Reference)							
	Ostrander (9)	Kennedy (10)	Kitchin (11)	Campbell (7)	Östör (8)	Furberg (12)	Casiglia (13)	Rotterdam Study
LAD, Code 2.1	18.4	6.5	8.5	NR	7.9	NR	13.1	8.9
Men	21.0		10.2		10.2		15.9	10.9
Women	16.2		7.1		5.6		11.4	7.5
RAD, Code 2.2	0.2	NR	0.8	NR	0.7	NR	NR	0.1
Men	0.3		1.9		0.8			0.1
Women	0.0		0.0		0.5			0.1
LVH, Code 3.1–3.3	10.1	14.0	9.7*	8.8	16.9	NR	10.0	11.9
Men	8.2		3.7	6.7	20.6		11.7	12.4
Women	11.5		7.1	10.2	13.1		8.9	11.6
LVH with ST-T	NR	6.3	NR	4.6	NR	4.2	NR	8.0
Men				2.9		4.3		7.4
Women				5.6		4.1		8.4
RVH, Code 3.2	NR	0.0	2.5	0.7	NR	NR	NR	0.0
Men			3.3	1.4				0.1
Women			1.9	0.3				0.0
ST segment items, Code 4.1–4.4	10.9	NR	10.1	6.2	10.6	NR	NR	20.3
Men	7.9		13.0	5.4	11.6			19.3
Women	13.4		24.0	6.7	9.7			20.9
T-wave items, Code 5.1–5.4	32.1	10.5**	27.0	15.3	24.4	6.3	23.6	30.9
Men	33.1		23.0	19.2	26.3	5.5	18.1	27.0
Women	31.3		30.0	12.9	22.6	6.8	27.0	33.6

NR, not reported; * Only code 3.1; ** ST-T combined Code 4.1 or 4.3 and Code 5.1 or 5.3.

Q-QS Patterns

The overall prevalence of Q-QS abnormalities, suggestive of myocardial infarction, in the elderly population varies between 4.5% and 15.7%. The prevalence ratio of minor and major infarct patterns is consistent, approximately 0.40, across all studies apart from the Rotterdam Study. Prevalence of Q-QS patterns, in particular minor Q-QS abnormalities, in the Rotterdam Study is higher than in the other studies. In all studies, Q-QS patterns are more frequent in men than in women, with prevalence clearly increasing with age in both sexes.

Table 4
Prevalence of Atrioventricular and Ventricular Conduction Defects, Extrasystoles, and Atrial Fibrillation in Eight Population-Based Studies in the Elderly

	First Author (Reference)							
	Ostrander (9)	Kennedy (10)	Kitchin (11)	Campbell (7)	Östör (8)	Furberg (12)	Casiglia (13)	Rotterdam Study
AV conduction defects, Code 6.1–6.3	NR	2.3	3.3	1.1	6.9	NR	NR	6.8
Men			3.7	1.5	8.7			8.0
Women			3.0	0.8	5.2			6.0
First degree AV block, Code 6.3	6.2	2.0	NR	0.9	6.8	5.3	3.9	6.8
Men	6.9			1.5	8.7	8.1	5.0	8.0
Women	5.6			0.6	5.0	3.2	3.2	6.0
LBBB, Code 7.1	1.7	2.5	0.6	1.4	1.6	1.7	3.9	2.9
Men	0.7		1.4	1.6	1.9	1.6	3.9	2.7
Women	2.5		0.0	1.2	1.3	1.8	3.9	3.0
RBBB, Code 7.2	2.0	3.5	2.3	1.8	2.3	4.3	7.4*	4.1
Men	3.0		2.3	2.8	3.6	6.8	10.8	6.5
Women	1.1		2.2	1.2	1.1	2.4	5.4	2.4
Incomplete RBBB, Code 7.3	2.1	2.8	1.5	1.4	1.7	NR	NR	2.8
Men	3.3		1.4	1.6	1.8			3.5
Women	1.1		1.5	1.3	1.5			2.4
Intraventricular block, Code 7.4	NR	NR	NR	0.5	0.8	2.7	NR	0.8
Men				0.8	1.2	4.7		1.2
Women				0.3	0.3	1.2		0.5
Extrasystole, Code 8.1	5.6	4.5	NR	3.1	3.1	NR	NR	3.7
Men	8.9			3.6	3.6			4.8
Women	2.8			2.5	2.5			3.0
Atrial fibrillation, Code 8.3	2.4	3.0	2.5	1.4	1.4	3.2	4.0	3.6
Men	2.6		2.3	1.3	1.3	4.0	3.8	4.0
Women	2.2		2.6	1.5	1.5	2.6	4.1	3.3

NR, not reported; * Code 7.2 and 7.3 combined.

QRS Axis Deviation

Ostrander et al[9,15] reported a prevalence of left axis deviation of 18% in men and women 60 years or over, whereas in other studies considerably lower prevalences are found. An increase in the prevalence of axis deviation with advancing age in both sexes is demonstrated in all studies, and men are more frequently affected than women.

Ventricular Hypertrophy

Major differences exist in the reported prevalence of left ventricular hypertrophy (LVH), which varies from 8.8% to 16.9%. Also, the presence of LVH with ST-T abnormalities varies considerably, from 4.2% to 8.0%. In 6 of the 8 studies, women appear to be more often affected by LVH than men. Only Ostor et al.[8] and Casiglia et al.[13] reported a higher prevalence of LVH in men. Right ventricular hypertrophy is rarely found and more refined criteria to detect minor abnormalities of the right ventricle have been proposed.[7]

ST-T Abnormalities

Also, the prevalence of ST-T wave abnormalities varies widely across studies. The prevalence of ST-segment items varies from 5.4% to 19.3% in men, and from 6.7% to 24.0% in women. Similarly, the prevalence of T-wave abnormalities varies from 5.5% to 33.1% in men and from 6.8% to 33.6% in women. The prevalence of ST-T abnormalities rapidly increases with age and no clear gender differences are present.

Conduction Defects

First-degree atrioventricular (AV) block is by far the most common atrioventricular conduction defect, ranging from 0.9% to 6.8% in older subjects. A right bundle branch block occurs more frequently than a left bundle branch block (range 1.8% to 4.3% and 0.6% to 3.9%, respectively). Right bundle branch block and intraventricular block appear to be more frequent in men than in women. Such a difference does not exist for left bundle branch block.

Arrhythmias

The prevalence of cardiac arrhythmias increases with age. Atrial fibrillation, with a reported prevalence of 1.4% to 4.0%, is the most common cardiac arrhythmia.

Comments

Reported prevalences of most ECG abnormalities according to the Minnesota Code showed considerable variation between individual studies. Although all studies reviewed were performed in nonhospitalized and unselected populations, these studies differ with regard to the number of participants, age and gender distribution, and response rate. Apart from regional differences in the occurrence of cardiovascular diseases, different selection criteria may explain at least part of the variation in prevalence of ECG abnormalities. In addition, the period in which the studies were performed, during the 1960s to the 1990s, may be a source of variation. Although coding took place according to the Minnesota Code, differences in coding procedures, by one or more observers, by hand or computer, may also account for part of the variation. Interobserver and intraobserver variability in Minnesota Coding may be considerable.[10,16,17] The Rotterdam Study is the only study using an extensively validated computer program for ECG coding.[18,19]

Several ECG abnormalities according to the Minnesota Code, eg, Q-QS patterns, left axis deviation, left bundle branch block, high amplitude R-waves, ST-T abnormalities, and atrial fibrillation are established risk indicators of future cardiovascular events.[8,13,20–23] Diagnosis and prognosis of these and other ECG abnormalities is discussed next in more detail.

Diagnosis and Prognosis of Specific ECG Abnormalities

Myocardial Infarction

Myocardial infarction may occur with or without symptoms[24] and with or without lasting ECG abnormalities.[25,26] Especially in the elderly, patients with myocardial infarction often present themselves with atypical symptoms and signs.[14]

The proportion of myocardial infarctions that occur without typical symptoms and silent myocardial infarctions, ranges from 20% to 68% (Table 5). This proportion appears to be higher in women than in men. The prevalence of silent myocardial infarction (on average 4.6% in men and 3.5% in women in the Rotterdam Study) increases with age.[14]

The prognosis of silent myocardial infarction with regard to the occurrence of new coronary events, such as recurrent myocardial infarction, ventricular fibrillation, and sudden cardiac death, is similar to that of symptomatic myocardial infarction.[27–31] In the elderly, the absolute risk of new coronary events is usually high. For example, Aronow et al.[28] reported that during 4 years of follow-up new coronary events occurred in 65% of men and women with recognized myocardial infarc-

Table 5
Proportion of Proven Electrocardiographic Myocardial
Infarction That Occurs without Symptoms (Silent)
in the Elderly

First Author (Reference)	Prevalence (% (Number of Silent Events/ Total Number of Myocardial Infarctions))
Rodstein (37)	31% (16/52)
Aronow (38)	68% (78/115)
Furberg (12)	20% (147/744)
Nadelmann (27)	34% (25/72)
De Bruyne (14)	36% (127/353)

tion and in 56% of men and women with silent myocardial infarction. As the detection of silent myocardial infarction is completely dependent on the ECG, these findings may have important implications for the use of ECGs for cardiovascular screening of elderly patients in medical practice.

Non-Q-wave myocardial infarction, defined as symptomatic myocardial infarction without matching ECG abnormalities, but confirmed by raised cardiac enzyme levels or autopsy, may occur in 38% to 62% of all myocardial infarctions, depending on the Minnesota Code criteria used, and is more frequent in myocardial infarctions that occurred farther in the past.[26] In the Bronx Aging Study,[27] among men and women aged 75 to 85 years, 62% of the reported myocardial infarctions are non-Q-wave myocardial infarctions. In the Rotterdam Study, the prevalence of non-Q-wave myocardial infarction is 4.4% in men and 1.8% in women. Overall, 26% of all myocardial infarctions were non-Q-wave infarctions. The prognostic implications of non-Q-wave myocardial infarctions are similar to those of electrocardiographic myocardial infarctions.[32–36]

Left Ventricular Hypertrophy

Diagnosis of left ventricular hypertrophy measured by ECG has a poor sensitivity and predictive value in detecting echocardiographically determined left ventricular hypertrophy. In a report by Aronow et al,[39] the sensitivity of 5 different ECG criteria for left ventricular hypertrophy varies from 12% to 29%, the specificity ranges from 93% to 96%, and the positive predictive value ranges from 62% to 72%. In the Framingham Heart Study the sensitivity of ECG criteria of left ventricular hypertrophy (using R in aVL, S in V_3 and QRS duration) for echocardiographic left ventricular hypertrophy is 39% in men and 51% in women, at a specificity level of 95%.[40] An even poorer sensitivity has been reported when diabetes, a common comorbidity, is present.[41] Prevalence estimates of left ventricular hypertrophy by ECG are strongly influenced by the ECG criteria used.

Prognosis of left ventricular hypertrophy in the elderly is reported to be similar to that of silent myocardial infarction.[42] Subjects with left ventricular hypertrophy are at increased risk for coronary events, atherothrombotic brain infarctions, congestive heart failure, peripheral artery disease, ventricular arrhythmias, and total mortality.[32,42–46] Also, serial changes in electrocardiographic left ventricular hypertrophy have prognostic implications. Serial increase of left ventricular hypertrophy has a poorer prognosis and serial decrease of left ventricular hypertrophy has a better prognosis for cardiovascular disease.[32,47] Recent studies indicate that treatment of left ventricular hypertrophy can reduce the incidence of coronary heart disease.[48]

ST-T Wave Changes

In previous studies, ST-T wave changes, either isolated or in combination with other ischemic or hypertrophic changes, have been associated with coronary heart disease and sudden cardiac death in middle-aged populations,[22,49–59] as well as in elderly populations.[8,21,60–65] In middle-aged populations, the association of ST-T abnormalities has often been reported to be more pronounced in men than in women, but this difference seems to be absent in the elderly. Although ST-T abnormalities often are transient, they are independently associated with future coronary heart disease. In the Framingham Study in asymptomatic men and women nonspecific ST-T abnormalities were associated with a 2-fold risk for future cardiovascular events.[63] The risk associated with ST-T abnormalities is more pronounced in combination with other ECG abnormalities, such as pathological Q-waves, left ventricular hypertrophy, or intraventricular conduction defects. Repolarization disturbances on the ECG are multifactorial and may be associated with increasing age, myocardial ischemia, hypertension, ventricular hypertrophy, ventricular conduction defects, use of digitalis, autonomic dysfunction, and other pathophysiological processes.

Conduction Defects

Atrioventricular conduction time increases with age, due to changes both in the atrioventricular nodal and the His-Purkinje system.[66] In addition, atrioventricular block is associated with coronary ischemia, vagotonia, and digitalis use.[67] In contrast to younger populations, in which the presence of atrioventricular block is usually considered a benign condition, not associated with an increased risk for coronary heart disease,[68,69] in older populations an association of atrioventricular blocks with coronary heart disease has been reported in several studies.[70–72] Other studies in elderly patients report no association of atrioventricular block with coronary events.[73]

Left bundle branch block is uncommon in the absence of cardiovascular disease[74] and is associated with future coronary heart disease[65, 75] and all-cause mortality[22, 73] in elderly men and women. Right bundle branch block occurs more frequently than left bundle branch block. Only in 20% of subjects with right bundle branch block, are clinical and necropsy findings of coronary heart disease are present.[76] Contradictory results have been published on the risk associated with right bundle branch block in the elderly. An association with mortality was observed in a study by Caird et al[22] and an association with coronary events was present in the Framingham Study,[77] while no associations were found in several other studies.[62,73,78,79]

Intraventricular conduction defects, defined as a prolonged QRS duration (0.11 seconds) in the absence of left or right bundle branch block, has been reported to increase the incidence of total mortality[78] and cardiac events[73] in the elderly. In the Framingham Heart Study, elderly men and women with intraventricular conduction defect were at increased risk for coronary heart disease, although this was not statistically significant.[65]

Arrhythmias

The prevalence of atrial fibrillation increases with age[80] and is higher in those with overt cardiovascular disease.[12,81,82] Many studies have reported that chronic atrial fibrillation is independently associated with thromboembolic stroke.[83–86] Recently, an association of atrial fibrillation with dementia was reported.[87] In addition, atrial fibrillation was a risk factor for all-cause mortality in the Coronary Drug Project[78] and for cardiovascular mortality in the Framingham Heart Study.[80]

Premature ventricular complexes on the resting ECG were a risk factor for total mortality in the Coronary Drug Project[78] and for cardiovascular mortality in the Busselton Study.[62] In the elderly an increased risk of cardiovascular events associated with frequent ventricular premature beats on ambulatory ECGs has been reported several times.[88–90] However, no association with cardiac outcome was found between ventricular premature beats on the resting ECG in elderly in the Baltimore Longitudinal Study.[91] Using 1-minute rhythm strips, no association was found in subjects without clinical heart disease, but a strong association was present in elderly subjects with a history of clinical heart disease.[92] The latter finding suggests that ventricular premature complexes are markers of underlying ischemic heart disease.

New ECG Indicators of Autonomic Function and Repolarization

Prolonged QTc interval and decreased heart rate variability (HRV) have been put forward as indicators of autonomic balance.[93, 94] With increasing age, sympathetic activity increases relative to vagal activity.[95] Autonomic balance, in particular QTc interval and heart rate variability, is influenced by various physiological and pathophysiological conditions, such as respiration,[96] diabetic neuropathy,[97–100] left ventricular function,[101] and coronary heart disease.[102–105] Both risk indicators have been associated with a poor prognosis in patients after myocardial infarction.[106–112]

Recently, some studies on the prognostic value of prolonged QTc interval were performed in the general population, producing controversial results. In 3 Dutch studies a positive association of prolonged QTc with cardiac outcome was reported. In the Dutch Civil Servants Study,[113] men and women with prolonged heart-rate adjusted QT intervals had a 2-fold risk for death from coronary heart disease. In the Zutphen Study[114] among middle-aged and elderly men, 3-fold increased risks for cardiac mortality were reported. Also in the Rotterdam Study, among men and women aged 55 years or older, about a 2-fold increased risk for cardiac mortality in those with prolonged QTc was reported.[115] However, no association was found between QTc interval and cardiac outcome in the Framingham Study[116] and the Bronx Aging Study.[71]

Results from population-based studies concerning the risk associated with decreased HRV are more consistent. In middle-aged men and women, decreased HRV was associated with a poorer cardiac prognosis in 3 studies.[117–119] An increased risk for all-cause mortality associated with decreased HRV was found in elderly men and women in the Framingham Study[120] and in elderly men in the Zutphen Study.[121] However, no association of decreased HRV with both cardiac and all-cause mortality was found in the Bronx Aging Study.[71] Surprisingly, in this study an association of increased HRV with cardiac events was present in women. A similar association was reported in elderly men in the Zutphen Study. Recently, the Rotterdam Study reported an association of both decreased and increased HRV with cardiac death in elderly men and women. In the latter study, it has been suggested that the risk associated with increased HRV may be due to sinus node dysfunction, rather than autonomic dysfunction.[115]

Two new indicators of ventricular repolarization have been put forward as predictors of cardiac outcome in the elderly. First, interlead variability of the length of the QT interval in the standard ECG, defined as QT dispersion, was found to be a strong independent predictor of cardiac mortality in older men and women.[122] Increased QT dispersion was associated with a more than 2-fold increased risk of cardiac death. Although it has been suggested that QT dispersion reflects regional differences in ventricular repolarization, this explanation has been criticized and the underlying mechanism of QTc dispersion remains largely unclear.

Finally, the electrical T axis has been put forward as a general marker of repolarization abnormality, indicative of subclinical myocardial damage.[115] In the Rotterdam Study a 4-fold risk for cardiac and sudden cardiac death was found in older men and women with an abnormal T axis. In this study, T axis was a stronger risk indicator than a history of myocardial infarction or diabetes mellitus.

Comments

Reports from literature show that the ECG contains a wealth of both etiologic and prognostic information. However, many studies use their own definitions of ECG diagnoses, and thus, results from different studies show wide variation and cannot easily be compared. In addition, characteristics of subjects included in individual studies differ. Measurement techniques of intervals and amplitudes need to be standardized, to allow results from epidemiological studies to be applicable in medical practice. Since computer programs with good performance have become available,[2] they offer an efficient, inexpensive, and, in particular, a standardized way to interpret ECGs.

Conclusions

The prevalence of abnormal ECG findings is relatively high in the elderly, increases with age and is higher in men than in women. Most ECG findings that are often markers of coronary heart disease or other disease processes, are associated with future coronary events. However, diagnostic criteria show wide variation among studies, and standardization is urgently needed. Computer programs for ECG analysis may offer a solution The significance of conventional and new ECG risk indicators in elderly men and women needs to be confirmed and the predictive value of ECG findings, in addition to established cardiovascular risk indicators, needs to be determined. Although in younger subjects without heart disease the ECG is not considered a useful tool for screening purposes,[123] the ECG may well be valuable to identify elderly subjects at risk for future coronary heart disease, because both prevalence of ECG abnormalities and incidence of cardiac disease are higher at older age.

References

1. Fye BW: A history of the origin, evolution, and impact of electrocardiography. *Am J Cardiol* 73:937–949, 1995.
2. Willems JL, Abreu-Lima C, Arnaud P, et al: The diagnostic performance of computer programs for the interpretation of electrocardiograms. *N Engl J Med* 325:1767–1773, 1991.
3. Prineas RJ, Crow RS, Blackburn H: *the Minnesota Code Manual of Electrocardiographic Findings: Standards and Procedures for Measurement and Classification.* Wright J, editor, Boston: Littlejohn M, 1982.
4. Rautaharju PM: Electrocardiography in epidemiology and clinical trials.

In: Macfarlane PW, Lawrie TDV, eds. *Comprehensive Electrocardiography. Theory and Practice in Health and Disease.* First edition. Oxford, Pergamon Press, 1989, pp 1219–1266.

5. Hoogervorst HJ, Hoes AW, Grobbee DE: Electrocardiographic abnormalities in the elderly: Findings in population-based studies. *Cardiol Elderly* 4;2:21–27, 1994.

6. Aronow WS: Prevalence and prognosis of electrocardiographic findings of intraventricular conduction abnormalities, unrecognized Q-wave myocardial infarction, and left ventricular hypertrophy in the elderly. *Cardiol Elderly* 5:9–13, 1997.

7. Campbell A, Caird FI, Jackson TF: Prevalence of abnormalities of electrocardiogram in old people. *Br Heart J* 36:1005–1011, 1974.

8. Ostor E, Schnohr P, Jensen G, et al: Electrocardiographic findings and their association with mortality in the Copenhagen City Heart Study. *Eur Heart J* 2:317–328, 1981.

9. Ostrander LD, Brandt RL, Kjelsberg MO, et al: Electrocardiographic findings among the adult population of a natural community, Tecumseh, Michigan. *Circulation* 31:888–898, 1965.

10. Kennedy RD, Caird FI: The application of the Minnesota code to population studies of the electrocardiogram in the elderly. *Gerontol Clin* 14:5–16, 1972.

11. Kitchin AH, Lowther CP, Milne JS: Prevalence of clinical and electrocardiographic evidence of ischaemic heart disease in the older population. *Br Heart J* 35:946–953, 1973

12. Furberg CD, Manolio TA, Psaty BM, et al: Major electrocardiographic abnormalities in persons aged 65 years and older (the Cardiovascular Health Study). Cardiovascular Health Study Collaborative Research Group. *Am J Cardiol* 69:1329–1335, 1992

13. Casiglia E, Spolaore P, Ginocchio G, et al: Mortality in relation to Minnesota code items in elderly subjects. Sex-related differences in a cardiovascular study in the elderly. *Jpn Heart J* 34:567–577, 1993

14. De Bruyne MC, Mosterd A, Hoes AW, et al: Prevalence, determinants, and misclassification of myocardial infarction in the elderly. *Epidemiology* 8:495–500, 1997.

15. Ostrander LD, Jr: Left axis deviation: Prevalence, associated conditions, and prognosis. An epidemiologic study. *Ann Intern Med* 75:23–28, 1971

16. Bjornson J, Hjermann I, Leren P: Reproducibility of the ECG classification system of the Minnesota code in the study of patients with coronary heart disease. *Acta Med Scand* 193:211–214, 1973

17. Elgrishi I, Ducimetiere P, Richard JL. Reproducibility of analysis of the electrocardiogram in epidemiology using the 'Minnesota code'. *Br J Prev Soc Med* 24:197–200, 1970.

18. Kors JA, Van Herpen G, Wu J, et al: Validation of a new computer program for Minnesota Coding. *J Electrocardiol* 29:83–88, 1996

19. Van Bemmel JH, Kors JA, Van Herpen G. Methodology of the modular ECG analysis system MEANS. *Methods Inf Med* 29:346–353, 1990

20. Casiglia E, Spolaore P, Ginocchio G, et al: Predictors of mortality in very old subjects aged 80 years or over. *Eur J Epidemiol* 9:577–586, 1993

21. Tervahauta M, Pekkanen J, Punsar S, et al: Resting electrocardiographic abnormalities as predictors of coronary events and total mortality among elderly men. *Am J Med* 100:641–645, 1996

22. Caird FI, Campbell A, Jackson TF. Significance of abnormalities of electrocardiogram in old people. *Br Heart J* 36:1012–1018, 1974

23. Rajala S, Haavisto M, Kaltiala K, et al: ECG findings and survival in very old people. Eur Heart J 6:247–252, 1985.
24. Kannel WB, McNamara PM, Feinleib M, et al: The unrecognized myocardial infarction. Fourteen-year follow-up experience in the Framingham study. Geriatrics 25:75–87, 1970
25. Pyorala K, Kentala E. Disappearance of Minnesota Code Q-QS patterns in the first year after myocardial infarction. Ann Clin Res 6:137–141, 1974
26. Uusitupa M, Pyorala K, Raunio H, et al: Sensitivity and specificity of Minnesota Code Q-QS abnormalities in the diagnosis of myocardial infarction verified at autopsy. Am Heart J 1983.
27. Nadelmann J, Frishman WH, Ooi WL, et al: Prevalence, incidence and prognosis of recognized and unrecognized myocardial infarction in persons aged 75 years or older: The Bronx Aging Study. Am J Cardiol 66: 533–537, 1990
28. Aronow WS: New coronary events at four-year follow-up in elderly patients with recognized or unrecognized myocardial infarction. Am J Cardiol 63:621–622, 1989
29. Kannel WB, Abbott RD: Incidence and prognosis of unrecognized myocardial infarction. An update on the Framingham study. N Engl J Med 311: 1144–1147, 1984.
30. Yano K, MacLean CJ: The incidence and prognosis of unrecognized myocardial infarction in the Honolulu, Hawaii, Heart Program. Arch Intern Med 149:1528–1532, 1989.
31. Vokonas PS, Kannel WB, Cupples LA. Incidence and prognosis of unrecognized mycardial infarction in the elderly. The Framingham Study. J Am Coll Cardiol 11 (suppl. A):51, 1988.
32. Kahn S, Frishman WH, Weissman S, et al: Left ventricular hypertrophy on electrocardiogram: Prognostic implications from a 10-year cohort study of older subjects. A report from the Bronx Longitudinal Aging Study. J Am Geriatr Soc 44:524–529, 1996.
33. Karlson BW, Herlitz J, Richter A, et al: Prognosis in acute myocardial infarction in relation to development of Q waves. Clin Cardiol 14:875–880, 1991.
34. Karlson BW, Herlitz J, Emanuelsson H, et al: One-year mortality rate after discharge from hospital in relation to whether or not a confirmed myocardial infarction was developed. Int J Cardiol 32:381–388, 1991.
35. Molstad P: Prognostic significance of type and location of a first myocardial infarction. J Intern Med 233:393–399, 1993.
36. Edlavitch SA, Crow R, Burke GL, et al: Secular trends in Q wave and non-Q wave acute myocardial infarction. The Minnesota Heart Survey. Circulation 83:492–503, 1991.
37. Rodstein M: The characteristics of nonfatal myocardial infarction in the aged. Arch Intern Med 98:84–90, 1956.
38. Aronow WS, Starling L, Etienne F, et al: Unrecognized Q-wave myocardial infarction in patients older than 64 years in a long-term health-care facility. Am J Cardiol 56:483, 1985.
39. Aronow WS, Schwartz KS, Koenigsberg M. Value of five electrocardiographic criteria correlated with echocardiographic left ventricular hypertrophy in elderly patients. Am J Noninvasive Cardiol 1:152–154, 1987.
40. Norman JE, Levy D. Improved electrocardiographic detection of echocardiographic left ventricular hypertrophy: Results of a correlated data base approach. J Am Coll Cardiol 26:1022–1029, 1995.

41. Gerritsen TA, Bak AAA, Jonker JJC, et al: Poor performance of the electrocardogram in detection of left ventricular hypertrophy in diabetic patients with hypertension. Submitted for publication.

42. Kannel WB, Dannenberg AL, Levy D. Population implications of electrocardiographic left ventricular hypertrophy. *Am J Cardiol* 60:85I-93I, 1987.

43. Levy D: Left ventricular hypertrophy. Epidemiological insights from the Framingham Heart Study. *Drugs* 35:1–5, 1988.

44. Levy D, Anderson KM, Savage DD, et al: Risk of ventricular arrhythmias in left ventricular hypertrophy: The Framingham Heart Study. *Am J Cardiol* 60:560–565, 1987.

45. Aronow WS: Usefulness of echocardiographic and electrocardiographic left ventricular hypertrophy in predicting new cardiac events and atherothrombotic brain infarction in elderly patients with systemic hypertension or coronary artery disease. *Am J Noninvasive Cardiol* 3:367–370, 1989.

46. Aronow WS, Ahn C, Kronzon I, et al: Congestive heart failure, coronary events, and atherothrombotic brain infarction in elderly blacks and whites with systemic hypertension and with and without echocardiographic and electrocardiographic evidence of left ventricular hypertrophy. *Am J Cardiol* 67, 1991.

47. Levy D, Salomon M, D'Agostino R, et al: Prognostic implications of baseline electrocardiographic features and their serial changes in subjects with left ventricular hypertrophy. *Circulation* 90:1786–1793, 1994.

48. Cruickshank JM, Lewis J, Moore V, et al: Reversibility of left ventricular hypertrophy by differing types of antihypertensive therapy. *J Hum Hypertens* 6:85–90, 1992.

49. Sigurdsson E, Sigfusson N, Sigvaldason H, et al: Silent ST-T changes in an epidemiologic cohort study—a marker of hypertension or coronary heart disease, or both: The Reykjavik study. *J Am Coll Cardiol* 27:1140–1147, 1996.

50. Schouten EG, Dekker JM, Pool J, et al: Well shaped ST segment and risk of cardiovascular mortality. *BMJ* 304:356–359, 1992.

51. Whincup PH, Wannamethee G, Macfarlane PW, et al: Resting electrocardiogram and risk of coronary heart disease in middle-aged British men. *J Cardiovasc Risk* 2:533–543, 1995.

52. Liao YL, Liu KA, Dyer A, et al: Major and minor electrocardiographic abnormalities and risk of death from coronary heart disease, cardiovascular diseases and all causes in men and women. *J Am Coll Cardiol* 12:1494–1500, 1988.

53. Liao Y, Liu K, Dyer A, et al: Sex differential in the relationship of electrocardiographic ST-T abnormalities to risk of coronary death: 11.5 year follow-up findings of the Chicago Heart Association Detection Project in Industry. *Circulation* 75:347–352, 1987.

54. Knutsen R, Knutsen SF, Curb JD, et al: The predictive value of resting electrocardiograms for 12-year incidence of coronary heart disease in the Honolulu Heart Program. *J Clin Epidemiol* 41:293–302, 1988.

55. Sutherland SE, Gazes PC, Keil JE, et al: Electrocardiographic abnormalities and 30-year mortality among white and black men of the Charleston Heart Study. *Circulation* 88:2685–2692, 1993.

56. Bartel A, Heyden S, Tyroler HA, et al: Electrocardiographic predictors of coronary heart disease. *Arch Intern Med* 128:929–937, 1971.

57. Rabkin SW, Mathewson FL, Tate RB: The electrocardiogram in apparently healthy men and the risk of sudden death. *Br Heart J* 47:546–552, 1982.
58. Rose G, Baxter PJ, Reid DD, et al: Prevalence and prognosis of electrocardiographic findings in middle-aged men. *Br Heart J* 40:636–643, 1978.
59. Kreger BE, Cupples LA, Kannel WB: The electrocardiogram in prediction of sudden death: Framingham Study experience. *Am Heart J* 113: 377–382, 1987.
60. Mihalick MJ, Fisch C: Electrocardiographic findings in the aged. *Am Heart J* 87:117–128. 1974.
61. Fruergaard P, Launbjerg J, Jacobsen HL, et al: Seven-year prognostic value of the electrocardiogram at rest and an exercise test in patients admitted for, but without, confirmed myocardial infarction. *Eur Heart J* 4:499–504, 1993.
62. Cullen K, Stenhouse NS, Wearne KL, et al: Electrocardiograms and 13 year cardiovascular mortality in the Busselton study. *Br Heart J* 47: 209–212, 1982.
63. Kannel WB, Anderson K, McGee DL, et al: Nonspecific electrocardiographic abnormality as a predictor of coronary heart disease: The Framingham Study. *Am Heart J* 113:370–376, 1987.
64. Aronow WS: Correlation of ischemic ST-segment depression on the resting electrocardiogram with new cardiac events in 1,106 patients over 62 years of age. *Am J Cardiol* 64:232–233, 1989.
65. Kannel WB: Common electrocardiographic markers for subsequent clinical coronary events. *Circulation* 75:II25–27, 1987.
66. Crijns HJGM, Van Gelder IC; Age-related changes in electrophysiology of the atrioventricular node and electrocardiographic manifestations. *Cardiol Elderly* 5:3–8, 1997.
67. Rodstein M, Brown M, Wolloch L: First-degree atrioventricular heart block in the aged. *Geriatrics* 23:159–165, 1968.
68. Mymin D, Mathewson FA, Tate RB, et al: The natural history of primary first-degree atrioventricular heart block. *N Engl J Med* 315:1183–1187, 1986.
69. Erickson EE, Lev M: Aging changes in the human atrioventricular node, bundle, and bundle branches. *J Gerontol* 7:1–12, 1952.
70. Blackburn H, Taylor HL, Keys A: Coronary heart disease in Seven Countries: XVI. The electrocardiogam in predicton of five-year coronary heart disease incidence among men aged forty through fifty-nine. *Circulation* 41&42 (suppl I):154–161, 1970.
71. Bernstein JM, Frishman WH, Jen Chang C: Value of ECG P-R and Q-Tc interval prolongation and heart rate variability for predicting cardiovascular morbidity and mortality in the elderly: the Bronx Aging Study. *Cardiol Elderly* 5:31–41, 1997.
72. Clark ANG, Craven AH: PR interval in the aged. *Age Ageing* 10:157–164, 1981.
73. Aronow WS. Correlation of arrhythmias and conduction defects on the resting electrocardiogram with new cardiac events in 1,153 elderly patients. *Am J Noninvasive Cardiol* 5:88–90, 1991.
74. Kreger BE, Anderson KM, Kannel WB. Prevalence of intraventricular block in the general population: the Framingham Study. *Am Heart J* 117: 903–910, 1989.
75. Schneider JF, Thomas HE, Kreger BE, et al: Newly acquired left bundle-branch block: the Framingham study. *Ann Intern Med* 90:303–310, 1979.

76. Roberts WC: Morphological features of the elderly heart. In: Tresch DD, Aronow WS, eds. *Cardiovascular Disease in the Elderly Patient*. New York: Marcel Dekker, 1994, pp 17–42.
77. Schneider JF, Thomas HE, Kreger BE, et al: Newly acquired right bundle-branch block: The Framingham Study. *Ann Intern Med* 92:37–44, 1980.
78. The Coronary Drug Project: The prognostic importance of the electrocardiogram after myocardial infarction. Ann Intern Med 77:677–689, 1972.
79. Fleg JL, Das DN, Lakatta EG: Right bundle branch block: Long term prognosis in apparently healthy men. *J Am Coll Cardiol* 1:387–392, 1983.
80. Kannel WB, Abbott RD, Savage DD, et al: Epidemiologic features of chronic atrial fibrillation. The Framingham Study. *N Engl J Med* 306: 1018–1022, 1982.
81. Podrid PJ. Arrhythmias in the elderly subject. Cardiol Elderly 5:18–21, 1997.
82. Lip GY, Beevers DG. ABC of atrial fibrillation. History, epidemiology, and importance of atrial fibrillation [published erratum appears in *BMJ* Jan 312(7022):49, 1996]. *BMJ* 311:1361–1363, 1995.
83. Wolf PA, Dawber TR, Thomas HE, et al: Epidemiologic assessment of chronic atrial fibrillation and risk of stroke: The Framingham study. *Neurology* 28:973–977, 1978.
84. Wolf PA, D'Agostino R, Belanger AJ, et al: Probability of stroke: a risk profile from the Framingham Study. *Stroke* 22:312–318, 1991.
85. Aronow WS:. Usefulness of the resting electrocardiogram in the elderly. *Compr Ther* 18:11–16, 1992.
86. Boysen G, Nyboe J, Appleyard M, et al: Stroke incidence and risk factors for stroke in Copenhagen, Denmark. *Stroke* 19:1345–1353, 1988.
87. Ott A, Breteler MMB, De Bruyne MC, et al: Atrial fibrillation and dementia in a population-based study. The Rotterdam Study. *Stroke* 28:316–321, 1997.
88. Frishmen WH, Heiman M, Karpenos A, et al: Twenty-four hour ambulatory electrocardiography in elderly subjects: Prevalence of various arrhythmias and prognostic implications (report from the Bronx Longitudinal Aging Study). *Am Heart J* 132:297–302, 1996.
89. Martin A, Benbow L, Butrous GS, et al: Five year follow-up of 101 elderly subjects by means of long-term ambulatory cardiac monitoring. *Eur Heart J* 5:592–596, 1984.
90. Raiha IJ, Piha SJ, Seppanen A, et al: Predictive value of continuous ambulatory electrocardiographic monitoring in elderly people. *BMJ* 309: 1263–1267, 1994.
91. Fleg JL, Kennedy HL. Long-term prognostic signficance of ambulatory electrocardiographic findings in apparently healthy subjects ≥ 60 years of age. *Am J Cardiol* 70:748–751, 1992.
92. Aronow WS, Epsein S, Mercando AD: Usefulness of complex ventricular arrhythmias detected by 24-hour ambulatory electrocardiogram and by electrocardiograms with one-minute rhythm strips in predicting new coronary events in elderly patients with and without heart disease. *J Cardiovasc Technol* 10:21–25, 1991.
93. Zipes DP: The long QT interval syndrome. A Rosetta stone for sympathetic related ventricular tachyarrhythmias. *Circulation* 84:1414–1419, 1991.
94. Task Force of the European Society of Cardiology and the North American Society of Pacing and Electrophysiology: Heart rate variability. Standards of measurement, physiological interpretation, and clinical use. *Eur Heart J* 17:354–381, 1996.

95. Ziegler MG, Lake CR, Kopin IJ: Plasma noradrenaline increases with age. *Nature* 261:333–335, 1976.
96. Angelone A, Coulter NAJ; Respiratory sinus arrhythmia: A frequency dependent phenomenon. *J Appl Physiol* 19:479–482, 1964.
97. Wei K, Dorian P, Newman D, et al: Association between QT dispersion and autonomic dysfunction in patients with diabetes mellitus. *J Am Coll Cardiol* 26:859–863, 1995.
98. Liao D, Cai J, Brancati FL, et al: Association of vagal tone with serum insulin, glucose, and diabetes mellitus—The ARIC Study. *Diabetes Res Clin Pract* 30:211–221, 1995.
99. Ewing DJ, Neilson JM, Travis P. New method for assessing cardiac parasympathetic activity using 24 hour electrocardiograms. *Br Heart J* 52: 396–402, 1984.
100. Bellavere F, Ferri M, Guarini L, et al: Prolonged QT period in diabetic autonomic neuropathy: A possible role in sudden cardiac death? *Br Heart J* 59:379–383, 1988.
101. Van Hoogenhuyze D, Weinstein N, Martin GJ, et al: Reproducibility and relation to mean heart rate of heart rate variability in normal subjects and in patients with congestive heart failure secondary to coronary artery disease. *Am J Cardiol* 68:1668–1676, 1991.
102. Wolf MM, Varigos GA, Hunt D, et al: Sinus arrhythmia in acute myocardial infarction. *Med J Aust* 2:52–53, 1978.
103. Lombardi F, Sandrone G, Pernpruner S, et al: Heart rate variability as an index of sympathovagal interaction after acute myocardial infarction. *Am J Cardiol* 60:1239–1245, 1987.
104. Huikuri HV, Niemela MJ, Ojala S, et al: Circadian rhythms of frequency domain measures of heart rate variability in healthy subjects and patients with coronary artery disease. Effects of arousal and upright posture. *Circulation* 90:121–126, 1994.
105. Rautaharju PM, Manolio TA, Psaty BM, et al: Correlates of QT prolongation in older adults (the Cardiovascular Health Study). Cardiovascular Health Study Collaborative Research Group. *Am J Cardiol* 73:999–1002, 1994.
106. Bigger JJ, Fleiss JL, Rolnitzky LM, et al: Frequency domain measures of heart period variability to assess risk late after myocardial infarction [published erratum appears in *J Am Coll Cardiol* 21(6):1537, 1993]. *J Am Coll Cardiol* 21:729–736, 1993.
107. Cripps TR, Malik M, Farrell TG, et al: Prognostic value of reduced heart rate variability after myocardial infarction: Clinical evaluation of a new analysis method. *Br Heart J* 65:14–19, 1991.
108. Farrell TG, Bashir Y, Cripps T, et al: Risk stratification for arrhythmic events in postinfarction patients based on heart rate variability, ambulatory electrocardiographic variables and the signal-averaged electrocardiogram. *J Am Coll Cardiol* 18:687–697, 1991.
109. Kjellgren O, Gomes JA. Heart rate variability and baroreflex sensitivity in myocardial infarction. *Am Heart J* 125:204–215, 1993.
110. Singh N, Mironov D, Armstrong PW, et al: Heart rate variability assessment early after acute myocardial infarction. Pathophysiological and prognostic correlates. GUSTO ECG Substudy Investigators. *Circulation* 93:1388–1395, 1996.
111. Ahnve S: QT interval prolongation in acute myocardial infarction. *Eur Heart J* 6(suppl D):85–95, 1985.

112. Schwartz PJ, Wolf S: QT interval prolongation as predictor of sudden death in patients with myocardial infarction. *Circulation* 57:1074–1077, 1978.
113. Schouten EG, Dekker JM, Meppelink P, et al: QT interval prolongation predicts cardiovascular mortality in an apparently healthy population. *Circulation* 84:1516–1523, 1991.
114. Dekker JM, Schouten EG, Klootwijk P, et al: Association between QT interval and coronary heart disease in middle-aged and elderly men. The Zutphen Study. *Circulation* 90:779–785, 1994.
115. De Bruyne MC: The electrocardiogram in the elderly. Diagnostic and prognostic studies. Thesis, Erasmus University Rotterdam, The Netherlands, 1997.
116. Goldberg RJ, Bengtson J, Chen ZY, et al: Duration of the QT interval and total and cardiovascular mortality in healthy persons (The Framingham Heart Study experience). *Am J Cardiol* 67:55–58, 1991.
117. Tibblin G, Eriksson CG, Bjuro T, et al: Heart rate and heart rate variability as a risk factor for the development of ischaemic heart disease (IHD) in the "Men Born in 1913 Study" - a ten years follow-up. IRCS Medical Science 3:95, 1975.
118. Tsuji H, Larson MG, Venditti FJ, et al: Impact of reduced heart rate variability on risk for cardiac events. The Framingham Heart Study. *Circulation* 94:2850–2855, 1994.
119. Liao D, Cai J, Rosamond WD, et al: Cardiac autonomic function and incident coronary heart disease: A population-based case-cohort study. The ARIC Study. *Am J Epidemiol* 145:696–706, 1997.
120. Tsuji H, Venditti F, Manders ES, et al: Reduced heart rate variability and mortality risk in an elderly cohort. The Framingham Heart Study. *Circulation* 90:878–883, 1994.
121. Dekker JM, Schouten EG, Klootwijk P, Pool J, Swenne CA, Kromhout D. Heart rate variability from short electrocardiographic recordings predicts mortality from all causes in middle-aged and elderly men. The Zutphen Study. *Am J Epidemiol* 145:899–908, 1997.
122. QTc dispersion predicts cardiac mortality in the elderly. *Circulation* 1998
123. Sox HJ, Garber AM, Littenberg B: The resting electrocardiogram as a screening test. A clinical analysis. *Ann Intern Med* 111:489–502, 1989.

Part 2

Diseases of the Heart and Pulmonary Vasculature

Chapter 6

Infective Endocarditis

Emily J. Erbelding, Dale N. Gerding, Elliot Chesler

In the last few decades there have been important changes in the demography, incidence, epidemiology, and clinical presentation of infective endocarditis. This has become a disease with a predilection for the elderly, among whom the clinical presentation is frequently ambiguous and the diagnosis missed at initial clinical presentation in up to 60% of cases.[1-3] In many instances there is confusion with other conditions, and the so-called "classic" findings (fever, splinter hemorrhages, changing murmurs, etc.) previously found in young patients with obvious rheumatic heart disease are uncommon in the elderly.

Some reviewers have reported that the pattern of infective endocarditis in the elderly is not different from that found in the young. However, such findings are based on a retrospective analysis of charts, and therefore, have limited relevance to everyday practice at the bedside. Although uncommon, the disease is important because of a quoted mortality rate of 45% in the elderly, compared with 32% in the middle aged and 9% in the young.[4-6] Those features germane to geriatric practice are discussed herein.

Trends in Demography, Epidemiology, and Incidence

Age

In many countries, populations are growing older, the elderly are living longer, and the mortality rate over age 80 years is falling. In the

From *Clinical Cardiology in the Elderly. Second Edition,* edited by Elliot Chesler. © 1999, Futura Publishing Company, Armonk, NY.

United States the population above the age of 80 years is expected to double by the year 2000.[7] Currently, therefore, there is a large reservoir of distinctive geriatric valvular pathology that will continually expand.

A significant trend toward an increasing age of patients with endocarditis has been well documented in clinical series, with most cases occurring above the age of 60 years.[1] A population-based study of infective endocarditis in Olmsted County, Minnesota, showed a steep rise in incidence of infective endocarditis with advancing years (0.4 cases per 100,000 person-years below the age of 20 years; increasing to 2.0 in the group aged 40 to 49 years; 15.2 in the group 70 to 79 years and 30.7 for age 80 years and older).[8] This trend is likely to continue, with the exception of the large cohort of intravenous drug abusers younger than age 40 years.[9,10]

Decreased Incidence of Rheumatic Fever

The striking decrease in the incidence of rheumatic fever and its related valve damage has shifted the incidence of infective endocarditis from the young to the old age group. There are fewer young people with rheumatic valvular disease susceptible to infective endocarditis and those who do have valve disease survive longer because of improved medical and surgical treatment.

Nosocomial Endocarditis

Nosocomial infections with bacteremia are increasing in prevalence, particularly gram-positive organisms, and endocarditis is an unusual, but serious complication. Both normal and abnormal native valves may be infected, but prosthetic endocarditis is more frequent. The most common portals for bacteremia are intravenous lines, catheters, and pacemaker leads. Surgical instrumentation of the genitourinary and gastrointestinal tracts and cardiac surgery are next in order of frequency.

Most series show that the majority of cases of nosocomial endocarditis occur in patients above age 60 years. This is not surprising considering the number of hospital beds occupied by the elderly and the instrumentation they are prone to receive. Left-sided valves are most commonly infected and *Staphylococcus aureus* is the usual organism. The mortality is significantly higher than community acquired infection (40% vs. 18%).[11]

Prosthetic Endocarditis

Cardiac surgery is performed with increasing frequency in the elderly. Aortic valve replacement for aortic stenosis is commonplace in

Table 1
Frequency of Infective Endocarditis in Teaching Hospitals

Institution	Period	No. Cases	Cases per Annum
Harvard Medical School, Boston, Mass[25]	1970–1977	63	8
St. Thomas's Hospital Med. School, London, U.K.[41]	1970–1979	104	10
Wayne State University, Detroit, Mich[10]	1968–1986	417	22
Montefiore Hospital, Albert Einstein University, New York[5]	1970–1977	56	7
Mayo Clinic, Rochester, Minn[42]	1970–1987	674	37
University of Tennessee, Memphis, Tenn[43]	1980–1984	63	12

the sixth and seventh decades and is also prevalent in octogenarians. Of the 191 patients age 80 years or more operated on at the Mayo Clinic between 1982 and 1986, 65% had valve replacement or repair, mostly for aortic stenosis.[12]

It is not surprising, therefore, that in some centers a cardiac valvular prosthesis is the most common predisposing basis for infective endocarditis and that the majority of the patients are elderly.[13] This reflects a change in the epidemiology of infective endocarditis, although there may be variations in the spectrum of the disease encountered at various institutions because of referral bias.[14,15]

Incidence

Despite the changes described above, infective endocarditis is an uncommon disease even in major teaching hospitals and referral centers (Table 1). The infrequency of admissions to large teaching hospitals is further illustrated by our own experience (Table 2). In a population-based study in neighboring Olmsted County Minnesota, 78 episodes of

Table 2
Incidence of Infective Endocarditis at Minneapolis Veterans Affairs Hospital

Year	Hospital Admissions	Endocarditis
1988	7795	16
1989	8088	16
1990	8216	17
1991	8465	24

infective endocarditis occurred in the period 1950–1981, yielding a mean annual incidence rate of only 3.8 per 100,000 person-years.[8] These numbers may be lower if relapses and re-infections were excluded. It is obvious, therefore, that despite changes in demography and epidemiology, infective endocarditis remains an uncommon disease even in teaching hospitals. Furthermore, because individual cases are usually seen by many physicians in consultation, few have intimate experience of the disease first hand, factors that must surely contribute to difficulties and delays in diagnosis to be discussed later.

Underlying Valvular Pathology

Clinical diagnosis of the type of valvular disease in the elderly is generally inaccurate. Study of autopsy material is much more informative, particularly when reviewed by a cardiac pathologist.[16] Although minor underlying valve disease may be obscured by the inflammatory process, it is usually possible to determine whether some prior abnormality was present.

In the Jesse E. Edwards Registry of Cardiovascular Disease, United Hospital, St. Paul, Minnesota, 100 specimens showed evidence of healed or active infective endocarditis in autopsies among persons above age 60 years during the period 1960–1990. The first 42 cases reported by Thell et al[3] (1960–1974) are compared with a further 58 cases encountered between 1974–1990[17] (Figure 1). These findings have important clinical implications:

1. Normal valves: No underlying cardiac disease was identifiable in approximately one third of cases, and this did not appear to change significantly through the years.

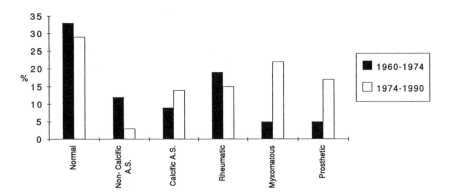

Figure 1: *Underlying valvular disease in 100 cases of bacterial endocarditis 1960 to 1990 in patients over age 60 years. The Jesse E. Edwards Registry of Cardiovascular Pathology.[17]*

2. Myxomatous mitral valves: These were involved next in order of frequency and the diagnosis has been made much more frequently in recent years. The most likely reason is that pathologists are more aware of the subtleties of this entity and there is less confusion with rheumatic heart disease.[18]

3. Prosthetic Valves: A similar trend was found in the incidence of prosthetic valve involvement, a change no doubt related to the epidemiological factors discussed previously.

4. Aortic valve disease: This as a group was next in order of frequency and includes calcific aortic stenosis and noncalcified congenital bicuspid or unicuspid valves.

5. Rheumatic valve disease: This was the smallest group and usually involved the mitral valve.

Unusual Valvular Pathology

In the above series amyloid infiltration of the tricuspid valve was the nidus in 1 case. Mitral annular calcification is common among the elderly but fortunately is rarely the site of infective endocarditis.[19] The condition is common and the incidence increases with advancing age. It is more than twice as common in women compared to men. Well-documented cases appear to be a result of infection superimposed on calcific material ulcerating through the base of the posterior leaflet.

Causative Organisms

The bacteria that most frequently cause endocarditis in the elderly are streptococci, staphylococci, and enterococci that are now classified separately from the streptococci. These 3 groups also dominate in the younger population although specific isolates appear with greater frequency among the elderly. A recent French comparative analysis of bacterial isolates from blood cultures demonstrated that gram-positive cocci of gastrointestinal tract origin (enterococci and Group D streptococci) were isolated significantly more frequently in endocarditis in the elderly compared to younger patients.[20] In older series, streptococci and enterococci have accounted for 40% to 45% of total cases of infective endocarditis in patients older than age 60 years. The viridans group of streptococci is responsible for more than 50% of these cases, a finding similar to that found in younger patients.[2,4] Almost unique to the geriatric population, however, is the nonenterococcal Group D streptococcus, or *Streptococcus bovis*, as a pathogen in this disease (16% of total streptococcal isolates). The association of *Streptococcus bovis* bacteremia and

underlying malignancy of the gastrointestinal tract, particularly adenocarcinoma of the colon, has been well described.[21]

The enterococcal species were formerly classified with Group D
streptococci and in most series represent a subgroup of the streptococcal
isolates. They now are reclassified as an independent genus. Enterococci are responsible for 10% to 13% of all cases of endocarditis in patients older than age 60 years. As might be expected, enterococcal bacteremia and endocarditis are most commonly seen in middle-aged to
elderly men, most of whom having had a prior urinary tract infection
or urologic procedure. Sources less commonly documented include he-
patobiliary or other gastrointestinal infections, often with polymicrob-
ial bacteremia, and rarely, from colonization of burns and diabetic or
decubitus ulcers.[22]

Staphylococci are the second largest group of pathogens causing
endocarditis in patients over age 60 years. Again, the proportion is
similar to that noted in younger patients. Of the staphylococci, *S. aureus* was the single most common isolate (21%–28% of cases), with coagulase-negative staphylococci comprising 15%.[2,4] These coagulase-negative species are typically reported to predominate in that subgroup of
middle-aged to elderly patients with infections of prosthetic valves, but
it is important to note that they can also infect native valves, particularly among the elderly, who in one series from Israel accounted for 7
of 7 reported patients.[23]

More unusual organisms, such as gram-negative bacteria, diphthe-
roids, and fungi are uncommon in all age groups. Collectively, they
account for about 3%–6% of all cases of endocarditis in patients older
than age 60 years.[2,4]

Predisposing Events

In all age groups, a portal of entry for infection often cannot be
identified retrospectively. When a source of infective endocarditis was
identified in one reported series, invasive vascular procedures, or a
recent history of an intravenous catheterization were the most common
predisposing events in patients older than age 60 years (17% of cases)
whereas these procedures accounted for less than 5% of predisposing
events in younger patients.[4] The next most common portals of entry
identified were a dental procedure (13%), skin lesions (11%), anorectal
disease (9%) and a recent urinary tract procedure (6%) in the preceding
2 months. A nosocomial source of infection was found in 23% of all
cases; 40% of all cases for which a source of infection was identified.
This trend towards nosocomially acquired infective endocarditis has
also been reported in a smaller series focusing on the elderly population.[24]

Laboratory Findings

Many features of the usual clinical laboratory profile are abnormal in infective endocarditis, although most are nonspecific and consistent with any chronic inflammatory process. A normocytic anemia and a leukocytosis are frequently present, with a mean hematocrit of 36% and a median leukocyte count of 12,700/mm.[3,25] The erythrocyte sedimentation rate is elevated in more than 90% of cases,[23,24] with a mean value of 57mm/hr. An abnormal urinalysis is also frequent with microscopic hematuria reported in 25%–55%, and red blood cell casts in freshly voided urine in 12% of cases.[1,4] Other nonspecific laboratory parameters consistent with chronic inflammation include a positive rheumatoid factor (24%–50%), hypergammaglobulinemia and hypocomplementemia (47%).[25–27] Values for these relatively nonspecific clinical laboratory tests did not differ significantly when those patients older than age 60 years were compared with other series reporting patients of all ages with infective endocarditis.[4]

Blood culture is the single most important laboratory test in the diagnosis of infective endocarditis. Continuous bacteremia is a key feature of the disease, although it may be of relatively low magnitude and fluctuate quantitatively over time. Of 205 cases of infective endocarditis reviewed at New York Hospital-Cornell Medical Center, 91% of patients had every blood culture positive (5 cc in each of 2 vials). Of the cases of streptococcal endocarditis, the first culture was positive in 96% of cases, and 98% were positive by the second culture. With nonstreptococcal organisms, the first culture was positive in 82% of cases, and 1 of the first 2 cultures was positive in all cases. Antibiotic therapy within the preceding 2 weeks decreased the incidence of positive blood cultures.[28] Based upon these data, 3 sets of blood cultures are nearly always adequate, either to identify a causative organism in a patient with infective endocarditis, or to rule out the disease in a patient not taking antibiotics.

Definition of Infective Endocarditis

Elderly persons are more susceptible to sepsis than the young, and more prone to bacteremia, particularly when hospitalized. It is important therefore to distinguish between infective endocarditis and other bacteremic infections in patients with coincidental heart disease. The definition proposed by Von Reyn et al[26] is helpful in making this distinction.

Definite Endocarditis

Direct evidence of infective endocarditis based on histology from surgery or autopsy, or on bacteriology (Gram stain or culture) of valvular vegetations or peripheral embolus.

Probable Endocarditis

A. Persistently positive blood cultures plus 1 of the following:

1. New regurgitant murmur, or
2. Predisposing heart disease and vascular phenomena

B. Negative or intermittently positive blood cultures plus all 3 of the following:

1. Fever
2. New regurgitant murmur, and
3. Vascular phenomena

Possible Endocarditis

A. Persistently positive blood cultures plus 1 of the following:

1. Predisposing heart disease, or
2. Vascular phenomena

B. Negative or intermittently positive blood cultures plus all 3 of the following:

1. Fever
2. Predisposing heart disease, and
3. Vascular phenomena

C. For *Streptococcus viridans* cases only: at least 2 positive blood cultures without an extracardiac source, and fever.

Clinical Features

Infective endocarditis is difficult to diagnose and the subtleties of its presentation cannot be solved with an algorithm. In most clinical series the clinical suspicion for the presence of infective endocarditis is low and the diagnosis is suspected in fewer than 40% of cases.[3] An initial diagnostic suspicion for endocarditis is much more likely to be correct in younger patients. Not infrequently, the disease masquerades as cerebro-vascular accident, unexplained congestive heart failure or uremia. Neoplasms such as lymphoma and hypernephroma, cardiac myxomas, polymalgia rheumatica and marantic endocarditis are frequent among the elderly and share many clinical and laboratory features. Recognition would probably be enhanced by appreciating that while fever is commonly present, murmurs may be absent.

Fever

This is the commonest clue and is present in more than 90% of cases. When congestive cardiac failure, stroke, transient ischemic attacks, mental confusion, renal failure, or severe back pain present for the first time and are accompanied by fever, the diagnosis of infective endocarditis should be immediately suspected. Unfortunately, presenting symptoms are often vague and significance of fever is frequently overlooked.

Murmur

The presence of a murmur or "changing" murmur is frequently the cornerstone of diagnosis in the physician's mind when confronted by a possible case of endocarditis. This is one of the factors responsible for difficulty and delay in diagnosis. In the elderly, aortic ejection murmurs are ubiquitous because of the frequency of senile aortic sclerosis, a condition not particularly prone to endocarditis without calcific stenosis.[29,30] The murmur of senile sclerosis is exceedingly difficult to distinguish from that of aortic stenosis. Also, the classic "anacroti'" pulse found in the young, is absent in the elderly because of a non-distensible, rigid vascular bed.[31,32] The electrocardiogram and chest x-ray are not helpful in making the distinction.[33] Furthermore, the murmur of aortic stenosis may disappear when congestive heart failure supervenes. Because infective endocarditis affects normal valves in at least 30% of cases, the presence or absence of a murmur should not sway the diagnosis one way or the other. Generally, however, the diagnosis is made more frequently when a murmur is present than when absent (54% vs. 9% in 1 series).[3]

For the geriatric cardiologist and the pathologist, the question as to what is a "normal valve" in geriatric practice is interesting. Above age 60 years it is almost the norm for echocardiography to demonstrate minor degrees of thickening of the left heart valves—particularly the aortic valve. Furthermore, such valves frequently have minor degrees of regurgitation detected by color flow Doppler. This has been termed "Doppler disease" because the technique is so sensitive, but is nevertheless a site of turbulence and a possible nidus for adherence of circulating organisms on what is otherwise a structurally normal and clinically silent valve.

Neurological Manifestations

These are found in approximately 40% of cases in the elderly (compared to 21% of all patients in 1 large series[34] and often dominate the clinical presentation. The presentation closely resembles the effects of senile cerebral arteriosclerosis and transient ischemic attacks, which are so common in geriatric practice.[35]

Cerebral Ischemia

Brain ischemia is the most common cause of stroke in patients with endocarditis.[34] Embolism commonly involves the branches of the middle cerebral arteries producing cerebral infarction. The posterior circulation is involved less frequently.

Transient Ischemic Attacks

Multiple transient ischemic attacks (TIAs) are an ominous sign that frequently presages cerebral hemorrhage.

Intracranial Hemorrhage

Rupture of a mycotic aneurysm may lead to subarachnoid or intra-cerebral bleeding and this may be the presenting sign of infective endo-carditis, particularly in *S. aureus* endocarditis.[34] Such aneurysms are usually situated in the terminal branches of the middle cerebral artery. Their rupture is often preceded by severe unrelenting headache that when accompanied by visual disturbance and a high erythrocyte sedi-mentation rate (ESR) may mimic the presentation of temporal arteritis.

Encephalopathy and Neuropsychiatric Disorder

These are probably a result of micro-abscesses and present with symptoms ranging from apathy and impaired concentration to frank psychiatric disorder with hallucinations, paranoia and severe confu-sion.

Acute Low Back Pain

Low back pain is common in the elderly. When it is of acute onset, accompanied by fever, leukocytosis and increased ESR, the diagnosis of infective endocarditis and vertebral osteomyelitis or discitis should be seriously entertained, particularly when there is evidence of radicu-lopathy. In one review, low back pain was the presenting symptom in 23% of patients with endocarditis.[36] We have encountered cases of acute lumbar discitis admitted to the neurosurgery service when the underly-ing cause was infective endocarditis of the mitral valve. These patients should be carefully auscultated and blood cultures obtained. When spine computed tomographic (CT) scan or magnetic resonance imaging (MRI) fail to show a local cause or blood cultures are positive, echocardiography should be performed.

Cardiac Findings

Congestive heart failure is the most common presenting feature and complication of the disease. The causes of heart failure are valve perforation, chordal rupture, infective myocarditis, and coronary embolism. Among patients with prosthetic valves there are additional mechanisms. Aortic prosthetic endocarditis is frequently complicated by dehiscence of the annulus due to abscess formation. This results in regurgitation much more commonly than with native aortic valve endocarditis. Frequently, dehiscence is accompanied by left bundle branch, or complete heart block owing to invasion of the conduction tissues. Prosthetic mitral endocarditis, in contrast to aortic valve endocarditis is complicated by obstruction rather than regurgitation.[14]

The combination of fever and congestive heart failure in an elderly patient should immediately raise strong suspicion of infective endocarditis, whether there is a murmur or not. Auscultation is of limited help. Not infrequently, the holosystolic murmur of mitral valve prolapse does not change in intensity with the development of endocarditis. In fact, it may become softer when the chordae rupture and severe cardiac failure with low cardiac output ensues. The same may happen in the case of mild aortic regurgitation with a soft early diastolic murmur. When there is sudden aortic valve disruption as a result of endocarditis there is equilibration of aortic and left ventricular diastolic pressures and the murmur may disappear. Under these circumstances, careful consideration should be given to predisposing causes of bacteremia (nosocomial infection of an intravenous device, instrumentation of the genitourinary tract, surgical or dental procedures). Blood cultures and echocardiography should be performed.

Echocardiography plays an important role in the diagnosis of infective endocarditis and detection of its complications. There are limitations to the transthoracic technique that have been overcome by transesophageal echocardiography (TEE). The aortic valve in elderly persons frequently shows evidence of "senile sclerosis" and may be markedly thickened, calcified and therefore, highly echogenic. Also, the aortic root shows senile dilatation. These changes make detection of the aortic annulus, vegetations, and perforation of leaflets difficult. These problems are enhanced when there is an aortic or mitral valve prosthesis. Such technical difficulties have been largely overcome with the advent of TEE that provides improved definition.[37] TEE should be used whenever there is a strong suspicion of infective endocarditis and also before re-operation in cases of prosthetic valve endocarditis. In conjunction with color flow Doppler, TEE is invaluable in locating fistulae, abscesses and disruption of the aortic annulus. In skilled hands it obviates the need for invasive cardiac catheterization and angiography and facilitates early diagnosis.

Renal Abnormalities

Hematuria, proteinuria, and pyelonephritis are found at the same rate and order of frequency as in the young. There are probably no specific features peculiar to the elderly.

Cutaneous Abnormalities

Splinter hemorrhages are found in approximately 16% of elderly persons compared to 19%–66% of the young. The notion that they may therefore be more specific if present in the elderly because they are less frequent, is not supported by clinical studies. In the elderly splinter hemorrhages are associated with a wide variety of medical conditions making it an unhelpful physical sign. They appear to be commonly associated with use of a walking aid. Osler's Nodes and Janeway lesions are uncommon in all age groups and there are no features peculiar to the elderly.[38]

Treatment

Medical

Prior to the initiation of antibiotic therapy, 3 blood cultures should be obtained in a patient suspected of having endocarditis. If the presentation is that of acute infective endocarditis, empiric antibiotic therapy should be initiated immediately for the most likely organisms, particularly S. aureus. If the presentation is subacute and the patient is clinically stable, there is no need to initiate empiric antibiotic therapy immediately but if 3 blood cultures have been obtained and the patient has not taken prior antibiotics (which could cause failure to detect bacteria in blood cultures), there is little to be gained from waiting.

Treatment regimens with established success for infective endocarditis are shown in Tables 3 and 4.[39] These options are applicable to all age groups, but features peculiar to the elderly population might favor certain choices. Departures from these regimens of proven efficacy are not recommended. Pre-existing renal insufficiency or hearing impairment should preclude use of an aminoglycoside in treating endocarditis only when there are effective alternatives. If an aminoglycoside is indicated, streptomycin and gentamicin historically have been considered equally effective choices, however, presently gentamicin is preferable in most elderly patients. Monitoring of gentamicin is widely available

Table 3
Established Therapy for Native Valve Streptococcal and Enterococcal Endocarditis*

Organism	Regimen	Duration
Viridans streptococci (penicillin susceptible, MIC ≤ 0.1 mcg/mL)	1. Penicillin G 12–18 mil U/24 hr IV either continuously or in six equally divided doses	4 wks
	2. Penicillin G (above dose)	2 wks
	plus	
or	**Gentamicin 1 mg/kg IV/IM q8h	2 wks
Streptococcus bovis (penicillin-susceptible, MIC ≤0.1 mcg/mL)	3. Ceftriaxone sodium 2.0 gm IV/IM once daily	4 wks
	4. ***Vancomycin hydrochloride 30 mg/kg IV q24h in two equally divided doses, not to exceed 2gm/24h unless serum levels are monitored	4 wks
Viridans streptococci (penicillin MIC >0.1 mcg/mL and ≤0.5 mcg/mL)	1. Penicillin 18 mil U/24 hr IV either continuously or in six equally divided doses	4 wks
	plus	
	**Gentamicin 1 mg/kg IV/IM q8h	2 wks
or		
Streptococcus bovis (penicillin MIC >0.1 mcg/mL and ≤0.5 mcg/mL)	2. ***Vancomycin hydrochloride 30 mg/kg IV q24h in two equally divided doses, not to exceed 2 gm/24h unless serum levels are monitored.	4 wks

See footnotes from Table 4.

so that there is a greater chance of detecting over or underdosing. Streptomycin monitoring is not readily available, and thus the higher risk of vestibular cranial nerve VIII toxicity may not be preventable during a long course of therapy. Both hearing loss and loss of vestibular function are debilitating in the elderly and both can be irreversible. The goal of aminoglycoside dosing should be synergistic levels (serum peaks of 3 µg/mL for gentamicin and 12 µg/mL for streptomycin) rather than the higher levels required for treating other infections. Renal function should be monitored at least 3 times weekly regardless of dose. Although once-daily dosing of aminoglycosides in patients with normal renal function has become standard in many centers, this practice is not recommended in the treatment of endocarditis because of uncertainty of maintaining a continuous bactericidal effect and lack of clinical outcome data in endocarditis.

Table 4
Established Therapy for Staphylococcal Endocarditis*

Organism	Regimen	Duration
Staphylococci, native valve Methicillin-sensitive	1. Nafcillin (or Oxacillin) 2gm IV q4h *plus (optional)*	4–6 wk.
	**Gentamicin 1 mg/kg IV/IM q8h	3–5 days
	2. Cefazolin 2gm IV q8h	4–6 wk.
	or Cephalothin 2gm IV q4h *plus (optional)*	4–6 wk.
	**Gentamicin 1 mg/kg IV/IM q8h	3–5 days
Methicillin-resistant	1. ***Vancomycin 30 mg/kg IV q24h in two equally divided doses not to exceed 2 gm/24h unless serum levels are monitored	4–6 wk.
Staphylococci, retained prosthetic material Methicillin-sensitive	1. Nafcillin (or Oxacillin) 2 gm IV q4h	≥6 wk.
	plus **Gentamicin 1 mg/kg IV/IM q8h	2 wk.
	plus ****Rifampin 300mg po q8h	≥6 wk.
Methicillin-resistant	1. ***Vancomycin 30 mg/kg IV q24h in two equally divided doses not to exceed 2 gm/24h unless serum levels are monitored. *plus*	≥6 wk.
	**Gentamicin 1 mg/kg IV/IM q8h *plus*	2 wk.
	****Rifampin 300mg po q8h	≥6 wk.

* Dosages recommended are for patients with normal renal function.

** Dose of gentamicin recommended should be based on ideal body weight if the patient is obese. For gentamicin resistant staphylococci another susceptible aminoglycoside should be used.

*** Infusion duration should be no less than 1 hr. to avoid "Red Man" syndrome associated with rapid infusion. Adjust dosing intervals based on renal function.

**** Rifampin is included for cases of coagulase-negative staphylococcal prosthetic valve infections; benefit is not established for native valve methicillin-resistant *S. aureus* endocarditis and is unknown for prosthetic valve methicillin-resistant *S. aureus* endocarditis

Surgical

Operative intervention is an option, even in octogenerians. However, the timing of valve replacement is usually the most difficult decision. Ideally, prompt effective antibiotic treatment should lead to resolution of bacteremia, renal failure and systemic embolism. Most cases of penicillin-sensitive streptococcal endocarditis will respond in this way. However, cardiac failure following valve perforation is an indication for immediate operation, irrespective of the duration of antibiotic treatment. Early operation is advocated for fungal endocarditis, aortic endocarditis with root abscess and for prosthetic endocarditis.[10] Although no prospective randomized trials are available, surgical therapy of prosthetic valve endocarditis appears to be more efficacious than medical management and should be given every consideration in the elderly if the patient is considered a surgical candidate.[40] Valve replacement should be considered when there is repeated cerebral embolism and the CT scan shows that infarction is not hemorrhagic.[41] Homograft replacement of the aortic root and valve is the preferred choice for prosthetic endocarditis, and also for aortic endocarditis complicated by annular destruction because homograft tissue is more resistant to future infection.[13,42]

Prognosis

There has been a general perception that elderly patients with endocarditis have increased mortality because of delay in diagnosis, increased rates of nosocomial infections, and a greater number of underlying medical conditions such as renal failure, chronic liver disease and chronic obstructive pulmonary disease. This may no longer be true because of earlier diagnosis and less hesitation by cardiac surgeons to operate on older patients. A recent study found that use of TEE resulted in earlier diagnosis. The one-year mortality (26%) among patients over age 70 years was not significantly different from the younger subjects, and the elderly had surgery as often (65%) as the younger subjects.[43]

Prevention

There has not been a controlled trial demonstrating that prophylactic antibiotic treatment reduces the risk of developing infective endocarditis. However, based on indirect evidence of benefit, it has become established practice to prescribe prophylactic antibiotics prior to procedures likely to induce bacteremia in high-risk patients. The risk of iatrogenic endocarditis resulting from a procedure varies according to the type of cardiac lesion present and the likelihood of bacteremia related to the procedure; this calculated risk must exceed the risk of a serious antibiotic reaction in order for antibiotic prophylaxis to be beneficial. Cardiac lesions commonly encountered in the geriatric population are classified according to degree of risk in Table 5. Prophylactic antibiotics are not recommended in those conditions associated with low or negligible risk.

Procedures for which antibiotic prophylaxis is recommended based upon risks of associated bacteremia are listed in Table 6.[44,45] Recommended antibiotic regimens are outlined in Table 7.[46] Choice of a spe-

Table 5
Risk of Endocarditis in the Elderly According to Cardiac Lesion

Highest Risk	Intermediate Risk	Low or Negligible Risk
prosthetic valves	mitral valve prolapse with murmur	coronary artery bypass grafts
prior episode of endocarditis	calcific aortic sclerosis	pacemakers
aortic stenosis	nonvalvular cardiac prosthetic material	mitral valve prolapse without murmur
mitral insufficiency	asymmetric septal hypertrophy	syphilitic aortitis

cific regimen should be based on the ability of a patient to take oral medication and the history of a hypersensitivity reaction to the penicillins. For dental procedures drugs are targeted against *Streptococcus viridans*. For gastrointestinal or urogenital procedures, therapy is directed against the enterococci because even though bacteremia from gram-negatives and anaerobes may occur, the risk of endocarditis from the latter organisms is lower. In the case of implanted or prosthetic

Table 6
Common Procedures and Use of Endocarditis Prophylaxis

Antibiotic prophylaxis recommended	Antibiotic prophylaxis not recommended
Dental procedures likely to cause bleeding	Cardiac catheterization including balloon angioplasty
Surgical procedures of upper respiratory tract likely to cause bleeding	Flexible bronchoscopy
Rigid bronchoscopy	Upper endoscopy $+/-$ biopsy
Esophageal dilatation or sclerotherapy	Transesophageal echocardiography
Biliary or intestinal surgery	Colonoscopy $+/-$ biopsy
Endoscopic retrograde cholangiography with biliary obstruction	Endotracheal intubation
Urologic procedures	Urethral catheterization without infection
Urethral catheterization with active urinary tract infection	Barium enema
Urethral dilatation	Vaginal delivery
Cystoscopy	Cesarean section
Prostatic surgery	
Incision and drainage of infected tissue	Implantation of cardiac pacemakers, defibrillators, and coronary artery stents

Table 7
Recommended Prophylactic Regimens for Endocarditis Prevention in Adults

Procedure	Regimen
1. Dental, oral, respiratory tract, or esophageal	Amoxicillin 2 gm po 1 hr before procedure *or* *Ampicillin 2 gm IM/IV within 30 minutes before procedure *or* **Clindamycin 600 mg po 1 hr before procedure *or* **Cephalexin or Cefadroxil 2 gm po 1 hr before procedure *or* **Azithromycin or Clarithromycin 500 mg po 1 hr before procedure
2. Genitourinary or gastrointestinal (excluding esophageal)	*Ampicillin 2 gm IM/IV, plus Gentamicin 1.5 mg/kg (up to 120 mg) within 30 minutes before procedure; 6 hr later, Ampicillin 1 gm IM/IV or Amoxicillin 1 gm po *or* **Vancomycin 1 gm IV over 1–2 hrs plus Gentamicin 1.5 mg/kg IM/IV (not to exceed 120 mg). Gentamicin to be infused/injected within 30 minutes before procedure

* Unable to take oral medications.

** Allergic to penicillin. Avoid Cephalosporins if the Penicillin allergy was an immediate-type reaction or anaphylaxis to penicillins. For patients allergic to Penicillin *and* unable to take oral medication, Clindamycin 600 mg IV or Cefazolin 1gm IM/IV within 30 minutes before procedure is recommended for dental, oral, respiratory tract or esophageal procedures.

cardiac devices such as pacemakers and cardiac valves, prophylaxis is directed against skin organisms, primarily the staphylococci.

References

1. Cantrell M, Yoshikawa T: Infective endocarditis in the aging patient. *Gerontology* 30:316, 1984.
2. Applefield M, Hornick R: Infective endocarditis in patients over age 60. *Am Heart J* 88:90, 1974.
3. Thell R, Martin F, Edwards J: Bacterial endocarditis in subjects 60 years of age and older. *Circulation* 51:174, 1975.

4. Terpenning M, Buggy B, Kauffman C: Infective endocarditis: Clinical features in young and elderly patients. *Am J Med* 83:626, 1987.
5. Robbins N, DeMaria A, Miller M: Infective endocarditis in the elderly. 73:1335, 1980.
6. Friedlander A, Yoshikawa T: Pathogenesis, management, and prevention of infective endocarditis in the elderly dental patient. *Oral Surg Oral Med Oral Pathol* 69:177, 1990.
7. Cassel C, Brody JA: Demography, epidemiology and aging. In: Cassel C, et al (eds): *Geriatric Medicine*. New York, NY, Springer-Verlag, 1990, p. 16.
8. Griffin M, Wilson W, Edwards W, et al: Infective endocarditis, Olmsted County, Minnesota, 1950 through 1981. *JAMA* 254:1199, 1985.
9. Gantz N: Geriatric endocarditis: Avoiding the trend toward mismanagement. *Geriatrics* 46:66, 1991.
10. Arbulu A, Asfaw I: Management of infective endocarditis: Seventeen years' experience. *Ann Thorac Surg* 43:144, 1987.
11. Chen S, Dwyer D, Sorrell T: A comparison of hospital and community-acquired infective endocarditis. *Am J Cardiol* 70:1449, 1992.
12. Freeman W, Schaff H, O'Brien P, et al: Cardiac surgery in the octogenarian: Perioperative outcome and clinical follow-up. *J Am Coll Cardiol* 18:29, 1991.
13. Glazier J, Verwilghen J, Donaldson R, Ross D: Treatment of complicated prosthetic aortic valve endocarditis with annular abscess formation by homograft aortic root replacement. *J Am Coll Cardiol* 17:1177, 1991.
14. Arnett E, Roberts W: Prosthetic valve endocarditis. *Am J Cardiol* 38:281, 1976.
15. Steckelberg J, Melton L, Ilstrup D, et al: Influence of referral bias on the apparent clinical spectrum of infective endocarditis. *Am J Med* 88:582, 1990.
16. Pomerance A: Cardiac pathology in the elderly. In: Brast AN (ed): *Geriatric Cardiology*. Philadelphia, PA, FA Davis, 1986, pp. 9–54.
17. Chesler E, Titus J, Edwards J: Unpublished observations. 1992.
18. Chesler E, Gornick CC: Maladies attributed to myxomatous mitral valve. *Circulation* 83:328, 1991.
19. Pomerance A: Pathological and clinical study of calcification of the mitral valve ring. *J Clin Pathol* 23:354, 1970.
20. Selton-Suty C, Hoen B, Grentzinger A, et al: Clinical and bacteriological characteristics of infective endocarditis in the elderly. *Heart* 77:260, 1997.
21. Klein R, Recco R, Catalano M, et al: Association of Streptococcus bovis with carcinoma of the colon. *N Engl J Med* 297:800, 1977.
22. Maki D, Agger W: Enterococcal bacteremia: Clinical features, the risk of endocarditis, and management. *Medicine* 67:248, 1988.
23. Arber N, Militianu A, Ben-Yehuda A, et al. Native valve *Staphylococcus epidermidis* endocarditis: report of seven cases and review of the literature. *Am J Med* 90:758, 1991.
24. Terpenning M, Buggy B, Kaufman C: Hospital-acquired infective endocarditis. *Arch Intern Med* 148:1601, 1988.
25. Pelletier L, Petersdorf R: Infective endocarditis: A review of 125 cases from the University of Washington Hospitals. *Medicine* 56:287, 1977.
26. Von Reyn CF, Levy BS, Arbeit RD, et al: Infective endocarditis: An analysis based on strict case definitions. *Ann Intern Med* 94:505, 1981.
27. Lerner P, Weinstein L: Infective endocarditis in the antibiotic era. *N Engl J Med* 274:199, 1966.

28. Werner A, Cobbs G, Kaye D, et al: Studies on the bacteremia of bacterial endocarditis. *JAMA* 202:199, 1967.
29. Pomerance A: Pathogenesis of aortic stenosis and its relation to age. *Br Heart J* 34:569, 1972.
30. Berman N: Valvular heart disease in the elderly. *Mt Sinai J Med* 52:594, 1985.
31. Flohr KH, Weir EK, Chesler E: Diagnosis of aortic stenosis in older age groups using external carotid pulse recording and phonocardiography. *Br Heart J* 45:577, 1981.
32. Davision T, Friedman S: Significance of systolic murmurs in the aged. *N Engl J Med* 279:225, 1968.
33. Fisch C: Electrocardiogram of nonagenarians. *Geriatrics* 24:89, 1969.
34. Hart RG, Foster JW, Luther MF, Kanter MC. Stroke in infective endocarditis. *Stroke* 21:695, 1990.
35. Jones H, Siekert R: Neurological manifestations of infective endocarditis. *Brain* 112:1295, 1989.
36. Buchman A: *Streptococcus viridans* osteomyelitis with endocarditis presenting as acute onset lower back pain. *J Emerg Med* 8:291, 1989.
37. Taams M, Gussenhoven E, Bos E, et al.: Enhanced morphological diagnosis in infective endocarditis by transoesophageal echocardiography. *Br Heart J* 63:109, 1990.
38. Young J, Mulley G: Splinter haemorrhages in the elderly. *Age Ageing* 16: 101, 1987.
39. Wilson RW, Karchmer AW, Dajani AS, et al. Antibiotic treatment of adults with infective endocarditis due to streptococci, enterococci, staphylococci, and HACEK microorganisms. *JAMA* 274:1706, 1995.
40. Yu VL, Fang GD, Keys TF, et al: Prosthetic valve endocarditis: superiority of surgical valve replacement versus medical therapy only. *Ann Thorac Surg* 58:1073, 1994.
41. Ting W, Silverman N, Levitsky S: Valve replacement in patients with endocarditis and cerebral septic emboli. *Ann Thorac Surg* 51:18, 1991.
42. Tuna I, Orszulak T, Schaff H, Danielson G: Results of homograft aortic valve replacement for active endocarditis. *Ann Thorac Surg* 49:619, 1990.
43. Werner GS, Schulz R, Fuchs JB, et al: Infective endocarditis in the elderly in the era of transesophageal echocardiography: Clinical features and prognosis compared with younger patients. *Am J Med* 100:90, 1996.
44. Durack D: Current issues in prevention of infective endocarditis. *Am J Med* 78:149, 1985.
45. Dajani AS, Taubert KA, Wilson W, et al: Prevention of bacterial endocarditis. *JAMA* 277:1794, 1997.
46. Levine DP, Fromm BS, Reddy BR. Slow response to vancomycin or vancomycin plus rifampin in methicillin-resistant *Staphylococcus aureus* endocarditis. *Ann Intern Med* 115:274, 1991.
47. Moulsdale M, Eykyn S, Phillips I: Infective endocarditis, 1970–1979 A study of culture-positive cases in St. Thomas' Hospital. 195:315, 1980.
48. Steckelberg J: Personal communication. 1992.
49. McKinsey D, Ratts T, Bisno A: Underlying cardiac lesions in adults with infective endocarditis. *Am J Med* 82:681, 1987.

Chapter 7

Pulmonary Hypertension

Stephen L. Archer, E. Kenneth Weir

Pulmonary hypertension (PHT) in the elderly is usually a hemodynamic complication of left ventricular failure or chronic lung disease, conditions that dominate the clinical picture. Occasionally, PHT leading to isolated right ventricular failure is the only presenting feature and the mechanism may be obscure. Recognition of the cause is important because life-threatening conditions such as chronic thromboembolism are potentially curable and need to be distinguished from primary PHT, which has a very different prognosis.

Definition

The pulmonary circulation is normally a low-pressure system. Pulmonary artery pressure drops rapidly at the time of birth and reaches adult levels around the end of the first week of life. Between childhood and middle-age, the mean pulmonary arterial pressure is about 14 mm Hg.[1] It increases slightly after the age of 60 years to 16 ± 3 (SD) mm Hg. In order to establish a cutoff for the diagnosis of unequivocal PHT, the NIH Primary Pulmonary Hypertension Registry decided to include patients whose mean pulmonary artery pressure at rest was more than 25 mm Hg.[2]

Change in Pulmonary Vascular Resistance with Age

Pulmonary vascular resistance index (mean pulmonary artery pressure-mean pulmonary artery wedge pressure/cardiac index mm

From *Clinical Cardiology in the Elderly. Second Edition,* edited by Elliot Chesler. © 1999, Futura Publishing Company, Armonk, NY.

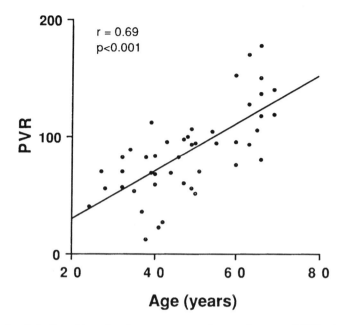

Figure 1: *Relationship of pulmonary vascular resistance (PVR, dynes / sec / cm⁻⁵) to increasing age in 47 normal subjects. Reproduced with permission from Davidson W, Fee E: Influence of aging on pulmonary hemodynamics in a population free of coronary artery disease. Am J Cardiol 65:1454–1458, 1990.*

Hg/L/min/m^2) ranges from 1.4 ± 0.7 (SD) units in childhood to 1.8 ± 0.7 units in middle-age and 2.6 ± 1.0 units over 60 years of age. A recent study of normal volunteers confirms that pulmonary vascular resistance increases as age progresses (Figure 1).[3]

The morphological basis for this increase in resistance has been examined in an autopsy study that excluded patients with heart or lung disease.[4] The amount of intimal abnormality increased with age in all sizes of artery. In those older than age 60 years, an increase in the area of the intima of the smallest arteries could reduce the lumen by up to 32%. In this study smoking was not found to be a related factor, but it has been incriminated by others.[5]

Based on an analysis of chest x-rays, it has been suggested that the prevalence of "moderate" (> 25 mm Hg) and "severe" (> 30 mm Hg) PHT in the 65–74 year age range might be as high as 25% and 20%, respectively.[6] However, when it is remembered that the upper limit of the normal mean pulmonary artery pressure (mean ± 2 SD) over age 60 is 22 mm Hg, a value of around 26 mm Hg might be considered mild PHT. Age-adjusted normal ranges for pulmonary artery pressure and resistance should be used more frequently.

Effect of Exercise on Pulmonary Hemodynamics

In normal young adults, supine exercise results in a modest rise in pulmonary artery wedge pressure and a slightly greater rise in mean pulmonary artery pressure.[1] The resulting small increase in transpulmonary gradient is offset by a rise in cardiac output so that pulmonary vascular resistance is usually unchanged between rest and exercise.

In older, but also normal, subjects (61 to 83 years of age), one third of the wedge pressure measurements made during exercise in one study exceeded 30 mm Hg.[7] The mean pulmonary artery pressure increased passively with this marked rise in wedge pressure (Figure 2), so that the

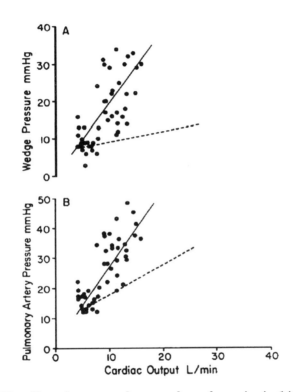

Figure 2: *The effect of age on pulmonary hemodynamics in 14 healthy men, 61–83 years old. Shown here are 52 measurements of wedge pressure (upper panel A) and of pulmonary arterial pressure (lower panel B) with increasing cardiac output from rest to supine exercise. The solid regression lines for these data are compared with the dotted regression lines for young men and women. The more rapid rise in wedge pressure in the older men is reflected by the steeper rise in pulmonary arterial pressure during exercise. Reproduced with permission from Reeves J, Grover R, Dempsey J: Pulmonary circulation during exercise. In* Pulmonary Vascular Physiology and Pathophysiology. *EK Weir, JT Reeves (eds). New York, Marcel Dekker, 1989.*

transpulmonary gradient did not change. The rise in wedge pressure is probably secondary to a decrease in left ventricular compliance in older subjects. In another report,[8] patients between ages 50 and 69 years were observed to have a slight increase in pulmonary vascular resistance during supine exercise.

These data indicate that the principal hemodynamic change with supine exercise in the older normal person is an increase in wedge pressure, with subsequent, mostly passive, changes in pulmonary artery pressure.

Pathophysiology

PHT is a complication of many diseases with varying pathophysiology. The early conceptual framework developed by Wood[9] is still useful. He subdivided PHT into (1) passive: related to elevated left heart filling pressures; (2) hyperkinetic: secondary to increased blood flow through the lungs, (3) obstructive or obliterative: associated with either intravascular obstruction such as emboli or thrombosis; or loss of vessels as in interstitial pulmonary fibrosis; (4) vasoconstrictive: this mechanism rarely occurs in isolation but may provide a "reactive" element superimposed on the other causes.

Elevated Left Heart Filling Pressures

This is the most frequent cause of significant PHT in the elderly. Pulmonary arterial remodeling and vasoconstriction are frequently superimposed on the passive increase in pulmonary artery pressure and contribute to the pulmonary hypertension.[10] Thus there are 3 components to the pathophysiology. Lowering the high downstream pressure usually results in a rapid fall in pulmonary arterial pressure as the passive and vasoconstrictor (reactive) elements are reversed.[11]

Conditions affecting the left heart that are particularly frequent in the elderly include left ventricular dysfunction secondary to coronary artery disease, systemic hypertension, cardiomyopathy (eg, amyloid), and valvular disease (especially calcific aortic stenosis and mitral regurgitation).

Older patients with systemic hypertension (> 65 years) have higher pulmonary arterial pressures and resistances than those who are younger.[12] This is a similar observation to that which was discussed earlier in the normal population.[3,4,8] PHT is important, not so much because it requires treatment separate from the underlying condition, but because it is a predictor of recurrent hospitalization and death among patients with ischemic or idiopathic cardiomyopathy.[13] Prior to cardiac transplantation, a pulmonary vascular resistance in excess of 2.5 mm Hg/L per minute despite nitroprusside, signals a poor prognosis after transplantation.[14]

High-Flow Pulmonary Hypertension

PHT that occurs as a result of a left to right shunt through a ventricular septal defect, patent ductus arteriosus, or more complex congenital anomaly is usually diagnosed in childhood. While most patients are also diagnosed earlier in life, in the case of atrial septal defect, symptoms and pulmonary artery pressure increase progressively with age,[15] and an occasional person presents only when elderly. Perloff[16] reported two such patients at ages 87 and 94 years, the first had a pulmonary artery pressure of 60/25 mm Hg.

In the 1960s, Wood[9] stated that ". . . 12% of uncomplicated cases of atrial septal defect and 15% of those with the Eisenmenger syndrome were in persons between 50 and 75 years of age." The pathology of pulmonary hypertension associated with atrial septal defect is that of plexogenic pulmonary arteriopathy with intimal proliferation, concentric fibrosis and plexiform lesions.[17] Thrombosis may occur in both small[17] and large[18] pulmonary arteries. It is likely that an impairment of endothelial-dependent vasodilatation also contributes to the development of pulmonary hypertension.[19]

Obstructive and Obliterative Pulmonary Hypertension

Pulmonary vascular obstruction is common to many forms of PHT. It may take the form of intraluminal obstruction, as in pulmonary embolism, or encroachment on the lumen, as seen when remodeling involves intimal proliferation and fibrosis.

Most of the etiologies listed in Table 1 fall under the "obstructive" heading. Pulmonary fibrosis, as a cause of PHT, comes under the "oblit-

---

Table 1
Pulmonary Hypertension Secondary to Pulmonary Vascular Disease in the Elderly: Obstructive

A. Recurrent or massive pulmonary emboli
B. Extrinsic compression of pulmonary arteries
C. Tumor "microemboli"
D. Schistosomiasis
E. Thrombocytosis
F. Pulmonary lymphangiomyomatosis
G. Pulmonary vascular amyloid
H. Toxic oil syndrome
I. Collagen-vascular disease (scleroderma, mixed connective tissue disease, systemic lupus erythematosus)
J. Primary pulmonary hypertension (PPH)
K. Portal hypertension associated with PPH

Table 2
Pulmonary Hypertension Secondary to Pulmonary Airway and Parenchymal Disease: Obliterative

A. Chronic obstructive lung disease
B. Cystic fibrosis
C. Severe pulmonary fibrosis
   i. Sarcoidosis and other granulomatous lung diseases
   ii. Diffuse interstitial fibrosis (including radiation, Hamman-Rich syndrome, idiopathic, etc.)
   iii. Pneumoconiosis
D. Adult respiratory distress syndrome
E. Pneumonectomy

erative" heading, along with the other conditions in Table 2. In both tables only those conditions likely to be seen in the elderly are included. It is important to remember, however, that in some diseases, PHT may be induced by several mechanisms. In the case of high-flow PHT, high-flow itself (hyperkinetic), vasoconstriction (reactive), and remodeling (obstructive) are operative factors.

Pulmonary Embolism

Pulmonary thromboembolism is probably the purest form of pulmonary vascular obstruction. It is frequent in the elderly because of immobilization and comorbid factors such as hip fractures, malignancy, and heart failure. In one autopsy study of nursing home residents aged 64 years and older, 8% died as a result of pulmonary embolism.[20] Pulmonary embolism has been reported in 20% of autopsies performed on patients over 70 years of age.[21] Thromboembolism is an important cause of chronic PHT, not so much because of its frequency but because, unlike most forms of PHT, it can be reversed. When emboli obstruct the proximal pulmonary arteries and become organized, thromboendarterectomy can be an effective treatment, even in older patients.

It has been estimated that approximately 450 of the 500,000 patients who experience pulmonary embolism each year, go on to develop chronic PHT.[22] It is unusual to find evidence of specific coagulopathies; about 10% of patients with chronic thromboembolic PHT have a lupus anticoagulant and less than 1% have protein C, protein S or antithrombin III deficiency.[22]

Extrinsic Compression of Pulmonary Arteries

It is particularly important in older patients to consider other causes of proximal pulmonary artery obstruction such as compression by tumors or fibrosing mediastinitis.[23] Even congenital absence of 1 pulmonary artery may simulate thrombotic occlusion; angiography or angioscopy can make the correct diagnosis.

Tumor Microembolism

Microangiopathy induced by microscopic tumor emboli should be considered when a patient with carcinoma, usually adenocarcinoma, develops pulmonary hypertension.[24] The tumor induces local activation of coagulation and also induces intimal proliferation. In 1 patient with a breast carcinoma, the pulmonary artery pressure was 120/56 mm Hg, with a mean pressure of 80 mm Hg.[25] In another, who had a right atrial myxoma, the pulmonary artery pressure was 74/29 mm Hg, with a mean pressure of 46 mm Hg.[26]

Unusual Causes of Pulmonary Hypertension in the Elderly

Schistosomiasis is a common cause of PHT in Egypt and Brazil, but is rarely seen in the United States. Embolization of the ova to the pulmonary arteries stimulates intimal proliferation, fibrosis, and even plexogenic arteriopathy.[17]

Other rare causes of PHT include thrombocytosis (in a 72-year-old man with myeloid metaplasia),[27] intravascular lymphomatosis (as a manifestation of a B cell lymphoma in a 79-year-old man),[28] severe diffuse pulmonary vascular amyloidosis (in a 65-year-old woman),[29] and toxic oil syndrome reported to cause pulmonary vascular disease in patients up to the age of 58 years.[30]

Among the collagen-vascular diseases, scleroderma is similar in many respects, both clinically and histologically, to primary pulmonary hypertension. The prevalence of significant PHT in scleroderma has been assessed to be between 9% and 16%.[31,32] Intimal fibroelastosis has been described, particularly in the CREST variant of scleroderma.[33] The cells involved in the intimal proliferation of the renal arteries in scleroderma have ultrastructural features of smooth muscle,[34] in common with the intimal cells of the pulmonary arteries seen in primary PHT.[35] The finding of increased levels of factor VIII/von Willebrand factor and β-thromboglobulin in the plasma of scleroderma patients also suggests endothelial involvement and platelet activation.[36] PHT has been reported, although less commonly, in systemic lupus erythematosus,[37,38] mixed connective tissue disease,[39] rheumatoid arthritis,[40] dermatomyositis,[41] and polymyositis.[42]

Primary Pulmonary Hypertension

Primary pulmonary hypertension (PPH) is usually considered to be a disease of young people, especially women. However, in the NIH

PPH registry, 9% of patients were over age 60 years and 1 was 81.[2] A recent series of 63 patients with PHT, age 65 years or older, included 8 in whom pulmonary hypertension could not be explained by other conditions.[43] Only 1 patient survived more than 25 months. Phipps et al[44] reported 2 cases of primary PHT in elderly patients.

The histopathology of PPH includes 3 main subsets: plexogenic arteriopathy (including concentric fibrosis and medial hypertrophy), thrombotic lesions in the small pulmonary arteries, and veno-occlusive disease.[45] Pulmonary capillary hemangiomatosis is sometimes considered to be a fourth subset. It is not clear whether plexogenic arteriopathy and the microthrombotic form of PPH are 2 separate entities or 2 ends of a single spectrum. The latter seems more likely.[46] The etiology of all forms of PPH is still obscure; when the pathophysiology is understood, effective treatment will be easier to devise.

Portal Hypertension

Patients with portal hypertension (PHT) even in the absence of cirrhosis, have an increased incidence of pulmonary hypertension with a histological picture of plexogenic arteriopathy or thrombotic lesions in the small arteries.[47] McDonnell et al[48] found that the incidence of pulmonary hypertension among patients with cirrhosis at autopsy was higher than among patients without cirrhosis (0.73 and 0.13%, respectively).[48] None of the 9 patients with unexplained PHT were elderly (ages 21–52 years), however, 3 of 12 patients with portal and pulmonary hypertension in another series were over age 60 years.[49] It is not clear whether some substance normally metabolized by the liver causes endothelial dysfunction in the pulmonary artery endothelium, leading to cellular proliferation and thrombosis.

Chronic Obstructive Pulmonary Disease

Although chronic obstructive pulmonary disease (COPD) is included in Table 2, when PHT occurs in these patients, it is secondary to a combination of obliteration, vasoconstriction, and obstruction. Obstruction to flow is caused by development of longitudinal muscle in the intima of muscular pulmonary arteries and the extension of longitudinal muscle into the small, normally nonmuscularized, arteries.[50] These changes correlate best with decrease in the forced expiratory volume in 1 second (FEV_1).

PHT at rest is relatively unusual in COPD. The mean pulmonary artery pressure was only equal to, or greater than 20 mm Hg, in 31 of 151 patients (21%) in one series.[51] However, 99 of these patients (66%) had a mean pressure of 30 mm Hg, or greater, on quite mild exercise. Even modest levels of PHT (pulmonary arterial mean pressure > 20 mm Hg) are reported to imply a poor prognosis,[52] (50% mortality in 4 years) although this is not uniformly observed.[53] In the first of these studies, increasing age had a substantial effect on survival; after 7 years, 62% of those under the age of 60 years were alive compared to only 33% of those over 60 years.[54] It is likely that PHT is a marker for a poor prognosis in COPD, rather than being the actual cause of death. The same is probably true for the PHT that may occur in adult respiratory distress syndrome (ARDS).[55] It has been suggested that the retention of salt and water in cor pulmonale is the result of a low systemic arterial pressure and resistance, not a consequence of decreased cardiac output or right ventricular function.[56] Focusing on the relatively mild PHT in these conditions may be a case of "blaming the messenger."

Pulmonary Fibrosis

The pulmonary vascular hemodynamics of idiopathic pulmonary fibrosis have been reported in a group of patients with a mean age of 58 years (the oldest being 83 years).[52] As in COPD, the resting mean pulmonary artery pressure was relatively low (22 ± 8 SD mm Hg), whereas with exercise it increased markedly (45 ± 16 mm Hg). The authors suggested that the observation of exercise-induced hypoxemia in these patients indicates that hypoxic pulmonary vasoconstriction may have been involved,[52] but it seems as likely that the hypoxemia is secondary to increased shunting of desaturated blood in the lungs.

Hypoxia and/or Hypercapnia

The more common causes of hypoxic and/or hypercapnic PHT in the elderly are shown in Table 3. Pulmonary vasoconstriction has been intensively studied in acute hypoxic PHT. One of the basic mechanisms that determines pulmonary vascular smooth muscle tone is the response to changes in oxygen tension. In the carotid body type 1 cell, it

---

Table 3
Pulmonary Hypertension Secondary to Hypoxia and/or Hypercapnia

A. High altitude residence
B. Primary hypoventilation
   1. sleep-induced disorders of breathing
   2. obesity-hypoventilation syndrome
   3. primary alveolar hypoventilation
C. Neuromuscular disorders
   1. myasthenia gravis
   2. poliomyelitis
D. Mechanical hypoventilation, eg, kyphoscoliosis

has been shown that hypoxia inhibits an outward potassium current and thus causes depolarization of the cell membrane.[57] Calcium entry through the voltage-dependent channel then signals a change in oxygen tension. It has recently been found that a similar mechanism exists in the pulmonary vascular smooth muscle.[58] An outward potassium current is present across the membrane of these cells, which is inhibited by hypoxia. It is possible that this mechanism is also involved in the vasoconstriction present in other types of PHT. The more chronic forms of hypoxic PHT involve both vasoconstriction and remodeling of the small pulmonary arteries, with increased medial thickness and development of longitudinal muscle in the intima.

High Altitude

Patients who have had previous episodes of high-altitude pulmonary edema (HAPE) have greater pulmonary vascular responses to hypoxia than controls.[59] Pulmonary arterial pressure in 8 such subjects increased from 17 ± 3 mm Hg to 34 ± 7 mm Hg in response to 10% inspired oxygen. Pulmonary vascular resistance also doubled. There are no data on the susceptibility of older people to HAPE, but they are less prone to develop acute mountain sickness,[60] which may be a prodrome of HAPE.

Sleep Apnea

A recent report indicates that sleep apnea is more common than previously recognized, occurring in 9% of middle-age women and 24% of middle-age men in the general population.[61] Moderate and severe scores for apnea and hypopnea are more common in women age 50 to 60 years than among younger women. Older patients were not studied.

The presence of hypoxemia and hypercapnia during the day,[62] and hypoxemia ($< 90\%$ O_2 saturation) at night[63] are associated with mild to moderate PHT when measured during the day. Again, it is unlikely that the PHT is severe enough to be life threatening.

Symptoms

The symptoms of PHT are usually vague (eg, fatigue, dyspnea, reduced exercise capacity) and often attributed to psychosomatic illness or other noncardiac disease. Delayed or incorrect diagnosis is further promoted by the infrequency of PHT and its tendency to be associated with nonspecific physical findings. Consequently, accurate diagnosis is often delayed for years.[64-67] This delay occurs regardless of the type of PHT, but is more pronounced in the elderly in whom fatigue and dyspnea are more readily attributed to chronic cardiopulmonary disease or the effects of "aging."

Symptoms of PHT do not usually occur until pulmonary artery pressure has doubled.[7] Dyspnea is an almost universal complaint of patients with any form of PHT[64-68] except for those with PHT due to sleep apnea and results from a combination of factors such as altered lung mechanics, reflex mechanisms, and hypoxemia. Interstitial lung disease, with reduced lung compliance and hypoxemia, is another cause of dyspnea in pulmonary hypertension, especially in patients with connective tissue disease. In patients with passive PHT, elevation of pulmonary capillary pressure and infiltration of fluid into the perivascular space may stimulate the J receptors, promoting dyspnea.

Fatigue may reflect reduced cardiac output and impaired oxygen delivery at rest, as well as inability to increase cardiac output with exercise. The rise in pulmonary artery pressure and resistance that occurs with exercise in the PHT probably contributes to exercise intolerance and fatigue.

Syncope occurs in one third of patients with primary PHT, but is rare in patients with cor pulmonale, unless they have coexistent cough-induced syncope. Patients may experience syncope when they exercise (eg, climbing stairs) or perform maneuvers that alter venous return (eg, bending over to tie their shoes). In the elderly, syncope is often multifactorial and, related to the inability of the obstructed pulmonary vascular bed to accommodate the increases in cardiac output necessary to sustain cerebral blood flow in the face of systemic vasodilatation, as well as unrelated causes (eg, carotid disease).

Chest pain in pulmonary hypertension may be pleuritic or have a dull character, suggesting angina. Potential mechanisms for chest pain in PHT include right ventricular ischemia and distention of the pulmonary arteries.

Rarely, patients may develop hoarseness (Ortner's syndrome) when the left recurrent laryngeal nerve is compressed in its course between the aorta and an enlarged pulmonary artery.[9,68] Ortner's syndrome was reported in up to 6–8% of patients with severe chronic pulmonary hypertension in older series, but is less prevalent in recent series.[64,66,67,69]

Hemoptysis occurs in many types of pulmonary hypertension. Moser et al[65] noted a history of hemoptysis in 53% of patients undergoing thromboendarterectomy for thromboembolic PHT. In the elderly patient with PHT, hemoptysis should not be attributed to the PHT until other common conditions such as bronchitis and lung cancer have been excluded.

Noninvasive Assessment of the Pulmonary Circulation

Electrocardiography

Electrocardiography is a specific, but nonsensitive means of diagnosing right ventricular hypertrophy (RVH).[70] There are many criteria

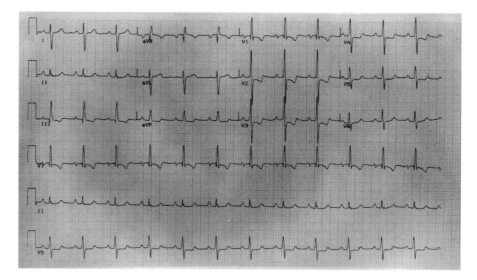

Figure 3: *Twelve-lead electrocardiogram. This ECG shows the characteristic findings of right ventricular hypertrophy and pulmonary hypertension including right axis deviation and dominant R wave in leads V_1 and V_2. The ST segment depression in V_1–V_3 is called a right ventricular strain pattern. This ECG was obtained from a patient with severe, thromboembolic pulmonary hypertension.*

proposed to identify RVH (Figure 3). In the elderly, RVH may exist without significant pulmonary hypertension or ECG changes, particularly in patients with systemic hypertension and aortic stenosis. Coexistent illnesses, common in the elderly, such as posterior myocardial infarction, and left posterior fascicular block may reduce the specificity of the ECG. These conditions cause right axis deviation and/or a predominant R in lead V_1. Posterior infarction can usually be detected in association with evidence of associated inferior infarction, ie, Q waves in the inferior leads.

Because RVH usually is associated with pulmonary hypertension, the ECG correlates somewhat with pulmonary hemodynamics, especially in advanced disease. Nonetheless, a normal ECG does not exclude mild or moderate pulmonary hypertension.

Chest Roentgenogram

The chest roentgenogram (CXR), like the ECG, is a convenient and widely available screening test for pulmonary hypertension. There are numerous signs, including enlargement of the pulmonary arteries, loss of peripheral vascular markings, and right heart enlargement. In the elderly, the CXR may show bullae or hyperinflation in patients with cor pulmonale. The most widely used roentgenographic criteria for diagnosing pulmonary hypertension are based, directly or indirectly, on pulmonary artery size.[71-73] The simplest criteria is to measure the descending right pulmonary artery (normal width: 12.1 ± 1.2 mm).[73] The CXR appears quite sensitive for PHT when studied in populations with a high prevalence of the disease; however, in a geriatric population, the CXR is of modest utility, except in severe disease. Furthermore, radiographic techniques may detect PHT, but are less useful in predicting a specific pressure in an individual.

Computerized Tomography

Using computerized tomography (CT) scans, pulmonary artery size has been compared with pulmonary artery pressure and resistance in 6 patients with cor pulmonale and 18 with primary or thromboembolic pulmonary hypertension.[72,74] Among patients with pulmonary vascular hypertension, arterial size was correlated with PVR but not pulmonary artery pressure.[74] Reduced arterial compliance in pulmonary vascular hypertension might account for the lack of correlation between vessel size and pressure.[74] Pulmonary vascular compliance is reduced in pulmonary vascular hypertension[75] but is normal in patients with cor pulmonale.[76] The pulmonary arteries in primary and thromboembolic PHT display more intimal fibrosis than is seen in cor pulmonale. Even if pulmonary size on CT does not universally predict pressure, it reflects pulmonary vascular resistance and cardiac output, thus providing useful clinical information.[74] The diameter of the main pulmonary artery, corrected for body surface area, in patients with pulmonary hypertension (pressure 65 ± 10 mm Hg) was 36 ± 6 mm.

Echocardiography

The echocardiogram is rarely normal in patients with severe pulmonary hypertension.[77] The important findings are enlargement of the right ventricular chamber and thickening of its walls detected by M-mode using two-dimensional techniques (Figure 4). Normal subjects have a right ventricular wall thickness of 2–4 mm.[78,79] Estimation of pulmonary artery pressure is accomplished by Doppler techniques.[78-86]

Pulsed Doppler

The normal pulmonary artery flow velocity is 81 ± 17 cm/sec and occurs with an acceleration time of 121 ± 27 sec. In pulmonary hypertension there is a more rapid acceleration of pulmonary flow velocity,

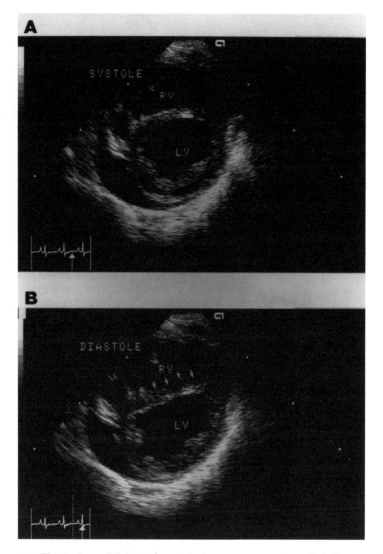

Figure 4: *Flattening of the interventricular septum: a sign of right ventricular pressure-volume overload. **Panel A:** This systolic frame shows a short-axis parasternal view of the right and left ventricles (LV and RV). There is mild flattening of the circular appearance of the LV. The right ventricle is hypertrophied and dilated. **Panel B:** The diastolic frame shows marked deviation of the septum. This appearance is consistent with a right ventricular end diastolic pressure which exceeds that in the LV.*

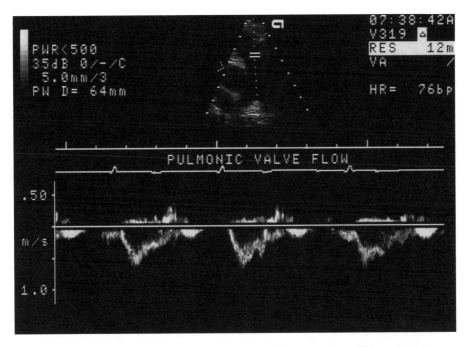

Figure 5: *Pulsed Doppler in severe pulmonary hypertension. This pulsed Doppler shows the classic short acceleration time and diminished peak velocity of pulmonary hypertension. The late systolic notching results from reflected waves returning from the noncompliant peripheral pulmonary vasculature.*

with or without early systolic deceleration. Figure 5 shows the classic pulmonary Doppler findings of severe pulmonary hypertension, ie, reduced pulmonary systolic flow velocity, short acceleration time, and "notching." There is a good correlation between acceleration time and mean pulmonary artery pressure.[86–91]

Continuous Wave Doppler

Color-guided imaging with continuous wave Doppler using tricuspid regurgitant jet velocity is the best method for noninvasive measurement of pulmonary artery pressure. Using the simplified, modified Bernoulli's equation: Systolic PAP = $4V^2$ + RAP, where V is the velocity of the tricuspid regurgitation jet, it is possible to estimate pressure quickly and accurately (Figure 6). Tricuspid regurgitation is common in normal individuals and increases in prevalence and severity as pulmonary artery pressures increase.[91–93] Berger et al.[91] found tricuspid regurgitation in approximately 39 of 49 patients with systolic pulmonary artery pressures < 35 mm Hg and 26 of 27 patients with pressures

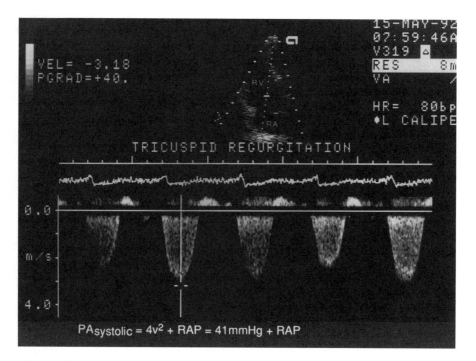

Figure 6: *Calculation of pulmonary artery systolic pressure using Bernoulli's equation. This still frame shows imaging, continuous wave Doppler measurement of a tricuspid regurgitation signal. In the upper panel the continuous wave Doppler probe is aligned across the tricuspid valve. The tricuspid regurgitation envelopes in the lower panel display normal respiratory variation. The systolic velocity of the jet (3.18 m/s) is entered into the modified Bernoulli Equation and a systolic pulmonary artery pressure is calculated (see Equation at bottom of figure). The right atrial pressure (RAP) may be estimated by observing the change in dimension of the inferior vena cava with inspiration on a subcostal view, or by measurement of jugular venous distension at the bedside.*

> 50 mm Hg and noted an excellent correlation between Doppler estimates and catheter measurements of pulmonary artery systolic pressure (r = 0.97). Yock and Popp[94] used the modified Bernoulli's equation to estimate right ventricular systolic pressures in patients with clinical signs of pulmonary hypertension. They were able to measure the velocity of tricuspid regurgitation in 54 of 62 patients and found a good correlation between the Doppler and catheter pressures, as has been validated by numerous authors.[95–98]

Magnetic Resonance Imaging

Magnetic resonance imaging (MRI) permits volumetric flow measurement in the major pulmonary arteries. There are many advantages of this technique in the elderly, including avoidance of intravenous contrast and a high probability of obtaining an adequate image, even in patients with lung disease. However, scan times remain significantly longer than those for CT scanning, cost is high, and unlike echocardiography, pressures cannot be accurately measured.[99]

Thallium Scintigraphy

Although thallium-201 scintigraphy is used clinically for the diagnosis of left ventricular ischemia, exercise thallium testing is occasionally performed in elderly patients whose PHT is masquerading as heart failure or angina. While thallium scintigraphy is not a routine part of our evaluation of the patient with pulmonary hypertension, it is important that the clinician realize the potential significance of right ventricular thallium uptake when this is observed during exercise testing. Thallium scintigraphy was found to be more sensitive for right ventricular pressure-volume overload than the ECG, CXR, or echocardiogram.[100–103]

Pulmonary Function Tests

Pulmonary function tests are usually abnormal in patients with PHT, regardless of the cause. Patients with thromboembolic and primary pulmonary hypertension often have mild restrictive or obstructive patterns noted on spirometry. Interpretation of the lung function tests is particularly difficult in patients with connective tissue disease. PHT patients with collagen vascular disease tend to have more severe lung disease than a cohort with primary PHT: diffusing capacity (DLCO) (11.9 ± 1.5 and 17.6 ± 0.6 mL/min/mm Hg, respectively), FEV_1 (1.9 ± 0.1 and 2.6 ± 0.1 L/s, respectively), FVC (2.4 ± 0.1 and 3.3 ± 0.1 L, respectively).[104]

Cardiac Catheterization

Catheterization of the pulmonary artery is the gold standard for measurement of pulmonary artery pressure and is usually required to establish a diagnosis of PHT. The goals of right heart catheterization include measurement of pressure, flow, and resistance and to establish the type of PHT.

Normally, the difference between mean pulmonary artery and wedge pressures is 3–10 mm Hg[1]; the hallmark of pulmonary vascular disease is a larger gradient. This may be due to fixed vascular obstruction in an obliterated vascular bed, increased pulmonary vascular tone, or a combination of these factors. Only a third of patients with primary

PHT respond to vasodilators, suggesting that the majority of the increase in pulmonary vascular resistance (PVR) in most patients is the result of fixed anatomic vascular disease, rather than vasospasm.

These findings contrast dramatically with those of left ventricular failure, where pulmonary artery diastolic and wedge pressures are similar. In such patients, total pulmonary resistance, which ignores left atrial or "wedge" pressure, is elevated but pulmonary vascular resistance is near normal.

Technical Considerations

The goal of right heart catheterization in the assessment of PHT is to measure pressure in all chambers, estimate left atrial pressure by obtaining a wedge pressure, and measure cardiac output. When there is a question of a shunt we measure O_2 saturation in the aorta and all right heart chambers and use indocyanine green "dye curves" to localize and quantify the shunt. We perform right heart catheterization using a femoral vein approach, usually under fluoroscopic guidance with a balloon flotation catheter.

Right heart catheterization carries increased risks in patients with PHT. The risks may be divided into three categories: (1) vasovagal reactions during vascular access, (2) placing a catheter in the pulmonary artery (rupture, arrhythmia), (3) medications (eg, negative inotropic effects, vasodilatation with hypotension).

Patients with PHT are intolerant of vasovagal reactions. Whether due to a drug reaction or vagal reflex, the dysfunctional right ventricle and obstructed pulmonary vascular bed may not support the normal increase in left heart output that accompanies systemic vasodilatation and a simple vasovagal reaction may lead to a cycle of bradycardia, hypotension, acidosis, and death. Rhodes et al[102] reported a 19% mortality rate related to catheterization in a study of 16 consecutive patients with primary PHT. All the deaths in this small study occurred in patients with poor exercise tolerance and the authors advocated that catheterization be avoided in such patients. In the accompanying editorial, Brundage[103] emphasized the need for meticulous prevention of pain and vasovagal reactions. It is noteworthy that there were no deaths during diagnostic catheterization of the National Institutes of Health (NIH) registry study in which 187 patients (mostly functional class III–IV) had right heart catheterization.[104]

Specific Types of Pulmonary Hypertension

Thromboembolic Pulmonary Hypertension

History

Patients with thromboembolic PHT may have a history of deep venous thrombosis or pleuritic chest pain.[22,105] Although the incidence of clinically recognized thromboembolism, prior to the diagnosis of PHT is low,[81] more than half of these patients have had an episode that, in retrospect, is consistent with venous thrombosis or acute pulmonary embolism.[22,105] Screening question for trauma, immobility, pleurisy, hemoptysis, or "pneumonia" may be useful.

Laboratory Examination

A minority of patients with thromboembolic PHT have abnormal coagulation. Roughly 10% of patients have lupus "anticoagulant" without clinical evidence of systemic lupus erythematosus.[22] The other known procoagulant abnormalities (protein C, protein S or antithrombin III deficiency) occur in less than 1% of these patients.

Ventilation Perfusion Scan

Ventilation/perfusion scans (V/Q) are widely used in assessing patients with pulmonary hypertension to exclude a thromboembolic etiology. Virtually all patients with thromboembolic pulmonary hypertension have one or more high-probability scans with segmental or large perfusion defects (Figure 7).

The major risk of V/Q scans in pulmonary hypertension is misinterpretation. Patients with primary pulmonary hypertension often have diffuse, inhomogenous perfusion scans which are interpreted as "low probability." This may lead to unnecessary angiography. Although death has been reported within minutes of injecting the small technetium-labeled (75 μm) albumin macroaggregates that are used as flow markers this is exceedingly rare.[106] This complication has occurred in patients with severe pulmonary hypertension and may represent the inability of a severely obstructed vascular bed to deal with a shower of

Post.   L.P.O.   L. Lat.

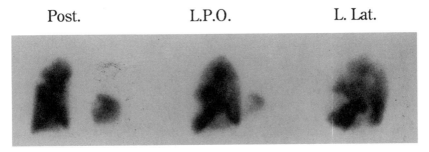

Figure 7: *Lung perfusion scan showing several segmental defects and nonperfusion of the right upper and middle lobes, virtually diagnostic of pulmonary thromboembolism.*

microemboli. Nonetheless, a V/Q scan is "safe" and should be included in the evaluation of every patient with unexplained pulmonary hypertension.

V/Q scans tend to underestimate the amount of thrombus present in the patients with thromboembolic pulmonary hypertension. The scan can be used to guide angiography when a high probability localized defect is identified.

Pulmonary Angiography

Pulmonary angiography is primarily used to exclude the presence of chronic pulmonary emboli but may also detect peripheral pulmonary artery stenoses, arteriovenous fistulae, and obliterative pulmonary vascular disease. Although pulmonary angiography is often avoided in pulmonary hypertension because of a perceived risk, it is a safe procedure with minimal morbidity or mortality. The incremental risk of injection of contrast, beyond the risk of placing a catheter merely to measure pressures, is relatively small. The individuals most at risk for complications of pulmonary angiography are those with elevated right ventricular end-diastolic pressures (>20 mm Hg) or overt right heart failure.

Generally, the right and left pulmonary arteries, or subdivisions, are injected selectively. Selective pulmonary angiography minimizes dye dilution, reduces overlap of opacified vessels and ensures opacification of embolized vessels.[107]

Images are acquired biplane (anteroposterior and 30 left anterior oblique) using either cut-film or cine. An acute embolism is diagnosed by the presence of either an intraluminal filling defect or an abrupt "cutoff" of a vessel. However, in chronic thromboembolic pulmonary hypertension the embolus may be incorporated into the vessel wall and the angiographic signs may be subtle. Because primary pulmonary hypertension is a diagnosis of exclusion, many patients with primary pulmonary hypertension have had pulmonary angiography. The classic appearance of the pulmonary angiogram in primary pulmonary hypertension is the combination of dilated proximal arteries and "pruning" of smaller, peripheral pulmonary arteries.

Wedge Angiography

While conventional angiography images the large vessels, "wedge angiography" can be used to study the microvasculature. This technique is primarily used to assess the anatomy of the small pulmonary arteries and capillary bed. Small amounts of contrast are injected slowly, distal to the inflated balloon of an end-hole, balloon flotation catheter that is "wedged." Magnified angiograms are obtained. In the normal lung the subsegmental pulmonary arteries are plump and smooth and there is a distal "blush" produced by the microcirculation.

Narrowing of the vessel and reduction in the size of the microvascular bed occurs with progressive pulmonary vascular disease,[108] detected as a loss of capillary "blush." Findings on wedge angiography correlate fairly well with histological assessment of the pulmonary vasculature on lung biopsy.[109]

The risks of pulmonary angiography are not dramatically increased in the elderly. Stein et al[110] compared the results of pulmonary angiography in 72 patients older than 70 years of age with 2 younger cohorts (<40 and 40–69 years). The rate of major complications in the elderly (1.0%) was not different than in the 562 younger patients (1.1%).[110] However, the elderly had a higher incidence of contrast-induced nephropathy (3%) than younger patients (0.7%).

Pulmonary Angioscopy

Shure et al[111] have extensive experience with angioscopy in patients with unexplained pulmonary hypertension and equivocal pulmonary angiograms and have demonstrated scalloping of the vessel wall with intimal irregularities, pitted masses, bands and webs consistent with recanalization of thrombus. These findings are often not evident on a pulmonary angiogram and, in their small series, fiberoptic angioscopy changed the diagnosis in 4 patients with pulmonary hypertension.[111] Unusual diseases that mimic thromboembolic pulmonary hypertension angiographically, such as congenital absence of the pulmonary artery and fibrosing mediastinitis, may be identified by angioscopy.

Computed Tomography

CT scans have also been used to differentiate thromboembolic from primary pulmonary hypertension.[112] In addition to avoiding the need for catheterization, the CT scan allows characterization of tissue density. The tomographic assessment of tissue density permits one to distinguish clot from vessel wall. The CT scan may be helpful in the crucial assessment of whether the thrombi are sufficiently proximal to permit thromboendarterectomy.[112]

Cor Pulmonale

Cor pulmonale and right ventricular hypertrophy associated with chronic lung disease, is associated with a high mortality (45% 2-year survival).[113] Pulmonary hypertension is usually a late manifestation of parenchymal pulmonary disease, and therefore, a history of asthma, bronchitis, or recurrent pneumonia is generally evident. Keller et al[114] reported a series of 31 patients with PHT associated with COPD.[114]

The mean age of these patients, 59 ± 6 years, is typical of patients with cor pulmonale.

Pulmonary fibrosis is more likely to cause significant pulmonary hypertension than COPD and a history of exposure to toxins, such as beryllium and asbestos that may cause fibrosis should be sought. Sleep apnea, one of the more treatable causes of pulmonary hypertension, should be actively pursued. We routinely inquire about daytime hypersomnolence and nocturnal apnea.

Laboratory

The finding of polycythemia is compatible with, but not diagnostic of, pulmonary hypertension in patients with chronic lung disease. Excessive elevations of hemoglobin increase pulmonary vascular resistance and phlebotomy may be beneficial in selected patients. The pulmonary hypertensive patient with cyanotic heart disease often has thrombocytopenia as well as polycythemia. Arterial blood gases are usually abnormal in patients with cor pulmonale. In chronic obstructive lung disease a Po_2 less than 60 mm Hg and PCo_2 greater than 40 mm Hg are thought to be threshold values for the development of pulmonary hypertension.[114] Milder hypoxemia is typically present in primary pulmonary hypertension as well, but is almost always associated with hypocapnia.[2,69]

Primary PHT

Primary PHT is a diagnosis of exclusion. Although it usually occurs in individuals in the 3rd and 4th decades, the elderly are occasionally affected. The presenting symptoms (dyspnea, chest pain, fatigue) and laboratory findings in these elderly patients (age greater than 65 years) were similar to those in younger patients with primary PHT.[43]

Connective Tissue Disease/Raynaud's Phenomenon

Pulmonary hypertension is relatively common in scleroderma,[32] systemic lupus,[115] and mixed connective tissue disease[116] and has been noted on rare occasions in patients with rheumatoid arthritis.[117] Therefore, one should solicit a history of arthritis, pleuritis, skin rashes, and dysphagia when evaluating an elderly patient with unexplained PHT. Raynaud's syndrome is common in patients with connective tissue disease, in the absence of pulmonary hypertension, but was also present in 24% of primary pulmonary hypertensives in the NIH registry. Raynaud's phenomenon does not occur with increased frequency in high-flow pulmonary hypertension, cor pulmonale, or thromboembolic pulmonary hypertension.[118] A history of Raynaud's phenomenon in a patient with pulmonary hypertension strongly suggests a diagnosis of primary pulmonary hypertension. Patients with primary pulmonary hypertension often have a positive fluorescent antinuclear antibody assay (FANA). The positive FANA in primary pulmonary hypertension usually occurs without evidence of rheumatologic diseases (arthritis, pleuritis, skin rash). However, patients with CREST syndrome,[119] systemic lupus erythematosus and, to a lesser extent, rheumatoid arthritis[117] are at increased risk of developing pulmonary hypertension. Unfortunately, patients with connective tissue disorders often have abnormal FANAs without pulmonary hypertension. The FANA and other markers of autoimmunity may provide a clue to the etiology of primary pulmonary hypertension.

Cirrhosis and Pulmonary Hypertension

Patients with cirrhosis have a low, but increased, frequency of pulmonary hypertension, which resembles primary pulmonary hypertension. The review of systems should document a patient's history of alcohol intake, cirrhosis or jaundice.

Treatment

Just as there are multiple etiologies for pulmonary hypertension, so are there as many treatments. Frequently pulmonary hypertension will respond to correction of the underlying problem. For instance, if the mitral valve is replaced because of mitral stenosis, the passive and reactive components of pulmonary hypertension will resolve rapidly.[120] Primary pulmonary hypertension will be considered first because it poses many of the problems of treating pulmonary hypertension in general in the geriatric population.

Primary Pulmonary Hypertension

Oxygen

Most PPH patients are not severely hypoxemic at rest.[2] Those who are, or who become desaturated on exertion, may benefit from supplemental oxygen. Oxygen is also advisable for hypoxemic patients when flying. Patients who are desaturated because of a right to left shunt through a patent foramen ovale are unlikely to show improvement. Smokers should be helped to quit, because carbon monoxide reduces the oxygen-carrying capacity of the blood and oxygen delivery is impaired if the cardiac output is fixed. PPH may be more common at high altitude.[121] In any case, vasoconstriction caused by hypoxia is likely to be deleterious and patients should be advised to move to lower altitude if possible.

Anticoagulation

In PPH, thrombin activity is often increased, as demonstrated by elevated levels of fibrinopeptide A in the plasma and a decrease in the half-life of fibrinogen.[122,123] Thrombi are frequently present in the small pulmonary arteries of patients who died as a result of plexogenic pulmonary hypertension, as well as those who have the "microthrombotic" form.[124] For these reasons, as well as the risk of pulmonary embolism in a fairly sedentary population, anticoagulation has been advised. In a retrospective, nonrandomized study reported by Fuster et al,[125] patients who were anticoagulated lived longer than those who were not. This trend is supported by a recent prospective study in which anticoagulants appeared to improve survival, although again the use of anticoagulants was not randomized.[126]

It is important to remember the risk of bleeding when anticoagulants are used in the elderly. In one report the cumulative risk of major bleeding in outpatients older than age 65 years was 18% and 35% at 1 and 4 years, respectively.[127] Part of the problem is the fact that elderly patients require less warfarin than younger patients to achieve the same level of anticoagulation.[128] Another factor that makes control of anticoagulation more difficult is the variability of reference thromboplastins. The prothrombin time ratio is the patient's PT divided by the control PT. If the WHO reference thromboplastin is used, then the ratio is called the international normalized ratio (INR). When anticoagulation is being controlled, except for mechanical valves, the INR should be in the 2 to 3 range.[129] Aspirin and nonsteroidal anti-inflammatory agents should be avoided when older patients take oral anticoagulants.

Vasodilators

The benefits of vasodilators in terms of improved left ventricular function have been recognized for many years. Unfortunately, vasodilator agents also cause systemic vasodilatation. The prevalence of orthostatic hypotension in a population of elderly people living in the community, who do not take vasodilator therapy is 6.4%.[130] In those who are placed on vasodilators in order to treat PPH, the prevalence would be much higher. When systemic vasodilatation does occur in the presence of a patent foramen ovale, increased right to left shunting of blood may lead to hypoxemia.

When a vasodilator is administered to PPH patients there are several possible hemodynamic responses. The optimal response is a fall in both pulmonary arterial pressure and resistance, without symptomatic systemic hypotension; the worst response is symptomatic systemic hypotension, without an improvement in pulmonary artery pressure or resistance. Probably the most common response is an increase in cardiac output, with only a minimal change in pulmonary artery pressure, causing a fall in pulmonary vascular resistance, usually without significant systemic hypotension. Because of the dangers of systemic hypotension and hypoxemia, intensive monitoring of pulmonary and systemic arterial pressures, cardiac output and blood gases is mandatory when vasodilators are first administered to a PPH patient.[131,132] This is particularly important in the elderly who may be more at risk because of coexistent coronary or cerebrovascular disease. In order to further reduce risk, the use of short-acting vasodilators, such as prostacyclin,[133,134] prostaglandin E_1,[135] adenosine,[136] acetylcholine,[137] and nitric oxide[138] as an initial test may be helpful. Unfortunately, prostaglandin E_1 does not accurately predict responsiveness to calcium blockers.[135] It may also cause significant systemic hypotension and hypoxemia. Adenosine is available and because its half-life is so short it has to be administered via a right atrial or right ventricular port, rather than intravenously. This rapid metabolism has the benefit that it has virtually no effect on the systemic arterial pressure.[136] Pulmonary arterial pressure (Figure 8) and resistance decrease in a dose-dependent manner. There is a significant correlation between the fall in pulmonary vascular resistance induced by adenosine and that resulting from

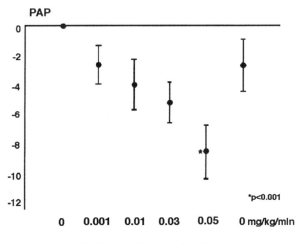

Adenosine infusion

Figure 8: *The decrease in pulmonary artery pressure (PAP) caused by increasing rates of adenosine infusion in seven patients with primary pulmonary hypertension. Values are shown as mean + SEM percent change from baseline. Reproduced with permission of the American Heart Association from Morgan J, McCormack D, Griffiths M, et al: Adenosine as a vasodilator in primary pulmonary hypertension.* Circulation *84:1145–1149, 1991.*

oral nifedipine.[139] In patients who responded to high-dose oral calcium blockers, adenosine caused a further decrease in pulmonary artery pressure and resistance.[140] In catheterization laboratories that do not have access to prostacyclin or nitric oxide, this may be the drug of choice for acute trials of responsiveness.

High-dose calcium channel blockers (nifedipine and diltiazem) have also been used for acute vasodilator challenge.[141] These have the disadvantage of not being short-acting and therefore could be more dangerous if systemic hypotension ensues, as in 2 of 47 patients reported. The major advantage is that if the calcium blocker is effective acutely, it can be used long term.[126] The hemodynamic response to the first dose (nifedipine, 20 mg or diltiazem, 60 mg) is compared to the effect of the maximal dose tolerated in Figures 9 and 10).

Chronic Vasodilator Treatment

Patients who respond to an acute vasodilator challenge by lowering pulmonary vascular resistance more than 30% tend to do better than those who show little or no fall in resistance.[142] It is not apparent whether the better outcome of the "responders" is due to subsequent

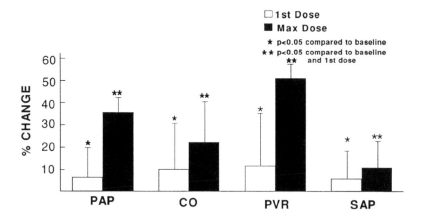

Figure 9: *The percent reduction in mean pulmonary artery pressure (PAP), pulmonary vascular resistance (PVR), and mean systemic arterial pressure (SAP) and increase in cardiac output (CO) are shown for patients with primary pulmonary hypertension characterized as pressure responders; those who had a 20% reduction in mean pulmonary artery pressure and a similar or greater reduction in PVR. The effects of the maximal (Max) doses on each variable were significantly (P < 0.05) greater than those of the first dose. Reprinted with permission from the American College of Cardiology: Rich S, Kaufmann E: High dose titration of calcium channel blocking agents for primary pulmonary hypertension: Guidelines for short-term drug testing. J Am Coll Cardiol 18: 1323–1327, 1991.*

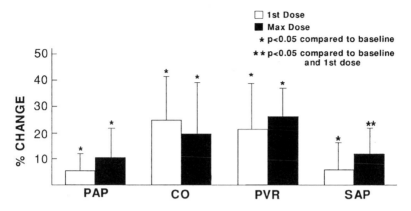

Figure 10: *The percent reduction in mean pulmonary artery pressure (PAP), pulmonary vascular resistance (PVR) and systemic arterial pressure (SAP), and increase in cardiac output (CO) are shown for patients with primary pulmonary hypertension characterized as resistance responders; those who had a 20% reduction in PVR but less than 20% in PAP. Reprinted with permission from the American College of Cardiology: Rich S, Kaufmann E: High dose titration of calcium channel blocking agents for primary pulmonary hypertension: Guidelines for short-term drug testing.* J Am Coll Cardiol *18:1323–1327, 1991.*

treatment or just means that the acute test can identify patients with a better prognosis. However, a follow-up of patients treated long-term with high-dose calcium channel blockers (nifedipine or diltiazem) suggests that this treatment both improves hemodynamics (Figure 11) and prolongs life (Figure 12).[126] It is important to note that verapamil should not be used because of its negative inotropic effect. The results of chronic treatment with nifedipine or diltiazem in those patients (26%), who responded acutely to these agents with a fall in both pulmonary artery pressure and resistance, has been encouraging.[126] It is less clear whether patients who respond acutely with only a fall in pulmonary vascular resistance should be treated chronically. If they tolerate the medication without orthostatic dizziness, hypoxemia, or signs of fluid accumulation, it should probably be given as the antiplatelet and antiproliferative effects may be beneficial. A clinical trial is necessary to resolve this question. Long-term vasodilator therapy with calcium blockers should not be used if the acute challenge results in an increase in pulmonary arterial pressure, a fall in cardiac output or worsening hypoxemia.

Continuous intravenous infusion of prostacyclin can produce sustained hemodynamic and symptomatic improvement in some patients without hypoxemia, even in the absence of an acute hemodynamic response, presumably through effects on platelets and on cell proliferation.[143–145] It is useful both as long-term therapy and as a "bridge" in patients awaiting lung transplantation. Patients may require an

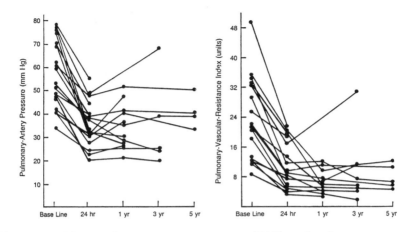

Figure 11: *Mean pulmonary artery pressure (PAP) and pulmonary vascular resistance index (PVRI) in the patients who had favorable responses to high-dose calcium blocker treatment (more than 20% decrease in PAP and PVRI). Values shown were measured at baseline, after the initial assessment of the effectiveness of the drug, and then periodically for up to 5 years. Reproduced with permission of Rich S, Kaufmann E, Levy P: The effect of high doses of calcium-channel blockers on survival in primary pulmonary hypertension. N Engl J Med 327:76–81, 1992.*

increased dose over time and septicemia or accidental interruption of infusion can be problems related to the external pump. There is now considerable interest in the administration of prostacyclin analogs by aerosol,[146] nitric oxide donors by aerosol and the oral administration of phosphodiesterase inhibitors to enhance levels of cGMP.

Lung Transplantation

The role of invasive therapy such as prostacyclin infusion, or lung transplantation, in older patients is questionable. Initially heart-lung transplantation was performed for both PPH and Eisenmenger syndrome but more recently single lung transplantation has been used successfully in PPH, even when right ventricular function is poor.[147] Currently the upper age limit for single lung transplantation is about 60 years. While old age is not an absolute contraindication to major intrathoracic surgery,[148] it is wise to remember the following advice: "it is neither humane or rational to undertake dangerous and unpleasant interventions in patients, whatever their age, in whom the benefits may be marginal."[149]

The immediate hemodynamic advantages of lung transplantation have to be weighed against the problems associated with immunosuppresive therapy, rejection and obliterative bronchiolitis. Another limiting factor is the availability of lungs for transplantation. The issues involved in lung transplantation are the subject of a recent report.[150]

Other Forms of Therapy in Pulmonary Hypertension

The considerations discussed above in deciding the best approach to treatment in PPH, also apply in general to other forms of pulmonary hypertension, with a few exceptions which will be mentioned. As stated earlier, secondary pulmonary hypertension is most effectively treated by correction of the primary problem, eg, mitral valve replacement for mitral stenosis.

Pulmonary Thromboendarterectomy

In the last 15 years, endarterectomy has proved to be an effective treatment for chronic thromboembolic pulmonary hypertension, induced by organized emboli in the proximal pulmonary arteries.[151] One center alone has performed over 800 such operations, including pa-

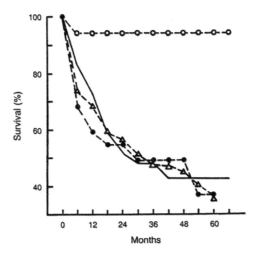

Figure 12: *Kaplan-Meier estimates of survival among patients who responded to treatment (open circles), those who did not respond (solid line), patients enrolled in the NIH Registry who were treated at the University of Illinois (solid circles), and the NIH Registry cohort (triangles). The percentages were calculated every 6 months for 5½ years. The rate of survival was significantly better in the patients who responded (P = 0.003) than in the other groups. "Response" is defined in the legend to Figure 11. Reproduced with permission of Rich S, Kaufmann E, Levy P: The effect of high doses of calcium-channel blockers on survival in primary pulmonary hypertension. N Engl J Med 327:76–81, 1992.*

tients up to age 84 years. With improvement in technique, circulatory arrest now lasts less than 20 minutes for each lung and consequently postoperative delirium is uncommon. Right ventricular dysfunction is no longer a contraindication to surgery. Overall mortality was 11.4% in the first 149 patients and was not related to age.[151] A filter is placed in the inferior vena cava either before or during surgery (Figure 13). For patients who are not candidates for surgery, long-term anticoagulation can lead to an improvement in oxygenation and in the number of lung segments perfused as detected by lung scan.[152] This observation may be helpful in the management of elderly patients, who may have other diseases that contraindicate surgery. It seems unlikely that vasodilators will be advantageous in this group. In view of the mortality associated with pulmonary embolism and thromboendarterectomy, prevention is more efficient than treatment. It is widely accepted that subcutaneous heparin reduces mortality in both medical[153] and surgical[154] patients, but less widely practiced.

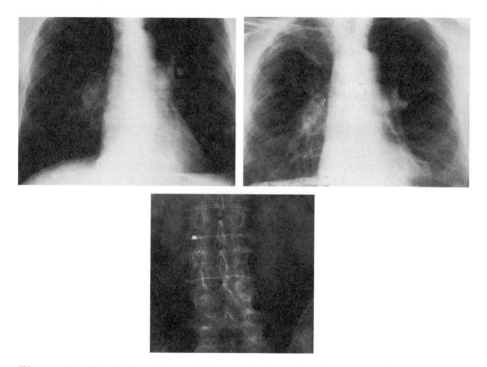

Figure 13: *Top left* and *top right* panels show the chest x-ray of a man age 75 years before and after thromboendarterectomy. Increased vascular markings can be seen postoperatively, especially in the right lower lobe. The bottom panel shows the inferior vena cava umbrella in place in the same patient.

Closure of Atrial Septal Defect

Among patients over the age of 60 years, surgical closure of an atrial septal defect (ASD) can be advised if the pulmonary to systemic blood flow-ratio is high and the pulmonary artery pressure only moderately elevated.[155] Another guideline for patients with pulmonary hypertension is that they can undergo successful surgery if the total pulmonary vascular resistance index is less than 1200 dyne/sec/cm^{-5}/m^2.[156] Despite surgery, patients who are older at the time of surgery (>41 years), are at long-term risk of developing, or continuing, atrial dysrhythmias.[157] Stroke is a related hazard. Fortunately, improvements in transcatheter techniques make it likely that surgery will no longer be necessary for the closure of secundum ASD.

Chronic Obstructive Pulmonary Disease

Pulmonary hypertension is a marker of a poor prognosis in COPD, but is not usually the cause of death. Consequently, efforts to reduce pulmonary hypertension by the use of vasodilators are probably ill advised.[158] The use of long-term oxygen therapy at home (>15 hours/day) has been shown to improve survival in patients with severe COPD and also has a very modest beneficial effect on pulmonary artery pressure.[159–161]

Histological examination of the pulmonary arteries of those who showed a hemodynamic improvement in response to oxygen and those who did not, was unable to recognize a difference.[162] Both had marked thickening of both intima and media. At present the treatment of pulmonary hypertension should not be a priority in the older patient with COPD.

ARDS

Some patients with ARDS develop severe hypoxemia, pulmonary hypertension, and right ventricular failure. In these individuals the ability to decrease right ventricular afterload by the use of vasodilators may be helpful. The acute administration of prostacyclin has been reported to reduce mean pulmonary arterial pressure in nine ARDS patients (18–68 years) from 36 ± 6 to 29 ± 4 mm Hg, associated with a 35% increase in cardiac output.[163] Despite increased intrapulmonary shunting, the rise in mixed venous oxygen content caused a 35% increase in systemic oxygen delivery. The efficacy of prostaglandin E$_1$ in improving survival, when infused over at least 6 days, has been studied in ARDS.[164] Although prostaglandin E$_1$ increased oxygen delivery and consumption, it did not increase survival, possibly because it was given relatively late in the course of events.

Nitric oxide would theoretically be a good pulmonary vasodilator to use in ARDS because, as discussed earlier, it does not act on nonventilated parts of the lung and increase intrapulmonary shunting. In 9 patients, inhalation of nitric oxide (18 ppm) reduced mean pulmonary arterial pressure from 37 ± 3 (SEM) to 30 ± 2 mm Hg and improved arterial oxygenation.[165] Prostacyclin in these patients also reduced pulmonary arterial pressure but reduced arterial oxygenation. Long-term inhalation of nitric oxide (3–53 days) continued to be effective in reducing pressure and improving oxygen exchange. The effect of nitric oxide on survival in ARDS remains to be determined.

Conclusion

Pulmonary hypertension is a significant clinical problem in the elderly. Some causes of pulmonary hypertension (eg, thromboembolic and cor pulmonale) are more common in an older population, while others are less common (eg, Eisenmenger's complex). The treatment of pulmonary hypertension in the elderly is similar to that of the younger patient and must begin with a search for reversible causes. Echocardiography provides the means for the noninvasive assessment of pulmonary artery pressure and right ventricular function, in addition to addressing several possible etiologies. The use of new vasodilators (nitric oxide) and new dosing regimens for old vasodilators (high-dose calcium channel blockers) give hope for better results of treatment. Significant breakthroughs in therapy will accompany the development of a selective inhibitor of intimal proliferation and fibrosis. Despite our enthusiasm for new techniques and treatments, it is especially important in the elderly that these innovations not be generally applied until they are proven to have a benefit.

References

1. Reeves JT, Groves BM: Approach to the patient with pulmonary hypertension. In. EK Weir, JT Reeves (eds): *Pulmonary Hypertension.* Mount Kisco, New York, Futura Publishing Company, Inc., 1984, 1–44.
2. Rich S, Dantzker D, Ayres S, et al: Primary pulmonary hypertension. A national prospective study. *Ann Intern Med* 107:216–223, 1987.
3. Davidson W, Fee E: Influence of aging on pulmonary hemodynamics in a population free of coronary artery disease. *Am J Cardiol* 65:1454–1458, 1990.
4. Fernie J, Lamb D: Effects of age and smoking on intima of muscular pulmonary arteries. *J Clin Pathol* 39:1204–1208, 1986.
5. Hale K, Niewoehner D, Cosio M: Morphologic changes in the muscular pulmonary arteries: Relationship to cigarette smoking, airway disease, and emphysema. *Am Rev Respir Dis* 122:273–278, 1980.
6. Rich S, Chomka E, Hasara L, et al: The prevalence of pulmonary hypertension in the United States. *Chest* 96:236–241, 1989.

7. Reeves J, Grover R, Dempsey J: Pulmonary circulation during exercise. In EK Weir, JT Reeves (eds): *Pulmonary Vascular Physiology and Pathophysiology*. New York, Marcel Dekker, 1989.

8. Ehrsam R, Perruchoud A, Oberholzer M, et al: Influence of age on pulmonary haemodynamics at rest and during supine exercise. *Clin Sci* 65: 653–660, 1983.

9. Wood P: *Diseases of the Heart and Circulation*. London, Eyre and Spottiswoode, 1968.

10. Dexter L: Pulmonary vascular disease in acquired heart disease. In KM Moser (ed): *Pulmonary Vascular Diseases*. New York, NY, Marcel Dekker, 1979, p 427–488.

11. Foltz B, Hessel E, Ivey T: The early course of pulmonary hypertension in patients undergoing mitral valve replacement with cardioplegic arrest. *J Thorac Cardiovasc Surg* 88:238–247, 1984.

12. Ghali J, Liao Y, Cooper R: Changes in pulmonary hemodynamics with aging in a predominantly hypertensive population. *Am J Cardiol* 70: 367–370, 1992.

13. Abramson S, Burke J, Kelly J, et al: Pulmonary hypertension predicts mortality and morbidity in patients with dilated cardiomyopathy. *Ann Intern Med* 116:888–895, 1992.

14. Costard-Jackle A, Fowler M: Influence of preoperative pulmonary artery pressure on mortality after heart transplantation testing of potential reversibility of pulmonary hypertension with nitroprusside is useful in defining a high risk group. *J Am Coll Cardiol* 19:48–54, 1992.

15. Hamilton W, Hafajee C, Dalen J, et al: *Atrial Septal Defect Secundum: Clinical Profile with Physiologic Correlates in Children and Adults*. Philadelphia, F.A. Davis Co, 1979, p 276.

16. Perloff J: Ostium secundum atrial septal defect—Survival for 87 and 94 years. *Am J Cardiol* 53:388–389, 1984.

17. Wagenvoort C: Lung biopsies and pulmonary vascular disease. In EK Weir, JT Reeves (eds): *Pulmonary Hypertension*. Mount Kisco, NY, Futura Publishing Company, 1984, 393–432.

18. Schamroth C, Sareli P, Popcock W, et al: Pulmonary arterial thrombosis in secundum atrial septal defect. *Am J Cardiol* 60:1152–1156, 1987.

19. Celermajer D, Cullen S, Deanfield J: Impairment of endothelium-dependent pulmonary artery relaxation in children with congenital heart disease and abnormal pulmonary hemodynamics. *Circulation* 87:440–446, 1993.

20. Gross J, Neufeld R, Libow L, et al: Autopsy study of the elderly institutionalized patient. Review of 234 autopsies. *Arch Intern Med* 148:173–176, 1988.

21. Coon W: The spectrum of pulmonary embolism, twenty years later. *Arch Surg* 111:398–402, 1976.

22. Moser K, Auger W, Fedullo P, et al: Chronic thromboembolic pulmonary hypertension: clinical picture and surgical treatment. *Eur Respir J* 5: 334–342, 1992.

23. Arnett N, Basoc J, Macher A, et al: Fibrosing mediastinitis causing pulmonary arterial hypertension without pulmonary venous hypertension. *Am J Med* 63:634–643, 1977.

24. von Herbay A, Iues A, Waldherr R, et al: Pulmonary tumor thrombotic microangiopathy with pulmonary hypertension. *Cancer* 66:587–592, 1990.

25. Fanta C, Compton C: Microscopic tumour emboli to the lungs: A hidden cause of dyspnoea and pulmonary hypertension. *Thorax* 43:794–795, 1979.
26. Heck Jr H, Gross C, Houghton J: Long-term severe pulmonary hypertension associated with right atrial myxoma. *Chest* 102:301–303, 1992.
27. Marvin K, Spellberg R: Pulmonary hypertension secondary to thrombocytosis in a patient with myeloid metaplasia. *Chest* 103:642–644, 1993.
28. Snyder L, Harmon K, Estensen R: Intravascular lymphomatosis (malignant angioendotheliomatosis) presenting as pulmonary hypertension. *Chest* 96:1199, 1989.
29. Shiue S-T, McNally D: Pulmonary hypertension from prominent vascular involvement in diffuse amyloidosis. *Arch Int Med* 148:687–689, 1988.
30. Gomez-Sanchez M, Saenz de la Calzada C, Gomez-Pajuelo C: Clinical and pathological manifestations of pulmonary vascular disease in the toxic oil syndrome. *J Am Coll Cardiol* 18:1539–1545, 1991.
31. Stupi A, Steen V, Owens G, et al: Pulmonary hypertension in the CREST variant of systemic sclerosis. *Arthritis Rheum* 29:515–524, 1986.
32. Ungerer R, Tashkin D, Furst D, et al: Prevalence and clinical correlates of pulmonary arterial hypertension in progressive systemic sclerosis. *Am J Med* 75:65–74, 1983.
33. Yousem S: The pulmonary pathologic manifestations of the CREST syndrome. *Human Pathol* 21:467–474, 1990.
34. Sinclair RA, Antonovych TT, Mostofi FK: Renal proliferative arteriopathies and associated glomerular changes. A light and electron microscopic study. *Hum Pathol* 7:565–573, 1976.
35. Heath D, Smith P, Gosney J, et al: The pathology of the early and late states of primary pulmonary hypertension. *Br Heart J* 58:204–213, 1987.
36. Kahaleh M, Osborn I, LeRoy E: Increased factor VIII/von Willebrand factor antigen and von Willebrand factor activity in scleroderma and in Raynaud phenomenon. *Ann Intern Med* 94:482–484, 1981.
37. Mahowald M, Weir E, Ridley D, et al: Pulmonary hypertension in systemic lupus erythematosus: Effect of vasodilators on pulmonary hemoydynamics. *J Rheumatol* 12:773–777, 1985.
38. Nair S, Askari A, Popelka C, et al: Pulmonary hypertension and systemic lupus erythematosus. *Arch Intern Med* 140:109–111, 1980.
39. Jones M, Osterholm R, Wilson R, et al: Fatal pulmonary hypertension and resolving immune-complex glomerulonephritis in mixed connective tissue disease. *Am J Med* 65:855–863, 1978.
40. Gardner D, Onthie J, Macleod J, et al: Pulmonary hypertension in rheumatoid arthritis. Report of a case with intimal sclerosis of the pulmonary and digital arteries. *Scot Med J* 2:183–185, 1957.
41. Caldwell I, Aitchison J: Pulmonary hypertension in dermatomyositis. *Br Heart J* 18:273–277, 1956.
42. Bunch T, Tancredi R, Lie J: Pulmonary hypertension in polymyositis. *Chest* 79:105–107, 1981.
43. Braman SS, Eby E, Kuhn C, et al: Primary pulmonary hypertension in the elderly. *Arch Intern Med* 151:2433–2438, 1991.
44. Phipps B, Wong B, Chang CHJ, et al: Unexplained severe pulmonary hypertension in the older age group. *Chest* 84:399–402, 1983.
45. Pietra G, Edwards W, Kay J, et al: Histopathology of primary pulmonary hypertension. *Circulation* 80:1198–1206, 1989.
46. Weir E, Archer S, Edwards J: Chronic primary and secondary thromboembolic pulmonary hypertension. *Chest* 93:149S–154S, 1988.

47. Robalino B, Moodie D: Association between primary pulmonary hypertension and portal hypertension: Analysis of its pathophysiology and clinical, laboratory and hemodynamic manifestations. *J Am Coll Cardiol* 17: 492–498, 1991.
48. McDonnell PJ, Toye PA, Hutchins GM: Primary pulmonary hypertension and cirrhosis: Are they related? *Am Rev Respir Dis* 127:437–441, 1983.
49. Edwards B, Weir E, Edwards JEE, et al: Coexistent pulmonary and portal hypertension: Morphologic and clinical features. *J Am Coll Cardiol* 10: 1233–1238, 1987.
50. Wilkinson M, Langhorne C, Heath D, et al: A pathophysiological study of 10 cases of hypoxic cor pumonale. *Quart J Med* 66:65–87, 1988.
51. Oswald-Mammosser M, Apprill M, Bachez P, et al: Pulmonary hemodynamics in chronic obstructive pulmonary disease of the emphysematous type. *Respiration* 58:304–310, 1991.
52. Weitzenblum E, Ehrhart M, Rasaholinjanahary J, et al: Pulmonary hemodynamics in idiopathic pulmonary fibrosis and other interstitial pulmonary diseases. *Respiration* 44:118–127, 1983.
53. Kawakami Y, Kishi F, Yamamoto H, et al: Relation of oxygen delivery, mixed venous oxygenation and pulmonary hemodynamics to prognosis in chronic obstructive pulmonary disease. *N Engl J Med* 308:1045–1049, 1983.
54. Weitzenblum E, Hirth C, Ducolone A, et al: Prognostic value of pulmonary artery pressure in chronic obstructive lung disease. *Thorax* 36:752–758, 1981.
55. Hsieh H, Lee C, Chuang C: Low oxygenation index and pulmonary artery hypertension in predicting early death from adult respiratory distress syndrome (ARDS). *J Form Med Assoc* 89:443–449, 1990.
56. Anand I, Chandrashekhar Y, Ferrari R, et al: Pathogenesis of congestive state in chronic obstructive pulmonary disease. *Circulation* 86:12–21, 1992.
57. Lopez-Barneo J, Lopez-Lopez J, Urena J, et al: Chemotransduction in the carotid body: K+ current modulated by P_{O_2} in type I chemoreceptor cells. *Science* 242:580–582, 1988.
58. Weir E, Archer S: The mechanism of acute hypoxic pulmonary vasoconstriction: The tale of two channels. *FASEB J* 9:183–189, 1995.
59. Yagi H, Yamada H, Kobayashi T, et al: Doppler assessment of pulmonary hypertension induced by hypoxic breathing in subjects susceptible to high altitude pulmonary edema. *Am Rev Respir Dis* 142:796–801, 1990.
60. Honigman B, Theis M, Koziol-McLain J, et al: Acute mountain sickness in a general tourist population at moderate altitudes. *Ann Intern Med* 118:587–592, 1993.
61. Young T, Palta M, Dempsey J, et al: The occurrence of sleep-disordered breathing among middle-aged adults. *N Engl J Med* 328:1230–1235, 1993.
62. Krieger J, Sforza E, Apprill M, et al: Pulmonary hypertension, hypoxemia, and hypercapnia in obstructive sleep apnea patients. *Chest* 96:729–737, 1989.
63. Levi-Valensi P, Weitzenblum E, Rida Z, et al: Sleep-related oxygen desaturation and daytime pulmonary haemodynamics in COPD patients. *Eur Respir J* 5:301–307, 1992.
64. D'Alonzo GE, Bower JS, Dantzker DR: Differentiation of patients with primary and thromboembolic pulmonary hypertension. *Chest* 85: 457–461, 1984.

65. Moser K, Spragg R, Utley J, et al: Chronic thrombotic obstruction of major pulmonary arteries. *Ann Intern Med* 99:299–305, 1983.
66. Moser KM, Daily PO, Peterson K, et al: Thromboendarterectomy for chronic, major-vessel thromboembolic pulmonary hypertension. *Ann Intern Med* 107:560–565, 1987.
67. Moser KM, Daly PO, Peterson KL: Management of chronic unresolved large vessel thromboembolism. In JA Will, CA Dawson, EK Weir, CK Buckner (eds): *The Pulmonary Circulation in Health and Disease.* Orlando, Florida, Academic Press, 1987, pp 533–554.
68. Voekel NF, Reeves JT: Primary pulmonary hypertension. In Lenfant C, Moser K (ed): *Pulmonary Vascular Disease.* New York, Marcel Dekker, 1979.
69. Rich S: Epidemiologic and clinical characteristics of primary pulmonary hypertension. In Will JA, Dawson CA, Weir EK, Buckner CK (ed): *The Pulmonary Circulation in Health and Disease.* Orlando, Florida, Academic Press, 1987, pp 499–509.
70. Lehtonen J, Sutinen S: Electrocardiographic criteria for the diagnosis of right ventricular hypertrophy verified at autopsy. *Chest* 93:839–842, 1988.
71. Viamonte M, Parks RE, Barrera F: Roentgenographic prediction of pulmonary hypertension in mitral stenosis. *Am J Roentgenol* 87:936–947, 1962.
72. Kanemoto N, Furuya H, Etoh T, et al: Chest roentgenograms in primary pulmonary hypertension. *Chest* 76:45–49, 1979.
73. Change CH: The normal roentgenographic measurement of the right descending pulmonary artery in 1085 cases. *Am J Roentgenol* 87:929–935, 1962.
74. Moore N, Scott J, Flower C, et al: The relationship between pulmonary artery pressure and pulmonary artery diameter in pulmonary hypertension. 39:486–489, 1988.
75. Reuben SR, Butler J, Lee GJ: Pulmonary arterial compliance in health and disease. *Br Heart J* 33:147, 1971.
76. Enson Y, Schmidt DH, Ferrer MI, et al: The effect of acutely induced hypervolemia on resistance to pulmonary blood flow and pulmonary arterial complicance in patients with chronic obstructive lung disease. *Am J Med* 57:395–401, 1974.
77. Salvaterra CG, Brundage BH, Rubin LJ: Is the early diagnosis of pulmonary hypertension possible, useful, and cost-effective. In EK Weir, SL Archer, JT Reeves (eds): *The Diagnosis and Treatment of Pulmonary Hypertension.* Mount Kisco, NY, Futura Publishing Company, 1992, pp 3–12.
78. Nanda N, Gramiak R, Robinson T, et al: Echocardiographic evaluation of pulmonary hypertension. *Circulation* 50:575, 1974.
79. Lew W, Karliner J: Assessment of pulmonary valve echogram in normal subjects and in patients with pulmonary arterial hypertension. *Br Heart J* 42:147–161, 1979.
80. Acquatella H, Schiller N, Sharpe D, et al: Lack of correlation between echocardiographic pulmonary valve morphology and simultaneous pulmonary arterial pressure. *Am J Cardiol* 43:946–950, 1979.
81. Okamoto M, Miyatake K, Kinoshite N, et al: Analysis of blood flow in pulmonary hypertension with the pulsed Doppler flowmeter combined with cross-sectional echocardiography. *Br Heart J* 51:407–415, 1984.
82. Park B, Dittrich H, Polikar R, et al: Echocardiographic evidence of pericardial effusion in severe chronic pulmonary hypertension. *Am J Cardiol* 63:143–145, 1989.

83. Bauman W, Wann L, Childress R, et al: Mid systolic notching of the pulmonary valve in the absence of pulmonary hypertension. *Am J Cardiol* 43: 1049–1052, 1979.
84. Tsuda T, Sawayama T, Kawai N, et al: Echocardiographic measurement of right ventricular wall thickness in adults by anterior approach. *Br Heart J* 44:55–61, 1980.
85. Gottdiener J, Gay J, Maron B, et al: Increased right ventricular wall thickness in left ventricular pressure overload: Echocardiographic determination of hypertrophic response of the "nonstressed" ventricle. *J Am Coll Cardiol* 6:550–555, 1985.
86. Levine R, Gibson T, Aretz T, et al: Echocardiographic measurement of right ventricular volume. *Circulation* 69:497–505, 1984.
87. Wilson N, Goldberg SJ, Dickinson DF: Normal intracardiac and great artery blood velocity measurements by pulsed Doppler echocardiography. *Br Heart J* 53:451–458, 1985.
88. Kitabatake A, Inoue M, Asao M, et al: Noninvasive evaluation of pulmonary hypertension by a pulsed Doppler technique. *Circulation* 68: 302–309, 1984.
89. Mahan G, Dabestani A, Gardin J, et al: Estimation of pulmonary artery pressure by pulsed Doppler echocardiography (abstract). *Circulation* 68 (Suppl III):III-367, 1983.
90. Chan K, Currie P, Seward J, et al: Comparison of three Doppler ultrasound methods in the prediction of pulmonary artery pressure. *J Am Coll Cardiol* 9:549–554, 1987.
91. Berger M, Hect S, Van Tosh A, et al: Pulsed and continuous wave Doppler echocardiographic assessment of valvular regurgitation in normal subjects. *J Am Coll Cardiol* 13:1540–1545, 1989.
92. Choong C, Abascal V, Weyman J, et al: Prevalence of valvular regurgitation by Doppler echocardiography in patients with structurally normal hearts by two dimensional echocardiography. *Am Heart J* 117:636–642, 1989.
93. Morrison D, Ovitt T, Hammermeister K, et al: Functional tricuspid regurgitation and right ventricular dysfunction in pulmonary hypertension. *Am J Cardiol* 62:108–112, 1988.
94. Yock P, Popp R: Noninvasive estimation of right ventricular systolic pressure by Doppler ultrasound in patients with tricuspid regurgitation. *Circulation* 70:657–662, 1984.
95. Currie P, Seward J, Chan K-L: Continuous wave Doppler determination of right ventricular pressure: A simultaneous Doppler-catheterization study in 127 patients. *J Am Coll Cardiol* 6:750–756, 1985.
96. Saal A, Otto C, Janko C, et al: Measurement of pulmonary systolic pressure in adults with tricuspid regurgitation using high pulse repetition frequency Doppler (abstract). *Circulation* 70(Suppl II):II-117, 1984.
97. Masuyama T, Kodama K, Kitabatake A, et al: Continuous-wave Doppler echocardiographic detection of pulmonary regurgitation and its application to noninvasive estimation of pulmonary artery pressure. *Circulation* 74:484–492, 1986.
98. Kircher B, Himelman R, Schiller N: Right atrial pressure estimation from respiratory behavior of the inferior vena cava. *Circulation* 78:2196, 1988.
99. Bogren H, Klipstein R, Mohiaddin R, et al: Pulmonary artery distensibility and blood flow patterns: A magnetic resonance study of normal subjects and of patients with pulmonary arterial hypertension. *Am Heart J* 118:990–999, 1989.

100. Cohen HA, Baird MG, Ronleau JR, et al: Thallium-201 myocardial imaging in patients with pulmonary hypertension. *Circulation* 54:790, 1976.
101. Khaja F, Alam M, Goldstein S, et al: Diagnostic value of visualization of the right ventricle using thallium-201 myocardial imaging. *Circulation* 59:182–188, 1979.
102. Rhodes J, Barst R, Garafano R, et al: Hemodynamic correlates of exercise function in patients with primary pulmonary hypertension. *J Am Coll Cardiol* 18:1738–1744, 1991.
103. Brundage B: Exercise testing in primary pulmonary hypertension: A valuable diagnostic tool. *J Am Coll Cardiol* 18:1745, 1991.
104. D'Alonzo GE, Barst RJ, Levy PS: Survival in patients with primary pulmonary hypertension. *Ann Intern Med* 115:343–349, 1991.
105. Moser KM, Fedullo PF, Auger WR: Results of pulmonary thromboendarterectomy for chronic, major-vessel thromboembolic pulmonary hypertension. In EK Weir, SL Archer, JT Reeves (eds): *The Diagnosis and Treatment of Pulmonary Hypertension.* Mount Kisco, N.Y., Futura Publishing Company, 1992, pp 331–329.
106. Child J, Wolfe J, Tashkin D, et al: Fatal lung scan in a case of pulmonary hypertension due to obliterative pulmonary vascular disease. *Chest* 67: 308–309, 1975.
107. Bookstein JJ: Segmental arteriography in pulmonary embolism. *Radiology* 93:1007–1012, 1969.
108. Schrijen F, Jezek V: Hemodynamic and pulmonary wedge angiography findings in chronic bronchopulmonary disease. *Scand J Resp Dis* 58: 151–158, 1977.
109. Rabinovitch M, Keane JF, Fellows KE, et al: Quantitative analysis of the pulmonary wedge angiogram in congenital heart defects: Correlation with hemodynamic data and morphometric findings in lung biopsy tissue. *Circulation* 63:152–164, 1981.
110. Stein P, Athanasoulis C, Alavi A, et al: Complications and validity of pulmonary angiography in acute pulmonary embolism. *Circulation* 85: 462–468, 1992.
111. Shure D, Gregoratos G, Moser KM: Fiberoptic angioscopy: Role in the diagnosis of chronic pulmonary arterial obstruction. *Ann Int Med* 103: 844–850, 1985.
112. Kereiakes D, Herfkens R, Brundage B, et al: Computerized tomography in chronic thromboembolic pulmonary hypertension. *Am Heart J* 106: 1432–1436, 1983.
113. McNee W: The clinical importance of right ventricular function in pulmonary hypertension. In EK Weir, SL Archer, JT Reeves (eds): *The Diagnosis and Treatment of Pulmonary Hypertension.* Mount Kisco, NY., Futura Publishing Company 1992, pp 13–40.
114. Keller CA, Shepard JW, Chun DS, et al: Pulmonary hypertension in obstructive pulmonary disease: Multivariate analysis. *Chest* 90:185–192, 1986.
115. Santini D, Fox D, Kloner RA, et al: Pulmonary hypertension in systemic lupus erythematosus: Hemodynamics and effects of vasodilator therapy. *Clin Cardiol* 3:406–411, 1980.
116. Wiener-Kronish JP, Solinger AM, Warnock ML, et al: Severe pulmonary involvement in mixed connective tissue disease. *Am Rev Resp Dis* 124: 499–503, 1981.
117. Young I, Ford S, Ford P: The association of pulmonary hypertension with rheumatoid arthritis. *J Rheumatol* 16:1266–1269, 1989.

118. Chapman P, Bateman E, Benatar: Prognostic and therapeutic considerations in clinical primary pulmonary hypertension. *Res Med* 84:485–494, 1990.
119. LeRoy E: Pulmonary hypertension: The bete noire of the diffuse connective tissue diseases. *Am J Med* 90:539–540, 1991.
120. Braunwald E, Braunwald N, Ross J, et al: Effects of mitral-valve replacement on the pulmonary vascular dynamics of patients with pulmonary hypertension. *N Engl J Med* 273:509–514, 1965.
121. Khoury G, Hawes C: Primary pulmonary hypertension in children living at high altitude. *J Pediat* 62:177–182, 1963.
122. Eisenberg P, Lucore C, Kaufman L, et al: Fibrinopeptide A levels indicative of pulmonary vascular thrombosis in patients with primary pulmonary hypertension. *Circulation* 82:841–847, 1990.
123. Langleben D, Moroz L, McGregor M, et al: Decreased half-life of fibrinogen in primary pulmonary hypertension. *Thromb Res* 40:577–580, 1985.
124. Wagenvoort C, Wagenvoort N: A pathologic study of the lung vessels in 156 clinically diagnosed cases. *Circulation* 42:1163–1184, 1970.
125. Fuster V, Steele P, Edwards W, et al: Primary pulmonary hypertension: Natural history and the importance of thrombosis. *Circulation* 70: 580–587, 1984.
126. Rich S, Kaufmann E, Levy P: The effect of high doses of calcium-channel blockers on survival in primary pulmonary hypertension. *N Engl J Med* 327:76–81, 1992.
127. Landefeld C, Goldman L: Major bleeding in outpatients treated with warfarin: incidence and prediction by factors known at the start of outpatient therapy. *Am J Med* 87:144–152, 1989.
128. Gurwitz J, Avorn J, Ross-Degnan D, et al: Aging and the anticoagulant response to warfarin therapy. *Ann Intern Med* 116:901–904, 1992.
129. Hirsh J, Dalen J, Deykin D, et al: Oral anticoagulants: Mechanism of action, clinical effectiveness, and optimal therapeutic range. *Chest* 102: 312S–326S, 1992.
130. Mader S, Josephson K, Rubenstein L: Low prevalence of postural hypotension among community-dwelling elderly. *JAMA* 258:1511–1514, 1987.
131. Palevsky H, Schloo B, Pietra G, et al: Vascular structure, morphometry, and responsiveness to vasodilator agents. *Circulation* 80:1207–1221, 1989.
132. Weir E, Rubin L, Ayres S: The acute administration of vasodilators in primary pulmonary hypertension. *Am Rev Respir Dis* 140:1623–1630, 1989.
133. Rubin L, Groves B, Reeves J, et al: Prostacyclin-induced pulmonary vasodilatation in primary pulmonary hypertension. *Circulation* 66:334–338, 1982.
134. Jones K, Higenbottam T, Wallwork J: Pulmonary vasodilation with prostacyclin in primary and secondary pulmonary hypertension. *Chest* 96: 784–789, 1989.
135. Halpern S, Shah P, Lehrman S, et al: Prostaglandin E1 as a screening vasodilator in primary pulmonary hypertension. *Chest* 92:686–691, 1987.
136. Morgan J, McCormack D, Griffiths M, et al: Adenosine as a vasodilator in primary pulmonary hypertension. *Circulation* 84:1145–1149, 1991.
137. Palevsky H, Long W, Crow J, et al: Prostacyclin and acetylcholine as screening agents for acute pulmonary vasodilator responsiveness in primary pulmonary hypertension. *Circulation* 82:2018–2026, 1990.

138. Pepke Z, Higerbottan T, Dirk-Xuan A, et al: Inhaled nitric oxide as a cause of selective pulmonary vasodilatation in pulmonary hypertension. *Lancet* 338:1173–1174, 1991.
139. Schrader B, Inbar S, Kaufmann L, et al: Comparison of the effects of adenosine and nifedipine in pulmonary hypertension. *J Am Coll Cardiol* 19:1060–1064, 1992.
140. Inbar S, Schrader B, Kaufmann E, et al: Effects of adenosine in combination with calcium channel blockers in patients with primary pulmonary hypertension. *J Am Coll Cardiol* 21:413–418, 1993.
141. Rich S, Kaufmann E: High dose titration of calcium channel blocking agents for primary pulmonary hypertension: Guidelines for short-term drug testing. *J Am Coll Cardiol* 18:1323–1327, 1991.
142. Reeves J, Groves B, Turkevich D: The case for treatment of selected patients with primary pulmonary hypertension. *Am Rev Respir Dis* 134: 342–346, 1986.
143. Jones D, Higenbottam T, Wallwork J: Treatment of primary pulmonary hypertension with intravenous epoprosternol (prostacyclin). *Br Heart J* 57:270–278, 1987.
144. Barst R, Rubin L, Long W, et al: A comparison of continuous intravenous epoprostenol (prostacyclin) with conventional therapy for primary pulmonary hypertension. *N Engl J Med* 334:296–301, 1996.
145. McLaughlin V, Genthner D, Panella M, et al: Reduction in pulmonary vascular resistance with long-term epoprostenol (protacyclin) therapy in primary pulmonary hypertension. *N Engl J Med* 338:273–277, 1998.
146. Olschewski H, Walmrath D, Schermuly R, et al: Aerosolized prostacyclin and iloprost in severe pulmonary hypertension. *Ann Int Med* 124: 820–824, 1996.
147. Frist W, Carmichael L, Loyd J, et al: Transplantation for pulmonary hypertension. *Transplantation Proceedings* 25:1159–1161, 1993.
148. Horvath K, DiSesa V, Peigh P, et al: Favorable results of coronary artery bypass grafting in patients older than 75 years. *J Thorac Cardiovasc Surg* 99:92–96, 1990.
149. Lessof M, Evans J, Joy M, et al: Cardiological intervention in elderly patients. *J Royal Coll Physicians London* 25:197–205, 1991.
150. Goldstein R, Wolt ATS: Lung transplantation. *Am Thoracic Society* 147: 772–776, 1993.
151. Daily P, Dembitzky W, Iversen S, et al: Current early results of pulmonary thromboendarterectomy for chronic pulmonary embolism. *Eur J Cardiothorac Surg* 4:117–123, 1990.
152. Palla A, Formichi B, Morales A, et al: Follow-up of patients affected by chronic thromboembolic pulmonary hypertension: Clinical and functional features. *Eur Respir J* 5(Suppl 15):40s, 1992.
153. Halkin H, Goldberg J, Modan M: Reduction of mortality in general medical in-patients by low-dose heparin prophylaxis. *Ann Intern Med* 96: 561–565, 1982.
154. Collins R, Scrimgeour A, Yusuf S: Reduction in fatal pulmonary embolism and venous thrombosis by perioperative administration of subcutaneous heparin: Overview of results of randomized trials in general, orthopedic, and urologic surgery. *N Engl J Med* 318:1162–1173, 1988.
155. St. John Sutton M, Tajik A, McGoon D: Atrial septal defect in patients ages 60 years or older: Operative results and long-term postoperative follow-up. *Circulation* 64:402–409, 1981.

156. Steele P, Fuster V, Cohen M, et al: Isolated atrial septal defect with pulmonary vascular obstructive disease: Long-term follow-up and prediction of outcome after surgical correction. *Circulation* 76:1037–1042, 1987.
157. Murphy J, Gersh B, Phil D, et al: Long-term outcome after surgical repair of isolated atrial septal defect. *N Engl J Med* 323:1645–1650, 1990.
158. Naeije R: Should pulmonary hypertension be treated in chronic obstructive pulmonary disease. In EK Weir, SL Archer, JT Reeves (eds): *The Diagnosis and Treatment of Pulmonary Hypertension.* Mount Kisco, NY, Futura Publishing Company, 1992, pp 209–239.
159. Stuart-Harris C, Bishop J, Clark T, et al: Long term domiciliary oxygen therapy in chronic hypoxic cor pulmonale complicating chronic bronchitis and emphysema. *Lancet* 28:681–685, 1981.
160. Timms R, Khaja F, Williams G: Hemodynamic response to oxygen therapy in chronic obstructive pulmonary disease. *Ann Intern Med* 102:29–36, 1985.
161. Weitzenblum E, Oswald M, Mirhom R, et al: Evolution of pulmonary haemodynamics in COLD patients under long-term oxygen therapy. *Eur Respir J* 7:669s–673s, 1989.
162. Wright J, Petty T, Thurlbeck W: Analysis of the structure of the muscular pulmonary arteries in patients with pulmonary hypertension and COPD: National Institutes of Health nocturnal oxygen therapy trial. *Lung* 170:109–124, 1992.
163. Radermacher P, Santak B, Wust H, et al: Prostacyclin for the treatment of pulmonary hypertension in the adult respiratory distress syndrome: Effects on pulmonary capillary pressure and ventilation-perfusion distributions. *Anesthesiology* 72:238–244, 1990.
164. Silverman H, Slotman G, Bone R, et al: Effects of prostaglandin E1 on oxygen delivery and consumption in patients with the adult respiratory distress syndrome. *Chest* 98:405–410, 1990.
165. Rossaint R, Falke K, Lopez F, et al: Inhaled nitric oxide for the adult respiratory distress syndrome. *N Engl J Med* 328:399–405, 1993.

Chapter 8

Diagnosis of Valve Disease in the Elderly

Stephen L. Archer, Elliot Chesler

Valve disease is the third most frequently cause of congestive heart failure in the elderly, exceeded in prevalence only by myocardial ischemia and systemic hypertension. The clinical presentation of valve disease in the elderly is strikingly different to that of the young.[1] Among the elderly, valve disease is often a mosaic composed of infective endocarditis, hypertensive and ischemic cardiomyopathy, amyloidosis and even congenital malformation, whereas in the young, valve disease is usually isolated and the diagnosis straightforward. Also, the assessment of valve disease in the elderly is complicated by the concurrence of other medical disorders, such as chronic lung disease and cancer, and effects of "normal" cardiovascular aging. Clinical examination is important, but because of limitations to be described, there should be little hesitation in turning to echocardiography for assistance in the diagnosis of valvular lesions, assessment of their hemodynamic severity and evaluation of left ventricular function.

Difficulties in Assessment of Elderly Patients with Valvular Disease

History

The goal of history taking is to accurately assess overall functional capacity and estimate the extent to which cardiac disease impinges on

From *Clinical Cardiology in the Elderly. Second Edition,* edited by Elliot Chesler. © 1999, Futura Publishing Company, Armonk, NY.

the lifestyle of the elderly. Unfortunately, many elderly patients have a long history of multiple diseases and are often unable to provide an accurate chronological account of their various symptoms. Frequently, symptoms characteristic of cardiac disorder are obfuscated by nonspecific complaints and poor chronology, which makes diagnostic and therapeutic decisions difficult.

General Medical Conditions

Other diseases frequently coexist and require careful assessment:

Chronic Obstructive Pulmonary Disease

Chronic obstructive pulmonary disease frustrates precordial palpation and cardiac auscultation. Also, therapeutic problems arise when there is the combination of emphysema and cardiac disease. For example, bronchospasm may be induced by β-adrenergic inhibitors, whereas cardiac dysrhythmias may be precipitated by aminophylline. Emphysema is an important cause of morbidity and mortality in the elderly and may preclude operation in otherwise suitable candidates for valve replacement.

Chronic Renal Disease

Serum creatinine levels may be misleading in the elderly. Creatinine clearance declines with age and there may be renal impairment despite only mild elevation of the serum creatinine level. When the serum creatinine exceeds 1.5 mg/dL it is probably advisable to institute prophylactic hydration prior to cardiac catheterization.

Fluid overload due to renal disease may be erroneously diagnosed as congestive heart failure. The risk for cardiac surgery may be prohibitive when renal insufficiency is severe. Fluid overload may also complicate chronic hepatic cirrhosis.

Medications

The importance of an accurate account of the patient's medications deserves emphasis. Sodium retention and exacerbation of congestive cardiac failure may be precipitated by nonsteroidal anti-inflammatory drugs (NSAIDs) that are so frequently used for arthritis. Digitalis-toxic dysrhythmias may be induced by overdiuresis and addition of quinidine. Metformin may precipitate fatal lactic acidosis in diabetic patients with impaired renal function who receive a dye load during diagnostic angiography.

Thyrotoxicosis

The usual presentation is one of atrial fibrillation and heart failure without the typical ocular or other systemic manifestations. Absence of adrenergic signs may result in so called "apathetic" thyrotoxicosis of the elderly in which patients may present with fatigue, weight loss and atrial fibrillation. Thyrotropin (TSH) levels should routinely be measured in elderly patients with new onset atrial fibrillation. In the elderly, as in the young, hyperthyroidism is diagnosed by documenting an elevation of thyroxine (T_4) or depression of the TSH levels.

Clinical Presentation

Incidental Murmur

A frequent mode of presentation of valve disease in the elderly is when, at routine examination, a cardiac murmur is encountered. Some degree of senile sclerosis of the aortic valve is common among people above age 65 years and therefore, an aortic ejection systolic murmur is almost universal. The clinical distinction between aortic stenosis and aortic sclerosis is difficult but important since aortic stenosis is the most common form of valve disease requiring operation (Figure 1).

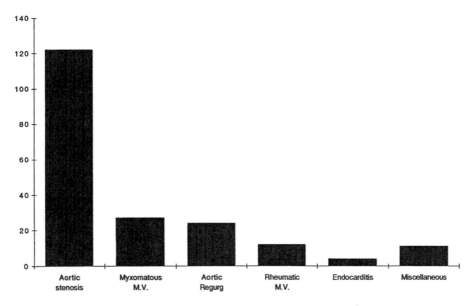

Figure 1: *Pathology of valve disease in 200 patients undergoing valve surgery at the Minneapolis, Veterans Administration Medical Center 1987–1990.*

Typically, the murmur in aortic sclerosis has an early peak and the second heart sound is normal whereas in severe aortic stenosis the murmur peaks in mid-late systole and the second heart sound is muted or absent. A holosystolic murmur resulting from various causes of mitral regurgitation is also a frequent finding. Aortic diastolic murmurs are less frequent and are a result of valvular regurgitation or ascending aortic aneurysm.

Heart Failure

Without a Murmur. Because 40% of cases of infective endocarditis involve normal valves, heart failure due to endocarditis may supervene without a murmur. Also, when aortic valve endocarditis results in sudden valve perforation, a pre-existing aortic diastolic murmur may disappear when there is sudden equalization of aortic diastolic and left ventricular end-diastolic pressures. Even in the absence of endocarditis, an aortic ejection systolic murmur may diminish in intensity or disappear when heart failure supervenes in a case of critical aortic stenosis.

With a Murmur. The more frequent causes of heart failure with a systolic murmur are: (1) aortic valve stenosis; (2) severe mitral regurgitation after spontaneous or infective rupture of the chordae; and (3) rheumatic mitral regurgitation. When the murmur is diastolic the usual cause is aortic regurgitation.

Syncope

Transient alteration of consciousness (presyncope) progressing to effort syncope occurs in about one third of symptomatic patients with aortic stenosis. However, syncope and near-syncope are common in the elderly without heart disease and the etiology is usually multifactorial.

Dysrhythmias

Atrial fibrillation is the most frequent dysrhythmia complicating valve disease. It may occur in severe mitral regurgitation of any cause. It is an ominous complication in severe aortic stenosis and may portend the development of congestive heart failure.

Cardiac Examination

Jugular Venous Pressure. The jugular venous pressure cannot be estimated from the external jugular veins because they are frequently kinked at their junction with the subclavian vessels. Similarly, the left innominate vein is often compressed by the aortic arch. Therefore, only the right internal jugular vein is reliable.[2]

Arterial Pulses

Slowing of the carotid upstroke in young patients is a reliable clinical sign of aortic stenosis. Among the elderly with severe aortic stenosis, however, the carotid upstroke is deceptively brisk because of diminished vascular compliance. External carotid pulse recordings have shown that the maximum rate of rise of the carotid pulse in elderly subjects is approximately 1270 mm Hg/sec, whereas for the young it is 920 mm Hg/sec. Among elderly patients with aortic stenosis, the maximum rate of rise falls to within the range for normal young so that the upstroke of the pulse feels normal; the classic "anacrotic" pulse is very unusual in the elderly.[3]

Auscultation

Ejection Systolic Murmurs: Aortic. The murmur of aortic stenosis is often heard best in the second right intercostal space, but it is not at all unusual to hear it best at the apex and left sternal border.[4] Typically, it is harsh but it may be musical or rasping so that even the most accomplished auscultator may have difficulty in distinguishing it from the murmurs of mitral regurgitation or hypertrophic cardiomyopathy. Loss of the aortic component of the second heart sound is a specific but insensitive sign of severe aortic stenosis.

Hypertrophic Cardiomyopathy. Hypertrophic cardiomyopathy is not infrequent in the elderly and may present with congestive heart failure, angina or syncope. Usually, a harsh ejection systolic murmur is best heard at the left sternal border in the left third intercostal space. As in the young the murmur may be confused with that of mitral regurgitation, which complicates hypertrophic cardiomyopathy in about one third of cases.[5]

Mitral Systolic Murmurs

Mitral Annular Calcification. Mitral annular calcification increases in prevalence with age and is more frequent in women. Mitral regurgitation is a result of splinting and distortion of the posterior mitral leaflet and failure of the rigid annulus to reduce its circumference in systole. Usually, regurgitation is mild and manifested by a soft holosystolic murmur localized at the apex.

Mitral Valve Prolapse

When mitral valve prolapse results from a myxomatous valve the presentation in the elderly may differ from that in the young in that the classic midsystolic click and late systolic murmur are infrequent. Because myxomatous degeneration is more severe the leaflets prolapse freely and the regurgitant orifice is large. Consequently, the leaflets are not restrained and do not "billow" so that the click caused by sudden arrest of superior leaflet excursion is absent. Among the elderly the murmur of mitral prolapse is usually holosystolic, rather than late or mid systolic, as in the young. The intensity and character of the murmur is variable but is best heard at the apex or left mid precordium when regurgitation is mild. Particularly in elderly men, however, mitral regurgitation may be severe and occasionally catastrophic when the chordae rupture.

When rupture of chordae tendinae complicates a myxomatous mitral valve the clinical picture may easily be confused with that of aortic stenosis. When chordae to the posterior leaflet rupture, the regurgitant jet is often directed anteriorly, striking the atrial septum adjacent to the aortic root so that the systolic murmur, like that of aortic stenosis, may be loudest in the second right intercostal space. When chordae to the anterior leaflet rupture, the regurgitant jet is directed to the posterior wall of the left atrium and the murmur is transmitted to the spine, or even the occiput. With both types of rupture, the systolic murmur is usually crescendo-decrescendo and terminates before the aortic component of the second heart sound. A third heart sound is common, the first heart sound is of normal or increased intensity and a mid diastolic murmur absent.

Rheumatic Mitral Regurgitation

Because there is thickening, shortening of leaflets, and some degree of commissural fusion in rheumatic mitral regurgitation, the auscultatory findings are quite different from those of mitral regurgitation complicating a myxomatous mitral valve. The first heart sound is soft, the holosystolic murmur ends after the second heart sound and there is a long rumbling mid-diastolic murmur.

Papillary Muscle Dysfunction

The papillary muscles are prone to dysfunction when they, and the contiguous left ventricular wall are affected by ischemia. The posterior papillary muscle (supplied by the posterior descending branch of the right coronary artery) is more commonly involved than the anterior papillary muscle. Varying degrees of mitral regurgitation may result.

When mild, the regurgitant murmur is late systolic and may mimic that of mitral valve prolapse; when more severe it is holosystolic and has to be differentiated from other causes of mitral regurgitation. These murmurs are common: some degree of mitral regurgitation occurs in approximately 30% of patients having coronary artery bypass surgery, most of which are a result of papillary muscle dysfunction.[6] While mitral regurgitation is common in the elderly patient with ischemic heart disease, it is usually mild and does not require mitral valve repair or replacement. Decisions regarding operative management of moderately severe, to severe lesions should be made on a case-by-case basis.

The clinical differentiation between aortic stenosis, mitral regurgitation and hypertrophic cardiomyopathy may be taxing in the young but can usually be resolved with the assistance of noninvasive maneuvers. However, these maneuvers are of limited value in the elderly who are frequently unable to cooperate with the Valsalva maneuver, inhalation of amyl nitrite, or rapid change from the standing to the squatting position. Furthermore, these maneuvers are of no help in differentiating between the murmurs of aortic sclerosis and aortic stenosis. Because even the milder forms of aortic sclerosis have some pressure gradient, the response to maneuvers is the same as that for aortic stenosis: that is both become louder with amyl nitrite and squatting and both soften with Valsalva maneuver and isometric hand grip.

The murmur of MVP may be confused with that of hypertrophic cardiomyopathy because both murmurs increase in intensity and duration with standing and decrease with squatting. However, the murmur of hypertrophic cardiomyopathy becomes louder following amyl nitrite inhalation whereas that of mitral regurgitation does not.

Electrocardiogram

The electrocardiogram may be difficult to interpret because nonspecific ST-T abnormalities are common and normal values for the elderly have not been clearly defined. Age-specific criteria for left ventricular hypertrophy are not available. Voltage in the limb and precordial leads decreases with age itself and because of coexistent emphysema. There is an increase in frequency of ectopic beats, prolongation of the P-R and Q-T intervals, bundle branch blocks, left fascicular blocks and pacemaker-induced left bundle branch block. Both emphysema and left anterior hemiblock are associated with poor R wave progression in the precordial leads which may falsely suggest a diagnosis of anterior myocardial infarction. The most frequent abnormalities are non-specific ST segment-T wave changes that result from hypokalemia or effects of digitalis, diuretics, antidepressants, and antidysrhythmic drugs.

The cumulative effect of these abnormalities deprives the electrocardiogram of some of its sensitivity and specificity in the elderly. For example, it is not unusual to encounter patients with critical aortic stenosis whose electrocardiogram shows normal voltage and nonspecific ST-T wave changes.

Chest X-Ray

In the absence of kyphoscoliosis, the chest x-ray may provide useful information about heart size and enlargement of specific chambers. Severe emphysema often prevents assessment of pulmonary venous hypertension. Among the young, poststenotic dilatation of the ascending aorta is a useful confirmatory sign of valvular aortic stenosis, even though it does not predict its severity; it is absent in hypertrophic cardiomyopathy. This radiological sign is of limited, if any value among the elderly because of the frequency of senile dilatation of the ascending aorta (see Chapter 1). It is important to distinguish between calcification of the mitral annulus and calcification of the aortic and mitral valvular leaflets. The absence of aortic valve calcification usually excludes severe aortic stenosis; when present it is of little value in distinguishing between calcific aortic sclerosis and significant aortic stenosis.

Echocardiography

Transthoracic echocardiography (TTE) greatly enhances the sensitivity and specificity of clinical examination in the diagnosis of valve disease in adults. In a study which compared echocardiography with physical examination (performed by a panel of experienced cardiologists), echocardiography made fewer diagnostic errors and was much more useful than clinical examination in determining the type of surgery needed. In fact, echocardiography was as accurate as cardiac catheterization in this study. [7] The incremental diagnostic gain from echocardiography is greatest for mitral and aortic stenosis (28% and 19%, respectively) and least for mitral regurgitation, where physical examination is excellent. [7] The ability to accurately measure pulmonary artery systolic pressure by Doppler echocardiography may obviate the need for right heart catheterization in some patients. The advent of transesophageal echocardiography is a major advance in diagnosis. It is particularly valuable for assessing whether valve replacement or repair is the better procedure for treating mitral regurgitation.

Changes in Echocardiographic Findings with Age

Valve Thickness

There are many changes in the heart that occur with age, including increases in heart weight and chamber dimensions. The mitral and aortic valves roughly double in thickness between 30 and 60 years of age.[8] The thickness of the cardiac valves, at autopsy, is unrelated to gender or heart size. Anticipation of gradual thickening and calcification of the senescent valve prevents false diagnosis of vegetations and valve stenosis. Patients under age 70 with aortic stenosis are most likely to have a calcified bicuspid valve; while those over age 70 usually have senile calcification of a trileaflet valve.[9] Among the elderly, rheumatic disease accounts for less than 20% of all aortic stenosis.

Changes in Doppler

Perhaps as a consequence of gradual thickening or "sclerosis" of left heart valves, there is a gradual decrease in aortic, but not pulmonic flow velocity with age. The pulmonic valve appears relatively free from the degenerative changes of normal aging. For normal individuals, age 21 to 30 years, aortic flow velocity is 93 ± 11 cm/s, as compared with 65 ± 12 cm/s for those age 61 to 70 years.[10] Valvular insufficiency is also more prevalent with age. Zavitsanos et al[11] studied 628 octogenarians and found mitral regurgitation in 61% (significant in 15%), aortic regurgitation in 51% (significant in 13%), and tricuspid regurgitation in 24% (significant in 6%) of subjects. These authors acknowledged the difficulty in distinguishing between disease as opposed to the natural consequence of aging. In a pulsed-Doppler study of normal individuals age 40 to 90 years, Akasaka[12] found that regurgitation increased in prevalence from age 50 years onward and was universal among octogenarians. The high prevalence of mild valvular insufficiency has been termed "Doppler disease" by some, indicating its lack of prognostic import. Judgment is required in interpreting and reporting mild or trace valve insufficiency in the elderly.

Diastolic filling of the left ventricle, measured as a ratio of peak atrial/early flow transmitral velocities (A/E ratio) also changes with age. The A/E ratio was 1.1 ± 0.3 in 10 healthy individuals age 62 to 73 years versus 0.5 ± 0.2 in 10 adults age 21 to 32 years ($P < 0.0001$).[13] The relative increase in velocity of the A wave is independent of sex, body size, left ventricular mass, blood pressure or heart rate.[13] Kitzmen et al[13] considered that altered diastolic flow may be a "primary biological effect of aging." An increased A/E ratio among the elderly is so frequent that diastolic dysfunction may almost be a "normal" variant.

Aortic Stenosis

Echocardiography measures mean gradient, valve area and left ventricular function. Otto and Pearlman[14] showed that echocardiography permits noninvasive determination of the need for aortic valve replacement with good sensitivity (98%) and specificity (89%). Furthermore, the echocardiogram is sufficiently reproducible to permit serial measurements of aortic valve area and left ventricular function, so that cardiac catheterization is deferred until the time of valve replacement and can usually be restricted to coronary angiography.

Measurement of Aortic Valve Gradient

The traditional method for measuring the transvalvular gradient in aortic stenosis is cardiac catheterization. This technique, whether accomplished by retrograde or transseptal catheterization or left ventricular puncture is time consuming, and risky. Patients with severe aortic stenosis have a much higher mortality (1%) from cardiac catheterization than the average patient undergoing diagnostic coronary angiography (<0.1%).

The echocardiographic technique for measuring transvalvular gradient based on the Bernoulli equation is widely accepted. [15] A continuous wave Doppler beam is directed across the aortic valve, often guided by both the two-dimensional image and a color Doppler representation of the stenotic jet. When the Doppler beam is parallel to the jet, a well-defined Doppler "envelope" is obtained (Figures 2 through 4). Color-guided Doppler greatly enhances the ease and accuracy of measuring-

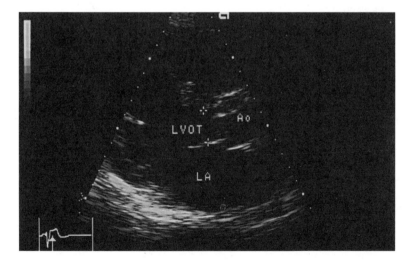

Figure 2: *Calculation of aortic valve area using continuity equation. A: Diameter of left ventricular outflow tract (LVOT) is measured in long axis parasternal view from anterior aspect of mitral leaflet to adjacent left ventricular aspect of ventricular septum. Area of the LVOT, calculated as $\pi r2$, was 3.3 cm^2. Ao, aorta; LA, left atrium.*

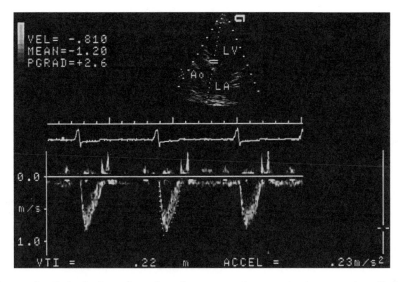

Figure 3: *Calculation of aortic valve area using continuity equation. Pulsed-Doppler measurements of subvalvular velocity, apical view. Velocity time integral (VTI) is 0.22 m.*

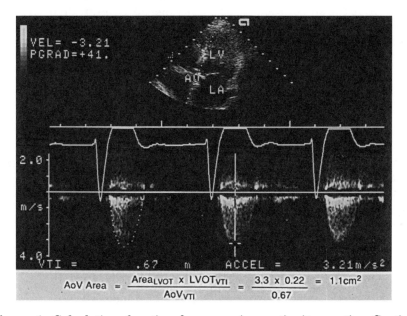

Figure 4: *Calculation of aortic valve area using continuity equation. Continuous wave Doppler measurement of transvalvular VTI = 0.67 m. Valve area is calculated using the continuity equation:* $\text{Area}_{AoV} = (\text{Area}_{LVOT} \times \text{LVOT}_{VTI}) / \text{AoV}_{VTI}$.

Table 1
Useful Formulae for Assessment of Valve Disease in the Elderly

Aortic Valve Area (Area$_{AoV}$)	$\text{Area}_{AoV} = \dfrac{\pi r^2 \times \text{VTI}_{LVOT}}{\text{VTI}_{AOV}}$
Continuity Equation	
Bernoulli's Equation†	$\Delta P = \frac{1}{2}\rho \times (V_2^2 - V_1^2)$
Mitral Valve Area MVA (cm^2)	$\text{MVA} = \dfrac{220}{\text{Pressure Halftime}_{(milliseconds)}}$
Pressure Half-time Method	
Pulmonary Artery Pressure (mm Hg)	$\text{PA systolic} = 4 \times V_{TR}^2 + \text{RA pressure}$
Modified Bernoulli's Equation	

VTI: velocity time integral; AoV: aortic valve; LVOT: left ventricular outflow tract; ΔP: pressure difference between chambers; V_2 and V_1: the velocities across and proximal to a stenotic valve; ρ: the mass density of blood (1.09×10^3 kg/m^3); if V_1 is negligible, relative to V_2, the equation is modified to: DP = $4V^2$; and †: in clinical practice, V_1 and blood viscosity are usually ignored, making the Bernoulli equation $\Delta P = 4V_2$.

the transaortic gradient by facilitating parallel alignment of the Doppler signal to the stenotic jet.[16] To reliably measure the gradient in aortic stenosis the valve must be interrogated from multiple windows. The maximal jet will usually be obtained from the apical or right parasternal views.

The Bernoulli equation is used to measure the aortic valve gradient (Table 1). The equation is used in modified form, eliminating subvalvular velocities, since these are usually close to 1m/s and do not impact on the calculated gradient. Among patients with high velocity flow in the left ventricular out-flow tract (LVOT) the LVOT velocity (V1) is subtracted from the transvalvular gradient (V2) to avoid overestimating the degree of valvular obstruction (Table 1). Otto et al[17] proposed a simple ratio of the velocity time integrals of LVOT to transaortic Doppler signals, as a measure of aortic stenosis. In their population (mean age 67 years) a ratio of velocity time integrals in the LVOT/aortic valve of <0.3 had a sensitivity of 97% for an aortic valve area of <1.0 cm^2.[17]

Doppler gradients correlate well with simultaneous catheter data (r = 0.93).[18] Initially, echocardiography equipment lacked the software to measure mean aortic gradient. This led to considerable confusion since echocardiographers reported peak instantaneous gradients (4V2), that were much greater than peak-to-peak or mean gradients measured by cardiac catheterization. The mean gradient is obtained by integrating the Doppler envelope throughout systole, a function now performed by software in virtually all ultrasound machines.

Gradients in Prosthetic Aortic Valves

Although the Bernoulli equation is applicable to prosthetic valves, there are several caveats. Local gradients and "pressure recovery" may cause overestimation of the net transvalvular gradient. Prosthetic valves have variable orifice velocity profiles and localized high gradients may be present in portions of the orifice that do not represent the net transvalvular gradient.[19] Local gradients may produce good quality, continuous wave Doppler signals which do not reflect the true, average transvalvular gradient.

Flow velocity is maximal in the prosthetic orifice and diminishes in the ascending aorta. The supravalvular decrease in flow velocities is associated with a rise in aortic pressure and thus a decrease in the transvalvular gradient (pressure recovery). Pressure recovery and localized gradients potentially cause overestimation of aortic gradients in Starr-Edwards and St. Jude valves; but these factors are rarely problematic in Hancock and Hall-Medtronic aortic prostheses.[20] Inaccurate estimation of gradient is sporadic, even in Starr-Edwards valves. We use fluoroscopy and transesophageal echocardiography (TEE) to demonstrate normal leaflet or poppet motion in cases where the Doppler suggests prosthetic obstruction but there is conflict with the clinical findings.

Calculation of Aortic Valve Area

Planimetry. Planimetry of the aortic valve area is rarely possible using transthoracic echocardiograms because of poor image quality, reverberation of echoes from calcific deposits and irregularity of the valve edges. This is particularly true in the case of senile aortic sclerosis where there is deposition of large masses of calcium in the cusps without commissural fusion. These deposits obscure leaflet motion and coaptation. However, much higher resolution is provided by TEE and it is often possible to planimeter the valve area.[21] To measure valve area by planimetry the aortic valve is imaged in the basal short axis view and leaflet excursion is reviewed in a cine loop.

Continuity Equation. Pressure and flow are the two major variables needed to estimate valve area, using the Gorlin formula in the catheterization laboratory, or the Doppler-based continuity equation (Figures 2 through 4) The continuity equation utilizes a Doppler estimate of flow and assumes that flow above and below the aortic valve is conserved (Table 1). Oh et al[22] showed that the continuity and Gorlin equations calculation of aortic valve area correlated well in 100 patients with aortic stenosis ($r = 0.8$). These authors concluded that among their elderly population (mean age 71 years), "cardiac catheterization will yield little additional information regarding patient management decisions."

Our practice is to perform echocardiography in every patient with suspected aortic stenosis prior to cardiac catheterization. When the echocardiogram shows severe aortic stenosis, and particularly when fluoroscopy demonstrates significant aortic valve calcification, catheterization of the left ventricle is avoided and the investigation is restricted to coronary angiography.

There are however, a number of problems associated with the continuity equation. The assumption that the LVOT area can be measured using the formula for the area of a circle (Table 1) may not always be true. More importantly, the elderly often have coexistent lung disease, making accurate measurement of the diameter of the LVOT difficult. Most men (age 60 years or more) have a LVOT diameter of 1.8–2.2 cm. Values that depart from this should be regarded with suspicion and careful attention paid to image quality and angulation when measurements are disparate. Small errors in measuring LVOT diameter result in large errors in calculation of valve area.

The continuity equation must also be used with caution in patients with small gradients and diminished left ventricular systolic performance, a situation encountered frequently among the elderly. Such patients are often found to have critical aortic stenosis, by continuity equation and Gorlin formula but may not have severe obstruction at operation. It may be that the continuity equation calculates the functional orifice of the valve, rather than the potential maximal orifice achieved by mechanical distention during systole. To address this problem some authors have advocated using dobutamine infusion at the time of echocardiography to transiently increase cardiac output. The echocardiographer should be circumspect in reporting critical aortic stenosis with peak velocities less than 3 m/sec and mean gradients less than 20 mm Hg.

Aortic Insufficiency

Several parameters are available for evaluation of severity of aortic regurgitation.

Color Flow

There are many criteria for the quantitation of aortic insufficiency by color Doppler, including measurement of length, breadth and area of the jet. The best criteria appears to be the echocardiographer's "overall" interpretation, which considers all these parameters. The single best measurement appears to be the width of the aortic insufficiency (AI) jet relative to that of the LVOT. Jets that occupy less than 24% or more

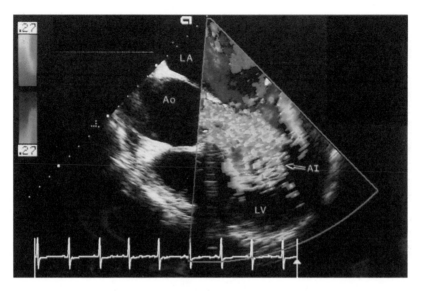

Figure 5: *Quantitating aortic insufficiency with TEE. Two-dimensional four-chamber view shows turbulent mosaic jet of aortic insufficiency (AI) filling entire LVOT. Ao: aorta; LV: left ventricle; LA: left atrium.*

than 65% of the LVOT are indicative of mild and severe AI, respectively.[23] We use the Q mode or color M-mode to measure the width of the jet relative to the LVOT (Figures 5 through 7). Once the long-axis parasternal image is optimized to demonstrate AI, the M-mode cursor is positioned perpendicular to the jet. The graphic display of diastolic turbulence is readily interpreted.

Acute AI

Premature closure of the mitral valve in diastole, before onset of the QRS complex,[24] and a short pressure half-time are reliable signs of sudden, severe AI. In these patients, echocardiography may be crucial as the murmur of AI may be absent and the patient too unstable for aortography.

Chronic Aortic Insufficiency

The diastolic slope of the continuous wave Doppler envelope is related to the severity of aortic insufficiency. Grayburn et al[25] found that slopes greater than 3 m/sec^2 correlated well with severe (3–4+) AI on aortography. However, this criterion is specific but insensitive, because many patients with severe, chronic AI have flat slopes (<2 m/sec^2).[25]

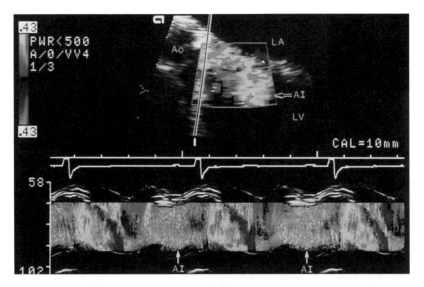

Figure 6: *Quantitating aortic insufficiency with TEE. Upper: Color M-mode Doppler shows M-mode cursor aligned across jet of AI. Lower: M-mode representation of AI jet (indicated by arrows) permits rapid determination of width of jet, relative to width of LVOT. In this case, the jet fills the entire LVOT, consistent with severe AI.*

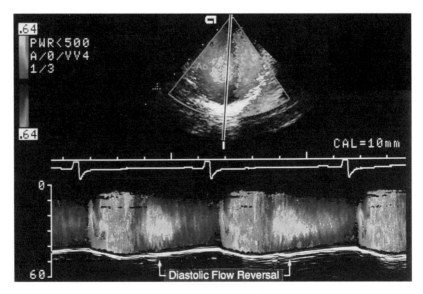

Figure 7: *Quantitating aortic insufficiency with TEE. Color Doppler M-mode of transverse aortic arch showing retrograde diastolic flow, consistent with severe AI.*

Most laboratories use the pressure half time, rather than the slope, as an indicator of the severity of AI. Although some laboratories consider this parameter quite reliable, we have found that severe chronic AI in elderly patients frequently occurs with a prolonged half-time (>500 m/sec). With aging, the left ventricle becomes less compliant as indicated by a decrease in ratio of the velocities of passive to active atrial filling. (E/A ratio).[13,26] Individuals with a decreased E/A ratio (< 1) tend to have artificially shortened $T_{1/2}$.[13] Thus, the severity of aortic insufficiency in the elderly may be easily misjudged.

Aortic Flow Reversal

Reversal of flow in the aorta is the basis for many of the physical signs of AI. Durozier's sign (an early diastolic bruit heard over the femoral arteries) is the auscultatory counterpart of reversal of blood flow detected by echocardiography. We have found that reversal of flow in the ascending aorta is a specific, albeit insensitive sign of significant AI (Figures 5 through 7). Normally, there is a small retrograde flow velocity at end-systole which closes the aortic valve. This is quite different from the prolonged and prominent early diastolic signal which is a result of aortic regurgitation. We routinely sample the ascending aorta (from the suprasternal window) for flow-reversal using color and pulsed Doppler in those cases when jet-width and $T_{1/2}$, are indeterminate. The presence of a short $T_{1/2}$, or prominent flow reversal suggests significant AI.

Hypertrophic Obstructive Cardiomyopathy

Although hypertrophic obstructive cardiomyopathy (HOCM) is considered a disease of young people, it is not uncommon among the elderly. Lewis and Maron[27] described a subset of patients (mean age 69 years) with asymmetric septal hypertrophy (ASH) and LVOT obstruction who became symptomatic late in life at an average age of 66 years). Elderly patients with HOCM are not particularly responsive to medical treatment. Lewis et al found that only 12 of 49 elderly HOCM patients were improved by conventional medical therapy at 1 year follow-up.

Elderly patients with HOCM display hyperdynamic left ventricular function and have a small LVOT diameter. Unlike younger patients with HOCM, the elderly often have prominent mitral annular calcification (MAC).[27] MAC was severe in 39 of 52 patients and may have contributed to narrowing of the LVOT. Relative to their younger counterparts with HOCM, older patients have less hypertrophy of the ventricular septum (mean septal thickness 21.5 mm), yet many responded to septal myomectomy.

Asymmetric Septal Hypertrophy

This is diagnosed when the ratio of the thickness of the septum relative to the posterior left ventricular wall exceeds 1.3/1.0. This ratio distinguishes HOCM from other causes of concentric hypertrophy. A sigmoid septum is common among the elderly and, when associated with concentric left ventricular hypertrophy, may simulate the appearance of HOCM. but, the septal/posterior wall ratio usually does not exceed 1.3/1.0.

LVOT Obstruction

The hallmark of obstructive cardiomyopathy is a gradient across the LVOT (>3 m/sec). Doppler interrogation of this gradient shows a characteristic late peak or "shark-tooth" morphology that distinguishes it from valvular obstruction. Demonstration of a gradient is important because patients with large gradients appear to benefit most from myomectomy. Consequently, when symptomatic patients do not have a resting gradient, we attempt to provoke dynamic obstruction, with inhalation of amyl nitrite or, less frequently, by infusion of isoproterenol. Although we have not had a complication from inhalation of amyl nitrite we avoid its use in patients who have a resting gradient of more than 3 m/sec.

Systolic Anterior Motion of the Mitral Valve

Systolic anterior motion of the mitral valve (SAM) is a hallmark finding of HOCM and is generally considered a result of entrainment of the anterior mitral leaflet by the high velocity blood flow through a narrowed LVOT (Venturi effect). It has also been proposed that anterior displacement of hypertrophied papillary muscles plays "a fundamental role in altering the balance of forces acting on the mitral leaflets and creating SAM".[28]

Mitral Annular Calcification

MAC is a deposition of calcium in the fibrous annulus of the mitral valve. It is common above age 65 years, particularly in women.[29] The possible importance of MAC as an individual contributor to cardiovascular morbidity is often obscured by its association with comorbid factors such as systolic murmurs, heart failure, heart block, atrial fibrillation and chronic renal failure. Nonetheless, studies using multiple logistic regression, in diseases such as stroke, have identified MAC as an independent risk factor.[30] Using TEE we have noted thrombus superimposed upon MAC on several occasions. Figures 8 through 10 shows a mobile thrombus on the posterior aspect of MAC that subsequently embolized or lysed without clinical mishap.

MAC is readily identified with M-mode or 2-dimensional echocardiography by its echodensity. The calcium typically causes reverberation of echoes and may obscure posterior structures. With 2-dimensional echocardiograms MAC is a characteristic C-shape, intense, echo-producing structure in the atrio-ventricular groove at the base of the posterior mitral leaflet.[31] Occasionally, calcification may extend beyond the annulus to involve the aortic root, in which case the calcification is circular.

Extensive MAC may obscure the posterior mitral leaflet and lead to underestimation of mitral regurgitation. In patients with severe MAC, the posterior mitral leaflet often appears thickened and immobile. In these cases, mitral stenosis can be excluded by TEE, which usually permits separation of the leaflets from MAC. The acoustic shadows posterior to MAC may obscure left atrial structure and Doppler signals in much the same way as a prosthetic valve. This is usually only a problem with severe MAC and can be overcome by examining the left atrium from behind with TEE. MAC may also make it difficult to assess motion of the inferior wall of the left ventricle, in the inferiorly angulated 4-chamber view.

Although valve dysfunction with MAC is usually mild, MAC may

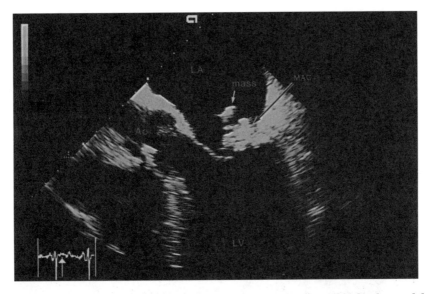

Figure 8: *Complications of mitral annular calcification (MAC) detected by TEE. Four-chamber view shows prominent echogenic mass of MAC with a mobile mass attached to its left atrial (LA) surface. LV: left ventricle.*

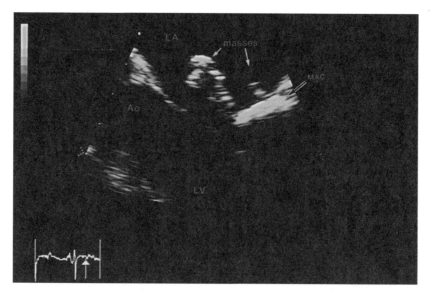

Figure 9: *Complications of MAC demonstrated by TEE. Close-up view showing two thrombi attached to MAC. Ao: aorta.*

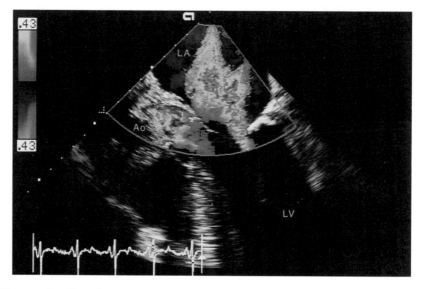

Figure 10: *Complications of MAC demonstrated by TEE. Color Doppler shows central jet of MR of moderate severity.*

occasionally be responsible for hemodynamically significant mitral stenosis or insufficiency. Labovitz et al found that 33% of 51 consecutive patients with MAC identified by echocardiography (mean age 70 years) had moderate to severe mitral regurgitation, while 8% had mitral stenosis (mitral valve area < 2.0 cm^2).[32] Heavy mitral annular calcification may make valve replacement difficult.

Mitral Regurgitation

Color Doppler contributes greatly to assessment of mitral regurgitation (MR) and correlates well with contrast ventriculography. Pulsed Doppler is useful in detecting mitral regurgitation,[33] but is more cumbersome and less graphic than color Doppler.[34] However, pulsed Doppler is helpful in assessing retrograde flow into the pulmonary veins and timing regurgitant jets.

Helmcke et al,[35] found an excellent correlation between color Doppler and contrast ventriculography estimation of the severity of mitral regurgitation. These authors found that the ratio of the area of the regurgitant jet to the left atrium, in the plane of maximum regurgitation, correlated with the severity of MR by ventriculography (r = 0.78). Jets that occupied less than 20% of the left atrium corresponded to mild MR; those over 40% to severe MR. The severity of MR on Doppler may also be quantitated by the distance the jet extends from the annulus. Miyatake et al[34] used an arbitrary scale (based on length of the jet from the annulus) less than 1.5 cm, 1.5 to 3.0 cm, 3 to 4.5 cm, and greater than 4.5 cm and showed these values correlated with 1–4+ MR respectively, on ventriculography (r = 0.87).

In everyday clinical practice we use visual estimates of jet area and length to estimate MR. With TEE a number of useful ancillary clues to the severity of MR can be obtained. These include the presence of generalized turbulence in the left atrium with color Doppler, elevated antegrade diastolic flow velocities across the mitral valve and retrograde flow into the pulmonary veins (Figures 11 through 13).

Distinction from Aortic Stenosis

Distinguishing insufficiency of the atrioventricular valves from aortic stenosis valves relies heavily on timing the onset of the Doppler signal relative to the surface ECG. Mitral and tricuspid insufficiency begins with the onset of isovolumetric systole; aortic stenosis starts 40 to 100 m/sec later, at the end of isovolumetric systole. This timing helps in distinguishing aortic stenosis from MR with the continuous wave Doppler signal. Similarly, the color envelope of MR usually precedes that of left ventricular ejection.

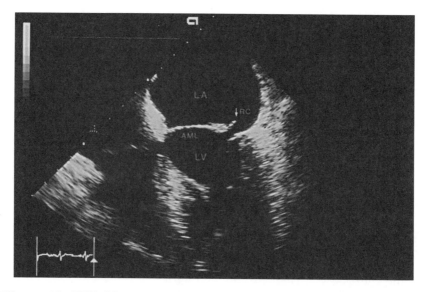

Figure 11: *TEE: Myxomatous mitral valve, prolapse of anterior leaflet, ruptured chordae. Four-chamber view shows enlarged left atrium (LA) with prolapse of anterior mitral leaflet (AML) and ruptured chordae (RC).*

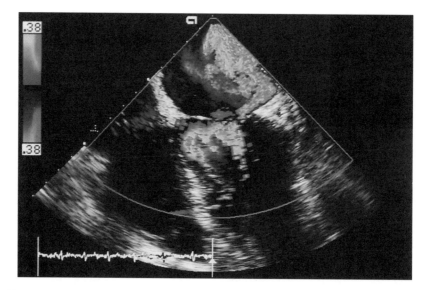

Figure 12: *TEE: Myxomatous mitral valve, prolapse of anterior leaflet, ruptured chordae. Color Doppler shows typical posteriorly-directed eccentric jet of MR that is the hallmark of anterior leaflet prolapse.*

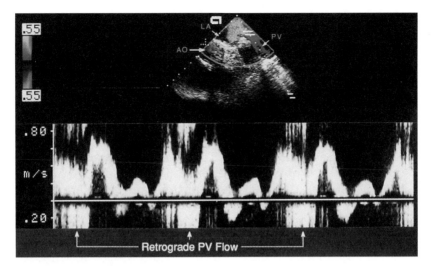

Figure 13: *TEE: Myxomatous mitral valve, prolapse of anterior leaflet, ruptured chordae. Retrograde flow (arrows) is detected in left upper lobe pulmonary vein (PV) using pulsed-Doppler.*

Mitral Valve Prolapse

Both M-mode and 2-dimensional techniques play important roles in the diagnosis and management of patients with mitral valve prolapse (MVP). Based on loose echocardiographic criteria the incidence of MVP has been variously reported at between 5% and 21% of the healthy population.[36] Such fallacies may be avoided by using at least 3 criteria for diagnosis.[37]

1. Clear echocardiographic evidence of leaflet redundancy and thickening with chordal lengthening compatible with myxomatous degeneration of the valve.

2. Some degree of mitral regurgitation.

3. Leaflet displacement superior to the high point of the saddle-shaped "three-dimensional" plane of the mitral annulus that has high points anteriorly and posteriorly.[38,39] Because of this configuration, the mitral leaflets frequently appear to prolapse when viewed in the apical 4-chamber view; overdiagnosis can be avoided by insisting that prolapse be visible on the long axis parasternal view.

4. The presence of calcified left atrial angle lesion above, and left ventricular endocardial friction lesions below the mitral annulus, are also useful corroborative signs of significant mitral valve prolapse.[40,41]

M-mode echocardiography has the limitation that the ultrasonic beam is narrow and provides only a so-called "ice-pick" view. The findings are:

1. Mid- or late systolic buckling: This sudden posterior displacement of the leaflets is quite characteristic of MVP and is useful for timing the onset of the "click" and murmur and there are few false-positives.

2. Holosystolic "hammocking": Holosystolic posterior displacement is not absolutely specific for MVP and may also occur when there is excessive cardiac movement as in pericardial effusion. Because a small amount of posterior movement of the normal mitral valve occurs during systole it has been suggested that the diagnosis only be made when this exceeds 2 mm. However, reliance on such discretionary M-mode criteria increases the number of false positives and the 2-dimensional echocardiogram should be the primary tool for the diagnosis of prolapse.

Two-Dimensional Echocardiography

Two-dimensional echocardiography provides much better spatial visualization of the leaflets, chordae, and papillary muscles and is particularly useful in diagnosis of ruptured chordae. The transesophageal technique is ideal for defining the anatomy more precisely and readily demonstrates failure of leaflet coaptation, lengthening and rupture of the chordae tendinae, and vegetations. The important changes are:

1. Thickening of leaflets and chordae with superior systolic displacement of segments of the valve into the left atrium above the plane of the mitral annulus. Using multiple views, it is possible to detect which portion of the leaflets are redundant and prolapsing.

2. Failure of leaflet coaptation with the edges frequently observed in several views.

3. A "whipping" motion of the leaflet and attached chordae observed when a sizable portion of a leaflet is detached.

4. Color flow Doppler clearly demonstrating eccentricity and direction of the jet depending upon which chordae have ruptured.

Surgery for MVP

The myxomatous valve is now the leading cause of MR in the United States. This follows a decline in the incidence of rheumatic fever and is also the result of a greater awareness of the condition by clinicians and pathologists. Signs of severe MR and heart failure supervene in a small proportion of patients with MVP and men above the age of 45 years are particularly prone to this complication. The average age in a series of 18 patients undergoing mitral repair at our institution was 61 ± 2 years and in more than 80% the underlying pathology was myxomatous mitral valve, with or without chordal rupture. Similar findings were noted in a series of 269 consecutive patients (mean age 60 years) undergoing mitral valve surgery at the Cleveland Clinic for pure mitral regurgitation. Myxomatous degeneration of the valve/chordae was causal in 63% of cases, compared to a 13% incidence of rheumatic disease.[42] In contrast, mitral stenosis and mixed lesions, are a result of rheumatic disease.[42]

While mitral anatomy, left atrial size, and functional status are important in predicting the outcome of surgical treatment, age is the most crucial prognostic factor.[43] Phillips et al[43] evaluated predictors of postoperative response to mitral valve replacement (MVR) in 105 patients undergoing surgery for pure MR (no coronary artery disease). Like Chavez et al,[42] they found that the primary pathology in this cohort was myxomatous mitral valve or ruptured chordae (79%); rheumatic disease accounted for only 20% of the cases.[43] These authors found that age greater than 60 years and ejection fraction (EF) less than 40% were the only variables that correlated with decreased survival at 3 years. This study emphasizes the importance of myxomatous mitral valve as a cause of MR in the elderly and identifies age as a major operative risk factor.

For the surgeon to consider mitral valve repair, the echocardiographer should provide information about chordal rupture or elongation, leaflet prolapse and annular dilatation.[44] This assessment is best made by TEE. The type of prolapse or chordal rupture determines the likelihood of success. Chavez et al[42] reported that 79% of patients with isolated posterior chordal rupture could be repaired, compared with only 40% of those with combined anterior and posterior chordal rupture. Sheikh et al[45] examined the role of pre- and intraoperative TEE in patients with valvular heart disease undergoing surgery and found that preoperative TEE changed the type of operation in 11% of cases. The most common findings missed in preoperative evaluation were severe insufficiency of another valve, or rupture of the mitral chordae.

Rupture of chordae may be readily identified by 2-dimensional TTE, but the transthoracic approach frequently underestimates the severity of MR because regurgitant jets tend to be eccentric and hug the wall of the left atrium. These eccentric jets are readily detected by TEE (Figures 11 through 13). Typically, posterior leaflet prolapse causes an anteriorly directed jet of MR and vice versa with prolapse of the anterior leaflet.[46] Although radiographic contrast ventriculography accurately quantifies mitral regurgitation we have found it less helpful in identifying the direction of the jet, and of minimal value in differentiating chordal elongation from rupture. The many varieties of mitral valve repair demand accurate preoperative diagnosis of mitral anatomy.

Echocardiographic Assessment After Mitral Repair

The role of echocardiography in the operative management of mitral regurgitation is 3-fold: (1) quantification of residual mitral insufficiency; (2) measurement of valve area; and (3) exclusion of postoperative SAM.

Although the intraoperative epicardial echocardiogram is equally accurate, TEE offers the advantage of a clear operative field. Some MR usually persists even with successful repair, but the severity can only be quantitated in the presence of adequate systemic blood pressure. Prior to closing the chest we often raise mean blood pressure to 70 to 90 mm Hg (by catecholamine infusion if necessary). Anything in excess of 2+ mitral regurgitation is an indication for immediate revision. Insertion of an annular ring and leaflet resection, common to most repairs, reduces the mitral valve area but rarely to less than 1.5 cm^2.

SAM has been reported in roughly 6% of patients undergoing mitral valve repair, although only a third of these have a gradient across the LVOT.[47] Grossi et al[47] reported that SAM was most common in patients having extensive resection of the posterior leaflet. Although SAM can lead to postoperative mitral insufficiency, Grossi et al[47] reported that medical management with negative inotropic drugs led to resolution of SAM in 47% of their patients and the gradient disappeared in all cases. Thus, the presence of SAM alone does not mean a repair must be revised.[47]

Mitral Stenosis

The primary goal of 2-dimensional echocardiography is to planimeter the valve area (from the short-axis parasternal window) and correlate this anatomic estimate of severity with Doppler measurement of valve stenosis (mean gradient, using the Bernoulli equation (Table 1), and valve area using the pressure half-time method). However, leaflet mobility, calcification, and chordal shortening, are also easily assessed and assist in the choice of therapeutic procedure.

Pressure Half-Time

Hatle et al[48] developed an empirical formula which correlated pressure half-time of the transmitral Doppler signal with valve area as measured by cardiac catheterization (Table 1). The principle underlying the formula is that pressure equalizes more rapidly between chambers, separated by a large, rather than a small orifice. Thus, in severe mitral stenosis the pressure half-time is prolonged. Although this calculation is affected by factors other than valve area (eg, transmitral gradient, compliance of the atria and ventricle) it is clinically useful. The many potential confounding factors that could invalidate the pressure half-time equation usually negate each other in the clinical setting with alterations in chamber compliance offsetting changes in pressure gradient.[49] However, in the presence of left ventricular hypertrophy, aortic insufficiency, and immediately after balloon mitral valvuloplasty, the half-time is shortened and this could lead to overestimation of mitral valve area.

Echocardiographic Score

Percutaneous balloon valvuloplasty, like surgical commissurotomy is most effective when the mitral leaflets are mobile and noncalcified, conditions not often present in the elderly. Abscal et al[50] found that a 4-point scoring system that included measurement of leaflet thickness, calcification, mobility and thickening of the subvalvular apparatus was the best predictor of the success for valvuloplasty. Occasional elderly patients may benefit from balloon valvuloplasty, but this requires careful screening. Vahanian found that the mean age of patients successfully treated by this technique was 41 ± 14 years (mean $\pm$ SD) versus 54 ± 17 years in those with poor results ($P < 0.001$).[51]

Papillary Muscle Dysfunction

Papillary muscle dysfunction is manifested by MR, echogenic papillary muscles, inferior regional wall motion abnormality and mitral annular dilatation. Izumi et al[6] found that asynergy of the myocardium or papillary muscle resulted in a jet of mitral regurgitation which originated from the ipsilateral side of the mitral orifice, whereas central jets of MR resulted primarily from annular dilatation. These authors found a direct relationship between left ventricular end-diastolic volume and annular dimension (annular dimensions ranged from 2 to 4 cm) in ischemic mitral regurgitation.[6]

Aortic Atherosclerosis

A new and important factor to consider in assessing stroke in the elderly is the presence of atherosclerotic debris in the aorta (Figures

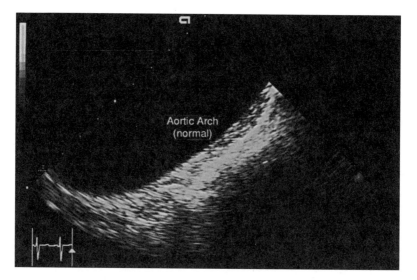

Figure 14: *Detection of atherosclerotic plaques in the aortic arch by transesophageal echocardiography (TEE). Normal aortic arch has smooth intima.*

14 through 16).[52,53] A significant number of intraoperative strokes result from embolization of aortic atherosclerotic debris among patients having cardiopulmonary bypass.[54] Atherosclerotic debris refers to protuberant, occasionally mobile, atherosclerotic plaques and overlying thrombus. Although the ascending thoracic aorta is usually spared, the arch is often involved (Figured 14 through 16). Thoracic atherosclerosis may be suspected preoperatively by the presence of excessive aortic calcification on chest roentgenogram. The surgeon traditionally palpates the aorta to avoid calcific plaques when placing the cannulae for bypass. Katz et al,[54] using TEE, found an incidence of protruding aortic atheromas of 18% in patients over 65 years of age undergoing cardiopulmonary bypass. They also showed that surgical palpation and chest roentgenogram were insensitive in detecting soft, mobile plaques, which were the type most likely to dislodge.

Atherosclerotic plaques may be dislodged at surgery by palpation, placement of cannulae for bypass or even insertion of the proximal anastamoses for vein bypass. Diagnostic catheterization also carries increased risk of embolization in these patients.[53] Our practice is to alter the site of aortic cannulation if plaque is detected in the ascending aorta; some groups even advocate debriding the aorta during complete cardiopulmonary arrest.[54] Further study is required to determine whether TEE of the aorta should be performed routinely in patients age 70 years or more who are being considered for cardiopulmonary bypass, particularly when there is evidence of carotid and iliofemoral disease.

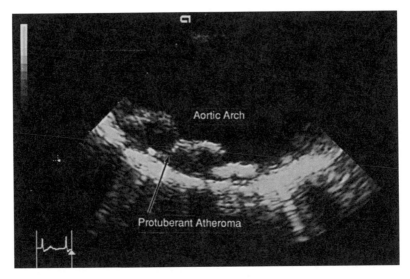

Figure 15: *Detection of atherosclerotic plaques in the aortic arch by transesophageal echocardiography (TEE). Protruberant nonmobile plaques in the arch are potential sources of emboli.*

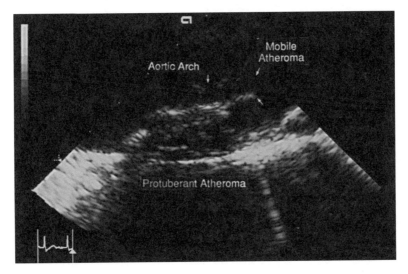

Figure 16: *Detection of atherosclerotic plaques in the aortic arch by transesophageal echocardiography (TEE). Large protruberant atheroma with serpentine mobile "tail."*

Aortic Aneurysm and Marfan's Syndrome

Marfan's syndrome is usually a disease of young people, and the mean age of death is 32 years; most deaths are a result of aortic dissection or rupture. There is, however, an older population with Marfan's (Figures 17 and 18). The Mayo Clinic reported a series of 28 patients with Marfan's syndrome diagnosed at mean age of 46 years.[55] Aortic insufficiency (AI) was found in 60% and mitral valve prolapse in 28%. Aortic root dilatation was common (76%) and usually associated with aortic insufficiency. Like young patients with Marfan's syndrome, this older group had a high incidence of morbid cardiac events, predominantly related to the aorta.[55] One patient died suddenly of aortic rupture and five had aortic dissection. It is noteworthy that deaths occurred in all functional classes and the only predictor of a good outcome was the presence of a normal size aorta on echocardiography.[55]

Idiopathic dilatation of the aorta is also a cause of AI in the older adult. Roman et al examined 102 patients with isolated, severe aortic insufficiency (mean age 47 years). They found that aortic dilatation was associated independently with age, but not with blood pressure.[56] Furthermore the mean age of patients with AI due to primary valve disease was 42 years compared to 59 years in those with idiopathic root dilatation ($P < 0.001$).

Larson et al[57] examined 161 patients with aortic dissection at autopsy. Hypertension was found to be a major risk factor for dissection

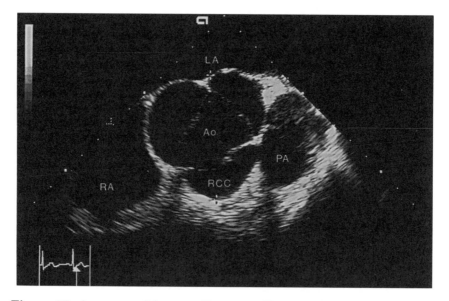

Figure 17: *Aneurysm of the ascending aorta. Transesophageal echocardiography (TEE): short-axis views of aortic valve. RA, right atrium; LA, left atrium; Ao, aorta; RCC, right coronary cusp; PA, pulmonary artery.*

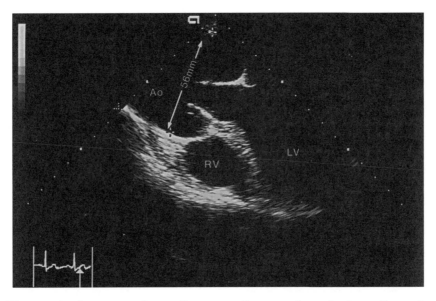

Figure 18: *Aneurysm of ascending aorta. Transesophageal echocardiography (TEE): long-axis view from the same patient in Figure 17 showing loss of sinotubular rideg. RV, right ventricle; LV, left ventricle.*

but the age at which dissection occurred was predicted by coexistent valve pathology. The mean age at dissection of patients with tricuspid, bicuspid and unicuspid aortic valves was 63, 55, and 40 years, respectively. The frequency and severity of cystic medial necrosis, blood pressure and heart weight did not vary significantly among the 3 morphologies of aortic valve. Bicuspid and unicuspid aortic valves were associated with 9- and 18-fold increases in risk of proximal aortic dissection.[57]

Transesophageal Echocardiography in the Elderly

There are no major alterations in basic technique required for safe performance of this procedure in the elderly.[58] However, the dose of anticholinergic agents and sedatives should be reduced. We monitor the electrocardiogram, blood pressure and oximetry during the procedure and have had no complications in our elderly patients. The common indications for TEE in the elderly include assessment of prosthetic valves, vegetations, embolic source, and aortic dissection. The remainder of TEEs are performed intraoperatively or when transthoracic images are inadequate. TEE is particularly helpful in defining left atrial pathology (Figures 19 and 20).

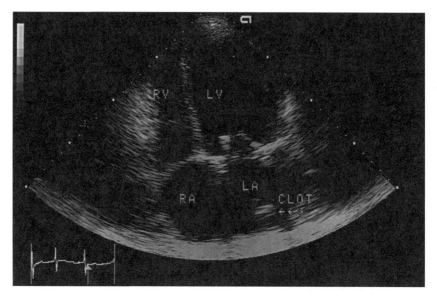

Figure 19: *Transesophageal echocardiography (TEE): prosthetic mitral valve. Four-chamber view showing echo-density posteriorly, in left atrium (LA) suggestive of thrombus.*

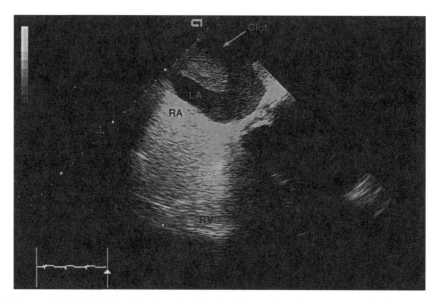

Figure 20: *TEE: Prosthetic mitral valve. Four-chamber view, bubble contrast study, opacifying right atrial (RA) and right ventricle (RV) demonstrating left atrial thrombus filling 80% of the chamber, including the appendage.*

Infective Endocarditis

The goals of echocardiography in assessing a patient with possible endocarditis are to detect vegetations and complications such as leaflet perforation.

Two-dimensional echocardiography can detect vegetations as small as 3 mm. M-Mode echocardiography is not as useful for detecting vegetations because of poor sensitivity and specificity. TTE has a diagnostic accuracy for vegetations of 70% to 80% and TEE approximately 90%. Mugge et al[59] compared TTE and TEE in 80 patients with proven endocarditis. TTE detected definite vegetations in 58% of patients compared to 90% with TEE. However, TEE determined that "definite" vegetations were present in 18 cases in which the anatomic findings revealed only microscopic bacterial colonies, clearly a fortuitous or "false," true-positive finding.

Many laboratories keep sensitivity for the diagnosis of vegetations high at the price of specificity. Furthermore, most measurements of sensitivity and specificity are made in patients who already have endocarditis. This high pretest probability of vegetations artificially elevates the sensitivity of the test. Among an elderly population, most focal masses on valves are not vegetations. Conversely, absence of vegetations on echocardiography does not exclude a diagnosis of endocarditis. Tape and Panzer performed a retrospective study to determine whether a high pretest suspicion of endocarditis biased interpretation of the echocardiogram. In 142 patients (mean age 57 years) they found that the more clinical features suggestive of endocarditis known prior to the echocardiogram, the higher the likelihood of a false-positive result.[60] They showed that when two or more clinical signs such as heart murmur and fever suggested endocarditis specificity decreased from 97% to 80%.

Unless there is a prior study for comparison, echocardiography is not readily able to diagnose vegetations when valves are severely deformed, particularly if chordae are ruptured and leaflets severely redundant. Most elderly individuals have echogenic, focal valve thickenings which could be misinterpreted as vegetations. Although acute vegetations are less echogenic than calcific degeneration seen in the elderly this interpretation is very subjective and also varies with the age of the vegetation. Vegetations may be sessile or mobile. Even sessile vegetations often shake or move independently of the valve. Vegetations are usually associated with signs of valve destruction or insufficiency.

It is generally believed that size of valvular vegetations is an important predictor of prognosis.[59] Larger vegetations have been reported to have a higher likelihood of receiving surgical treatment, embolizing, or causing heart failure when the aortic valve is affected.[60] Large vegetations (greater than 1 cm), particularly on the mitral valve, have a higher incidence of embolism than smaller vegetations.[59,61] However, vegetation size is not predictive of survival.[59] In most cases of infective endocarditis prognosis is determined by the severity of valve insufficiency. Jaffe et al[62] found that valve insufficiency, rather than vegetation size, was the best predictor of outcome in endocarditis. They found that when valvular regurgitation was mild, in-hospital mortality was low and the incidence of surgery small.[62]

Detection of an aortic root abscess or mycotic aneurysm reinforces the need for surgery and alters the type of surgery performed. Root abscesses can be detected by TTE and TEE. They are best seen on TTE in the parasternal views and appear as an echolucent chamber adjacent to the aorta.[63] Unlike annular erosion, there is no flow between the root abscess and the aorta. In patients with prosthetic valves, the normal crescentic lucency between the prosthesis and the aorta should not be mistaken for an abscess.

The chances of a medical cure of an aortic root abscess are poor and surgery is almost universally recommended. Most surgeons replace the valve and ascending aorta with a composite graft. Failure to make a preoperative diagnosis of root abscess can greatly complicate operation in patients where there is discontinuity of the ventricle and aorta. Preoperative diagnosis of root abscess ensures that an experienced surgeon performs the operation and procures the correct prosthesis.[63] The size of aortic prosthesis required is determined by measuring the internal dimension of the aortic root at the level of the annulus. This allows the surgeon to confidently "pre-clot" the prosthesis, saving valuable time on bypass. It is important to realize that root abscess may occur in patients who lack significant valve insufficiency.[62]

Marantic Endocarditis

Marantic, or nonbacterial, thrombotic endocarditis is found in approximately 1% of routine autopsies.[64] It is primarily a disease of the middle-aged and elderly. In a review of the literature more than 60% of cases occurred in patients over 60 years of age.[64] Marantic vegetations are usually located on the atrial surface of the mitral valve and the ventricular aspect of the aortic valve. They are usually multiple and small (less than 3 mm).

Marantic endocarditis is usually diagnosed postmortem, although a handful of echocardiographic reports exist.[65,66] Perhaps the diagnosis would be made more frequently if patients with conditions known to predispose to marantic endocarditis (cancer, burns, indwelling catheters, disseminated intravascular coagulation), especially those with systemic emboli, were systematically surveyed. However, the small size of these vegetations, together with the prevalence of nonspecific valve thickening in the elderly, make the diagnosis difficult.

Tricuspid Endocarditis

This entity is relatively rare among the elderly, because of the low prevalence of intravenous drug abuse. However, tricuspid endocarditis should be suspected among patients who have indwelling catheters and signs of endocarditis, and particularly among those with septic pulmonary emboli.

In general, tricuspid vegetations are large (1.7 ± 0.5 cm in one study),[67] but in contrast to left-sided endocarditis, size of vegetation is not predictive of prognosis. The prognosis of tricuspid endocarditis in the elderly is unknown.

References

1. Berman N: Valvular heart disease in the elderly. *Mt Sinai J Med* 52: 594–600, 1985.
2. Sleight P: Unilateral elevation of the internal jugular pulse. *Br Heart J* 24:726–730, 1962.
3. Flohr KH, Weir EK, Chesler E: Diagnosis of aortic stenosis in older age groups using external carotid pulse recording and phonocardiography. *Br Heart J* 45:577, 1981.
4. Davison T, Friedman S: Significance of systolic murmurs in the aged. *N Engl J Med* 279:225–230, 1968.
5. Criley J: Prolapsed mitral leaflet syndrome. *Cardiovasc Clin* 10:213, 1979.
6. Izumi S, Miyatake K, Beppu S, et al: Mechanism of mitral regurgitation in patients with myocardial infarction: A study using real-time two-dimensional Doppler flow imaging and echocardiography. *Circulation* 76: 777–785, 1987.
7. Jaffe W, Roche A, Coverdale H, et al: Clinical evaluation versus Doppler echocardiography in the quantitative assessment of valvular heart disease. *Circulation* 2:267–275, 1988.
8. Sahasakul Y, Edwards W, Naessens J, et al: Age-related changes in aortic and mitral valve thickness: Implication for two-dimensional echocardiography based on an autopsy study of 200 normal human hearts. *Am J Cardiol* 62:424–430, 1988.
9. Passik C, Ackermann D, Pluth J, et al: Temporal changes in the causes of aortic stenosis: A surgical pathologic study of 646 cases. *Mayo Clin Proc* 62:119–123, 1987.
10. Gardin J, Davidson D, Rohan M, et al: Relationship between age, body size, gender, and blood pressure and Doppler flow measurements in the aorta and pulmonary artery. *Am Heart J* 113:101–109, 1987.
11. Zavitsanos JP, Goldman AP, Kotler MN, et al: The echo Doppler spectrum of valvular abnormalities in the hospitalized octogenarian. *Clin Cardiol* 11:683–688, 1988.
12. Akasaka T, Yoshikawa J, Yoshida K, et al: Age-related valvular regurgitation: A study by pulsed Doppler echocardiography. *Circulation* 76:262–265, 1987.
13. Kitzman DW, Sheikh KH, Beere PA, et al: Age-related alterations of Doppler left ventricular filling indexes in normal subjects are independent of left ventricular mass, heart rate, contractility and loading conditions. *J Am Coll Cardiol* 18:1243–1250, 1991.
14. Otto C, Pearlman A: Doppler echocardiography in adults with symptomatic aortic stenosis. *Arch Intern Med* 148:2553–2560, 1988.
15. Hatle L, Angelsen B, Tromsdal A: Non-invasive assessment of aortic valve stenosis by Doppler ultrasound. *Br Heart J* 43:284–292, 1980.

16. Fan P-H, Kapur K, Nanda N: Color-guided Doppler echocardiographic assessment of aortic valve stenosis. *J Am Coll Cardiol* 12:441–449, 1988.
17. Otto C, Pearlman A, Comess K, et al: Determination of the stenotic aortic valve area in adults using Doppler echocardiography. *J Am Coll Cardiol* 7:509–517, 1986.
18. Smith M, Dawson P, Elion J, et al: Systematic correlation of continuous-wave Doppler and hemodynamic measurements in patients with aortic stenosis. *Am Heart J* 111:245–252, 1986.
19. Stewart SFC, Nast EP, Arabia FA, et al: Errors in pressure gradient measurement by continuous wave Doppler ultrasound: Type, size and age effects of bioprosthetic aortic valves. *J Am Coll Cardiol* 18:769–779, 1991.
20. Baumgartner H, Khan S, DeRobertis M, et al: Effect of prosthetic valve design on the Doppler-catheter gradient correlation: An in vitro study of normal St. Jude, Medtronic-Hall, Starr-Edwards and Hancock valves. *J Am Coll Cardiol* 19:324–332, 1992.
21. Hofmann T, Kasper W, Meinertz T, et al: Determination of aortic valve orifice area in aortic valve stenosis by two-dimensional transesophageal echocardiography. *Am J Cardiol* 59:330–335, 1987.
22. Oh J, Taliercio C, Holmes D, et al: Prediction of the severity of aortic stenosis by Doppler aortic valve area determination: Prospective Doppler-catheterization correlation in 100 patients. *J Am Coll Cardiol* 11:1227–1234, 1988.
23. Perry GJ, Helmcke F, Nanda N, et al: Evaluation of aortic insufficiency by color Doppler flow mapping. *J Am Coll Cardiol* 9:952–959, 1987.
24. Sareli P, Klein HO, Schamroth CL, et al: Contribution of echocardiography and immediate surgery to the management of severe aortic regurgitation from active infective endocarditis. *Am J Cardiol* 57(6):413, 1986.
25. Grayburn P, Handshoe R, Smith M, et al: Quantitative assessment of the hemodynamic consequences of aortic regurgitation by means of continuous wave Doppler recordings. *J Am Coll Cardiol* 10:135–141, 1987.
26. Vanoverschelde J, Taymans-Robert AR, Raphael DA, et al: Influence of transmitral filling dynamics on continuous-wave Doppler Assessment of aortic regurgitation by half-time methods. *Am J Cardiol* 64:614–619, 1989.
27. Lewis JF, Maron BJ: Elderly patients with hypertrophic cardiomyopathy: A subset with distinctive left ventricular morphology and progressive clinical course late in life. *J Am Coll Cardiol* 13:36–45, 1989.
28. Jiang L, Levine RA, King ME, et al: An integrated mechanism for systolic anterior motion of the mitral valve in hypertrophic cardiomyopathy based on echocardiographic observations. *Am Heart J* 113:633–644, 1987.
29. Papa L, Raniolo J, Schiff S, et al: Mitral annular calcification. *Postgrad Med* 71:63–66, 1982.
30. Benjamin E, Plehn J, D'Agostino R, et al: Mitral annular calcification and the risk of stroke in an elderly cohort. *N Engl J Med* 327:374–379, 1992.
31. Nair C, Thomson W, Ryschon K, et al: Long-term follow-up of patients with echocardiographically detected mitral annular calcium and comparison with age- and sex-matched control subjects. *Am J Cardiol* 63:465–470, 1989.
32. Labovitz A, Nelson J, Windhorst D, Kennedy H. and Williams G: Frequency of mitral valve dysfunction from mitral annular calcium as detected by Doppler echocardiography. *Am J Cardiol* 55:133–137, 1985.
33. Veyrat C, Ameur A, Bas S, et al: Pulsed Doppler echocardiographic indices for assessing mitral regurgitation. *Br Heart J* 51:130–138, 1984.

34. Miyatake K, Izumi S, Okamoto M, et al: Semiquantitative grading of severity of mitral regurgitation by real-time two-dimensional Doppler flow imaging technique. *J Am Coll Cardiol* 7:82–88, 1986.
35. Helmcke F, Nanda N, Hsiung M, et al: Color Doppler assessment of mitral regurgitation with orthogonal planes. *Circulation* 75:175–183, 1987.
36. Chesler EGCC: Maladies attributed to myxomatous mitral valve. *Circulation* 83:328, 1991.
37. Levine RA, Weyman AE: Mitral valve prolapse: A disease in search of, or created by, its definition. *Echocardiography* 1:3–14, 1984.
38. Levine RA, Triulzi MO, Harrigan P, et al: The relationship of mitral annular shape to the diagnosis of mitral valve prolapse. *Circulation* 75:756–767, 1987.
39. Levine RA, Stahogiannis E, Newell JB, et al: Reconsideration of echocardiographic standards for mitral valve prolapse: Lack of association between leaflet displacement isolated to the apical four chamber view and independent echocardiographic evidence of abnormality. *J Am Coll Cardiol* 11:1010–1019, 1988.
40. Chesler E, King RA, Edwards JE: The myxomatous mitral valve and sudden death. *Circulation* 67:632–639, 1983.
41. Chesler E, Gornick C, Edwards JE: Calcification of the mural endocardium of the left ventricle complicating the myxomatous mitral valve. *Am J Cardiol* 1196–1198, 1987.
42. Chavez A, Cosgrove D, Lytle B, et al: Applicability of mitral valvuloplasty techniques in a North American population. *Am J Cardiol* 62:253–256, 1988.
43. Phillips H, Levine F, Carter J, et al: Mitral valve replacement for isolated mitral regurgitation: Analysis of clinical course and late postoperative left ventricular ejection fraction. *Am J Cardiol* 48:647–654, 1981.
44. Carpentier A: Cardiac valve surgery: The "French correction." *J Thorac Cardiovasc Surg* 86:323–337, 1983.
45. Sheikh K, de Bruijn N, Rankin J, et al: The utility of transesophageal echocardiography and Doppler color flow imaging in patients undergoing cardiac valve surgery. *J Am Coll Cardiol* 15:363–372, 1990.
46. Czer L, Maurer G: Intraoperative echocardiography in mitral and tricuspid valve repair. *Echocardiography* 7:305–322, 1990.
47. Grossi EA, Galloway AC, Parish MA, et al: Experience with twenty-eight cases of systolic anterior motion after mitral valve reconstruction by Carpentier technique. *J Thorac Cardiovasc Surg* 103:466–470, 1992.
48. Hatle J, Angleson B: *Doppler Ultrasound in Cardiology: Physical Principles and Clinical Applications.* Philadelphia: Lea and Febiger, 1982.
49. Thomas J, Weyman A: Doppler mitral pressure half-time: A clinical tool in search of theoretical justification. *J Am Coll Cardiol* 10:923–929, 1987.
50. Abascal V, Wilkins G, Choong C, et al: Echocardiographic evaluation of mitral valve structure and function in patients followed for at least 6 months after percutaneous balloon mitral valvuloplasty. *J Am Coll Cardiol* 12:606–615, 1988.
51. Vahanian A, Michel P, Cormier B, et al: Results of percutaneous mitral commissurotomy in 200 patients. *Am J Cardiol* 63:847–852, 1989.
52. Amarenco P, Duyckaerts C, Tzourio C, et al: The prevalence of ulcerated plaques in the aortic arch in patients with stroke. *N Engl J Med* 326:221–225, 1992.
53. Karalis D, Chandrasekaran K, Victor M, et al: Recognition and embolic

potential of intraaortic atherosclerotic debris. *J Am Coll Cardiol* 17:73–78, 1991.

54. Katz E, Tunick P, Rusinek H, et al: Protruding aortic atheromas predict stroke in elderly patients undergoing cardiopulmonary bypass: Experience with intraoperative transesophageal echocardiography. *J Am Coll Cardiol* 20:70–77, 1992.

55. Chan K-L, Callahan J, Seward J, et al: Marfan syndrome diagnosed in patients 32 years of age or older. *Mayo Clin Proc* 62:589–594, 1987.

56. Roman M, Devereux R, Niles N, et al: Aortic root dilatation as a cause of isolated, severe aortic regurgitation. *Ann Intern Med* 106:800–807, 1987.

57. Larson E, Edwards W: Risk factors for aortic dissection: A necropsy study of 161 cases. *Am J Cardiol* 53:849–855, 1984.

58. Seward J, Khandheria B, Oh J, et al: Transesophageal echocardiography: Technique, anatomic correlations, implementation, and clinical applications. *Mayo Clin Proc* 63:649–680, 1988.

59. Mugge A, Daniel WG, Gunter F, et al: Echocardiography in infective endocarditis: Reassessment of prognostic implications of vegetation size determined by the transthoracic and the transesophageal approach. *J Am Coll Cardiol* 14:631–638, 1989.

60. Tape TG, Panzer RJ: Echocardiography, endocarditis and clinical information bias. *J Gen Intern Med* 1:300–304, 1986.

61. Wong D, Chandraratna AN, Wishnow RM, et al: Clinical implications of large vegetations in infectious endocarditis. *Arch Intern Med* 143: 1874–1877, 1983.

62. Jaffe WM, Morgan DE, Pearlman AS, et al: Infective endocarditis, 1983–1988: echocardiographic findings and factors influencing morbidity and mortality. *J Am Coll Cardiol* 15:1227–1233, 1990.

63. Saner HE, Asinger RW, Homans DC, et al: Two-dimensional echocardiographic Identification of complicated aortic root endocarditis: implications for surgery. *J Am Coll Cardiol* 10:859–868, 1987.

64. Lopez JA, Ross RS, Fishbein MC, et al: Nonbacterial thrombotic endocarditis: A review. *Am Heart J* 113:773–784, 1987.

65. Estevez CM, Corya BC: Serial echocardiographic abnormalities in nonbacterial thrombotic endocarditis of the mitral valve. *Chest* 69:801–804, 1976.

66. Siegel RJ, Ginzton LE, Flanagan K, et al: Marantic endocarditis. Diagnosis by 2-D echocardiography. *Chest* 80:118–119, 1981.

67. Manolis AS, Melita H: Echocardiographic and clinical correlates in drug addicts with infective endocarditis: Implications of vegetation size. *Arch Intern Med* 148:2461–2465, 1988.

Chapter 9

Presentation and Evaluation of Ischemic Heart Disease

Henry D. McIntosh

Fear old age, for it does not come alone.
Plato

That our society is aging is an inescapable fact. With the passage of time, this change will become even more established. In 1987, there were approximately 2.7 million citizens older than 85 years in the United States.[1] In 1993, there were 3.5 million such aged Americans.[2] It is predicted that in the year 2030, there will be 16 million Americans older than 85 years.[1] But this aging phenomenon is occurring not only in the United States. It is occurring worldwide.

The importance of aging in our society was emphasized in October 1997 by 100 editors of medical journals worldwide joining together to highlight, in editorials in their respective journals, the theme of aging.[3] This unprecedented act was undertaken by these leaders of the medical/scientific community to share with their worldwide readership(s) their concern(s) about the significance that the changes that will/could result from the aging of the population may have on this planet.

During the time course of this century, life expectancy at birth has increased by more than 25 years in most countries throughout the universe. With improved control of infectious diseases in developing countries, coupled with improved sanitation, nutrition, declining fertility and maternal and infant mortality rates, more children survive to adulthood and succumb to adult diseases.[3]

One of the most striking features about the characteristics of the aging population in the United States is that the proportion of women has increased dramatically. Based on the data available from the U.S. Bureau of Statistics, from 1980 to 1986, there were 83 men aged 65 to

From *Clinical Cardiology in the Elderly. Second Edition,* edited by Elliot Chesler. © 1999, Futura Publishing Company, Armonk, NY.

69 years per 100 women of that age; but there were only 40 men per 100 women after the age of 85 years.[4] Life expectancy for men from birth in this country is now about 72 years. However, women can expect to live 79 years. Ninety-five percent of the women in the United States reach age 50 and of these halfcenturial women, nearly 25% will attain age 90.[5] Obviously, the absolute number of older Americans, both males and females, will increase greatly as the "baby boomers" (people born in 1946) attain the half-century mark.

Incidence of Ischemic Heart Disease

It is this older population that will experience and frequently succumb to ischemic heart disease (IHD) in the United States and other industrialized countries. Even in this decade, despite the technological advances, 1.25 million people experience an acute myocardial infarction each year in the United States. About 500,000 of these die, and about one-half of the deaths (250,000) are classified as occurring suddenly. Of those, about one-half (125,000) die before reaching a hospital emergency departement. By convention, death is considered to have occurred suddenly if it was unexpected, within 1 hour after the onset of symptoms and before the patient was admitted to the hospital ward, regardless if the patient had been already admitted to a hospital emergency department.[6] Over 80% of the deaths due to IHD now occur in individuals older than 65 years of age. In 1987, 57% of all patients hospitalized with an acute myocardial infarction (AMI) in the United States were aged 65 years or older.[6]

Castelli and associates[7] at Framingham reported in 1986 that whereas every fifth male had a coronary event before age 60, only every 17th woman had such an event by that age. Furthermore, Roberts[8] reported that at least 50% of the coronary events occurred in men before their 60th birthday, and 75% of the men destined to have a fatal coronary event had it before their 70th birthday.

But with efforts to modify recognized risk factors and follow a heart healthy lifestyle, the age of the first infarct in members of our society is regressing. Stamler[9] reported, based on data from Multiple Risk Factor Intervention Trial (MRFIT), that the 11,000 subjects in the lowest quintal of cholesterol (166 mg/dL) who had also the lower blood pressures (117/77) and who did not smoke, from the 1970s, compared to the other 350,000 men with less ideal risk factors, during the subsequent almost 12 years, had a 90% lower death rate from coronary heart disease (CHD), a 70% lower death rate from stroke, an 86% lower death rate from cardiovascular disease, a 30% lower cancer death rate, a 21.5% lower death rate from accidents and suicides, and a 54% decrease in total deaths.

Changes in the Heart due to Aging

But does advancing age per se predispose the individual to IHD? It would seem not. Roberts[10] reported in 1993 his findings from personally conducted postmortem examinations of 93 hearts from patients who died at greater than 90 years of age. Only 20 (21%) had had a clinical history of angina pectoris and/or AMI. Thirty-five of the 93 hearts (38%) did have evidence of an AMI. Calcific deposits and atherosclerotic plaques were present in an epicardial artery of 88 of the 93 (95%) hearts; 59 of the 93 (63%) had a more than 75% cross-sectional narrowing of at least one of the four major arteries. After the examination and with support of clinical data, death was attributed to a cardiac cause in 29 patients (31%), a noncardiac but vascular cause in 17 (18%), and a noncardiovascular cause in 47 (51%).

The challenge faced during the last decade or more and even now, by both clinicians and investigators, was/is to determine what changes in structure and function that occurred in the cardiovascular system was/are a result of aging and what was/are due to an acquired disease such as CHD that could have been prevented by therapy or lifestyle changes. Josephson and Fannin[11] (see Chapter 2) have emphasized that it is important not to attribute abnormalities or symptoms in elderly subjects categorically to "normal" aging.

Fleg[12] and associates at the Gerontology Research Center, Baltimore, Maryland, studied the cardiac anatomy and function by echocardiograms of 200 volunteers, aged 22 to 86 years, in whom CHD had been excluded by history and a stress thallium. It was found that in normotensive subjects, the posterior left ventricular (LV) wall thickness increased with advancing age. However, there was no change in LV diastolic or systolic dimension(s) related to age; nor did stroke volume (SV), heart rate or cardiac output change at rest solely because of age. There were changes, however, related to age in LV diastolic function. A blunting of the early diastolic peak filling rate as well as the peak in the A-wave velocity, representing late LV filling due to atrial contraction, was demonstrated by echocardiogram. But these changes in diastolic LV function were not attributed to reduction in physical activity associated with age because highly trained older endurance athletes demonstrated similar findings.[12]

Fleg[12] emphasized that Western cultures experience a gradual rise in systolic blood pressure (SBP) with age. In the Framingham population, SBP increased approximately 35 mm Hg in women and 25 mm Hg in men between the fourth and eighth decades.[13] But these changes did not result in so-called established hypertension. Diastolic blood pressure (DBP), in contrast, undergoes little alteration with age. A much smaller rise in SBP has been observed in less industrialized societies suggesting that behavioral factors, such as higher salt intake, physical inactivity and obesity, contribute to the age-associated rise in SBP in our society.[14]

Although the SV in older volunteers in the Baltimore Longitudinal Study of Aging (BLSA) was observed during exercise to be well maintained, LV emptying was reduced, ie, LV endsystolic volume (LVES) at maximal effort was larger and did not decrease as much in older subjects. Thus, the rise in LV ejection fraction (LVEF) from rest was blunted with age, resulting in a lower LVEF at maximal effort in older subjects. But there was a greater exercise-induced increase in LV end-diastolic (LVED) volume with advancing age. Fleg[12] attributed these changes of a blunted heart rate and LVEF response and augmented LV dilatation to a diminished functional response to β-adrenergic stimulation.

Rapaport[15] attributed the blunted heart rate response to a decrease in the total number of myocytes and pacemaker cells. He reported that the number of pacemaker cells in the sinoatrial (SA) node in an octogenarian is about 10% of the number present in a 20-year-old. He stated that these changes contribute to the increased incidence of SA node disease observed in the elderly. Titus and Edwards[16] reported that well-defined histopathologic changes in the structure of the SA node occur with aging without changes in the electrocardiogram (ECG) (see Chapter 1)

Not only are the number of myocytes decreased, but those present are reported to be enlarged. Rapaport[15] also reported that there is an increase in elastic tissue, collagen, amyloid and lipid depositions in the myocardium attributable to aging. One wonders if these changes contribute to the slight increase in posterior LV wall thickness observed by Fleg.[12] Could these changes also contribute to damage of the sensory autonomic fibers resulting in a higher pain threshold and a decrease in the perception of pain associated with myocardial ischemia that is common among the aged? This phenomenon will be discussed subsequently in greater detail.

Few Diseases in the Elderly are "Pure"

In the elderly, especially octogenarians, few diseases are isolated or "pure."[17] It is not unusual for individuals of that age to have had, in the previous half century or so, one or more illnesses which resulted in an alteration of function of the renal, gastrointestinal, pulmonary, musculoskeletal, hemopoietic, autonomic and the central nervous and/or other systems. Therefore, altered cardiac function due to IHD could contribute to new and/or increased symptomatic dysfunction of one of these previously impaired organs/systems. Furthermore, depressive and other emotional- based symptoms, frequently unrecognized by caregivers, are not uncommon in the elderly. Depression has been reported to precede a myocardial infarction in 35% to 50% of patients and be associated with an increased mortality and medical morbidity.[18]

Some patients may have cardiac scars of an arrested rheumatic process and only with the passage of years, if not decades, does/do the altered structural effect(s) become significant enough to result in functional disability. The impaired function of a congenital abnormality of the heart may also make its first clinical appearance in the aged. For example, aortic stenosis due to a congenital bicuspid aortic valve may first become symptomatic when this previously silent clinical impairment summates with the impairment resulting from IHD. Attention is directed to the discussion by Archer and Chesler[19] (see Chapter 8) on the effects of valvular heart disease in the elderly that might contribute to the clinical course of IHD.

The Elderly are Subject to Polypharmacy

Because of the likelihood of a previously experienced disease process having become chronic, at the time they experience IHD, many elderly patients may already be receiving multiple medications. Individuals older than age 65 are reported to purchase 50% of all drugs prescribed in this country. Those younger than 65 purchase an average of 4 prescription drugs per year, whereas those older than 65 purchase 11 prescription drugs per year.[20]

Rapaport[15] reported that nearly 25% community dwelling elderly are receiving potentially inappropriate drugs. Furthermore, 50% of deaths due to adverse reactions from medications are in patients over 60 years of age.

These adverse effects may be due to altered drug absorption due to altered gastric motility, modified drug distribution and/or lipid solubility because of less lean body mass and increased fat content of the elderly individual compared to younger individuals in whom the recommended dose was established; alterations of renal and/or hepatic function, etc., may also contribute to unexpected pharmacological effects.[21-23] Also, it must be remembered that, because of changes of short-term memory, etc., the elderly patient may not comply compulsively to the recommended dosage schedule.

It should, therefore, not be surprising that the usually expected clinical manifestation of new onset or worsening IHD could be modified significantly because of altered pharmacokinetics or pharmacodynamics of prescribed or over-the-counter medications taken by the elderly patient[22,23] (see Chapter 3).

Many Elderly Bear the Burden of Many Years of Unhealthy Living

Our aging society has been subjected to many years of urbanization, with its crowding, industrialization and resulting environmental pollution. Furthermore, many have become smokers and/or have been and may continue to be one of the millions of people exposed to tobacco smoke, not as an active smoker, but by inhalation of environmental tobacco smoke (ETS). The public health impact of ETS is considerable. Of the estimated 480,000 smoking-related deaths that occur every year in the United States, 53,000 have been attributed to ETS, making passive smoke the third leading preventable cause of death, after active smoking and alcohol use.[24] Many of these individuals become victims of IHD. There is a 52% higher risk of death from IHD among cigarette smokers, age 65 to 74 years, than among nonsmokers or ex-smokers. But it should be appreciated that this high death rate for smokers declines within 5 years of ceasing to smoke.[24]

Many in our society at all ages, but especially the elderly, became sedentary "couch potatoes," consuming diets high in calories, saturated fats, and sodium.[25–29]

In the Framingham Study, as people gained weight, a host of risk factors worsened.[29] The total cholesterol, low density lipoprotein (LDL) cholesterol and triglyceride levels rose, and the high density lipoprotein (HDL) cholesterol level decreased. Blood pressure levels rose, and blood sugar, uric acid, the size of the left ventricle, as determined echocardiographically, all worsened with weight gain.[25–30] The more people weigh, the higher the rates of atherosclerotic cardiovascular disease. After 8 years of obesity for men and 14 years for women, the Framingham data have shown that obesity becomes an independent risk factor for coronary artery disease (CAD).[29]

In many, paralleling the weight gain is a loss of muscle mass. Muscle strength in most persons is well preserved until they are about 45 years old. It then begins to decline about 5% to 10% for a decade. The average person will lose about 30% of muscle strength and 40% of muscle size between the second and seventh decades of life, which is a process called sarcopenia.[31] There is impressive evidence that participating in a physically-active lifestyle contributes significantly to a decreased risk of cardiovascular disease by attaining and maintaining a heart healthy weight, more nearly ideal lipids and blood pressure (BP), and by reducing the occurrence of cancer, as well as stroke, osteoporosis and arthritis.[27]

Approximately 50 million adults in the United States have hypertension; nearly three-quarters do not control the pressure below the ideal of 140/90 mm Hg.[13,32]

It is now known, contrary to claims in the past, that older people do not tolerate high BP better than do younger people. Indeed, Framingham has shown that the impact of hypertension is worse in elderly individuals, both on an absolute and a relative scale. Furthermore, it is now known that SBP is a better predictor of cardiovascular events than is DBP.[23]

A double-blind placebo controlled study, Systolic Hypertension in the Elderly Program (SHEP),[32] at the end of 5 years demonstrated, as a result of lowering SBP, a statistically significant reduction in CHD events, congestive heart failure (CHF), and overall cardiovascular disease. The initial treatment used was 12.5 mg of chlorthalidone, increased to 25 mg, if no response; atenolol was added in subjects who did not achieve goal BP. Each participant had a goal BP established as follows: persons with SBP 180 mm Hg or more had a goal reduction to less than 160 mm Hg, whereas, those with SBP of 160–179 mm Hg had a goal reduction of 20 mm Hg or more. Thus, a patient with a baseline SBP of 165 mm Hg had a goal of 145 mm Hg. All subjects at entry had a DBP less than 90 mm Hg and were 60 years of age or older.[32]

There is persuasive evidence accumulating that total cholesterol appears to be inversely correlated with mortality, not only in the average adult, but in the very old as well.[33] Elevated serum cholesterol concentration and low serum HDL cholesterol concentration are associated with an increased risk of acute coronary events and premature atherosclerosis even in the very old.[33,34] Total cholesterol/HDL cholesterol ratio was demonstrated, in 1983, based on a 26-year follow-up of participants in Framingham to be significantly related to CHD in men over 65 years of age. For each unit rise in the ratio, the odds ratio rises 1.14 and is the most powerful predictor in elderly women where the odds ratio increases 1.25 for each unit rise in the ratio over 4.0.[34] Based on a mean follow-up of 4.5 years, Frost et al[33] found that the data from SHEP demonstrated a significant relationship between total, non-HDL, and LDL cholesterol levels and the ratios of total, HDL and LDL to HDL cholesterol and the incidence of CHD. This study included 4736 men and women 60 years of age or older.

The possible role of lipoprotein(a) in the progression of CHD is beyond the scope of this discussion; also, homocystine[35,36] and an infectious agent such as chlamydia pneumonia.[37] But none of these, and others, can be discounted at this time, as possibly contributing significantly to the progression of coronary atherosclerosis.[38]

But it is generally accepted that, as a large segment of our aging society have for years and are continuing to subject their bodies to a physically inactive lifestyle, inhaling much direct and/or ETS, consuming an excessively fat and sodium-laden diet resulting in considerable obesity and developing and maintaining a low cholesterol/HDL ratio, hypertension and frequently acquiring diabetes, the epidemic of IHD will shift even more to the elderly.[24-26] Furthermore, it should be apparent that the incidence of IHD among elderly women is increasing and will continue to increase greatly. CAD now accounts for 70% to 80% of the deaths among both men and women younger than 65 years.[38] These changes have been defined by Dr. Ryan as the healthcare transition.[3]

Thus, with extensive CAD so common in the large and enlarging elderly population, astute clinicians will/must consider whether new symptoms, however vague and ill defined, experienced by an elderly individual might be initiated because of changes in cardiac function due to newly developed or worsening IHD.

Establishing the Diagnosis of IHD

The History, The Symptoms

The cornerstone to establishing the diagnosis of IHD in an elderly individual is to determine whether the symptoms with which the patient is complaining could be or have been due to inadequate myocardial blood flow or could have been the result of newly developed inadequate blood flow to a previously compromised organ/system as a result of new onset IHD. Thus, the importance of a carefully, thoughtfully obtained history cannot be overemphasized. Attention should be directed not only to ruling out the presence of the symptoms of classical IHD, i.e. angina pectoris, but also the premonitory symptoms of an acute coronary occlusion that have been reported by numerous clinicians, as occurring hours to days before the acute event.[39–43] Dack[40] in 1941 reported:

> The premonitory symptoms usually appeared within 24 hours prior to the acute attack, but in some cases they began 23 weeks before. The duration of symptoms varied from a few minutes to several hours. Although premonitory pain was usually intermittent or continuous, a pain-free period frequently intervened before the onset of acute occlusion. The anatomic basis for the premonitory symptoms is assumed to be a gradual occlusion of the lumen of the coronary artery by progressive or recurrent intramural hemorrhage or by primary thrombosis on a plaque which may take hours or days for completion.

Furthermore, it must be appreciated that the characteristic pain of myocardial ischemia has been reported to be not as frequent a presenting symptom in the elderly as in the young. Such an altered pattern of pain is particularly common in the old-old individual, that is the patient 85 years and older.[41–43] A number of studies have reported that chest pain alone was seen in only 25% to 43% of elderly patients. In a very carefully executed study, Bayer and associates[44] found that although chest pain was the most frequently reported symptom by patients subsequently diagnosed as having IHD, there was a decrease in the frequency of reports of chest pain with increasing age. It was reported by 79.4% of 243 patients age 70 to 74 years, but by only 37.5% of 88 patients above age 85 years. In these older patients, pain was replaced by shortness of breath as the most common presenting symptom. Dyspnea was the most common presenting complaint in 43 of 88 patients above 85 years. Muller et al[45] reported that in patients older than 85 years, chest pain was absent in 75% of those experiencing an AMI. It has also been suggested that many elderly patients are very sedentary and do not exercise vigorously enough to adequately stress the heart to the point of producing ischemic pain.[46] Others have suggested that short-term memory loss results in "forgetting the symptom."[47]

Rapaport,[15] in commenting on the physical activity at the time of pain, indicated that in patients under age 50, an AMI was more likely to be associated with concurrent exercise than in individuals older than 70 years of age. Similarly, when over 70, one is more likely to be in bed when suffering an infarction. This does not appear to be related to changes in circadian rhythm. It rather appears to reflect the lifestyle of elderly patients, many of whom, unfortunately, are likely to be inactive during much of the 24-hour period. Such inactivity may not be just because of a lack of desire to be active, but because of one or more musculoskeletal and/or other exercise limiting disabilities.

Rapaport[15] further indicated that the level of activity appears to influence outcome. He cited the report of Stewart et al,[48] who stated that patients who were exercising at the time of their infarct had approximately 40% less likelihood of in-hospital mortality compared to those whose onset occurred in bed or at rest.

Silent Ischemia

These observations would suggest that silent ischemia is not uncommon in the elderly. Furthermore, the absence of pain, as indicated, is more common in the elderly than in young individuals. But it should be remembered that patients with silent ischemia, on ambulatory electrocardiographic monitoring, regardless of age, may have a higher rate of cardiac events over time than patients without such demonstrated silent ischemia.[44-48]

Why should there be a decrease in the frequency of the perception of pain, or the intensity of perceived pain, associated with myocardial ischemia in older individuals? Although there is no conclusive explanation, it has been suggested that older patients have a higher pain threshold.[49] They could have experienced damage to the sensory and/or autonomic fibers from previous myocardial ischemia. Or they could have experienced cortical failure, or other neurological impairment, secondary to cerebrovascular disease (CVD). Some individuals could have developed autonomic dysfunction.[44] That autonomic dysfunction may be an important reason for the lower incidence in the perception of pain by elderly individuals is suggested by a decreased reporting of sweating, nausea, and vomiting by older patients. Bayer et al[44] reported that sweating and vomiting were uncommon without chest pain, and both were less frequently reported with increasing age. Neither of these signs/symptoms have been associated with silent ischemia. Finally, as previously suggested, the elderly could complain of less pain because many of them exercise much less frequently and less vigorously than younger patients. Or it might be because short-term memory is poor in many older patients and they easily forget the symptoms that they have had, even if experienced recently.[47]

Care should be exercised in administering nitroglycerin to such a patient, as might be done for diagnostic purposes to a young patient.

Friesinger[21] emphasized that older patients are notoriously more susceptible to the hypotension produced by nitroglycerin because of its effect on preload. This phenomenon is altered by the age- related diastolic dysfunction, described by Fleg[12] and a blunted baroreceptor response. Younger patients experience a reflex tachycardia in response to the associated reduction in blood pressure. But a similar compensatory change does not occur in older people.

Stunning and Hibernation of the Heart

As a result of increasing experience with thrombolytic therapy and other forms of interventional recanalization for the treatment of acute ischemic syndromes, coupled with the recognition that many patients with CAD experience spontaneous reperfusion after coronary spasm or thrombosis, there is increasing interest in the phenomena of myocardial stunning.[50–53] Myocardial stunning is the mechanical dysfunction of the myocardium that may be present for hours to days after an ischemic even, despite restoration of normal or near normal coronary flow and in the absence of irreversible myocardial damage. Bolli[53] demonstrated in dogs that the severity and/or of stunning duration of the ischemia is the major determinant of the severity. It is important to appreciate that stunning may, if not corrected promptly, contribute to morbidity and mortality. It is, according to Bolli,[50,51] probably the most frequent cause of myocardial dysfunction and the low cardiac output syndrome after otherwise successful coronary artery bypass grafting (CABG). It would appear that stunning of the myocardium can occur with episodes of silent ischemia.

Gheorghiade and Bonow[54] reported that recurrent episodes of myocardial ischemia, with resulting repetitive episodes of myocardial stunning, may contribute to the overall magnitude of LV dysfunction and heart failure symptoms. The techniques to diagnose this phenomenon will be discussed subsequently. But the best approach is to prevent stunning before it occurs. This can usually be accomplished by positive inotropic intervention(s).

Whereas the diagnosis of stunning requires the demonstration of dysfunctional myocardium with normal or near normal blood flow, hibernating myocardium is defined as persistent myocardial contractile dysfunction associated with reduced coronary flow and preserved myocardial viability. The myocardium has, therefore, downregulated to the point where the reduced oxygen supply can be tolerated for extended periods of time without cell death and without clinical or metabolic evidence of ischemia. Once coronary flow is restored, the dysfunction is completely reversed.[55,56] Thus, the diagnosis is established in patients in whom regional contractile abnormalities are detected during angina-free intervals associated with reduced perfusion which is caused by significant obstruction to flow that was corrected by coronary revascularization. The possibility that function may dramatically improve or even normalize after restoration of normal perfusion makes diagnosis of the condition highly desirable.[52] The use of positron emission tomography (PET), or thallium-201 computed tomography (CT) for this purpose will be discussed subsequently.

Although the diagnosis may be suspected, it cannot be established until after definitive therapy has been undertaken. But stunning could occur after the therapeutic effort correcting the hibernation and then subsequently regress.[56]

It is unknown whether or not stunning and/or hibernation is/are more or less common in the elderly compared with the younger population. Although discussed as separate independent phenomena, Ambrosios[52] emphasized that the two phenomena may be coexistent.

Symptoms Finally Concern the Patient

When characteristic angina is not the predominant presenting symptom in the elderly patient, there is, or are likely to be, one or more other symptoms of recent onset that cause concern, prompting the patient to seek early medical care. Dyspnea, as indicated, is very common. This may be caused by incipient, or even frank CHF or underlying pulmonary disease. There may be an increased frequency of weakness, giddiness, varying degrees of confusion, or even syncope. The latter may be precipitated by orthostatic hypotension that is common in the elderly. The hemodynamic sequelae of the orthostatic changes could be intensified by an unrecognized ischemic event. Atrial and ventricular premature ectopy, atrial fibrillation, or heart block are common in the elderly patient with IHD.

Older patients tend to have smaller myocardial infarctions (MIs) compared to younger patients. The latter are more likely to experience an infarct following closure of a major vessel. But by age 85 years, small vessels, even collaterals that may be more numerous, are crucially important; the closure of such a small vessel could produce an MI. Such closure, however, would likely involve only a small segment of myocardium. The Coronary Artery Surgery Study (CASS) reported that 53% of patients older than 85 years of age had triple-vessel disease.[57] Because an infarct in an older individual is likely to be small, they usually cause only minor electrocardiographic changes and minor enzyme elevations. There appear to be more non-Q-wave infarcts in the elderly compared with younger individuals. The total creatine phosphokinase (CPK) values may be normal, or only slightly elevated above normal, but the MB fractions may be moderately elevated.

As has been discussed, the presentation of an ischemic event in the elderly may also be altered and not suggestive of the classic presentation of such an event experienced by a younger patient. This is frequently because associated diseases may cause many symptoms, as previously noted, that are not classically seen with an IHD. As previously stated, elderly subjects rarely present the clinical or laboratory picture of pure diseases. Many patients with CAD also have hypertensive vascular disease, CHF, CVD, and peripheral vascular disease. They may also have diabetes, chronic obstructive lung disease, anemia, musculoskeletal disease, and gastrointestinal disorders.

The ischemic process may reduce cardiac output slightly and this could result in an accentuation of the symptoms resulting from another disease process. For example, until the patient sustained a reduced cardiac output, because of an IHD, aortic stenosis or other valvular defects of the heart that might be present, might have been asymptomatic. The acute event might produce a sufficient added hemodynamic burden to result in symptomatic CHF. Thus, the classic findings of IHD might be overshadowed by signs and symptoms of other processes.

CHD accounts for at least 365,000 deaths for women in the United States each year.[58] A recent study of over 5000 outpatients, cared for by family practitioners, demonstrated that the prevalence of chronic stable angina was greater in women than men. Although the onset of CAD becomes symptomatic at a later age in women than men, it is the most important cause of death over the entire life span of women.[58,59] Pepine[60] emphasized that because more women than men survive to an old age, mortality due to CHD for all ages combined is at least as great in women as in men. But unfortunately, because women traditionally have been under-represented in, or excluded from clinical studies of CAD, there is considerably less information about the specific use of diagnostic and treatment strategies in women.[61-62] The astute clinician must, therefore, have a high index of suspicion when seeing an elderly female with new onset of symptoms.

The Changing Action of Drugs

As previously discussed, an elderly patient is likely to be on a number of medications. He or she might be on the verge of becoming symptomatic from the interaction of one or more of several drugs just before an ischemic event. A reduced cardiac output following myocardial damage could significantly alter the metabolism of any one or more of a variety of commonly prescribed drugs. An AMI might be essentially silent except for the clinical manifestations of an excessive drug level(s). When a patient becomes intolerant to a previously tolerated drug regimen, the physician should consider the possibility that the patient might have sustained an AMI.

Consider the Entire Patient

Clearly, the need for a careful history, elicited thoughtfully and without haste from the elderly patient with new onset symptoms, cannot be overemphasized. It is important to carefully determine the risk factors, both inherited and acquired, that are borne by the individual, even though IHD might not be suspected as a result of a patient's initial complaints. This is particularly important if the patient is elderly and is a smoker, is sedentary and obese, and is hypertensive and has a low cholesterol/HDL ratio. The possibility of altered hemodynamics due to IHD causing the symptoms should be considered.

Because ischemia in the elderly is often clinically silent or associated with atypical symptoms, establishing the diagnosis will frequently depend on the results of thoughtfully selected and implemented tests. But each test should be implemented for a meaningful purpose to avoid wasteful and unnecessary expenditure of resources.

If it is decided that the patient has had a painless ischemic event, Freisinger[21] recommends determining, if possible, why the episode was painless. Was it because the signal for pain was altered? Was it because the patient exercised infrequently and without vigor? Does the patient suffer from a poor short-term memory? Or has the signal for pain been altered? Freisinger[21] further stated, "There is an extraordinary heterogeneity in the rate and manner in which people age, particularly past the age of 70. Thus, chronology is a relatively poor guide to physiological aging. It is absolutely critical to individualize care in older patients with any condition, but particularly of an acute MI."

The Physical Examination

When evaluating the physical condition of the patient, in addition to carefully carrying out the examination taught in medical school, one must determine the physiological age of the patient. This is far more important in the total evaluation than defining and focusing on the chronological age. Attention must be directed not only to the BP, heart rate and rhythm, and characteristics of the pulse, temperature, and rate and characteristics of respiration, but attention should be directed, as previously indicated, to the level of physical activity at the time of the event and the usual daily activities of the patient. Careful attention should be directed to the neck veins, the retinal vessels for signs of diabetes, the skin, subcutaneous tissue and the amount there is, and the muscle mass and relative strength. Careful attention should obviously be directed to the heart, its size and the impulse and the sounds that are generated as well as the arterial system, seeking evidence of possible obstruction and/or dilatation and the venous system for evidence of obstruction. The other organ systems should also be carefully evaluated with special attention being directed to recognizing newly developed dysfunction. It is particularly important to carefully evaluate the neurologic system and to document any neurological deficit(s) that may exist. Such a record would be particularly useful should the patient subsequently experience a neurological event. It might be important to know, as of a definite date, whether or not specific neurological impairments existed.

The ECG

The ECG is of key importance in attempting to establish the diagnosis of IHD. Although it may be normal in many patients with classic angina, Rothbaum[63] indicated that it might well be abnormal without ischemia. He furthermore indicated that 50% of patients older than 65 have an abnormal ECG and that the abnormalities are frequently due to noncoronary disease. Coodley[43] reported an incidence in similar patients of nonspecific ST-T changes in 26.1%, left axis deviation in 57%, first degree atrioventricular (AV) block in 9%, and complete AV block in 7.6%. Tresch and associates,[64] in a study of 2482 consecutive adult emergency medical service patients with chest pain, found that approximately 40% of the patients older than 70 years of age who had an AMI did not demonstrate typical ST elevation with the development of Q waves. Thus, they were classified as having non- Q-wave infarcts. In comparison, only 25% of the infarcts in patients 70 years or younger were so classified.

Rajala and associates,[65] after a careful study of persons older than 85 years, concluded that the specificity of the ECG changes for heart disease was not very high. However, the ECG may help in establishing a diagnosis of an arrhythmia. It is also of help if there are changes in comparison to the findings on recent tracings. Similar changes that occur in serial tracings during a symptomatic period may be of help in establishing a proper diagnosis. But it should be remembered that the standard 12- lead ECG inconsistently records electrical activity of the posterior wall and the right ventricle.

Older patients should be encouraged to carry a copy of a recent ECG and a summary of pertinent medical events and pertinent laboratory reports when traveling from the base of their routine medical care.

The Routine Laboratory Assessment

If the suspicion of an ischemic event is significant, serial cardiac enzymes may be helpful. As indicated previously, however, because the size of infarcts in the elderly are not as large as those commonly seen in younger individuals, the magnitude of changes may not be as great as seen in younger patients. The CPK-MB determination is widely used when an acute process is suspected. But it is not diagnostic until eight to 12 hours after the onset of symptoms. If the acute event is suspected to have occurred more than 48 hours before the evaluation, a lactate dehydrogenase (LDH) test with isoenzyme determination may be useful. Changes in percentages of fractions of isoenzymes derived from cardiac and skeletal muscle may be diagnostic. Cardiac- specific troponin I or T and improved assays for markers such as myoglobin, and the CPK-MB isoforms show promise as sensitive indicators of myocardial injury. Myoglobin becomes positive within 2 to 4 hours after the onset of symptoms and peaks 4 to 5 hours after onset of symptoms. They are becoming available in most laboratories.[66,67] Myoglobin has been reported as having a 100% sensitivity within 1.5 hours after admission, compared with 4 hours as was reported for CPK-MB.[68]

Furthermore, if an ischemic event is suspected and the value(s) for recently measured lipid markers is/are not known, serum for such determinations should be obtained with the drawing of the first sample for cardiac enzymes. For it has been demonstrated that within 24 hours of the onset of an AMI, the serum cholesterol will begin declining, and may decline as much as 30%. The level does not return to baseline value for 3 to 6 months.[69,70] Thus, if the lipid values are not obtained within the 24-hour window, neither the physician nor the patient will know how important lipid normalization therapy will be. This is most unfortunate because, when the patient is in the hospital with the acute symptoms of a heart attack and is receiving what could well be interpreted as "lifesaving" medications, he/she will be most receptive to recommendations regarding lipid management. Clearly, outlining a definitive, goal-oriented program will be more productive than telling the patient that he/she will be given advice regarding cholesterol, etc., in 3 to 6 months. If the patient was not fasting when the first sample for cardiac enzymes was obtained, a reliable second sample can be obtained when fasting within 24 hours of the onset of symptoms for little decline in the value occurs during that interval.

Obviously, the hemogram, urinalysis, and routine laboratory screen of organ function should be obtained. Such is important not only to rule out abnormal function, but to establish a current baseline for future use to detect newly developed abnormalities. Also, if the patient is taking a medication such as digoxin, coumadin, etc., the blood level or activity level should be determined.

The Chest X-Ray

The chest roentgenogram is of little value in establishing the diagnosis of IHD. Coronary artery calcifications, when present in an individual younger than age 60, are significant, but may be present in up to 90% of individuals older than 70 years of age.[38] There does appear to be a correlation between the extent of calcification and the severity of atherosclerosis. Ultrafast CT appears to be a very sensitive method to detect significant calcification and may well become useful clinically. But at present, it is not widely available, is costly and its clinical usefulness has not been established.

Although a roentgenogram may be of little value in diagnosing IHD, one should be taken if a recent study has not been performed. It could reveal a silent associated or unrelated but symptomatic disease process and it can give insight into the size of the heart and the state of the great vessels.

The Exercise Stress Test

An exercise stress test is one of the most frequently used modalities to detect IHD in the public at large. Exercise testing in the elderly, whether by treadmill or bicycle ergometry, when performed with acceptable standards, appears to retain the same diagnostic and prognostic value as demonstrated in younger patients. With care and prudent evaluation of the patient, it is as safe as in younger individuals. Frequently, however, such a procedure is impossible in the elderly because of physical or emotional limitations or lack of coordination. The test can frequently be satisfactorily accomplished, by accommodating the protocol to the limitations of the patient. Many elderly patients cannot accomplish the requirements of the standard Bruce protocol wherein both speed and elevation of the treadmill are increased simultaneously with each stage. This requires large increases in energy expenditure between successive stages. Many poorly conditioned elderly patients will terminate the effort prematurely. However, many such individuals can and will tolerate the Naughton, modified Bruce, or Balke protocols, which maintain a modest constant speed and increase only the percentage grade between stages. Bicycle exercise testing may be used in some patients who have difficulty walking. The test should start at a low work load and be increased by modest intervals. The optimal duration for an exercise stress test, whether walking or cycling, should be between 8 and 12 minutes. It should be emphasized that such a duration allows sufficient time to observe graded changes in heart rate, BP, and ST segment response while avoiding boredom, undue fatigue, or muscular discomfort. The results usually give the examiner an opportunity to determine the likelihood or not of significant IHD being present.[71,72]

Unfortunately, even with a cooperative patient, the test may not give the physician confidence to establish the presence or absence of significant ischemic disease. For example, the patient may have a left bundle branch block pattern or develop it with stress, or have nonspecific changes, even in the resting tracing.

Hilton et al[73] studied 120 patients 70 years of age or older with known or suspected CAD who had a Bruce protocol stress test with thallium-201 injection. These patients had a follow-up of 36 ± 12 months. There was a cardiac event rate of 10%, with 6 deaths from arrhythmia or heart failure, 5 fatal AMIs, and 1 nonfatal AMI. By univariant analysis, they found 3 variables associated with the development of a cardiac event: (1) maximum ST segment depression of 2.0 mm or greater (27% with an event vs. 6% without); (2) peak exercise beyond stage I of a Bruce protocol (18% event rate in those who could not get beyond stage I vs. 6% if they did); (3) the presence of a fixed or reversible thallium defect (18% event rate with vs. 2% without). The use of the isotope marker clearly improves the sensitivity and specificity of the standard stress test, but at considerable increased cost.

A number of studies indicate that an abnormal exercise ECG stress test has limited diagnostic accuracy in women.[72,73] A 5- to 20-fold greater occurrence of false-positive exercise ECG ST segments in women than in men have been described. Miller[74] reported that postinfarction studies of exercise ECG testing in the thrombolytic era have continued to under-represent women who made up only 15% to 20% of most study populations. He suggested that those findings might reflect the lack of physician confidence in the diagnostic and prognostic value of standard stress ECG analysis in women with known or suspected CAD.

An ECG stress test is useful, prior to discharge, after treatment for an AMI. The performance of the patient, i.e. duration, heart rate and ECG changes suggesting ischemia, or the occurrence of rhythm disturbances, is helpful in planning the postdischarge therapy. An abnormal response with limited duration might suggest the need for predischarge nuclear imaging studies and/or cardiac catheterization.

Echocardiography

Echocardiography is particularly well suited for use in elderly patients. Important diagnostic information about cardiac structural and functional abnormalities can be obtained without subjecting the patient to the risk of an invasive procedure. Echocardiography is also useful for following serially the progression of heart disease. The cost/ratio benefit, however, should be considered before ordering the test.

By means of M-mode echocardiography, LVED and LVES dimensions as well as intraventricular septal and posterior LV wall thickness can be obtained.

Two-dimensional M-mode echocardiography with color flow Doppler offers the ability to evaluate regional abnormalities of myocardial motion and LV global function. Demonstration of a normal LVEF ($\geq$50%) or an LVEF of <50% is of prognostic importanc and could influence therapeutic decisions. Aronow[75] reported that the 95% confidence limits of reproducibility of an LVEF obtained by quantitative two-dimensional echocardiography are $\pm$7%.

Doppler echocardiography is also useful in diagnosing LV diastolic dysfunction. It can also estimate pulmonary artery pressure and diagnose the presence, etiology and severity of aortic stenosis, aortic regurgitarion, mitral regurgitation and mitral stenosis as well as other forms of valvular disease and/or dysfunction, such as papillary muscle dysfunction as well as the rupture of the intraventricular septum. The technique can also detect LV segmental wall motion dysfunction and aneurysmal formation as well as LV and/or atrial thrombus formation.

Although exercise ECG is the time-honored technique for determining whether or not a person develops myocardial ischemia as a result of stress, it is frequently not highly specific for answering this question in a given patient. This is particularly the case in women. A 5- to 20-fold greater occurrence of false-positive ECG ST-segment responses have been reported in women.[76] Stress echocardiography appears a more reliable option. But echocardiography stress testing may be nondiagnostic in some women, as well as many middle aged elderly males, because it requires vigorous exercise. Also, unstable echocardiographic images may result from obesity, an elongated thorax, deep breathing, or excessive chest motion.[71,72]

But most of these problems can be obviated by stressing the heart pharmacologically rather than physiologically. Myocardial blood flow can be increased by an infusion of dipyridamole or dobutamine. Dobutamine stress echocardiography has been demonstrated to be a powerful predictor of subsequent cardiac events. Infusing dobutamine, starting with a low dose, 5 μg/kg per minute, and increasing this dose 5 μg/kg per minute up to 40 μg/kg per minute or to the dose producing significant symptoms and/or ECG abnormalities. The normal myocardial response shows enhanced function with dobutamine; the ischemic myocardium has enhanced function at low dose, and no change or worsening function at higher dose. The scarred myocardium has no enhanced function.[75,76] Clearly pharmacological stress with dobutamine infusion provides an important alternative to exercise echocardiography.

It must always be remembered that the quality of echocardiographic studies is dependent on the training, skill, and compulsiveness of the technician who obtains the data and the physician who interprets it. The body build, adiposity and cooperation of the patient also determine the quality of the images obtained. Beyond the scope of this discussion is the use of transesophageal echocardiography.

Radionuclide Perfusion Imaging

When the presence of myocardial ischemia, as a result of physical stress, cannot be documented/ruled out by standard treadmill testing, radionuclide perfusion imaging, using thallium-201 or technetium 99m sestamibi, may be useful. Such problems are not uncommon in women.[77-80] These techniques demonstrate, with radioactive isotopes, the distribution of myocardial blood flow. Thallium is distributed into the myocardial tissue immediately after intravenous injection. Its distribution is dependent on coronary blood flow and the ability of the myocardial cells to extract the thallium. Infarcted tissue, regardless of age, does not actively take up thallium and will appear as an area lacking in isotope on the scanner image. The technetium 99m is an isotope that is taken up by myocardium in proportion to blood flow. It has very limited redistribution with time. Therefore, the imaging can be performed several hours after the intravenous injection to determine the state of perfusion at the time of injection when the patient might have been symptomatic, but at the time of scanning the patient was asymptomatic.

Because redistribution of radioisotopes takes place proportionate to the myocardial blood flow, comparison of the distribution of the isotope during exercise with the distribution of the isotope at rest differentiates myocardial scar from viable myocardium.[78–80]

But the techniques are not without limitations. With nuclear imaging, the photons, located in the myocardium, escape through the thorax and breast tissue to reach the external camera detector surface. The attenuation or scatter of these photons by soft tissue and bone may create artifactual defects in the anterior-septal and anterior region that might be mistaken for perfusion abnormalities. Such defects are usually fixed but, in the female, especially one with large breasts, as well as a morbidly obese male, could appear to be reversible defects if the breast or adipose tissue position change between the stress and rest images.[59]

Osbakken[77] reported that thallium-201 has a lower sensitivity for CAD detection in women than in men (54% vs. 79%). Goodgold and associates[78] reported that among 840 patients with suspected CAD studied by thallium-201, 44 (11%) of 391 women were judged to have inadequate diagnostic images due to breast artifacts compared to only 7 (2%) of 449 men ($P < 0.05$). These suboptimal studies occurred despite the laboratory's experience with the use of breast "markers" to improve the diagnostic accuracy. Miller[74] reported that among women whose coronary angiograms are normal, rates of false-positive results with thallium based tests are ranged from 8% to 58%.

Concerns about the high rate of false-positive cardiac imaging tests using thallium- 201 led to the development of technetium 99m (Tc-99m) labeled myocardial perfusion agents. The Tc-99m sestamibi emits substantially higher levels of energy (140 KeV) than thallium-201. Therefore, photon scattering and attenuation is less of a problem and should yield improved, more reliable images. But with the sestamibi, two separate injections, usually 90 minutes apart, of the radiotracer are required to document perfusion status at rest and at peak stress during exercise or during infusion of a pharmacological stressor such as dipyridamole.

It would appear that the problem with false-positive thallium-201 tests in females has been greatly reduced by the single photon emission computed tomography (SPECT). Miller[74] reported that the cardiac event rates were extremely low in patients with a normal Tc-99m SPECT during a 2-year follow-up of 214 women and 1262 men (0.6% in women and 1.4% in men). In patients with at least one reversible defect on the SPECT, the cardiac event rate in women was 6.9% as compared with 10.9% in men ($P = $ NS).

It was shown by Maes and associates[80] that PET was more predictive of viability/nonviability and recovery of contractile function after revascularization than Tc-99m sestamibi SPECT, but the latter is more widely available and considerably less costly than PET.

If the patient is unable to exercise, myocardial blood flow can be increased by dobutamine, dipyridamole and/or adenosine.[71,72] They have the advantage, compared to exercise ECG stress, of demonstrating which myocardial territories are supplied by obstructed vessels. Also, with sestamibi, LV ejection fraction and measurements of LV wall motion can be obtained. In the study by Hilton et al[79] previously discussed, they found that on multivariant analysis, the combination of inability to attain a peak exercise beyond stage I and the presence of any thallium defect, carried a risk ratio of 5.3 at 1 year.

As a result of the persistence of Dr. Raymond Bahr,[81] Chest Pain Emergency Departments are becoming widespread. In a number of such centers, patients with a suspected but not proven acute AMI or acute coronary syndrome are injected with a tracer dose of Tc-99m as soon as they are triaged in the emergency department. The patient subsequently undergoes imaging, and the results of the SPECT perfusion image is used to determine the need for early intervention, or in the case of a normal study, for early noninvasive stress testing before discharge. Such an approach has been demonstrated by Tatum and associates[82] to be cost effective and improve patient care and patient convenience.

Ambulatory (Holter) Monitoring

By ambulatory ECG (Holter) monitoring, it may be possible to establish whether or not symptomatic and/or silent myocardial ischemia occurs as the patient participates in daily acts of living. Furthermore, it records the electrical signal from the heart under varying daily-life circumstances (ie, mental, environmental and physical stressors) that may provoke ischemia in certain individuals. Furthermore, it may record changes that might occur as a result of the circadian variation in heart rate and rhythm and cardiac ischemia. The patient should record the times of occurrence and the nature of unusual symptoms. Not only can the heart rate and rhythm be recorded, but also changes of ST segment which might reflect ischemia.

Such monitoring may be useful in contributing to the understanding of the significance of symptoms such as unexplained paroxysmal dyspnea that might reflect silent ischemia. A Scandinavian study reported a 4.4-fold increased coronary mortality in apparently healthy 68-year-old men who demonstrated silent myocardial ischemia on ambulatory monitoring.[83] Fleg[84] reported that over a 10-year mean follow-up of 98 clinically normal subjects in the Baltimore Longitudinal Study on Aging who underwent ambulatory 24-hour ECG recording, when aged 60 to 85 years, the subset of 16 with transient horizontal or slowly upsloping ST-segment depressions experienced nearly 4 times the rate of coronary events as those without such ST-segment shifts.

Aronow and Epstein[85] demonstrated by Holter monitoring silent ischemia in 34% of 185 nursing home residents (mean age 83 years). Such observations may contribute significantly to determining the function of the myocardium and help establish or not the diagnosis of ischemic heart disease.

Cardiac Catheterization and Angioplasty

Cardiac catheterization, with coronary angiography can define the coronary anatomy and the extent of vascular involvement, and the study can be performed with minimal risk in the elderly patient. However, Freisinger[21] pointed out that the physician's ability to predict prognosis solely on the coronary arteriographic findings in the elderly is somewhat limited.

Several studies have demonstrated that lesions frequently occur in previously normal sites.[86] Singh[87] reported that repeat coronary arteriograms, separated by a mean of 51 months in 52 patients receiving medical therapy, demonstrated that two-thirds of lesions were stable and only one-third showed progression. Thirty-seven new lesions developed during the period of observation. Little et al[88] studied a group of 42 consecutive patients before, and up to one month after, an AMI. Of the 42 patients, 29 had a newly occluded coronary artery and experience suggests that 13 of the patients, who did not have an occluded artery at the time of the study, might have had one demonstrated had they been studied earlier. Twenty-five of the 29 patients had at least one artery with more than 50% stenosis in the initial arteriogram. This, and other similar studies, strongly indicate that, in most instances, the cardiologist reviewing the coronary arteriogram of a patient in a stable condition cannot, with confidence, predict which lesions are critical and which vessels are likely to become suddenly occluded in the near future.

The patients' complaints, exercise tolerance, ventricular function, EF and comorbidity, rather than solely the altered coronary anatomy, are important determinants of prognosis. The older the patient, the more individualized the decision must be to undertake the procedure and possibly other invasive efforts. But this and other invasive procedures such as angioplasty and bypass surgery should not be arbitrarily withheld from even the very elderly with appropriate indications just because of age.[15]

Before coronary arteriography is undertaken in the elderly, or for that matter in any patient, the physician and the patient should have decided how the information obtained will be used. The elderly patient of 70 years who is physically well preserved should be interested not just in symptomatic improvement, that is, quality of life, but also longevity, or quantity of life. Whereas the elderly, who are older than age 85, even if fit, are not likely to benefit from invasive procedures to prolong life; they might benefit more from relief of symptoms and improvement of function. This might be obtained by medical means and, therefore, may make a need for knowledge of coronary anatomy unnecessary. This would clearly be true if the individual had already requested not to be resuscitated[89] (see Chapter 30). The caring physician should have discussed with an elderly patient what he or she wishes to do with his or her life before introducing a discussion about catheterization.

If there is any question whether the patient should have coronary arteriograms, the physician should not hesitate to recommend that a second opinion be obtained.[86] Unfortunately, the demonstration of lesions in the coronary anatomy frequently urges the beholder "to do something . . . .".[27] Mark Twain apparently recognized this phenomenon. He is alleged to have said, "To a man with a hammer, there are a lot of things that look like nails that need to be hammered."

But indeed there are lesions that could be "hammered" for the benefit of a patient with a balloon. There is increasing evidence suggesting that direct angioplasty may be superior to thrombolysis as urgent therapy for an AMI.[90,91] But such a decision regarding these specific therapies, as well as the use of stems, thrombectomy, antiplatelet and other specific pharmacologic therapy is beyond the scope of this document. Attention is directed to Chapters 10 through 13 of this book.

Pain-to-Door Time

Many investigators report that the elderly who experience symptoms subsequently diagnosed as due to IHD do not seek medical care as promptly as younger patients. In fact, few elderly arrive at an ED early enough to benefit from thrombolytic therapy. Friesinger and associates[21,91] studied 10,850 patients seen in the ED with chest pain judged to be due to myocardial ischemia. Unmistakable evidence of MI by serial clinical enzymatic, and ECG study was found in 1584 patients. Typical ST- segment elevation in the emergency department was less common in older patients than in the younger cohorts (31% in patients 75 years or older compared with 47% less than 75 years). But nearly 40% of patients 65 years or older who arrived in the emergency department with ST-segment elevation had had the onset of their chest pain 6 hours or more earlier, whereas, only 18% of patients less than 65 years with diagnostic ST-segment elevations arrived in the emergency department within 6 hours of the onset of pain.

Tresch and associates[92] found, in a study of 2482 adults with chest pain seen by paramedics, that the 998 70- to 79-year-olds and the 401 80-years or older delayed more than 6 hours seeking medical assistance compared with the 1484 younger patients who sought assistance less than 4 hours after the onset of pain. Forty percent of the older aged group had non-Q-wave infarcts compared to 23% in the younger group. The hospital mortality was 2 to 3 times higher in the elderly with an AMI compared to the younger patients. Weaver and associates[93] made similar observations in the community-wide study in Seattle, Washington.

Clearly, the patient should be counseled during the hospitalization and at the time of discharge, and when seen in follow-up visits as to the importance of remembering the symptoms that occurred before the recent event, and should they again be experienced, they should call immediately 911. I have found it helpful to liken the discussion regarding the serious nature of recurrent symptoms and the need for prompt emergency department evaluation to the warning given by flight attendants to the passengers on every flight about action to take when a crash of their airplane seemed imminent. I frequently show the patient a card, obtained from an airline, with a descriprion of the needed action when I am discussing possible recurrent ischemic symptoms with my patients. I tell most patients that should they experience the symptoms under discussion to sit down and take a single nitroglycerin tablet (unless contraindicated). If the symptoms persist for 3 minutes, take a second tablet. If the symptoms were still present and had been present for 5 minutes, despite 2 nitroglycerin tablets, the patient should call 911. After being certain the patient understands the instructions, I tell the patient that I do not expect such to occur—just like the Flight Attendant does not expect the airplane to crash—but they should be ready to carry out the plan should the need arise.

Unfortunately, there is little doubt that many patients do experience anxiety when they perceive the symptoms possibly due to IHD, and this anxiety fuels more anxiety—anxiety of having to rely on the health care system. The caring physician must appreciate the likelihood of such anxiety and work to prevent it.

Maintenance of Heart–Healthy Lifestyle

The complete therapy of the patient, in addition to those identified above, and other pharmacological efforts will be discussed in Chapters 9 through 13 of this text.

But most important is to emphasize the necessity of renewing what hopefully has been a longstanding practice of following or initiating a heart-healthy lifestyle. The goal of the physician, in all contacts with patients, should be directed toward stimulating the patient to become ultimately a physically and mentally young centenarian.

It should be emphasized that the evidence is overwhelming that even among elderly individuals with a mean age of 82 years, smoking, hypertension, diabetes mellitus, serum total cholesterol, HDL-cholesterol, and triglycerides were all independent risk factors for new coronary event.[94,95]

There is now evidence from the Post-CABG Trial[96] that lowering LDL less than 85 mg/dL by therapy with HMG-COA reductase inhibitor lovastatin and with cholestyramine, if required, there was less progression demonstrated by coronary arteriography and fewer revascularization procedures required. Similar salutary results were demonstrated in the Lipoprotein and Coronary Atherosclerosis Study (LCAS).[97] These studies both demonstrated that to get the desirable benefits, the cholesterol levels had to be monitored and the physician had to take a compulsive approach to getting patient compliance.

Summary

Fox[98] reported that the caring physician knows that he/she has not completed their responsibility to their patient when they have only outlined and prescribed the appropriate therapy. The physician must be confident that the patient will comply/adhere to the recommended therapy during the coming months/years. But the likelihood of noncompliance can exceed 50%. Sixty percent of rehospitalizations for CHF are due to nonadherence to diet or medication, or failure to heed signs of deterioration. A review of a random sample of more than 4000 discharge charts of Medicare patients with CHF revealed that fewer than half of the patients received usable instructions with their medications, diet or weight management.

But the cost of medications can have a large influence on compliance. In 110 indigent patients on Medicare, which does not cover the cost of chronic medication, the price of prescribed drugs amounted to one-third of their income. When the patients were assisted in obtaining their prescriptions free or at a low cost, the noncompliance rate fell from 52.6% to 13.5%. It is also noteworthy that patients who are depressed are poor compliers to the recommended therapy. Clearly "the best laid plans" can be of little value if they are not carried out by the patient. Therefore, the caring physician, really serious about the welfare of his/her patient(s), must maintain frequent contact with the patient through office visits and/or telephone calls personally or by an office assistant.

Dr. Jeanne Wei[99] reasoned that "aging really is more within our control than we might think it is. Even if we identify the longevity-relevant gene or genes, they will not significantly help people who don't take good care of themselves." We must be diligent and see that our patients do take good care of themselves and do follow a heart healthy lifestyle. Such a practice will decrease the likelihood of fatal CHD before the patient becomes a centenarian.

References

1. Page LB: Introductory remark. Presented at the 18th Bethesda Conference: Cardiovascular Disease in the Elderly. Wenger NK, chairperson. *J Am Coll Cardiol* 10:7A, 1987.
2. Champion EW: The oldest old. *N Engl J Med* 330:1819–1820, 1994.
3. Ryan TJ: Aging: Some additional considerations for the cardiovascular clinician. *Am J Geriatr Cardiol* 6(5):11–14, 1997.
4. US Bureau of Census: Estimates of the Population of the United States

by Age, Sex and Race: 1980 to 1986. Current Population Reports Series P-25, No 100; Washington, USGPO, 1987.

5. Olshansky SJ, Carnes BA, Cassel C: In search of Methuselah: Estimating the upper limits to human longevity. *Science* 250:634–640, 1990.

6. McIntosh HD: Early management of acute myocardial ischemic events. *J Florida Med Assoc* 82:87–91, 1995.

7. Castelli WP, Garrison RJ, Wilson PWF, et al: Incidence of coronary heart disease and lipoprotein cholesterol levels. The Framingham Heart Study. *JAMA* 256:2835–2840, 1986.

8. Roberts WC: Atherosclerotic risk factors—Are there ten or is there only one? *Am J Cardiol* 64:552–553, 1989.

9. Stamler J: Established major coronary risk factors. In: M Marmot, P Elliot (eds): *Coronary Heart Disease Epidemiology. From Etiology to Public Health*. New York: Oxford University Press; 1992, pp 45–66.

10. Roberts WC: Ninety-three hearts >90 years of age. *Am J Cardiol* 71:599–602, 1993.

11. Josephson RA, Fannin S: Physiology of the aging heart. In: E Chesler (ed): *Clinical Cardiology in The Elderly*. Armonk, NY: Futura Publishing Co, Inc, 1994, pp 37–62.

12. Fleg JL: Normative aging changes in cardiovascular structure and function. *Am J Geriatr Cardiol* 5(1):7–15, 1996.

13. Kannel WB: Host and environmental determinants of hypertension. Perspective from the Framingham Study. In: H Kesteloot, J Joossens (eds): *Epidemiology in Arterial Blood Pressure*. The Hague, Martinus Nijhoff, 1980, pp 265–295.

14. Avolio AP, Fa-Quan D, We-Qiang L, et al: Effects of aging on arterial distensibility in populations with high and low prevalence of hypertension: Comparison between urban and rural communities. *Circulation* 71:202–210, 1985.

15. Rapaport E: Myths and facts about coronary disease in the elderly. *Am J Geriatr Cardiol* 7(1):41–47, 1998.

16. Titus JL, Edwards JE: Pathology of the aging heart. In E Chesler (ed): *Clinical Cardiology in the Elderly*. Armonk, NY, Futura Publishing Company, Inc, 1994, pp 1–36.

17. McIntosh HD: Diagnostic differentials of co-existing diseases in the elderly patients with heart disease. *Am J Geriatr Cardiol* 5(1):41–44, 1996.

18. Schleifer SJ, Macari-Hinson MM, Coyle DA, et al: The nature and course of depression following myocardial infarction. *Arch Intern Med* 149:1785–1789, 1989.

19. Archer SL, Chesler E: Diagnosis of valvular heart disease in the elderly. In E Chesler (ed): *Clinical Cardiology in the Elderly*. Armonk, NY, Futura Publishing Company, Inc, 1994, pp 265–308.

20. Montamat SC, Cusack BJ, Vestal RE: Management of drug therapy in the elderly. *N Engl J Med* 321:303–310, 1989.

21. Friesinger GC: Coronary heart disease in the elderly: Management considerations. *Am J Geriatr Cardiol* 3(3):42–50, 1994.

22. Schwartz JB: Age-related pharmacodynamic changes in the elderly: Treatment considerations in heart failure. *Am J Geriatr Cardiol* 5(1):52–55, 1996.

23. Holtzman JL: Effect of age on the action and disposition of drugs used in the treatment of cardiovascular disease. In E Chesler (ed): *Clinical Cardiology in The Elderly*. Armonk, NY, Futura Publishing Company, Inc, 1994, pp 63–110.

24. Glantz SA, Parmley WW: Passive smoking and heart disease: Epidemiology, physiology and biochemistry. *Circulation* 83:1–12, 1991.
25. Aronow WS: Coronary disease in the elderly: What factors increase risk. *J Crit Ill* 8:59–69, 1993.
26. McIntosh HD: Geriatric cardiology: A subspecialty or mainstream for the twenty-first century. *Prog Cardiol* 3:117–125, 1990.
27. McIntosh HD: Risk factors for cardiovascular disease and death: A clinical perspective. *J Am Coll Cardiol* 14:24–30, 1989.
28. Castelli WP: Risk factors in the elderly: A view from Framingham. *Am J Geriatr Cardiol* 2(5):8–19, 1993.
29. Hubert HB, Feinleib M, McNamara PM, et al: Obesity as an independent risk factor for cardiovascular disease: A 26 year follow-up of participants in the Framingham Heart Study. *Circulation* 67:968–977, 1983.
30. Weverling-Rijnsburger AWE: Total cholesterol and risk of mortality in the oldest old. *Lancet* 350:1119–1123, 1997.
31. Nieman DC, Eichner ER: Can regular exercise slow the aging process? *Your Patient & Fitness* 10(1):6–17, 1995.
32. SHEP Cooperative Research Group. Prevention of stroke by antihypertensive drug treatment in older persons with isolated systolic hypertension. *JAMA* 265:3255–3264, 1991.
33. Forst PH, Davis BR, Burlando AJ: Serum lipids and incidence of coronary heart disease. Findings from the systolic hypertension in the elderly program. *Circulation* 94:2381–2388, 1996.
34. Wilson PWF, Kannel WB: Hypercholesterolemia and coronary risk in the elderly: The Framingham Study. *Am J Geriatr Cardiol* 2:52–56, 1993.
35. Remm EB, Willett WC, Hu FB, et al: Folate and vitamin B6 from diet and supplements in relation to risk of coronary heart disease among women. *JAMA* 279:359–364, 1998.
36. McCully KS: Homocysteine, folate, vitamin B6 and cardiovascular disease. *JAMA* 279:392–393, 1998.
37. Mason M: Are heart attacks contagious? *Hippocrates* (Dec):42–49, 1997.
38. Cannon LA, Marshall JM: Cardiac disease in the elderly population. *Clin Geriatr Med* 9:499–525, 1993.
39. Bahr RD, McIntosh HD: Reawakening awareness of the importance of prodromal symptoms in the shifting paradigm of early heart attack care (EHAC). *Clinician* 14:7–9, 1996.
40. Master AM, Dack S, Jaffe HL: Premonitory symptoms of acute coronary occlusion: A study of 260 cases. *Ann Intern Med* 14:1155–1164, 1941.
41. Solomon HA, Edwards AL, Killip T: Prodromata in acute myocardial infarction. *Circulation* 40:463–471, 1969.
42. McIntosh HD: Presentation and evaluation of ischemic heart disease. In: E Chesler (ed): *Clinical Cardiology in the Elderly*. Armonk, NY, Futura Publishing Company, Inc, 1994, pp 111–122.
43. Coodley EL: Clinical spectrum and diagnostic techniques of coronary heart disease in the elderly. *J Am Geriatr Soc* 36:447–450, 1988.
44. Bayer AJ, Chadha JS, Farag RR, et al: Changing presentation of myocardial infarction with increasing old age. *J Am Geriatr Soc* 34:263–270, 1986.
45. Muller RT, Gould LA, Betzu R, et al: Painless myocardial infarction in the elderly. *Am Heart J* 119:204–210, 1990.
46. Gottlieb SO, Weisfeidt ML, Ouyang P, et al: Silent ischemia as a marker for early unfavorable outcomes in patients with unstable angina. *N Engl J Med* 314:1214–1220, 1984.

47. Black DA: Mental state and presentation of myocardial infarction in the elderly. *Age Aging* 16:125–130, 1987.
48. Stewart RAH, Robertson MC, Wilkins GT, et al: Association between activity at onset of symptoms and outcome of acute myocardial infarction. *J Am Coll Cardiol* 29:250–253, 1997.
49. Miller PF, Sheps DS, Bragdon EE, et al: Aging and pain perception in ischemic heart disease. *Am Heart J* 120:22–30, 1990.
50. Bolli R: Mechanism of myocardial "stunning". *Circulation* 82:723–738, 1990.
51. Bolli R: Myocardial "stunning" in man. *Circulation* 86:1671–1691, 1992.
52. Ambrosio G, Perrone-Filardi P, Chiariello M: Myocardial hibernation and stunning: what is their practical significance. *J Myo Ischem* 6:19–32, 1994.
53. Bolli R, Zher WX, Thornly JL, et al: Time-course and determinants of recovery of function after reversible ischemia in unconscious dogs. *Am J Physiol* 254:H102-H114, 1988.
54. Gheorghiade M, Bonow RO: Chronic heart failure in the United States. A manifestation of coronary artery disease. *Circulation* 97:282–289, 1998.
55. Rahimtoola SH: The hibernating myocardium. *Am Heart J* 117:211–221, 1989.
56. Ross J Jr: Myocardial perfusion-contraction matching: Implications for coronary heart disease and hibernation. *Circulation* 83:1076–1083, 1991.
57. Gersh BJ, Krormal RH, Schaff HF, et al: Comparison of coronary artery bypass surgery and medical therapy in patients 65 years of age older. A nonrandomized study from the Coronary Artery Study (CASS) registry. *N Engl J Med* 313:217–225, 1985.
58. Pipine CJ, Abram J, Marks RG, et al, for the TIDES investigators: Characteristics of a contemporary population with angina pectoris. *Am J Cardiol* 74:226–231, 1994.
59. Pepine CJ, Lewis JF, Limacher MC, et al: Limitations of current diagnostic tests. *J Myo Ischem* 7:251–253, 1995.
60. Pepine CJ: IHD in women: Magnitude and scope of the problem. *J Myo Ischem* 7:235, 1995.
61. Wenger NK, Speroff L, Packard B: Cardiovascular health and disease in women. *N Engl J Med* 329:247–256, 1993.
62. Merkatz RB, Temple R, Feider K, et al: Women in clinical trials of new drugs: A change in Food and Drug Administration Policy. *N Engl J Med* 329:292–296, 1993.
63. Rothbaum DA: Coronary artery disease in geriatric cardiology. In JR Noble, DA Rothbaum (eds): *Cardiovascular Clinics*. Philadelphia, FA Davis Co, 1981, pp 105–117.
64. Tresch DD, Brady TP, Lawrence SW, et al: Comparison of elderly and young patients with out-of-hospital chest pain. *Arch Intern Med* 156:1089–1093, 1996.
65. Rajala SA, Ulla KM, Geiger MKM: Electrocardiogram, clinical findings, and chest x-ray in persons aged 85 or older. *Am J Cardiol* 55:1175–1181, 1985.
66. Adams JE, Schechtman KB, Landt Y, et al: Comparable detection of acute myocardial infarction by creatine kinase MG isoenzyme and cardiac Troponin I. *Clin Chem* 40:1291–1295, 1994.
67. Antman EM, Tanasijevic MJ, Thompson B, et al: Cardiac specific I levels predict the risk of mortality in patients with acute coronary syndromes. *N Engl J Med* 335:1342–1349, 1996.

68. Stack LB, Morgan JA, Hedges JR, et al: Advances in the use of ancillary diagnostic testing in the Emergency Department evaluation of chest pain. *Emerg Med Clin North Am* 13:713–732, 1995

69. Alexander W: Assessing post MI cholesterol. *Cardiol World News* Sept 15: 19, 1996.

70. International randomized trial comparing four thrombolytic strategies for acute myocardial infarction. The GUSTO Investigation. *N Engl J Med* 329: 673–680, 1993.

71. Gardin JM: The diagnostic utility of noninvasive tests in the office or outpatient evaluation of the elderly patient with congestive heart failure. *Am J Geriatr Cardiol* 5(1):34–40, 1996.

72. Sketch MN, Mohiuddin SM, Lynch JD, et al: Significant sex difference in the correlation of electrocardiographic exercise testing and coronary arteriograms. *Am J Cardiol* 36:169–173, 1975.

73. Barolsky SM, Gelber CA, Fauqui A, et al: Differences in electrocardiographic response to exercise of women and men: A non-Bayesian factor. *Circulation* 60:1021–1027, 1979.

74. Miller DD: Noninvasive diagnosis of CAD in women. *J Myo Ischem* 7: 263–267, 1995.

75. Aronow WS: Echocardiography should be performed in all healthy patients with congestive heart failure. *J Am Geriatr Soc* 42:1300–1302, 1994.

76. Fleg JL: Myocardial ischemia in the asymptomatic older patient. *Am J Geriatr Cardiol* 7(1):54–59, 198.

77. Osbakken MD: Exercise stress testing in women: Diagnostic dilemma. *Cardiovasc Clin* 19(3):187–194, 1989.

78. Goodgold HM, Rehder JG, Samuels LD, et al: Improved interpretation of exercise thallium-201 scintigraphy in women: Characterization of breast attenuation artifacts. *Radiology* 165:361–366, 1987.

79. Hilton TC, Shaw LJ, Chariman BR, et al: Prognostic significance of exercise thallium-201 testing in patients aged greater than or equal to 70 years with known or suspected coronary artery disease. *Am J Cardiol* 69:45–50, 1992.

80. Maes AF, Gorgers M, Fameng W, et al: Assessment of myocardial viability in chronic coronary artery disease using technetium-99m sestamibi SPECT: Correlation with histologic and positron emission tomographic studies and functional follow-up. *J Am Coll Cardiol* 29:62–72, 1997.

81. Bahr R: Growth in chest pain emergency departments throughout the United States: Cardiologist's spin on solving the heart attack problem. *Coron Artery Dis* 6(10):827–830, 1995.

82. Tatum JL, Jesse RL, Kontos MC, et al: A comprehensive strategy for the evaluation and triage of the chest pain patient. *Ann Emerg Med* 29: 116–125, 1997.

83. Hedblah B, Jwel-Molle S, Svensson K, et al: Increased mortality in men with ST segment depression during 24 hour ambulatory long-term ECG recording. *Br Heart J* 10:149–158, 1989.

84. Fleg JL, Kennedy HL: Long-term prognostic significance of ambulatory electrocardiographic findings in apparently healthy subjects ≥60 years of age. *Am J Cardiol* 70:748–751, 1992.

85. Aronow WS, Epstein S: Usefulness of silent myocardial ischemia detected by ambulatory events in elderly patients. *Am J Cardiol* 62:1295–1299, 1988.

86. McIntosh HD: Second opinions for aortocoronary bypass grafting are beneficial. *JAMA* 258:1644–1649, 1987.

87. Singh RN: Progression of coronary atherosclerosis. Clues to pathologies from serial coronary arteriography. *Br Heart J* 52:451–457, 1984.
88. Little WC, Constantinescu M, Applegate RJ, et al: Can coronary angiography predict the site of a subsequent myocardial infarction in patients with mild to moderate coronary artery disease? *Circulation* 78:157–163, 1988.
89. McIntosh HD: Attaining and maintaining autonomy. In Chesler E (ed): *Clinical Cardiology in the Elderly.* Armonk, NY, Futura Publishing Company, Inc, 1994, pp 547–564.
90. Michels KB, Yusef S: Does PTCA in acute myocardial infarction affect mortality and reinfarction rates? A quantitative overview (meta-analysis) of randomized clinical trials. *Circulation* 91:476–485, 1995.
91. Krumholz HM, Friesinger GC, Cook EF, et al: Relationship of age and eligibility for thrombolytic therapy and mortality among patients with suspected acute myocardial infarction. *J Am Geriatr Soc* 42:127–131, 1994.
92. Tresch DD, Brady WJ, Aiefderheidi TP, et al: Comparison of elderly and younger patients with out-of-hospital chest pain. *Arch Intern Med* 156: 1089–1093, 1996.
93. Weaver WD, Litwin PE, Martin JS, et al: Effect of age on use of thrombolytic therapy and mortality in acute myocardial infarction. *J Am Coll Cardiol* 18:657–662, 1991.
94. Stein PP: Hypercholesterolemia in the elderly: evaluation and treatment. *Am J Geriatr Cardiol* 6(3):33–41, 1997.
95. Aronow W, Herzig A, Etienne F, et al: 41 month follow-up of risk factors correlated with new coronary events in 708 elderly patients. *J Am Geriatr Soc* 37:501–506, 1989.
96. The Post Coronary Artery Bypass Graft Trial Inventigators: The effects of aggressive lowering of low-density lipoprotein, cholesterol levels and low-dose anticoagulant and obstructive changes in saphenous vein coronary artery bypass grafts. *N Engl J Med* 336:153–162, 1997.
97. Herd JA, Ballantyne CM, Farmer JA, et al: Effects of fluvastatin on coronary atherosclerosis in patients with mild to moderate cholesterol elevations. (Lipoprotein and Coronary Atherosclerosis Study [LCAS]). *Am J Cardiol* 80:278–286, 1997.
98. Fox R: Compliance, adherence, concordance. *Circulation* 97:127, 1998.
99. Lehrman S: Can the clock be slowed. *Harvard Health Letter* 20:1–3, 1995.

Chapter 10

Treatment of Acute Ischemic Heart Disease

Gordon L. Pierpont

A common method for summarizing therapeutic strategy in modern medicine is the branching algorithm, or "decision tree," that purports to lead to the correct approach depending on the answers to a series of questions. The questions each have a "yes" or "no" answer depending on the presence or absence of a clinical finding or results of a diagnostic study. Unfortunately, such decision trees are quite inadequate for defining a proper approach to the elderly patient who presents with unstable ischemic heart disease (IHD). Indeed, decision trees in such circumstances may even be hazardous, for 2 basic reasons.

First, algorithms require input that is black or white (positive or negative), without gradation. This is inappropriate because most clinical and laboratory information falls along a scale proceeding from normal, through borderline, to severely abnormal. By reducing such information to simply normal versus abnormal, valuable information may be lost. Second, decision trees are inappropriate in that they are too limited in the information they bring to bear on a problem. Most decision trees are attempts to simplify a problem and thus lead directly to a solution. They assume that the patient has but one problem to address, a situation that is uncommon among the elderly, who frequently have several concomitant medical problems.

Physicians must make decisions that are often difficult, and in unstable IHD they also need to be made promptly. Even though the final decision may be a simple yes or no (either give a drug or not, perform a procedure or not), nothing can substitute for balanced clinical reasoning in weighing all the complex factors before choosing a particu-

From *Clinical Cardiology in the Elderly. Second Edition,* edited by Elliot Chesler. © 1999, Futura Publishing Company, Armonk, NY.

lar course of action. The previous chapter emphasizes important differences in the presentation and evaluation of elderly patients compared to younger patients with ischemic heart disease. This chapter supplements that information by describing an approach to the clinical assessment of patients with unstable IHD that will help direct the choice of specific diagnostic and therapeutic options.

Clinical Assessment

A schematic diagram is presented in Figure 1 that can act as a framework for organizing a systematic approach to patients presenting with unstable IHD. Four key areas are identified that must be graded along a scale from absent to severe. These include severity of symptoms, amount of myocardium at risk, amount of myocardial damage, and amount of salvageable myocardium.

Symptoms

It is well recognized that symptoms of acute myocardial infarction (MI) can precede electrocardiographic changes. This makes assessment of symptoms of paramount importance during initial evaluation of patients with possible acute MI. The problem of confirming suspicious symptoms electrocardiographically is made more difficult in the elderly because of a higher incidence of baseline electrocardiographic (ECG) abnormalities that may be present, even in the absence of other evidence of heart disease.[1] Conduction defects and resting ST abnormalities decrease the sensitivity for detecting acute changes of MI. Left ventricular hypertrophy or a paced ventricular rhythm similarly can alter the ability to assess acute ECG changes. Indeed, recognizing that ECG evidence of acute MI may not always be present, the investigators for ISIS (International Study of Infarct Survival) entered patients into their clinical trials based solely on the physicians' assessment that symptoms were consistent with acute MI, even if the ECG was normal.[2-4]

Implicit in the process of determining severity of symptoms is application of clinical judgment on the nature of the symptoms. Severity of symptoms refers not to how much the pain hurts, but how likely the pain is to be of cardiac origin; and if the source is indeed cardiac, where it fits along the spectrum from angina to unstable angina to acute MI. A dull substernal pressure sensation associated with shortness of breath and diaphoresis of sudden onset and persisting for an hour would be considered severe; whereas an extremely sharp pain that occasionally shoots through the left side of the chest for a few seconds would unlikely be of cardiac origin and thus not be considered severe.

The classic symptoms of angina, infarction, and their variants, are

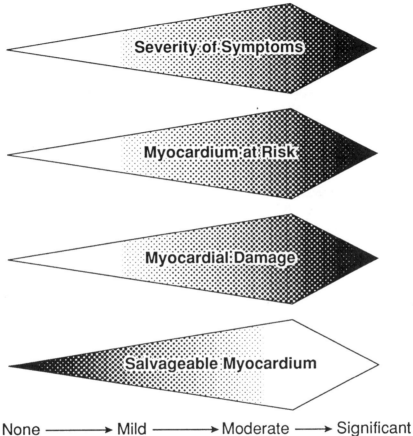

Figure 1: *Four key areas of assessment for patients with unstable ischemic heart disease.*

widely known and chapter 8 emphasizes the variety of ways the elderly can present with IHD. Subsequent sections in this chapter will recognize that there is a continuous spectrum of symptoms in unstable IHD that can make absolute distinctions between the different cardiac ischemic syndromes hazy. Indeed, recognizing the degree of confidence or uncertainty is an important part of assessing each key area. This allows the physician to choose a more appropriate "weight" to place on each bit of information in positioning the patient along the scales in Figure 1, and avoids forcing an artificial choice of either present or absent.

Myocardium at Risk

The tools immediately available for assessing myocardium acutely at risk are quite limited, and essentially include only the ECG. While coronary angiography is the "gold standard," it involves significant time delay, is invasive, and is not always readily available. Exercise tests can often provide valuable information on the extent and location of myocardium at risk, especially when thallium imaging is combined with electrocardiographic monitoring. However, these are not usually indicated on initial presentation of the patient with unstable IHD, be it acute MI or unstable angina. Echocardiography provides information on global and regional left ventricular function that can occasionally provide additional information about myocardium at risk. Finally, cardiac enzyme analysis can be performed rapidly in many hospitals to provide a good index of ongoing or recent myocardial damage. Unfortunately, even a relatively short delay in obtaining cardiac enzymes or an echocardiogram may not be affordable, and critical decisions regarding initial therapy often must proceed without the benefit of such studies.

As noted previously, the ECG does not always provide the desired information. However, this does not diminish its importance, particularly when an old tracing is available for comparison. ECG findings of particular importance are those that indicate greater amounts of myocardium involved in the acute process.[5] Table 1 presents several examples of important factors to consider. As will be emphasized subsequently, correlating the time course of the patient's symptoms with ECG changes can be critically important in making therapeutic decisions.

Physical signs may augment information obtained by ECG when assessing myocardium at risk. A transitory S_3 diastolic gallop heard during chest pain helps confirm cardiac origin of the symptoms and

---

Table 1
Examples of ECG Changes Used to Assess the Extent of Myocardium Involved (Acute Prognostic Indicators)

Less Ominous	⇒	More Ominous
Minimal ST elevation	⇒	Marked ST elevation
Changes in few leads	⇒	Multiple leads involved
Previously normal ECG	⇒	Previous damage evident
Inferior MI	⇒	Anterior MI
ST depression	⇒	ST elevation
No Q waves	⇒	Evolving Q waves
No conduction abnormality	⇒	New conduction defect
Inferior changes alone	⇒	Inferior MI + anterior ST 1
Normal sinus rhythm	⇒	Atrial fibrillation/flutter

suggests a significant amount of myocardium is involved. Hypotension with chest pain, or a new murmur of mitral insufficiency with chest pain, provide stronger evidence that a critically large area of myocardium is threatened. Both signs suggest that ischemia or infarction results in either inability to maintain baseline blood pressure, or malalignment of the mitral valve apparatus due to papillary muscle involvement. If ischemia or infarction persists at this level of severity, pulmonary edema may ensue.

Myocardial Damage

Determining the amount of myocardial damage, like most clinical assessments, also begins with the medical history. The nature and extent of previous heart disease can greatly influence the response to an acute episode of IHD. Evidence of previous MI, known congestive heart failure, or concomitant valvular heart disease must be sought to fully assess the effects of the acute event. Previous damage obviously makes any acute episode more ominous.

Physical examination is more likely to indicate the amount of myocardial damage than the amount of myocardium at risk. The presence and extent of rales in the chest, for example, was clearly shown by Killip et al[6] to have prognostic implications in acute MI. This information can be supplemented with evidence of neck vein distention, presence of a diffuse and/or sustained precordial impulse, an S_3 gallop, murmur of mitral insufficiency, or hypotension. Peripheral perfusion should be assessed by examining peripheral pulses, looking for cold, clammy, or mottled skin, or evidence of cerebral dysfunction.

The ECG is vitally important in assessing the amount of myocardial damage. If time allows, myocardial damage can also be determined by chest x-ray (cardiomegaly, pulmonary congestion or edema, pleural effusion), echocardiography, or radionuclide ventriculography. Plasma enzymes, particularly CPK-MB or troponin-I, are obviously of value in assessing ongoing myocardial damage. However, all of these studies must be put in perspective, and the order in which they are to be obtained prioritized. Important therapeutic decisions usually must be made before many potentially relevant studies are completed.

Salvageable Myocardium

Initial clinical assessment of the amount of myocardium that is salvageable also depends primarily on the history and ECG. The individual key areas of assessment are not independent of each other, and there is often significant overlap. Consider, for example, a patient presenting with severe but intermittent chest pain who demonstrates dramatic ST depression in all precordial leads during pain that rapidly normalizes as the pain is relieved by nitroglycerin. In this circumstance, if there is no evidence of myocardial damage, the diagnosis would be unstable angina, and the amount of myocardium at risk is potentially all salvageable. If, however, a patient presents with dyspnea, but no evidence of acute ischemia or infarction, the salvageable myocardium might be negligible, the amount of myocardial damage may be extensive, and the amount of myocardium at risk uncertain. Initial management in this latter instance would be oriented toward evaluation and treatment of congestive heart failure, with future studies to better assess myocardium at risk considered electively.

Assessing the amount of myocardium salvageable becomes most critical in patients considered to be suffering acute MI. In this instance, the salvageable myocardium will depend on the extent of myocardium involved with the acute process (ie, size of the vascular bed of the "culprit vessel") and the duration of the coronary occlusion.[7]

The rate of myocardial necrosis after coronary occlusion can be quite variable depending on the size of the vascular bed involved, the severity of the occlusion (complete or near complete), the extent of collateral circulation, and metabolic demands of the heart at the time. This makes it difficult to predict in an individual patient with acute MI exactly how much myocardium at risk is salvageable. Since reperfusion therapy can potentially open an acutely occluded vessel, an attempt must be made to ascertain the amount of salvageable myocardium despite these difficulties. As depicted in Figure 2, at the onset of coronary occlusion all the myocardium at risk would potentially be salvageable, but this decreases progressively with time. This diagram is theoretic, but supported nonetheless by extensive experimental data, including large clinical trials of lytic therapy in acute MI. Thus, in patients pre-

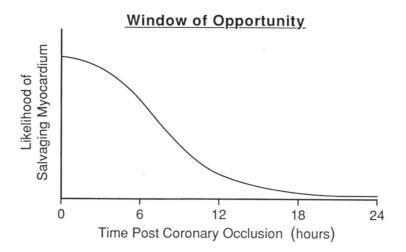

Figure 2: *The window of opportunity shows the likelihood of success with reperfusion decreasing over several hours following coronary occlusion.*

senting with IHD and evidence of continuing ischemia or infarction, the time from onset of symptoms is a major determinant in assessing the relative percentage of salvageable myocardium.

It is important to emphasize that after the patient is defined along the spectrum of each key area of assessment, the process does not stop. The initial assessment is likely to lead to therapeutic intervention that may alter many parameters, and additional diagnostic data may become available. By definition, unstable IHD has the potential to change or evolve rapidly. It is therefore of paramount importance that clinical surveillance continues until the patient is stabilized.

Therapy

Antiplatelet Therapy

The pathophysiology of unstable IHD usually involves thrombus formation at a sight of vascular injury, most often due to a fissure or rupture of atherosclerotic plaque. The severity of the resultant obstruction to myocardial blood flow helps determine the clinical diagnosis most likely to apply to the individual case, i.e. unstable angina, non Q-wave MI, Q- wave MI, etc.. Because clot is so frequently involved, it appears logical that antithrombotic agents or anti coagulants might be beneficial. However, the variety of agents available can make the decision of which agent or agents to use, and when and how to use them, quite complex. None the less, one therapeutic decision is easy. Aspirin has perhaps one of the most favorable risk/benefit and cost/benefit ratios of any medicine or procedure used in cardiology. It should be given immediately and continued chronically unless there is a clear contraindication.

As demonstrated in Figure 3, aspirin has been shown to save lives in patients with acute MI, and it is synergistic with lytic therapy.[3] The ISIS-2 study that so clearly demonstrated the benefits of aspirin in MI was preceded by several smaller studies that generally showed a trend toward benefit with aspirin, but the evidence was not decisive.[8] ISIS-2 had no age restrictions, and thus included many elderly subjects. Subgroup analysis in categories aged younger than 60, 60 to 69, and older than 70 years showed the benefit of aspirin in all 3 age groups, and the benefit of combining aspirin with streptokinase for acute MI.

Aspirin is also of proven benefit in unstable angina,[9-11] can help prevent occlusion of saphenous vein coronary artery bypass grafts,[12] and decreases the incidence of MI among patients with chronic stable angina.[13,14] The Swedish unstable angina study[10] and RISC study[12] were limited to men younger than age 70 years, but the 2 Veterans Administration cooperative studies[9,12] and 1 of the stable angina studies[13] had no age restriction for inclusion, while the other stable angina[14] study had an upper age limit of 80. Subgroup analysis by age was not

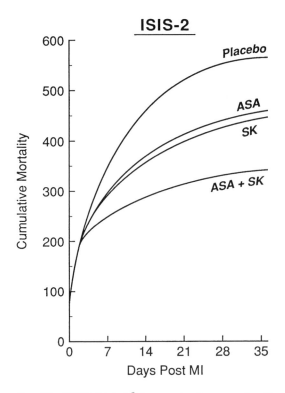

Figure 3: *Results of the ISIS-2 trial,[3] demonstrating survival benefit of aspirin (ASA) and streptokinase (SK) for treating acute MI, with additional benefit combining the 2 agents.*

reported in these latter 4 studies. However, there is no reason to suspect that the benefit of aspirin would be limited to younger patients. Because the efficacy of aspirin appears to be so universal, the decision to use it can be made early in clinical assessment of patients presenting with unstable IHD.

The dosage of oral aspirin used in the above studies ranged from 75 mg once daily to 325 mg 3 times a day. Aspirin inhibits platelet aggregation by blocking the enzyme cyclo-oxygenase responsible for conversion of arachidonic acid to thromboxane-A_2 in platelets. This effect is irreversible, and thus the physiological half-life of aspirin depends on the turnover rate of platelets. The life span of platelets is about 10 days, so bleeding time will return to normal in most people within this time period. Since thromboxane-A_2 induces platelet aggregation and vasoconstriction, less thromboxane-A_2 is beneficial. Cyclo-oxygenase also converts arachidonic acid in the vascular wall to prostaglandin-I_2 (prostacyclin), which inhibits platelet aggregation and is a vasodilator. Reducing prostaglandin-I_2 makes aspirin potentially harmful. Fortunately, the inhibition of thromboxane-A_2 appears to predominate at low dosages. This fact, plus evidence that adverse side effects of aspirin (primarily gastrointestinal bleeding) are dosage dependent,[15] provide strong impetus to keep the dosage of aspirin as low as possible. The most widely used preparations of aspirin usually contain 325 mg per dose, and there is no reason to use more than 325 mg/day. In the VA cooperative study of graft patency 325 mg 3 times a day was no more effective than 325 mg once a day.[12] A dose of 162 mg per day is well supported by ISIS-2,[3] and 75 mg a day was efficacious in the Swedish unstable angina study.[10] Clearly, more is not better when using aspirin in unstable ischemic heart disease.

Alternative antiplatelet therapy that has been used in IHD includes sulfinpyrazone, dipyridamole, ticlopidine, and glycoprotein IIb/IIIa inhibitors. Sulfinpyrazone was used by the Anturane Reinfarction Trial Research Group[16] in a randomized trial comparing sulfinpyrazone (200 mg, qid) to placebo to enhance survival after MI. Although this study reported a benefit in reducing subsequent cardiac mortality (9.5% per year vs. 4.9% with placebo), subsequent critical analysis of the conduct of the trial and interpretation of the results raised serious questions about the validity of the conclusions. As a result, the Federal Drug Administration did not approve the indication of preventing death post-MI for sulfinpyrazone. Results of a subsequent trial in Italy were inconsistent,[17] and a Canadian study[18] failed to demonstrate any benefit of sulfinpyrazone, either alone or combined with aspirin. At this time there is little indication for the use of sulfinpyrazone in unstable IHD.

Dipyridamole (Persantin) has been used in combination with aspirin following acute MI in 2 studies by the Persantin Aspirin Reinfarction Study Group.[19,20] These studies demonstrated beneficial effects of aspirin plus dipyridamole compared to placebo, but neither provided evidence that the combination was better than aspirin alone. Dipyridamole has not been shown to be of benefit used alone in any large scale trials, and thus has no role as antiplatelet therapy in unstable IHD.

Ticlopidine is a potent platelet inhibitor that acts through a mechanism different from that of aspirin, ie, by inhibiting the adenosine diphosphate pathway of platelet aggregation. A double blind randomized trial in Italy demonstrated beneficial effects of ticlopidine in patients with unstable angina[21,22] and ticlopidine decreased the morbidity due to ischemic heart disease in a Swedish study of patients with intermittent claudication.[23] A retrospective study from Japan,[24] specifically looking at secondary prevention in a group of older patients (older than age 60 years), suggested a beneficial effect of ticlopidine on survival after MI. However, ticlopidine is more expensive than aspirin, and has significant side effects that require close monitoring, including diarrhea, skin rash, gastrointestinal symptoms, and a reversible neutropenia. Ticlopidine has gained widespread use as adjunctive therapy to prevent early restenosis after coronary artery angioplasty, but is not preferred for primary treatment or prevention in unstable ischemic heart disease.

The glycoprotein IIb/IIIa receptors bind fibrinogen and other adhesive proteins to form cross-bridges between adjacent platelets, and this action constitutes the final common pathway of platelet aggregation, independent of the stimulus that initiates coagulation. Agents that block these receptors can thus be quite potent inhibitors of coagulation. As such, a number of glycoprotein inhibitors are under investigation for use in unstable ischemic heart disease, be it unstable angina or acute MI. The greatest experience with these agents has been in the prevention of early re-occlusion following percutaneous coronary angioplasty (PTCA). Several multicenter randomized trials have documented successful reduction in the number of ischemic events after PTCA using these agents.[28-31] Interestingly, the beneficial effects appear to persist long after the acute intervention.[32-33] At the time of this writing, intravenous abciximab (ReoPro™) is the only glycoprotein IIb/IIIa inhibitor approved for use in the United States by the Federal Drug Administration. Orally active glycoprotein IIb/IIIa antagonists are currently being evaluated in hopes of providing additional benefit following PTCA.[34,35]

Glycoprotein IIb/IIIa inhibitors have also been used as an adjunct to thrombolytic therapy in acute MI,[36] but have not yet gained an established role in this clinical setting. In unstable angina, a short term infusion of glycoprotein IIb/IIIa antagonist was shown to decrease the number and duration of ischemic episodes detectable on Holter monitor recording.[37] In a separate unstable angina study,[39] a longer duration infusion (3 to 5 days) using a different antagonist showed promise toward protecting against severe ischemic events and reduced the need for urgent revascularization. The incidence of death and infarction one month later was also reduced in this double blind, randomized trial. The risk of major bleeding complications with this type of drug has been shown to increase with age,[39] and additional data are clearly necessary before these agents can be considered for routine use in unstable ischemic heart disease.

Low-dosage aspirin is clearly the antiplatelet agent of choice. It should be used for patients of all ages independent of the presenting diagnosis in unstable ischemic heart disease. Despite the simplicity of this decision, elderly patients have frequently not received the benefit of aspirin therapy. Krumholz et al[40] found that about one-third of elderly patients with acute MI who had no contraindications to aspirin failed to receive it within 2 days of hospital admission, and those with the highest risk of death were the least likely to receive aspirin. Perhaps this type of failure to apply specific therapy helps explain, at least in part, the finding that older age groups have not benefited from the decrease in mortality associated with acute MI experienced by younger patients.[41] Treatment of elderly patients with acute coronary syndromes offers both a challenge and an opportunity.

Reperfusion Therapy

If initial assessment of the patient presenting with unstable IHD is consistent with acute MI, ie, there is a high likelihood a thrombus is completely or almost completely occlusive in a significant coronary artery, and if there is reasonable chance of salvaging myocardium, reperfusion therapy should be considered immediately. This may be achieved by either emergency coronary angioplasty or with thrombolytic drugs. Practical considerations often dictate which choice is better for any individual patient.

Thrombolytics

Yusuf et al[42] summarized 24 randomized trials of intravenous fibrinolytic therapy in acute MI performed before 1985. They concluded that the collective data indicated a highly significant (22% ± 5%, $P < 0.001$) reduction in the odds of death with intravenous thrombolytic therapy, an even larger reduction in the odds of reinfarction, and a frequency of serious adverse side effects much smaller than the absolute reduction in mortality (ie, a very favorable risk/benefit ratio). Subsequent trials, including ASSET,[43] AIMS,[44] GISSI,[45] and ISIS-2,[3] also confirmed the beneficial effect of lytic therapy in acute MI.

Some of the earlier, smaller trials (8 of 24) had upper age limits as entry criteria for the study, but the very large, and consequently statistically powerful, ISIS-2 (see Figure 3) did not. Subgroup analysis in ISIS-2 showed improved vascular mortality for those younger than 60 years of age (4.2% death with streptokinase vs. 5.8% with placebo), from 60 to 69 years (10.6% vs. 14.4%), and those 70 and older (18.2% vs. 21.6%). Thus the risk of dying of acute MI increased with aged, but the potential benefit of lytic therapy remained. The ASSET[43] and AIMS[44] trials had upper age limits for entry (75 and 70 years, respectively), but within these limits the older age groups also demonstrated beneficial response to lytic therapy. Moreover, thrombolytic therapy with streptokinase has been "cost effective" in elderly patients with suspected acute MI in a wide variety of clinical circumstances.[46] Consequently, lytic therapy is indicated *at any age*, and should be considered as soon as acute MI is suspected.

When thrombolytic therapy is considered in unstable IHD, the decision to administer the drug is more problematic than use of aspirin for several reasons. Thrombolytic therapy shares with aspirin a great potential benefit, but unlike low dosage aspirin, has a much higher risk of serious side effects, including stroke, major bleeding, anaphylaxis, and death. The cost of thrombolytic therapy can be quite significant, and the indications are narrower than for aspirin. Even though thrombus is often part of the pathophysiology of patients with unstable angina,[47,48] use of thrombolytics for unstable angina is still of uncertain benefit.[49,50] Many of the studies examining thrombolysis in unstable angina studied effects on coronary anatomy, and some also included response of symptoms and clinical course. Some studies with small numbers of patients have suggested a potential benefit,[51,52] but others have not,[53] and one trial was stopped early due to a negative trend toward outcome after thrombolysis.[54] Until more data are available, thrombolysis should be considered for all patients with acute MI, but restricted in unstable angina to cases where alternative measures have failed.

Even when the working diagnosis is acute MI, it must be recognized that not all acute MIs are caused by coronary thrombosis. Table 2 lists causes of MI in the elderly. Coronary thrombosis is certainly the most common cause of acute MI,[55] but alternative possibilities should be considered before giving thrombolytic therapy. Fortunately, most of the other causes provide clinical clues to their presence. Embolic phenomenon, for example, would be considered in patients with a predisposing factor such as a prosthetic heart valve, and systemic illness would likely be evident if infective endocarditis or arteritis were present.

This chapter emphasizes the need to assess severity of disease along a spectrum, and this approach also applies to assessing contraindications to therapy. Contraindications to lytic therapy can be absolute or relative. A patient having acute MI during blood transfusion for major gastrointestinal bleeding is obviously not a candidate for thrombolysis. Conversely, a history of bleeding duodenal ulcer occurring 10 years ago, without recurrence or interim symptoms, can probably be ignored. But intermediate levels of risk also occur, such as a bleeding duodenal ulcer within the last 6 months. How long after a total knee arthroplasty is it safe to give lytics? The answer is not always clear, but the contraindications must be assessed, and a relative risk placed on each factor present. Table 3 lists the types of problems that should be considered. The likelihood of having one or more of these risk factors increases with age, but age itself should not be considered a risk factor or contraindication to thrombolysis.

Once the relative risk of thrombolytic therapy is determined, the decision to proceed with lytic therapy is made by weighing the risk against the potential benefit as determined from the 4 key areas of assessment. Factors contributing heavily toward treating include: (1)

Table 2
Etiology of Acute Myocardial Ischemia
or Infarction in the Elderly

Coronary Artery Thrombosis
Critical Atherosclerotic Stenosis
Coronary Artery Embolism
Aortic or Coronary Artery Dissection
Trauma (including surgical)
Coronary Artery Spasm
Systemic Hypoxia
Coronary Arteritis
Critical Aortic Stenosis

Table 3
Absolute and Relative Contraindication
to Thrombolytic Therapy in the Elderly

Hemorrhagic stroke
Recent embolic stroke
Recent gastrointestinal or genitourinary bleed
Recent surgery or trauma
Intracranial or visceral cancer
Severe hepatic dysfunction
Bleeding diathesis
Severe uncontrolled hypertension
Cutaneous ulceration
Hemorrhagic retinopathy
Arteriovenous malformation
Recent arterial puncture
Allergy to thrombolytic drug
(consider alternate agent)

symptoms indicative of MI rather than unstable angina; (2) evidence of significant myocardium at risk; and (3) a high likelihood that the myocardium at risk is salvageable.

Thus, an 80-year-old man with classic crushing substernal chest pain of three hours duration and new inferior ST elevation without contraindications is a good candidate for lytic therapy. In contrast, consider the case of an octogenarian evaluated 6 months previously for mild anemia and a positive test for occult blood in his stools. No specific source of blood loss was found, and follow-up visits showed resolution of anemia and blood loss. Given this relative contraindication to lytic therapy, assessment should indicate a greater potential for benefit before administering a thrombolytic. Classic symptoms of MI for less than an hour, plus dramatic anterior lead ST elevation in the presence of hypotension would likely warrant lytic therapy despite the risk of gastrointestinal bleeding. On the other hand, if the symptoms were not classic, onset was 14 hours previously, and ECG changes consisted of slight inferior ST elevation, more conservative management might be appropriate. These two brief examples help demonstrate that the decision to use lytic therapy must consider all factors involved in managing the elderly patient.

Once the decision to use thrombolytic therapy has been made, it should be given expediently,[56] and all efforts should be made to ensure patient safety. For this reason, intravenous administration of thrombolytic agents is preferable to intracoronary administration. The potential benefit of intra-coronary administration is far outweighed by the greater ease and rapidity of the intravenous route.[42] This avoids the need to transfer to a local or remote cardiac catheterization laboratory.

The choice of thrombolytic agent has been intensely controversial in recent years. This is unfortunate because it detracts from the major decision that must be made, i.e. whether to use a lytic agent in the first place. Thrombolytic agents available for use in the USA include streptokinase (SK, kabikinase™), urokinase (UK, abbokinase™), recombinant tissue plasminogen activator (rTPA, activase™), recombinant plasminogen activator (rPA, retavase™), and anisoylated plasminogen streptokinase activator (APSAC, eminase™). There is good evidence that all these agents are successful in the treatment of acute MI. The major reason for controversy has been the tremendous difference in cost, best exemplified by the much greater expense of rTPA compared to SK. This has led to questions whether the greater cost is rewarded by major improvement in beneficial effects.

Early studies with rTPA suggested greater potential benefit because rTPA appeared to achieve higher patency rates of the infarct related artery compared to SK.[57,58] Allergic reactions were rare with rTPA, and anaphylactic reactions absent. However, in trials comparing rTPA to other thrombolytics, these potential benefits did not always translate into greater survival. The GISSI-2 trial[59] showed no difference in survival among 12,490 patients with acute MI randomized to either rTPA or SK. When an additional 8401 patients were added using the same protocol,[60] results were unchanged. Similarly, ISIS-3[4] showed no difference between rTPA, SK, and APSAC in 41,299 patients with acute MI. Two additional studies[61,62] failed to show any further improvement in left ventricular function when acute MI was treated with rTPA compared to SK. More recently, the investigators for the Global Utilization of Streptokinase and Tissue Plasminogen Activator for Occluded Coronary Arteries (GUSTO) trial demonstrated a small but significant improvement in survival of patients treated with rTPA compared to SK.[63] This trial randomized 41,021 patients suffering acute MI at 1081 hospitals in 15 countries to four different thrombolytic regimens, SK + subcutaneous heparin, SK + intravenous heparin, rTPA + intravenous heparin, and SK + rTPA + intravenous heparin. Results showed a 14% reduction in 30 day mortality (absolute mortality 6.3%) with rTPA compared to the two different regimens of SK (absolute mortality 7.2% and 7.4%, respectively), with no benefit of combining SK with rTPA (absolute mortality 7.0%). The benefit of rTPA over SK persisted at 1 year,[64] and was likely due to faster and more complete reperfusion.[65] The most recently approved thrombolytic (rPA) has been compared directly to rTPA with results indicating no clear superiority of one over the other.[66,67] Thus cost, ease of use, availability, and personal preference may all play a role in choice of thrombolytic agent. It should be re-emphasized that the major decision is whether to give a lytic agent or not, rather than which one to use.

Percutaneous Coronary Angioplasty

Immediate angioplasty (primary PTCA) provides an attractive alternative to thrombolytic therapy for acute MI. A systematic overview of studies comparing PTCA and thrombolytic therapy in patients with acute MI concluded that "primary PTCA may be more beneficial than thrombolytic therapy."[68] The most convincing study supporting use of primary PTCA for acute MI is the PAMI (Primary Angioplasty in Myocardial Infarction) study group.[69] This multicenter, randomized trial included 395 patients at 12 centers, and found in-hospital death or reinfarction to be lower in the PTCA group (5.1%) than the thrombolytic group (12.0%, $P = 0.02$). This study included 107 patients over age 75 (i.e. over one-fourth of those studied), so it is reasonable to surmise that any potential benefit of primary PTCA would be applicable to the elderly. Indeed, older patients may potentially benefit from primary PTCA during acute MI even in the presence of cardiogenic shock.[70]

It was noted above that practical considerations often dictate the choice of reperfusion therapy when acute MI is suspected. Figure 2 emphasized the importance of obtaining reperfusion as quickly as possible following the onset of symptoms. This timing is so important that thrombolytic therapy is now being administered pre-hospital by paramedics in some communities with favorable results.[71] Primary PTCA is therefore a preferred alternative to thrombolytics only if it can be attained without undue delay. This opinion is consistent with the practice guidelines provided by the ACC/AHA (American College of Cardiology/American Heart Association), who have commented that "there is serious concern that a routine policy of primary PTCA for patients with acute MI will result in unacceptable delays in achieving reperfusion in a substantial number of cases and less than optimal outcomes if performed by less than experienced operators."[72] Of course if there is a high risk of bleeding complications with thrombolytic therapy, primary PTCA may be the only reasonable option.

It must be emphasized that the considerations used when choosing PTCA as primary reperfusion therapy for acute MI do not apply for use of PTCA following thrombolytic therapy. The TIMI-IIA trial[73] demonstrated that routine aggressive use of PTCA after thrombolytic therapy for acute MI is not beneficial, and indeed that conservative strategy achieves equally good short and long term outcomes with less morbidity. A most reasonable approach is to avoid invasive procedures after thrombolytic therapy unless complications such as recurrent pain, new ischemic changes on electrocardiogram, or cardiogenic shock require intervention. The resolution and remodeling of the thrombosis can continue for several days after lytic therapy, during which time continued heparin may be beneficial. If the patient remains stable, re-assessment of the myocardium at risk can be made just prior to planned discharge, and intervention considered electively if warranted based on this assessment.

If the assessment of the patient on initial presentation is more consistant with unstable angina than acute MI, the role of coronary arteriography can be considered more electively. If symptoms are controlled and the patient stabilized with initial therapy, additional studies such as provocative thallium perfusion scans or echocardiography can help define the amount of myocardium at risk. Often results of these studies need to be interpreted with due consideration of known interventions. Many elderly patients presenting with unstable IHD will have had prior angiography, PTCA or coronary artery bypass surgery. If the coronary anatomy is known from prior studies, it will help set the threshold for further intervention. For example, if an area of ischemia seen on provocative testing appears to arise from a region of myocardium previously known to be supplied by bridging collaterals around a totally occluded proximal artery to small distal vessels, the threshold for intervention may be higher knowing that PTCA is not an option and the risk/benefit ration for surgery unfavorable. Alternatively, if the region of ischemia is supplied by a large vessel that was recently dilated by PTCA, re-occlusion would be considered likely, and the possibility of successful repeat intervention appear more favorable.

When severe symptoms persist despite aggressive medical therapy, angiography in anticipation of proceeding to PTCA or coronary artery bypass surgery may be almost unavoidable. These interventions are considered further in Chapters 10 and 12. Despite all of the tools currently available for treating IHD, it is possible that the patient may be at such high risk or low potential benefit (or both) that he/she is not a candidate for further intervention. It is then important to focus on appropriate measures to manage pain, assure emotional support, and provide methods for coping with disabilities, much as one would for patients with progressive cancer or other debilitating diseases no longer amenable to cure.

Anticoagulants

Heparin appears to be a logical choice for therapy in unstable IHD because of the prominent role thrombosis plays in the pathophysiology of acute MI and unstable angina. Surprisingly, beneficial effects of heparin in acute MI have been more difficult to demonstrate than with aspirin. No clinical trial has clearly shown heparin to enhance survival in acute MI, although a combined analysis of several studies does suggest a potential benefit.[74,75] Also, high-dosage heparin may help prevent left ventricular mural thrombus formation in anterior MI.[76] Because of the very clearly demonstrable benefit of lytic therapy, heparin is relegated to a secondary role as adjunctive therapy in the management of acute MI.

The ISIS-2 trial[3] so powerffully documented the beneficial effects of thrombolysis combined with aspirin in acute MI, that the follow-up ISIS-3 study[4] was designed in part to determine whether addition of heparin to aspirin plus thrombolysis could further improve survival. In this study, during the 7-day in-hospital heparin infusion period, there were slightly fewer deaths in the group receiving heparin (7.4% on heparin vs. 7.9% on placebo, $P = 0.06$). By 35 days, and again at 6 months of follow up, there was no difference in survival between those who had received heparin compared to those who did not. This small short-term benefit was achieved at a cost of a small but significant excess of strokes attributed to definite or probable cerebral hemorhage in the heparin group (0.56% on heparin compared to 0.40% on placebo, $P < 0.05$). The GISSI-2 trial[60] showed a marginal trend toward benefit from addition of heparin on reducing mortality during the period of heparin infusion. Combining these results suggests that there may be a small additional benefit by adding heparin to the combination of aspirin and lytic therapy for acute MI. Subgroup analysis to determine if those with advanced age might have a greater potential benefit, or alternatively have a greater risk of complications (especially intracranial bleeding) has not been reported.

Results of the ISIS-3 and GISSI-2 trials are emphasized here not only because they were large, and therefore very powerful cooperative studies, but also because of the end-points chosen for analysis. Death and major complications were the primary end-points in these trials; outcomes that are directly relevant to the goals of a physician treating patients, that is to prolong life and decrease morbidity.

Several smaller studies have used alternative end points that appear as logical therapeutic goals. Hsia et al,[77] for example, reported higher rates of coronary artery patency 7 to 24 hours after t-PA in patients who had received intravenous heparin compared to those that had received 80 mg of aspirin orally. These results were supported by the findings of Bleich et al.[78] The larger ECSG-6 trial[79] also showed a modest benefit on coronary artery patency by adding heparin when compared to aspirin alone in acute MI patients given lytic therapy. However, Topol et al[80] failed to demonstrate any beneficial effects of adjunctive heparin on coronary artery patency, and The National Heart Foundation of Australia Coronary Thrombolysis Group found no benefit to continued heparin beyond 24 hours after lytic therapy.[81] Integrating such results into clinical practice becomes problematic. A therapeutic regimen that lyses clot faster, or achieves higher patency rates is beneficial only if these events lead to greater survival, decreased disability, or relief of symptoms, with fewer major side effects. Analysis of these clinical trials may be further complicated by the possibility that results might differ with use of heparin depending on the particular lytic agent chosen, or the method and dosage of heparin used. For example, the ISIS-3 trial has been criticized because it used a subcutaneous heparin regimen (12,500 IU twice daily), rather that a more aggressive regimen of intravenous heparin. While it is certainly possible that a more intensive heparin regimen could prove beneficial, it is also possible that increased bleeding could result in an overall detrimental effect. The data from ISIS-3 and GISSI-2 suggest that even if alternative heparin regimens are more beneficial, the incremental improvement is likely to be small. The GUSTO trial quoted above used heparin in all of the regimens studied, and heparin has become a standard adjunct to lytic therapy despite the relatively small potential benefit that has been objectively demonstrated. Use of heparin in acute MI in the absence of indications for lytic therapy is of questionable value.

In unstable angina, although heparin infusion may decrease the frequency of chest pain and episodes of silent ischemia,[82] it cannot be expected to consistently relieve symptoms immediately. The rationale for using heparin in unstable angina is to prevent progression of thrombosis, allowing intrinsic thrombolysis to proceed, thus stabilizing the patient. Sansa et al[83] provided angiographic evidence that cross sectional area of the culprit vessel increases in response to heparin in patients with unstable angina. Stabilizing the culprit lesion could provide time for further evaluation of the amount of myocardium at risk, without interfering with the use of additional agents directed toward relief of symptoms. Clinical evidence that heparin succeeds in this way is provided by the study of Theroux et al[84] who documented that heparin decreases the incidence of MI during the acute phase of unstable angina. Furthermore, stopping heparin may lead to recurrence of unstable angina.[85] Finally, there is some evidence to suggest that heparin may enhance survival in patients with unstable angina.[86,87]

Thus, it is logical to use heparin in patients presenting with unstable angina. The optimal dosage and route of administration are not clear. However, since patients with unstable angina warrant initial monitoring in a coronary care unit,[88] intravenous access should be readily available, making this route convenient for initial therapy. The duration of treatment will depend to a large extent on the clinical course and results of efforts to assess myocardial damage and myocardium remaining at risk.

Hirudin is a direct thrombin inhibitor derived from leeches. It and its analogues are potent anticoagulants that have several theoretic advantages over heparin. They do not require a cofactor such as antithrombin III, are active against thrombin already bound to clot, and have no known natural inhibitors such as platelet factor 4. They have been studied in patients undergoing angioplasty to prevent restenosis by acute clots,[89-91] in patients presenting with acute coronary syndromes,[92] and as adjunctive therapy to thrombolysis in acute MI.[93] Their potential role in unstable IHD remains to be established. At this time lepirudin (Refludan™) is the only agent in this class approved by the Federal Drug Administration for use in the United States. It is indicated for anticoagulation in patients with heparin induce thrombocytopenia and associated thromboembolic disease in order to prevent further thromboembolic complications.

Nitrates

Nitrates are particularly useful in unstable IHD because they can provide diagnostic information at the same time that they are therapeutic. As noted previously, it is most important to determine as soon as possible whether the patient presenting with unstable IHD is suffering an acute MI. The ECG is critical in making the diagnosis. However, while ST elevation usually indicates acute MI, this may also occur as a manifestation of angina, and may occasionally be reversed with nitroglycerin. Alternatively, ST depression, while usually associated with acute ischemia, may also be a sign of MI. It is therefore often very useful to administer nitroglycerin (if there is no evident contraindication) as soon as the ECG has been recorded. The ECG leads can be left in place to allow easy confirmation of any changes in the tracing should symptoms respond to nitroglycerin. This procedure can be particularly useful in assessing the amount of myocardium at risk and the amount salvageable, thus helping to ascertain the potential benefit of proceeding with reperfusion therapy. Moreover, the rapid onset of sublingual nitroglycerin allows this test dose to be tried without serious delay.

Apart from a brief initial "test dose" of nitroglycerin, there may be some benefit from sustained use of nitrates in unstable IHD. Yusuf et al[94] reviewed randomized trials studying the effect of intravenous nitrates on mortality in acute MI. Taken separately, the individual trials were all too small to produce conclusive results. However, collectively the trials suggested a benefit of using both nitroglycerin and nitroprusside in reducing mortality, with the greatest reduction occurring during the first week of follow-up. This conclusion has not been supported by more recent large scale randomized trials. GISSI-3 failed to demonstrate any survival benefit of using glyceryl trinitrate (transdermal patch) at 6 weeks[95] or 6 months[96] after acute MI, and ISIS-4[97] similarly found no improvement in survival at 5 weeks post-MI using controlled release mononitrate. There is no evidence that nitrates prolong survival if the initial diagnosis is unstable angina rather than acute MI. However, if the initial response to nitroglycerin is beneficial in acute IHD, a continuous infusion is often efficacious for relief of symptoms.[98]

Many different nitrate preparations are available, but in unstable IHD nitroglycerin is the drug of choice, at least initially. Because its onset of action is so rapid, nitroglycerin can be used in the orally absorbed form (sublingual tablets or spray), or intravenously. The sublingual dose is quite standard (0.2-0.6 mg), and often worth trying even if the patient has already used it. It is not unusual to obtain a better response in the emergency department than that experienced by the patient before arrival because nitroglycerin tablets may deteriorate with time. Chewable isosorbide dinitrate is also rapidly absorbed, and provides a reasonable alternative.

Hypotension is the only significant side effect of nitroglycerin in the elderly, who are often more susceptible to vasodilator induced hypotension. Autonomic dysfunction or blunted autonomic reflexes are common among the elderly. This may be a result of concomitant diseases such as diabetes mellitus, or part of the normal aging process. It is well documented that circulating norepinephrine increases with age,[99–101] possibly because of reduced clearance from the circulation,[102] although increased sympathetic nerve activity with increased norepinephrine release into the circulation may also be a factor.[103] Increased adrenergic tone could be responsible for decreased tissue concentration of norepinephrine,[104] and, through receptor downregulation, may be responsible for the decreased cardiovascular responsiveness to adrenergic stimuli seen with aging.[105–107] These physiological alterations can be exacerbated by additional factors such as hypovolemia. Older patients are more likely to be taking diuretics for hypertension, heart failure, or renal dysfunction. It is also important to recognize that the risk of hypotension with the use of nitrates may be greater in inferior MI,[108] particularly when there is electrocardiographic or clinical evidence of right ventricular infarction.[109] Hypotension responds well to volume expansion and should be treated with intravenous fluids and stopping or decreasing the dosage of nitrates. Pressor agents should be used only if absolutely necessary to maintain an adequate blood pressure.

Headache is a common side effect of nitroglycerin, but usually responds well to mild analgesics. Nitrate tolerance can occur fairly rapidly, and within 24 hours may result in minimal physiological effect from a dosage that was initially adequate. This was well demonstrated by Elkayam et al[110] in patients with coronary artery disease and heart failure (Figure 4). Tolerance may be temporarily overcome by increasing the dosage, but plans should be made early to switch to oral therapy and a dosage schedule that will avoid tolerance. When symptoms cannot be relieved with nitrates, narcotic analgesia is indicated.

β-Adrenergic Receptor Antagonists

β-Blocking drugs have been used for decades to treat angina pectoris. In recent years, several large randomized clinical trials have demonstrated efficacy in the treatment of acute MI. A thorough review by Yusuf et al,[111] summarizes evidence showing that early intervention with β-blockers in acute MI helps relieve symptoms, limit infarct size, and reduce arrhythmias. If β-blockers are continued long term, the odds of death and reinfarction can be reduced by approximately 25%. It is thus reasonable to consider β-blockade in patients with unstable ischemic heart disease whether they are diagnosed as definite acute MI, unstable angina, or accelerating angina.

In acute MI, data on use of β-blockers can be divided into those studies using drug on initial presentation, and those where treatment is given several days to weeks after the acute event for secondary prevention. The greatest insight into use of β-blockers as an acute intervention in MI, and effects relative to age of the patient, can be obtained from ISIS-1.[2] In this study 16,027 patients admitted to 245 collaborating coronary care units for acute MI were randomized to either intravenous atenolol (followed by oral atenolol) or to placebo. Overall vascular mortality during the 7 day treatment period was improved by atenolol compared to placebo (Table 4). When analyzed by age, the greatest

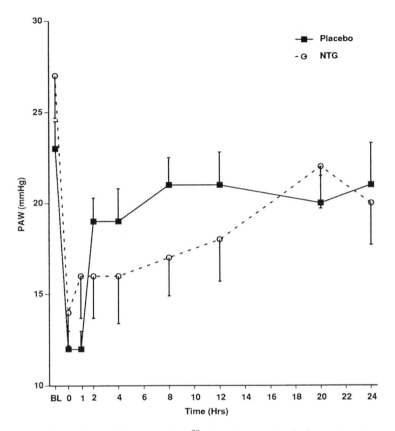

Figure 4: *Data from Elkayam, et al[69] showing tachyphylaxis to intravenous nitroglycerin. Pulmonary artery wedge pressure (PAW) is decreased by nitroglycerin (NTG) infusion in both placebo and active drug groups compared to baseline. Following the initial trial of nitroglycerin in both groups, the placebo group is switched to placebo, and PAW rises rapidly. However, in the group maintained on NTG, PAW also increases, albeit at a slower rate.*

improvement in survival with β-blocker was evident in the older age group.

Other early intervention trials did not necessarily analyze their data by age, but investigators for ISIS-1 combined their total mortality results with those of 27 other trials using intravenous β-blockers. As seen in table 4, the combined analysis supports the conclusion that early intervention with a β-blocker can improve survival in acute MI. It is interesting to speculate whether improved survival in response to β-blockers in the older age groups might be related to the changes in adrenergic nervous system function described in the previous section discussing nitrate therapy.

It is important to realize that ISIS-1 and the other trials summa-

Table 4
Vascular and Total Mortality in ISIS-1,[2] as well as Summarized
Results from 27 Other Intravenous Trials of β-Blockers in Acute MI*

		Vascular Deaths			All Deaths		
Trial	Age	β-Blocker	Placebo	p	β-Blocker	Placebo	p
ISIS-1	<55	29/2700 (1.1%)	32/2720 (1.2%)				
	55–64	104/2693 (3.9%)	107/2629 (4.0%)				
	>64	180/2644 (6.8%)	276/2578 (8.8%)				
	all	313/8037 (3.9%)	365/7990 (4.6%)	<0.04	317/8037 (3.9%)	367/7990 (4.6%)	<0.05
27 others	—				195/5778 (3.4%)	219/5731 (3.8%)	NS
Combined	—				513/13895 (3.7%)	586/13721 (4.3%)	<0.02

* Both sets of data are combined in the last row. Data are number of deaths divided by n, followed by the calculated percent.

rized in table 4 were made before general acceptance of the benefit of lytic therapy in acute MI. It is not yet clear whether combining immediate β-blockade with lytic therapy would be antagonistic, additive, or possibly even synergistic. Certainly, the 2 types of drugs are not a priori mutually exclusive. Given the importance of timing in determining the success of lytic therapy in acute MI (Figure 2) the most rational approach would be to decide whether to use lytic therapy before considering a β-blocker. If lytic therapy is administered, addition of a β-blocker can be elective. In many cases, this might not occur until after lytic therapy is complete. On the other hand, if the patient is hypertensive, or has tachycardia or both, and there are no contraindications to a β-blocker, there may be a benefit from earlier treatment. If lytic therapy is not indicated, the potential benefits of beta blockade should certainly be considered early in therapy.

Since β-blockade is generally efficacious in unstable IHD, the final decision to proceed or not will depend to a large extent on presence and importance of absolute or relative contraindications. It can be seen in Table 4 that the overall mortality for both β-blocker and placebo groups in the combined studies was (513 + 586)/(13895 + 13721) = 4.0%. This is lower than that observed in the large lytic trials such as GISSI[45] and ISIS-2,[3] where the combined mortality was 11.8% and 11% respectively. The duration of follow-up effects overall mortality, but the discrepancy between mortality in β-blocker trials compared to lytic trials can be explained in part by stricter eligibility criteria for the β-blocker trials. In ISIS-1, patients were excluded for: (1) heart rate persistently below 50 beats per minute; (2) systolic blood pressure below 100 mm

Hg; (3) second- or third-degree heart block; (4) severe heart failure; or (5) bronchospasm.

Similar exclusion criteria were present in the other β-blocker trials, and it is evident that many high risk patients were therefore excluded (particularly those with heart failure) who would not be excluded from the lytic trials. Thus comparing absolute results between different studies must be made with caution. The smaller overall mortality in the β-blocker trials leaves less room for therapy to have a positive impact.

Unfortunately, longer term secondary prevention trials following MI do not lend themselves well to analysis by age groups. As seen in Table 5, which summarizes 12 major long term post MI β-blocker trials, upper age limits for entry ranged from 65 to 75. Nonetheless, it is worth noting that β-blockade in these trials clearly improved survival. Moreover, despite the upper age limit, subgroup analysis by age revealed that the number of deaths and reinfarctions prevented by timolol treatment in the Norwegian Timolol Trial,[125] was twice as high in patients aged 65 to 75 years as in patients below 65 years of age. This finding was supported by subgroup analysis in the BHAT trial,[126] where propranolol reduced mortality in the 60 to 69 year age group by 33%. Thus older age alone should not preclude β-blockers.

Since β-blockers are negatively inotropic their use has been of particular concern in patients with left ventricular dysfunction, and it is worthwhile to assess how often they were discontinued because of heart failure. As can be seen in table 5, relatively few patients developed heart failure in the long term trials. Heart failure occurred with placebo (2.8%) almost as often as with active β-blocker (3.4%). Since patients

Table 5
Mortality and Incidence of Withdrawal due to Heart Failure in 12 Long-Term Trials of β-Blocker for Myocardial Infarction

Trial	Drug	Max. Age	Max. Duration	n		Heart Failure (%)		Total mortality (%)	
				Drug	Placebo	Drug	Placebo	Drug	Placebo
Wilhelmsson[71]	alprenolol	67	2 yr	114	116	0.9	0.9	6.1	12.1
Multicentre[72,73]	practolol	69	1 yr	1520	1533	4.1	3.6	3.2	5.1
Babel[74]	propranolol	70	9 mo	355	365	6.2	6.0	7.9	7.4
Norwegian[75]	timolol	75	33 mo	945	939	3.7	2.3	10.4	16.2
Hjalmarson[76]	metoprolol	74	90 day	698	697	0.6	1.0	5.7	8.9
Hansteen[77]	propranolol	70	1 yr	278	282	7.9	5.7	9.0	13.1
BHAT[78]	propranolol	69	4 yr	1916	1921	4.0	3.5	7.2	9.8
Julian[79]	sotalol	69	1 yr	873	583	0.9	0.3	7.3	8.9
Taylor[80]	oxprenolol	65	7 yr	632	471	1.6	1.3	9.5	10.2
Australian[81]	pindolol	69	2 yr	263	266	7.6	4.1	17.1	17.7
EIS[82]	oxprenolol	69	1 yr	858	883	3.1	2.4	6.6	5.1
Olsson[83]	metoprolol	69	3 yr	154	147	4.5	0.7	16.2	21.1
All combined				**8606**	**8203**	**3.4**	**2.8**	**7.4**	**9.5**

with MI suffer varying degrees of myocardial damage and dysfunction, it is important to realize that β-blockade should be contraindicated only when heart failure is severe. Subgroup analysis according to presence or absence of heart failure by history (ie, before randomization) in the BHAT study[127] confirms this assessment, since propranolol decreased total mortality equally in patients with (27%) and without (25%) a history of heart failure. Indeed, a β-blocker (carvedilol) has now been approved by the Federal Drug Administration specifically for treatment of mild to moderate congestive heart failure because of its ability to inhibit clinical progression.[128]

The presence of relative contraindications to β-blocker therapy, listed above, will tend to be more prevalent and/or more severe with advanced age. Thus a larger proportion of patients most likely to benefit from β-blockade (ie, older patients) present problems in therapeutic strategy because they may be more likely to suffer adverse side effects of the drugs. The decision to use a β-blocker is made a little easier by the availability of an intravenous agent with a very short half life (esmolol). Acute β-blockade can be tried in many borderline situations where the result might be uncertain. Esmolol can be accurately titrated to achieve the desired response, and if adverse effects occur, stopping the infusion allows rapid recovery. Indeed, the fairly consistent benefit demonstrated in multiple β-blocker trials using many different agents suggests that the choice of drug can be made by considering route of administration, drug kinetics, and ancillary properties such as β-receptor selectivity, cost, etc. with confidence that whichever drug is chosen will likely be equivalently efficacious.

Calcium Antagonists

Drugs classified as calcium antagonists comprise a heterogeneous group of compounds. Their structure can be very different, and it is not surprising that their hemodynamic and electrophysiological effects vary, as do their side effects. This variety makes it difficult to generalize about the role of calcium antagonists in therapy for unstable IHD.

Held et al[129] provided a systematic review of randomized trials of calcium antagonists in acute MI and unstable angina. After analyzing 19,000 patients in 28 randomized trials, they concluded that there was no evidence that calcium antagonists reduce the risk of initial or recurrent infarction, or death, when given routinely to patients with acute MI or unstable angina. Nor was there any difference found when analyzing by type of agent or time that treatment was started.

A subsequent update of this analysis[130] included an additional 3 long-term randomized trials of calcium antagonists in either stable angina pectoris or after MI. The authors appropriately concluded that evidence favoring use of calcium antagonists is much weaker than that indicating benefit of β-blockers or antiplatelet agents in reducing mortality or re-infarction in the acute phase or long term treatment of

MI. Indeed, adverse outcome is suggested with nifedipine, and perhaps other dihydropyridine calcium antagonists. However, calcium antagonists that lower heart rate may have a potential to reduce re-infarction. If there is clinical evidence of heart failure, calcium antagonists should be used with great caution, if at all.

Placing the collective data on calcium antagonists in perspective, it appears prudent to avoid their use in the acute phase of MI and limit their use to stable patients.

Angiotensin-Converting Enzyme Inhibitors

Angiotensin-converting enzyme (ACE) inhibitors are generally not useful in the early treatment of unstable ischemic heart disease because the potential for hypotension and other adverse effects outweigh any potential benefits. Use of ACE inhibitors as adjuvant therapy following acute events is discussed in the following section.

Adjuvant Therapy and Supportive Measures

One of the most important decisions to be made in managing elderly patients with unstable IHD, is how aggressive to be with invasive diagnostic, therapeutic, or supportive measures. Such decisions are becoming easier as living wills and advance health care directives are more widely used. However, blanket statements expressing a desire to avoid prolonged life-sustaining measures in terminal illness are often inadequate to address specific issues in acute unstable IHD. Because the first 48 hours following presentation with unstable IHD is the period during which patients are at greatest risk for complications, many of which are readily treatable, it is important to establish early the extent to which life saving measures are to be applied.

Most often it is insufficient to simply address whether a patient should be resuscitated, because such efforts include several distinct actions having quite differing potential implications for the patient's short-term comfort and long term outcome. Intubation and respiratory support is the most critical issue to consider. Since heart failure indicates a poor prognosis, it is important to assess whether emergency intubation and respiratory support are likely to change the course of events. A frank discussion with the patient and family and or friends will help ensure that the patient does not become inappropriately respirator dependent.

Treatment of other complications of unstable IHD does not carry the potentially adverse long term consequences of intubation. For example, successful electrical cardioversion of ventricular tachycardia or ventricular fibrillation can be achieved rapidly, and may have a good long-term outcome. When attempts to cardiovert life threatening arrhythmias are unsuccessful, it is helpful to have established guidelines for each patient regarding how far to continue, particularly whether to proceed with external cardiac massage. In the Minneapolis VA Medical Center CCU it is quite common to establish orders not to intubate or perform external cardiac massage, but to proceed with aggressive therapy short of these two measures. This therapy may include medical treatment of arrhythmias, electrical cardioversion of tachyarrhythmias, pacemaker therapy for bradyarrhythmias, and invasive hemodynamic monitoring to help guide therapy for heart failure. This approach helps ensure that a patient will not die of a remediable problem, and avoids an undesirable situation that prolongs dying rather than preserving life.

Because so many aspects of CCU care for the elderly must be individualized, use of "standing orders" should be minimized. There are, however, a few measures (along with electrocardiographic monitoring) that may be routinely applied to most patients. For example, because caffeine can be arrhythmogenic in susceptible individuals, it is reasonable to serve only decaffeinated coffee. However, requiring that drinks cannot be served either hot or cold is probably too conservative. Since patients with unstable IHD by definition may have sudden changes in clinical status, it is reasonable to limit intake on admission to clear liquids, to avoid having food in the stomach during a major procedure. Diet can be liberalized as these patients stabilize and chances of requiring acute interventions decrease.

Supplemental oxygen has never been shown to decrease mortality in patients with unstable IHD. However, it is not unusual for patients with acute MI to be mildly hypoxemic, even without clinical heart failure. [131] Since oxygen is low risk and may have some potential benefit for some patients, it is often used routinely, at least initially.[72]

Adequate relief of pain and anxiety is important. This can often be achieved with thrombolytic therapy, nitrates, oxygen, etc., which are designed to adequately perfuse and oxygenate ischemic myocardium. However, adequate analgesia should be promptly administered if initial efforts at pain relief are unsuccessful. Intravenous morphine remains the drug of choice for relieving the pain of acute MI.[72] Minor tranquilizers may have a supplemental role for the first few days following presentation.

Besides these general measures, certain complications of unstable IHD occur frequently enough to warrant consideration not only for treatment, but also for prophylaxis. Problems with cardiac rhythm have been particularly controversial concerning prophylactic therapy, not so much for unstable angina as in acute MI. This controversy includes both tachy- and brady- arrhythmias. Although supraventricular arrhythmias, particularly if rapid, can exacerbate ischemia, they are not usually acutely life threatening and do not require prophylaxis. More controversial is the question of prophylaxis of ventricular arrhythmias with lidocaine. A meta-analysis of 14 randomized trials for prophylactic lidocaine in suspected acute MI by MacMahon et al[132] suggests that treatment may reduce episodes of ventricular fibrillation by 33%, but provides no evidence for improved mortality. Because older patients may be more susceptible to side effects of lidocaine, prophylactic use is not recommended. The Guidelines for the Early Management of Patients with Acute Myocardial Infarction developed by the American College of Cardiology and American Heart Association Task Force on Assessment of Diagnostic and Therapeutic Cardiovascular Procedures[72] have listed lidocaine as usually indicated for patients with acute ischemia or infarction having premature ventricular complexes that are frequent (> 6/min); closely coupled (R on T); multiform; or occurring in bursts of three or more in tandem. However, this does not mean that lidocaine should always be used in the above situations. It is often reasonable to reserve lidocaine for patients with ventricular tachycardia or ventricular fibrillation, where it remains the drug of choice. When lidocaine produces undesirable side effects, or is ineffective, intravenous procainamide is a good alternative.

Bradyarrhythmias also should be treated in most cases as they occur, rather than prophylactically. External cardiac pacemakers are widely available, often as an integral part of a defibrillator. Because these units can be quite effective, and can be applied to patients with minimal delay, need for prophylactic temporary transvenous pacemakers have been diminished. External pacing can be uncomfortable, as the skeletal muscles of the chest wall are frequently stimulated, but this is rarely painful. External pacing is a temporary measure, and should generally be used only to maintain adequate heart rate while positioning a transvenous electrode. A discussion regarding specific indications for pacing, including in the setting of acute MI can be found in Chapter 14 on diagnosis and treatment of arrhythmias.

Prophylactic therapy for heart failure in unstable IHD has received less attention than prophylaxis for arrhythmias. However, a Veterans Administration cooperative study[133] examined use of nitroprusside in 812 patients with acute MI having pulmonary artery wedge pressures of at least 12 mm Hg. A 48-hour nitroprusside infusion failed to show any short (21-day) or long-term (13-week) survival benefit compared to placebo. It was concluded that nitroprusside should not be used routinely in acute MI when complicated by high left ventricular filling pressure. However, patients with persistent pump failure might benefit from the hemodynamic improvement provided by nitroprusside. The above study prospectively stratified by age (below or above 65), but results did not differ in the 2 subgroups.

Several randomized trials have examined the effects of ACE inhibitors in patients following acute MI. The rationale is that ACE inhibitors would prevent subsequent left ventricular remodeling, thus preventing or controlling heart failure and decreasing mortality. Consistent with current practice for large scale clinical trials, these studies are de-

Table 6
Studies of ACE Inhibitors After MI

Study	n	Drug	F/U (mo.)	Favored Rx
CONSENSUS II	6090	enalapril	6	neither
SAVE	2231	captopril	24–60	ACE-I
AIRE	2006	ramapril	>6	ACE-I
GISSI-3	19394	lisinopril	1.5 & 6	ACE-I
ISIS-4	58050	captopril	1	ACE-I
SMILE	1556	zofenopril	1.5 & 12	ACE-I
TRACE	1749	trandolapril	24–50	ACE-I
CATS	298	captopril	12	ACE-I
CCS-1	13634	captopril	1	*ACE-I

Abbreviations: n, number of patients in the trial; F/U (mo.), length of follow-up in months; favored Rx, the therapy preferred according to the conclusions of the study, either placebo, angiotensin converting enzyme inhibitor (ACE-I), or neither; *, not statistically significant.

scribed by acronyms. Table 6 summarizes pertinent data from these efforts, which constitute a total experience involving over 100,000 patients. These studies include many elderly patients, as only two of them (SAVE and SMILE) had upper age exclusion criteria, and they were both at age 80. In three of the studies (SAVE, AIRE, and TRACE) there had to be evidence of left ventricular dysfunction upon entry, but this was not required in the others. These studies had many variations in the methods used, but taken collectively they clearly favor using an ACE inhibitor following myocardial infarction, especially when there is evidence of left ventricular dysfunction. All but two of these studies (CATS, and CCS-1) presented subanalysis by age. In the CONSENSUS-II trial, older patients tended to do worse on ACE inhibitor than placebo. However, in SAVE, AIRE, GISSI-3, and TRACE, the older patients appeared to benefit even more from ACE inhibitors than younger patients, while ISIS-4 and SMILE had relatively neutral effects when comparing the response of older and younger age groups. Although older patients may be more susceptible to adverse side effects of ACE inhibitors than younger patients, these drugs should be considered as potentially beneficial long term therapy for all patients who have suffered MI independent of age.

Criteria for use of nitroprusside in the VA Cooperative Study,[133] required invasive hemodynamic monitoring of all potential candidates. Since a clear survival benefit for therapy was not demonstrated, the routine use of invasive hemodynamic monitoring was also of unproven benefit. Because invasive hemodynamic monitoring is uncomfortable, expensive, and has occasionally serious complications, it should only be used after carefully weighing the risk/ benefit ratio. The incidence of complications from invasive hemodynamic monitoring is too low to assess risk by age groups. However, a reasonable estimate of the risk of complications from hemodynamic monitoring in the elderly can be gained by examining data from the Minneapolis VA Medical Center, where the average age of patients admitted to the coronary care unit is very close to 65 years. The complications of invasive monitoring, including both medical and surgical services over the past 5 years, are shown in Table 7. The overall complication rate for balloon directed pulmonary artery catheters was 1 in 400, and for arterial lines was 1 in 200.

The figures in Table 6 can be used to weigh the risks of hemodynamic monitoring, but benefits are more difficult to predict. Invasive monitoring is clearly indicated in severe congestive heart failure, pulmonary edema, inadequate peripheral perfusion, labile systemic pressure, and cardiogenic shock. Balloon directed right heart catheterization can also assist in diagnosis of complications such as ventricular septal defect, papillary muscle rupture, right ventricular infarction, hypovolemia, and pericardial tamponade. Decisions regarding invasive hemodynamic monitoring must recognize the potential need for lytic therapy in acute MI. It is risky to initiate invasive monitoring when a patient has received thrombolytics, and it is difficult to justify delaying lytic therapy to establish invasive monitoring. It is worthwhile to remember that invasive monitoring helps guide potentially life saving therapy, but in itself does not cure anything. Initial therapy in unstable IHD must therefore be guided by clinical assessment, with confirmatory hemodynamic data obtained only after all other higher priority measures have been instituted.

Table 7
Complications of Invasive Hemodynamic Monitoring over a 6 year period (1986–1991) at the Minneapolis VAMC

Complication	Number	% of Complications	% of All Inserted
PULMONARY ARTERY CATHETERS (total inserted = 4415)			
Infection	5	45%	0.11%
Perforation	2	18%	0.05%
Embolus	1	9%	0.02%
Thrombus	1	9%	0.02%
Death	2	18%	0.05%
Total	11	100%	0.25%
INTRA-ARTERIAL CATHETERS (total inserted = 7905)			
Sepsis	2	4%	0.03%
Bleed	3	7%	0.04%
Ischemia	18	40%	0.23%
Parasthesias	5	11%	0.06%
Embolectomy	13	29%	0.16%
Other	4	9%	0.05%
Total	45	100%	0.57%

Despite optimal use of potent pharmacological agents guided by invasive hemodynamic monitoring, some patients will remain in refractory heart failure. Mechanical cardiac support may be the only way to maintain life. Left ventricular assist devices and intra-aortic balloon counterpulsation can provide temporary support for such patients. However, these devices are supportive, not curative. As such, they are rarely justified in geriatric patients. They should be considered only when there is a readily identifiable correctable condition with a clearly defined endpoint. An example might be a patient with ruptured papillary muscle complicating acute MI who has adequate residual left ventricular function to warrant consideration of mitral valve replacement. Mechanical support would be used only to maintain life while preparing for surgery. If angioplasty is the preferred intervention, but is very high risk, mechanical support during the procedure may be useful.[143,144] Intra-aortic balloon pumping in such situations remains the method of choice,[145] but it must also be recognized that complications of intra-aortic balloon counterpulsation increase with age.[146] In general, mechanical support should not be considered in elderly patients where decompensation is a result of massive left ventricular damage not reversible by medical means.

Just as some patients will remain in heart failure despite the best medical therapy, others may fail to stabilize due to signs or symptoms of recurrent or persistent ischemia. These patients can be considered for heart catheterization and possible reperfusion based on the considerations discussed in Chapters 11 and 12.

Discharge Planning

Preparing the elderly patient recovering from an episode of unstable ischemic heart disease for hospital discharge frequently requires a team approach. Nurses play a major role in readying a patient for self administered health care maintenance at home. A dietitian may contribute by implementing dietary instructions, and pharmacists can ensure that the patient knows and understands the medical regimen. The degree of services required from rehabilitation medicine personnel or social service workers can become considerable depending on the patient's physical, mental, social, and financial status. The role of the physician in coordinating the efforts of this team cannot be overemphasized.

Physician directed discharge planning begins with a re-evaluation of the 4 key areas of assessment described at the beginning of this chapter. The medical regimen chosen for continued outpatient therapy will depend to a large extent on such factors as whether or not there are residual areas of myocardium at risk for recurrent ischemia. If so, anti-anginals will be prescribed. If left ventricular function is compromised, therapy for chronic heart failure is needed. This process of pre-discharge assessment is usually aided considerably by exercise testing.

Pre-discharge testing need not be complex (i.e. radioactive imaging etc.), but low level exercise tests should be used to ensure that the patient can safely continue normal daily activities at home. Concomitant disabilities in the elderly can sometimes preclude formal treadmill or bicycle exercise; telemetric monitoring for arrhythmias while the patient is observed for symptoms while performing the activities of daily living may suffice.

Specific attention should be directed toward preventing recurrent ischemic events. Advanced age is not a rationale for failure to emphasize the need to stop smoking or to maintain a heart healthy diet. Management of lipid disorders in the elderly is discussed in Chapter 13.

The complexity of discharge planning is evident when it is recognized that multiple medications may be required. The potential combinations are too numerous to review in detail, but adverse drug interactions and over medication occur all too easily. Particular caution is necessary to avoid placing the patient in simple categories that dictate specific action without considering the whole picture.

A good example of overemphasis on categories is evident when patients are divided into Q wave and non-Q wave MI. As noted in Table 1, presence or absence of Q waves during acute MI can help in assessing prognosis, and contributes to knowledge about myocardial damage and myocardium at risk. However, analysis for Q-waves is not inclusive. Patients with electronic ventricular pacemakers or left bundle branch block, for example, are left out of this simple classification. Moreover, within each category (Q or non-Q) there is a spectrum of patients. While in general, non-Q wave MI's indicate less myocardial damage, this is not always true, and some patients with non-Q wave MI may have severe heart failure. Alternatively, some patients develop Q waves with only small amounts of myocardial damage. Thus placing a patient into a category of Q wave versus non-Q wave MI is unsatisfactory as a sole determinant of subsequent therapy. Specifically, it is inappropriate to make a recommendation such as "diltiazem is the only therapy of proven benefit for use after non-Q wave MI."[147] This statement was based in part on a review of the MDPIT trial,[148] which prospectively examined the effect of diltiazem on mortality and reinfarction following acute MI. Diltiazem was detrimental in those with pulmonary congestion or with low ejection fraction, but potentially beneficial in those with good ejection fraction. It is not surprising that patients with non-Q wave MI would be more likely to fall into the latter category, and therefore also show potential benefit. However, the more important variable is left ventricular function, not presence or absence of Q waves. The process of thoroughly evaluating and treating the elderly patient with unstable IHD can not be simplified.

In summary, it has been said that medical care of the elderly infarction patient is no different from that for a younger victim.[149] However, while it is true that the same diagnostic and therapeutic tools are considered for both young and old, great care must be taken to consider all aspects of the changes that occur with aging to ensure that each intervention used in elderly patients does more good than harm.

References

1. Coodley EL, Coodley G: Electrocardiographic changes associated with aging. In: EL Coodley (ed): *Geriatric Heart Disease*. Littleton, MA, PSG Publishing Co., 1985, p 182.
2. ISIS-1 Collaborative Group: randomized trial of intravenous atenolol among 16,027 cases of suspected acute myocardial infarction: ISIS-1. *Lancet* 2:57, 1986.
3. ISIS-2 Collaborative Group: Randomized trial of intravenous streptokinase, oral aspirin, both, or neither, among 17,187 cases of suspected acute myocardial infarction: ISIS-2. *Lancet* 2:349, 1988.
4. ISIS-3 Collaborative Group: ISIS-3: A randomized comparison of streptokinase vs tissue plasminogen activator vs anistreplase and of aspirin plus heparin vs aspirin alone among 41,299 cases of suspected acute myocardial infarction. *Lancet* 339:753, 1992.
5. Wellens HJJ, Conover MB: *The ECG in Emergency Decision Making*. W.B. Saunders, Philadelphia, 1992.
6. Killip T, Kimball JT: Treatment of myocardial infarction in a coronary care unit: A two year experience with 250 patients. *Am J Cardiol* 20:457, 1967.
7. Bar FW, Vermeer F, De Zwaan C, et al: Value of admission electrocardiogram in predicting outcome of thrombolytic therapy in acute myocardial infarction: A randomized trial conducted by the Netherlands Interuniversity Cardiology Institute. *Am J Cardiol* 59:6, 1987.
8. Resnekov L, Chediak J, Hirsh J, et al: Antithrombotic agents in coronary disease. *Chest* 89:54S, 1986.
9. Lewis HD, Davis JW, Archibald DG, et al: Protective effects of aspirin against acute myocardial infarction and death in men with unstable angina: Results of a Veterans Administration Cooperative Study. *N Engl J Med* 309:396, 1983.
10. Wallentin LC and The Research Group on Instability in Coronary Artery Disease in Southeast Sweden: Aspirin (75 mg/day) After an episode of unstable coronary artery disease: long-term effects on the risk for myocardial infarction, occurance of severe angina, and the need for revascularization. *J Am Coll Cardiol* 18:1587, 1991.
11. The RISC Group. Risk of myocardial infarction and death during treatment with low dose aspirin and intravenous heparin in men with unstable coronary artery disease. *Lancet* 336:827, 1990.
12. Goldman S, Copeland J, Moritz T, et al: improvement in early saphenous vein graft patency after coronary artery bypass surgery with antiplatelet therapy: Results of a Veterans Administration Cooperative Study. *Circulation* 77:1324, 1988.
13. Ridker PM, Manson JE, Gaziano JM, et al: Low-dose aspirin therapy for chronic stable angina: A randomized, placebo-controlled clinical trial. *Ann Intern Med* 114:835, 1991.
14. Juul-Moller S, Edvardsson N, Jahnmatz B, et al: Double-blind trial of aspirin in primary prevention of myocardial infarction in patients with stable chronic angina pectoris. *Lancet* 340:1421, 1992.

15. Levy M: Aspirin use in patients with major upper gastrointestinal bleeding and peptic-ulcer disease. *N Engl J Med* 290:1158, 1974.
16. The Anturane Reinfarction Trial Research Group: Sulfinpyrazone in the prevention of cardiac death after myocardial infarction: The Anturane Reinfarction Trial. *N Engl J Med* 298:289, 1978.
17. Report from the Anturane Reinfarction Italian Study: Sulfinpyrazone in post-myocardial infarction. *Lancet* 1:237, 1982.
18. Cairns JA, Gent M, Singer J, et al: Aspirin, sulfinpyrazone, or both in unstable angina: Results of a Canadian multicenter trial. *N Engl J Med* 313:1369, 1985
19. The Persantin-Aspirin Reinfarction Study Research Group: Persantine and aspirin in coronary heart disease. *Circulation* 62:449, 1980.
20. Klimt CR, Knatterud GL, Stamler J, et al: Persantine-aspirin reinfarction study. Part II. Secondary coronary prevention with persantine and aspirin. *J Am Coll Cardiol* 7:251, 1986.
21. Balsano F, Rizzon P, Violi F, et al: Antiplatelet Treatment with Triclopidine in Unstable Angina: A Controlled Multicenter Clinical Trial. Circulation 82:17, 1990.
22. Scrutino D, Lagioia R, Rizzon P, et al: Triclopidine treatment for patients with unstable angina at rest: A Further analysis of the study of triclopidine in unstable angina. *Eur Heart J* 12:G27, 1991.
23. Janzon L, Bergqvist D, Boberg J, et al: Prevention of myocardial infarction and stroke in patients with intermittent claudication; Effects of triclopidine. Results from STIMS, The Swedish Triclopidine Multicentre Study. *J Intern Med* 227:301, 1990.
24. Sakai M, Kuboki K, Maeda S, et al: Effect of antiplatelet and anticoagulant therapy on secondary prevention and long-term prognosis after acute myocardial infarction in aged patients. *Jpn J Geriatrics* 29:29, 1992.
25. Schomig A, Neumann F-J, Kastrati A, et al: A randomized comparison of antiplatelet and anticoagulant therapy in the placement of coronary artery stents. *N Engl J Med* 334:1084, 1996.
26. Hall P, Nakamura S, Maiello L, et al: A randomized comparison of combined ticlopidine and aspirin therapy versus aspirin therapy alone after successful intravascular ultrasound-guided stent implantation. *Circulation* 93:215, 1996.
27. Neumann F-J, Gawax M, Dickfeld T, et al: Antiplatelet effect of ticlopidine after coronary stenting. *J Am Coll Cardiol* 29:1515, 1997.
28. The EPIC Investigators: Use of a monoclonal antibody directed against the platelet glycoprotein IIb/IIIa receptor in high-risk coronary angioplasty. *N Engl J Med* 330:956, 1994.
29. The EPILOG Investigators: Platelet glycoprotein IIb/IIIa receptor blockade and low-dose heparin during percutaneous coronary revascularization. *N Engl J Med* 336:1689, 1997.
30. The CAPTURE Investigators: Randomised placebo-controlled trial of abciximab before and during coronary intervention in refractory unstable angina: The CAPTURE study. *Lancet* 349:1429–1435, 1997.
31. The IMPACT-II Investigators: Randomised placebo-controlled trial of effect of eptifibatide on complications of percutaneous coronary intervention: IMPACT-II. *Lancet* 349:1422, 1997.
32. Topol E, Califf R, Weisman H, et al: Randomised trial of coronary intervention with antibody against platelet IIb/IIIa integrin for reduction of clinical restenosis: Results at six months. Lancet 343:881, 1994.

33. Topol E, Ferguson J, Weisman H, et al: Long-term protection from myocardial ischemic events in a randomized trial of brief integrin β_3 blockade with percutaneous coronary intervention. *JAMA* 278:479, 1997.

34. Simpfendorfer C, Kottke-Marchant K, Lowrie M, et al: First chronic oral platelet glycoprotein IIb/IIIa Integrin blockade. *Circulation* 96:76, 1997.

35. Kereiakes D, Runyon J, Kleiman N, et al: Differential dose-response to oral xemilofiban after antecedent intravenous abciximab. *Circulation* 94:906, 1996.

36. Ohman E, Kleiman N, Gacioch G, et al: Combined accelerated tissue-plasminogen activator and platelet glycoprotein IIb/IIIa integrin receptor blockade with integrilin in acute myocardial infarction. *Circulation* 95:846, 1997.

37. Schulman S, Goldschmidt-Clermont P, Topol E, et al: Effects of integrelin, a platelet glycoprotein IIb/IIIa receptor antagonist, in unstable angina. *Circulation* 94:2083, 1996.

38. Theroux P, Kouz S, Roy L, et al: Platelet membrane receptor glycoprotein IIb/IIIa antagonism in unstable angina. *Circulation* 94:809, 1996.

39. Aguirre F, Topol E, Ferguson J, et al: Bleeding complications with the chimeric antibody to platelet glycoprotein IIb/IIIa integrin in patients undergoing percutaneous coronary intervention. *Circulation* 91:2882, 1995.

40. Krumholz H, Radford M, Ellerbeck E, et al: Aspirin in the treatment of acute myocardial infarction in elderly medicare beneficiaries. *Circulation* 92:2841, 1995.

41. Gurwitz J, Goldberg R, Chen Z, et al: Recent trends in hospital mortality of acute myocardial infarction: The Worcester Heart Attack Study. *Arch Intern Med* 154:2202, 1994.

42. Yusuf S, Collins R, Petro R, et. al.: Intravenous and intracoronary fibrinolytic therapy in acute myocardial infarction: Overview of Results on mortality, reinfarction and side-effects from 33 randomized controlled trials. *Eur Heart J* 6:556, 1985.

43. Wilcox RG, Von Der Lippe G, Olsson CG, et. al.: Trial of tissue plasminogen activator for mortality reduction in acute myocardial infarction: Anglo-Scandinavian Study of Early Thrombolysis (ASSET). *Lancet* 2:525, 1988.

44. AIMS Trial Study Group: Long-term effects of intravenous anistreplase in acute myocardial infarction: Final report of the AIMS Study. *Lancet* 335:427, 1990.

45. Gruppo Italiano per lo Studio della Streptochinasi Nell'Infarcto Miocardico (GISSI): Effectiveness of intravenous thrombolytic treatment in acute myocardial infarction. *Lancet* 1:397, 1986.

46. Krumholz H, Pasternak R, Weinstein M, et al: Cost effectiveness of thrombolytic therapy with streptokinase in elderly patients with suspected acute myocardial infarction. *N Engl J Med* 327:7, 1992.

47. Sherman CT, Litvack F, Grundfest W, et. al.: Coronary Angioscopy in Patients with Unstable Angina Pectoris. *N Engl J Med* 315:913, 1986.

48. Freeman MR, Williams AE, Chisholm RJ, et al: Intracoronary thrombus and complex morphology in unstable angina: Relation to Timing of angiography and in-hospital cardiac events. *Circulation* 80:17, 1989.

49. Ambrose JA, Alexopoulos D: Thrombolysis in unstable angina: Will beneficial effects of thrombolytic therapy in myocardial infarction apply to patients with unstable angina? *J Am Coll Cardiol* 13:1666, 1989.

50. Rutherford JD: Unstable angina and thrombolysis. *Chest* 97:156S, 1990.
51. Lawrence JR, Shepherd JT, Bone I, et al: Fibrinolytic therapy in Unstable angina pectoris: A controlled clinical Trial. *Thromb Res* 17:767, 1980.
52. Saran RK, Bhandari K, Narain VS, et al: Intravenous streptokinase in the management of a subset of patients with unstable angina: A randomized controlled trial. *Int J Cardiol* 28:209, 1990.
53. Bär FW, Verheugt FW, Materne P, et al: Thrombolysis in patients with unstable angina improves the angiographic but not the clinical outcome: Results of UNASEM, a multicenter, randomized, placebo-controlled, clinical trial with anistreplase. *Circulation* 86:131, 1992.
54. Schreiber TL, Rizik D, White C, et al: Randomized trial of thrombolysis versus heparin in unstable angina. *Circulation* 86:1407, 1992.
55. DeWood MA, Spores J, Notske R, et al: Prevelance of total coronary occlusion during the early hours of transmural myocardial infarction. *N Engl J Med* 303:897, 1980.
56. Sharkey SW, Brunette DD, Ruiz E, et al: An analysis of time delays preceding thrombolysis for acute myocardial infarction. JAMA 262:3171, 1989.
57. Sheehan FH, Braunwald E, Canner P, et al: The effect of intravenous thrombolytic therapy on left ventricular function: A Report on Tissue-Type Plasminogen Activator and Streptokinase from the Thrombosis in Myocardial Infarction (TIMI Phase I) Trial. *Circulation* 75:817, 1987.
58. Magnani B, for the PAIMS Investigators: Plasminogen Activator Italian Multicenter Study (PAIMS): Comparison of intravenous recombinant single-chain human tissue-type plasminogen activator (rt-PA) with intravenous streptokinase in acute myocardial infarction. *J Am Coll Cardiol* 13: 19, 1989.
59. Gruppo Italiano per lo Studio della Sopravvivenza Nell' Infarto Miocardico: GISSI-2: A factorial randomized trial of alteplase versus streptokinase and heparin versus no heparin among 12,490 patients with acute myocardial infarction. *Lancet* 336:65, 1990.
60. The International Study Group: In-hospital mortality and clinical course of 20,891 patients with suspected acute myocardial infarction randomized between alteplase and streptokinase with or without heparin. *Lancet* 336: 71, 1990.
61. Verstraete M, Bernard R, Bory M, et al: Randomized trial of intravenous recombinant tissue-type plasminogen activator versus intravenous streptokinase in acute myocardial infarction: Report from the European Cooperative Study Group for Recombinant Tissue-Type Plasminogen Activator. *Lancet* 1:842, 1985.
62. White HD, Rivers JT, Maslowski AH, et al: Effect of intravenous streptokinase as compared with that of tissue plasminogen activator on left ventricular function after first myocardial infarction. *N Engl J Med* 320:817, 1989.
63. The GUSTO Investigators: An international randomized trial comparing four thrombolytic strategies for acute myocardial infarction. *N Engl J Med* 329:673, 1993.
64. Califf R, White H, Van de Werf F, et al: One-year results from the global utilization of streptokinase and TPA for occluded coronary arteries (GUSTO-I) trial. *Circulation* 94:1233, 1996.
65. The GUSTO Angiographic Investivators. The effects tissue plasminogen activator, streptokinase, or both on coronary-artery patency, ventricular

function, and survival after acute myocardial infarction. *N Engl J Med* 329:1615, 1993.

66. Bode C, Smalling R, Berg G, et al: Randomized comparison of coronary thrombolysis achieved with double-bolus reteplase (recombinant plasminogen activator) and front-loaded, accelerated alteplase (recombinant tissue plasminogen activator) in patients with acute myocardial infarction. *Circulation* 94:891, 1996.

67. Cody R: Results from late breaking clinical trials sessions at ACC '97. *J Am Coll Cardiol* 30:1, 1997.

68. Michels K, Yusuf S: Does PTCA in acute myocardial infarction affect mortality and reinfarction rates? A quantitative overview (meta-analysis) of the randomized clinical trials. *Circulation* 91:476, 1995.

69. Grines C, Browne K, Marco J, et al: A comparison of immediate angioplasty with thrombolytic therapy for acute myocardial infarction. *N Engl J Med* 328:67, 1993.

70. Carter L, Stephan W, Cavero P, et al: Advanced age is not a contraindication for primary infarct angioplasty in patients with cardiogenic shock. *J Am Coll Cardiol* 956:205A, 1995.

71. The European Myocardial Infarction Project Group: Prehospital thrombolytic therapy in patients with suspected acute myocardial infarction. *N Engl J Med* 329:383, 1993.

72. American College of Cardiology/American Heart Association Task Force on Assessment of Diagnostic and Therapeutic Cardiovascular Procedures (Subcommittee to Develop Guidelines for the Early Management of Patients with Acute Myocardial Infarction): Guidelines for the early management of patients with acute myocardial infarction. *J Am Coll Cardiol* 16:249, 1990.

73. Rogers W, Baim D, Gore J, et al: Comparison of immediate invasive, delayed invasive, and conservative strategies after tissue-type plasminogen activator. *Circulation* 81:1457, 1990.

74. Lopez LM, Mehta JL: Anticoagulation in coronary heart disease: Heparin and warfarin trials. *Cardiovasc Clin* 18:215, 1987.

75. MacMahon S, Collins R, Knight C, et al: Reduction in major morbidity and mortality by heparin in acute myocardial infarction. *Circulation* 78: II-98, 1988.

76. Turpie AGG, Robinson JG, Doyle DJ, et al: Comparison of high-dose with low-dose subcutaneous heparin to prevent left ventricular mural thrombus in patients with acute transmural anterior myocardial infarction. *N Engl J Med* 320:352, 1989

77. Hsia J, Hamilton WP, Kleiman N, et al: A comparison between heparin and low-dose aspirin as adjunctive therapy with tissue plasminogen activator for acute myocardial infarction. *N Engl J Med* 323:1433, 1990.

78. Bleich SD, Nichols TC, Schumacher RR, et al: Effect of heparin on coronary artery patency after thrombolysis with tissue plasminogen activator in acute myocardial infarction. *Am J Cardiol* 66:1412, 1990.

79. de Bono DP, Simoons ML, Tijssen J, et al: Effect of Early intravenous heparin on coronary patency, infarct size, and bleeding complications after alteplase thrombolysis: Results of a randomized double blind European cooperative study group trial. *Br Heart J* 67:122, 1992.

80. Topol EJ, George BS, Kereiakes DJ, et al: A randomized controlled trial of intravenous tissue plasminogen activator and early intravenous heparin in acute myocardial infarction. Circulation 79:281, 1989.

81. Thompson PL, Aylward PE, Federman J, et al: A Randomized comparison of intravenous heparin with oral aspirin and dipyridomole 24 hours after recombinant tissue-type plasminogen activator for acute myocardial infarction. *Circulation* 83:1534, 1991.

82. Serneri GGN, Gensini GF, Poggesi L, et al: Effect of heparin, aspirin, or alteplase in reduction of myocardial ischaemia in refractory unstable angina. *Lancet* 335:615, 1990.

83. Sansa M, Cernigliaro C, Campi A, et al: Effects of urokinase and heparin on minimal cross-sectional area of culprit narrowing in unstable angina pectoris. *Am J Cardiol* 68:451, 1991.

84. Theroux P, Ouimet H, McCans J, et al: Aspirin, heparin, or both to treat acute unstable angina. *N Engl J Med* 319:1105, 1988.

85. Theroux P, Waters D, Lam J, et al: Reactivation of unstable angina after discontinuation of heparin. *N Engl J Med* 327:141, 1992.

86. Telford AM, Wilson C: Trial of heparin versus atenolol in prevention of myocardial infarction in intermediate coronary syndrome. *Lancet* 1:1225, 1981.

87. Williams DO, Kirby MG, McPherson K, et al: Anticoagulation treatment in unstable angina. *Br J Clin Pract* 40:114, 1986.

88. Amsterdam EA, Lee G, Mason DT: Management of unstable angina: Current status and new perspectives. *Am Heart J* 102:144,1981.

89. Topol E, Bonan R, Jewitt D, et al: Use of a direct antithrombin, hirulog, in place of heparin during coronary angioplasty. *Circulation* 87:1622, 1993.

90. Serruys P, Herrman J-P, Simon R, et al: A comparison of hirudin with heparin in the prevention of restenosis after coronary angioplasty. *N Engl J Med* 333:757, 1995.

91. Bittl J, Strony J, Brinker J, et al: Treatment with bivalirudin (hirulog) as compared with heparin during coronary angioplasty for unstable or postinfarction angina. *N Engl J Med* 333:764, 1995.

92. The GUSTO IIa Investigators. Randomized trial of intravenous heparin versus recombinant hirudin for acute coronary syndromes. *Circulation* 90:1631, 1994.

93. Antman E: Hirudin in acute myocardial infarction. Safety report from the thrombosis and thrombin inhibition in myocardial infarction (TIMI) 9A trial. *Circulation* 90:1624, 1994.

94. Yusuf S, Collins R, MacMahon S, et al: Effect of Intravenous nitrates on mortality in acute myocardial infarction: An overview of the randomized trials. *Lancet* 1:1088, 1988.

95. The GISSI-2 Group. GISSI-3: effects of lisinopril and transdermal glyceryl trinitrate singly and together on 6-week mortality and ventricular function after acute myocardial infarction. *Lancet* 343:1115, 1994.

96. The GISSI-3 Group. Six-month effects of early treatment with lisinopril and transdermal glyceryl trinitrate singly and together withdrawn six weeks after acute myocardial infarction: The GISSI-3 trial. *J Am Coll Cardiol* 27:337, 1996.

97. The ISIS-4 Group. ISIS-4: A randomised factorial trial assessing early oral captopril, oral mononitrate, and intravenous magnesium sulphate in 58 050 patients with suspected acute myocardial infarction. *Lancet* 345: 669, 1995.

98. Mikolich JR, Nicoloff NB, Robinson PH, et al: Relief of refractory angina with continuous intravenous infusion of nitroglycerin. *Chest* 77:375, 1980.

99. Ziegler MG, Lake CR, Kopin IJ: Plasma noradrenaline increases with age. *Nature* 261:333, 1976.

100. Jones DH, Hamilton CA, Reid JL: Plasma noradrenaline, age and blood pressure: A population study. *Clin Sci Mol Med* 55:73s, 1978.
101. Saar N, Gordon RD: Variability of plasma catecholamine levels: Age, duration of posture, and time of day. *Br J Pharmacol* 8:353, 1979.
102. Esler M, Skews H, Leonard P, et al: Age-dependence of noradrenaline kinetics in normal subjects. *Clin Sci* 60:217, 1981.
103. Rubin PC, Scott PJW, McLean K, et al: Noradrenaline release and clearance in relation to age and blood pressure in man. *Eur J Clin Invest* 12:121, 1982.
104. Neubauer B, Christensen NJ: The decrease in noradrenaline concentration in the posterior tibial artery with age. *Gerontology* 24:299, 1978.
105. Lakatta EG: Age-Related Alterations in the Cardiovascular Response to Adrenergic Mediated Stress. *Fed Proc* 39:3173, 1980.
106. Bertel O, Bühler FR, Kiowski W, et al: Decreased beta-adrenoreceptor responsiveness as related to age, blood pressure, and plasma catecholamines in patients with essential hypertension. *Hypertension* 2:130, 1980.
107. Krall JF, Connelly M, Weisbart R, et al: Age-related elevation of plasma catecholamine concentration and reduced responsiveness of lymphocyte adenylate cyclase. *J Clin Endocrinol Metab* 52:863, 1981.
108. Come PC, Pitt B: Nitroglycerin-induced severe hypotension and bradycardia in patients with acute myocardial infarction. *Circulation* 54:624, 1976.
109. Ferguson JJ, Diver DJ, Boldt M, et al: Significance of nitroglycerin-induced hypotension with inferior wall acute myocardial infarction. *Am J Cardiol* 64:311, 1989.
110. Elkayam U, Kulick D, McIntosh N, et al: Incidence of early tolerance to hemodynamic effects of continuous infusion of nitroglycerin in patients with coronary artery disease and heart failure. *Circulation* 76:577, 1987.
111. Yusuf S, Peto R, Lewis J, et al: Beta blockade during and after myocardial infarction: An overview of the randomized trials. *Prog Cardiovasc Dis* 27:335, 1985.
112. Wilhelmsson C, Vedin JA, Wilhelmsen L, et al: Reduction of sudden deaths after myocardial infarction by treatment with alprenolol. *Lancet* 2:1157, 1974.
113. Multicentre International Study: Improvement in prognosis of myocardial infarction by long-term beta-adrenoreceptor blockade using practolol. *Br Med J* 3:735, 1975.
114. Multicentre International Study: Supplementary report: Reduction in mortality after myocardial infarction with long-term beta-adrenoceptor blockade. *Br Med J* 2:419, 1977.
115. Baber NS, Evans DW, Howitt G, et al: Multicentre post-infarction trial of propranolol in 49 hospitals in the United Kingdom, Italy, and Yugoslavia. *Br Heart J* 44:96, 1980.
116. Norwegian Multicenter Study Group: Timolol-induced reduction in mortality and reinfarction in patients surviving acute myocardial infarction. *N Engl J Med* 304:801, 1981.
117. Hjalmarson A, Elmfeldt D, Herlitz J, et al: Effect on Mortality of metoprolol in acute myocardial infarction. *Lancet* 2:823, 1981.
118. Hansteen V, Moinichen E, Lorensten E, et al: One Year's treatment with propranolol after myocardial infarction: Preliminary Report of Norwegian Multicentre Trial. *Br Med J* 284:155, 1982.
119. β-Blocker Heart Attack Trial Research Group: A randomized trial of propranolol in patients with acute myocardial infarction I. Mortality Results. *JAMA* 247:1707, 1982.

120. Julian DG, Prescott RJ, Jackson FS, et al: Controlled trial of sotalol for one year after myocardial infarction. *Lancet* 1:1142, 1982.
121. Taylor SH, Silke B, Ebbutt A, et al: A Long-term prevention study with oxprenolol in coronary heart disease. *N Engl J Med* 307:1293, 1982.
122. Australian and Swedish Pindolol Study Group: The Effect of Pindolol on the Two Years Mortality After Complicated Myocardial Infarction. *Eur Heart J* 4:367, 1983.
123. European Infarct Study Group: European Infarct Study (E.I.S.): A secondary prevention study with slow-release oxprenolol after myocardial infarction: Morbidity and mortality. *Eur Heart J* 5:189, 1984.
124. Olsson G, Rehnqvist N, Sjögren A, et al: long-term treatment with metoprolol after myocardial infarction: Effect on 3 year mortality and morbidity. *J Am Coll Cardiol* 5:1428, 1985.
125. Gundersen T: Secondary prevention after myocardial infarction: Subgroup analysis of patients at risk in the Norwegian Timolol Multicenter Study. *Clin Cardiol* 8:253, 1985.
126. Hawkins CM, Richardson DW, Vokonas PS: Effect of propranolol in reducing mortality in older myocardial infarction patients: The Beta-Blocker Heart Attack Trial Experience. *Circulation* 67:I-94, 1983.
127. Chadda K, Goldstein S, Byington R, et al: Effect of propranolol after acute myocardial infarction in patients with congestive heart failure. *Circulation* 73:503, 1986.
128. Colucci W, Packer M, Bristow M, et al: Carvedilol inhibits clinical progression in patients with mild symptoms of heart failure. *Circulation* 94:2800, 1996.
129. Held PH, Yusuf S, Furberg CD: Calcium channel blockers in acute myocardial infarction and unstable angina: An overview. *Br Med J* 299:1187, 1989.
130. Yusuf S, Held P, Furberg C: Update of effects of calcium antagonists in myocardial infarction or angina in light of the Second Danish Verapamil Infarction Trial (DAVIT-II) and other recent studies. *Am J Cardiol* 67: 1295, 1991.
131. Fillmore SJ, Shapiro M, Killip T: Arterial oxygen tension in acute myocardial infarction. Serial analysis of clinical state and blood gas changes. *Am Heart J* 79:620, 1970.
132. MacMahon S, Collins R, Peto R, et al: Effects of Prophylactic lidocaine in suspected acute myocardial infarction: An overview of results from the randomized, controlled trials. *JAMA* 260:1910, 1988.
133. Cohn JN, Franciosa JA, Francis GS, et al: Effect of short-term infusion of sodium nitroprusside on mortality rate in acute myocardial infarction complicated by left ventricular failure: Results of a Veterans Administration Cooperative Study. *N Engl J Med* 306:1129, 1982.
134. Swedberg K, Held P, Kjekshus J, et al: Effects of the Early administration of enalapril on mortality in patients with acute myocardial infarction: Results of the Cooperative New Scandinavian Enalapril Survival Study II (CONSENSUS II). *N Engl J Med* 327:678, 1992.
135. Moye L, Pfeffer M, Braunwald E. Rationale, design and baseline characteristics of the survival and ventricular enlargement trial. *Am J Cardiol* 68:70D, 1991
136. Pfeffer MA, Braunwald E, Moye LA, et al: Effect of captopril on mortality and morbidity in patients with left ventricular dysfunction after myocardial infarction: Results of the Survival and Ventricular Enlargement Trial. *N Engl J Med* 327:669, 1992.

137. The AIRE Study Investigators. Effect of ramipril on mortality and morbidity of survivors of acute myocardial infarction with clinical evidence of heart failure. *Lancet* 342:821, 1993.
138. Ambrosioni E, Borghi C, Magnani B. The effect of the angiotensin-converting-enzyme inhibitor zofenopril on mortality and morbidity after anterior myocardial infarction. *N Engl J Med* 332:80, 1995.
139. Kober L, Torp-Pedersen C, Carlsen J, et al: A clinical trial of the angiotensin-converting-enzyme inhibitior trandolapril in patients with left ventricular dysfunction after myocardial infarction. *N Engl J Med* 333:1670, 1995.
140. Kingma J, van Gilst W, Peels C, et al: Acute intervention with captopril during thrombolysis in patients with first anterior myocardial infarction. *Eur Heart J* 15:898, 1994.
141. van Gilst W, Kingma H, Peels K, et al: Which patient benefits from early angiotensin-converting enzyme inhibition after myocardial infarction? *J Am Coll Cardiol* 28:114, 1996.
142. The CCS-1 Group. Oral captopril versus placebo among 13 634 patients with suspected acute myocardial infarction: interim report from the Chinese cardiac study (CCS-1). *Lancet* 345:686, 1995.
143. Kahn J, Rutherford B, McConahay D, et al: Supported "high risk" coronary angioplasty using intraaortic balloon pump counterpulsation. *J Am Coll Cardiol* 15:1151, 1990.
144. Ishihara M, Sato H, Tateishi H, et al: Intraaortic balloon pumping as the postangioplasty strategy in acute myocardial infarction. *Am Heart J* 122:385, 1991.
145. Pierpont, GL: Mechanical support of the failing circulation in acute coronary insufficiency and myocardial infarction. In: GS Francis, JS Alpert (eds): *Modern Coronary Care*. Boston, MA, Little, Brown and Co., 1990, p. 267.
146. Goldberger M, Tabak SW, Shah PK: Clinical Experience with intra-aortic balloon counterpulsation in 112 consecutive patients. *Am Heart J* 111:497, 1986.
147. Boden WE: Management of non-Q-wave myocardial infarction: Role of diltiazem versus β-blocker therapy. *J Cardiovasc Pharmacol* 16:S55, 1990.
148. Multicenter Diltiazem Postinfarction Trial Research Group: The effect of diltiazem on mortality and reinfarction after myocardial infarction. *N Engl J Med* 319:385, 1988.
149. Limacher MC: Clinical features of coronary heart disease in the elderly. In: DT Lowenthal (ed). Geriatric Cardiology. Philadelphia, PA, FA Davis Co., 1992, p. 63.

Chapter 11

Cardiac Procedure Use and Outcome of Elderly Patients with Acute Myocardial Infarction

Steven M. Wright, Jennifer Daley,
George E. Thibault

In 1998, an estimated 1.1 million Americans will have a new or recurrent coronary event, and about one third of them will die.[1] Acute myocardial infarction (AMI) is the leading cause of death in the United States. Although life expectancy after an AMI is increasing, mortality and morbidity after AMI are still significant. Poor prognosis is particularly marked for AMI patients over age 65 and reported trends in decreasing mortality after AMI have not been equivalent for patients under and over age 65.

The development of new medical technologies and the introduction of new drugs have contributed to significant improvements in the diagnosis and management of AMI. Significant reductions in morbidity and mortality have been demonstrated by advances in medical therapies including β-blockers,[2-5] thrombolysis,[6-8] aspirin,[9] anticoagulants,[10-14] and angiotensin-converting enzyme inhibitors.[15-17] Technological improvements in coronary bypass surgery including cardioplegia, anesthesia, and increasing use of mammary artery grafts may have de-

This research was supported by the Department of Veterans Affairs (VA) Health Services Research and Development Service Grant no. PPR/HSRD 94-001. Dr. Daley was a Senior Research Associate in the Career Development Program in Health Service Research and Development in the VA when these studies were conducted.

From *Clinical Cardiology in the Elderly. Second Edition,* edited by Elliot Chesler. © 1999, Futura Publishing Company, Armonk, NY.

creased operative mortality.[18] In addition to technological improvement, the number of diagnostic and therapeutic procedures performed has signifcantly increased and has been associated with a decrease in AMI fatalities and overall coronary deaths.[19,20] This rapid evolution in the treatment of AMI, however, has been accompanied by evidence of signifcant variation in the management of AMI, raising questions about the effectiveness and costs of different practice patterns.

In this chapter, we examine the utilization of procedures and the medical outcome for elderly patients hospitalized with AMI. We report results derived from administrative databases that contain information on AMI hospitalizations, use of procedures, and patient survival.

Because detailed longitudinal data are uniquely available in the Department of Veterans Affairs (VA) health care system, we use the veteran patient as a model to identify trends in variation in the use of procedures and outcomes. VA administrative data can also be linked to Medicare administrative data so we can also compare the use of cardiac procedures by elderly veterans using VA, Medicare services, or both. Finally, we examine the association between procedure use and mortality in the VA, Medicare, and Canadian health systems.

Variations in Practice Patterns and Effectiveness of Care

Seminal observations of John Wennberg, Robert Brook, and other investigators in the 1970s and 1980s focused attention on marked variations in medical practices across geographic regions.[21] Since then, there has been tremendous interest in reports of geographic variation[22,23] in clinical practice for many types of conditions,[24-26] in many types of institutions,[27,28] and among different populations.[29,30] These observed variations have led researchers and clinicians to study the effectiveness of medical care through outcomes research. Outcomes research involves linking the process of care received by patients who have a particular condition to outcomes of care (eg, mortality, morbidity, functional status, quality of life). Process of care refers to what health care providers do to, or for, patients. The process of care in AMI can refer to diagnostic or therapeutic interventions such as the use of coronary angiography, angioplasty, bypass surgery or the use of pharmacological therapy.

Randomized clinical trials (RCTs) are often viewed as the standard for evaluating what clinical interventions work best. This methodologic approach examines the efficacy of medical interventions when applied under ideal conditions. RCTs are both time consuming and expensive. They are often limited to subpopulations that may not be representative of the all patients with a particular condition in the general population. As an alternative to RCTs, population-based observational outcome studies provide an important method for examining what works well in real world practice settings rather than through controlled experiments. This approach examines the effectiveness of medical care. These studies may use large administrative databases that identify patient populations, measure process of care variables, and ascertain outcomes. These data sources have obvious cost and time savings over primary data collection, can characterize large groups of patients more representative of the general population, and are relatively easy to access. Outcome studies can be used to quantify variation in practice patterns among systems of care, subpopulations such as the elderly, and for specific diseases such as AMI. They also can be used to make important resource allocation decisions and assess the quality of care.

Administrative databases, however, are not a perfect alternative to RCTs. Data in these databases are collected for purpose other than effectiveness research (ie, billing and reimbursement, workload planning) and thus findings may be confounded by selection biases that are dealt with in RCTs by randomization. These databases lack important information about clinical factors that may be related to the process and outcomes of care. It is sometimes diffcult to identify diagnoses, comorbidities and severity of illness because of the imprecision and inaccuracy of the International Classification of Diseases, Ninth Revision, Clinical Modification (ICD-9-CVI) codes.

Elderly Veterans with AMI

The VA is one of the largest direct-delivery health care systems in the country with an extensive network of hospitals, outpatient clinics, domiciliaries, and nursing homes.[31] In the fiscal year 1997, the VA provided these services to 2.6 million of the nation's 26 million veterans. Although the overall veteran population has been declining for nearly 15 years, the number of elderly veterans (defined as those 65 and older) has increased rapidly and will peak at 9.3 million in the year 2000 as Korean Conflict-era veterans reach age 65, and again peak at 9 million in the mid- 2010s as Vietnam-era veterans turn 65.[32,33]

Between 1988 and 1997, there were 72,276 VA hospitalizations for the principal diagnosis of AMl (ICD-9-CM code 410). The yearly proportion of elderly veterans hospitalized for AMI steadily increased from 47% in 1988 to 54% in 1997 (total between 1988 and 1997, 38,232). Veterans with AMI were initially hospitalized in one of three types of VA medical centers (VAMCs): basic service (no coronary angiography or revascularization services available onsite); catheterization-only (only coronary angiography available onsite services); and cardiac surgery (coronary angiography and revascularization services available onsite). These hospitals are part of an integrated delivery svstem that provides a wide array of cardiac services to patients hospitalized for AMI. Veterans who are initially admitted to VAMCs without onsite services are transferred or referred, as needed, to a VAMC that does have the requisite services available onsite; they may receive such services in a non-VA hospital depending on distance, patient and/or doctor preferences, and the medical status of the veteran. Because VA and Medicare databases can be linked, we can specifically assess the extent to which elderly AMI veterans who were initially admitted to a VAMC then crossed over to nonfederal hospitals to undergo a cardiac procedure.

Examining variations in the treatment and outcomes of veterans with AMI has been the primary mission of the Center for the Study of Practice Patterns in Veterans with Acute Myocardial Infarction. The AMI Center conducts health services research designed to inform current and future clinical and policy discussions about effective treatment of veterans with AMI. The Center has conducted extensive analyses of variation and trends in procedure utilization and outcomes using national discharge abstract files maintained by the VA. These secondary data files, called the Patient Treatment File or PTF, contain diagnostic, treatment, and patient demographic information on all veterans who used VA inpatient or outpatient services. Using these data files, the AMI Center created a national, longitudinal database of all veterans hospitalized with AMI in VAMCs between 1988 and 1997. VA data from recent years (1992 to 1995) have been also linked with the Medicare inpatient database to assess use of cardiac procedures and outcomes in nonfederal hospitals for elderly veterans who were also users of the VA medical system (VA users).

Growth of Cardiac Procedures and Improving Survival

There has been striking growth in the use of cardiac procedures in the VA health care system. For veterans of all ages hospitalized with AMI between 1988 and 1994, the rate of coronary angiography increased by 30% (38.3% to 50.0%), coronary angioplasty increased by 176% (5.4% to 14.9%), and bypass surgery increased by 50% (7.2% to 11.1%).[34] The growth in procedure use was most pronounced among elderly veterans. Their rate of procedure use increased for coronary angiography by 43.4% (28.3% to 40.6%), coronary angioplasty 224.2% (3.3% to 10.8%), and bypass surgery 76.1% (5.2% to 9.1%). There has also been substantial growth in the use of these procedures in the nonveteran population. One study of U.S. hospitals that performed myocardial revascularization procedures covered by Medicare found that between 1987 and 1990 the rate of coronary angioplasty increased by 55% (24.4 per 10,000 in 1990) and the rate of bypass surgery increased 18% (34.4 per 10,000 in 1990).[19] Another study examining a population of elderly Medicare patients hospitalized for AMI between 1987 and 1990 reported that the rates of coronary angiography increased by 38% (24% to 33%), bypass surgery increased by 38% (8% to 11%), and coronary angioplasty increased by 100% (5% to 10%).[35]

Growth in the rates of procedure use was also different for patients initially admitted to the different types of VAMCs.[34] Onsite availability of cardiac technology is associated with greater use of cardiac procedures,[36,37] even after adjusting for important clinical characteristics of patients.[38,39] Trend analyses indicate that the growth in the use of procedures was generally greater in VAMCs without onsite technology (ie, basic service hospital) compared to VAMCs with onsite technology (ie, cardiac catheterization-only and cardiac surgery hospitals). An increasing proportion of elderly veterans experiencing an AMI received initial care at basic service hospitals were transferred to other VAMCs for cardiac procedures. It is believed that the increasing procedure rates between 1988 and 1994 were the results of improvements in system protocols for interhospital transfer and better integration between different types of VAMCs.[40,41] Although the association between the use and availability of cardiac procedures also exist in the non-VA sector, no studies have evaluated whether these trends are similar in that health care sector.

There was also a significant decline in mortality rates of AMI veterans hospitalized during this same period. Similar temporal trends in short-term survival rates among non-VA patients hospitalized with AMI have been shown.[42–46] The rate of decline, however, was greater for veterans under age 65 than elderly veterans. The 30-day mortality rate for elderly veterans decreased by 25.9% (21.2% to 15.7%) compared to 32.5% (9.6% to 6.4%) for younger veterans. The 1-year mortality rate for elderly veterans decreased by 17.8% (35.9% to 29.5%) compared to 31.1% (17.7% to 12.2%) for younger veterans. These fndings are consistent with observations in the non-VA patient population. In the Worcester Heart Attack Study, in-hospital mortality rates of patients hospitalized with AMI between 1988 and 1990 decreased by 52% (6.2% to 3.0%) for patients less than age 65 compared to 11% (15.9% to 14.2%) for patients 65 to 74 and 13% (33.5% to 29.2%) for patients 75 years or older.[47] Although studies have suggested that the use of cardiovascular tests, procedures, and drug therapies with known survival benefits decline with advancing age,[48–50] the reasons for the observed differences between younger and older patients are not known.

Use of VA and Medicare by Veterans with AMI

We examined cardiac procedure use and outcomes in Medicare and VA from 1992 to 1995.[51] We identifed elderly veterans who had previously used VA inpatient or outpatient services (VA users) and were initially hospitalized with a principal diagnosis of AMI in either Medicare or VA. Because VA users age 65 and older are dually eligible to receive Medicare and VA services, they provide a unique opportunity to examine the management of AMI in two systems of care in a patient population with similar sociodemographic characteristics. We identifed VA users who were hospitalized with AMI in either a VAMC or nonfederal Medicare hospital (N = 52,827). We examined where VA users were initially hospitalized and then compared rates of cardiac procedure use and mortality by the initial svstem of care.

We found that 69% of VA users who were hospitalized for AMI were initially admitted to a nonfederal Medicare hospital as opposed to a VAMC. We speculate that access to more than 6000 Medicare hospitals, the longer distance to the closest VAMC versus a nonfederal hospital, and characteristics of emergency transport services may account for the greater proportion of VA users with AMI being hospitalized in Medicare hospitals. VA users had signifcantly higher rates of procedure use when hospitalized in a nonfederal hospital compared to a VAMC. Rates were higher for coronary angiography (54.2% vs. 40.7%); for coronary angioplasty (18.1% vs. 10.2%), and for bypass surgery (18.4% vs. 10.7%). We do not know whether these higher rates reflect inappropriate use of cardiac procedures in Medicare hospitals, barriers limiting access to cardiac procedures in the VA, or some combination of both.

Our examination of the outcomes of elderly VA users initially hospitalized in VA or Medicare show that unadjusted mortality rates were signifcantly different for the two systems of care. Mortality was lower for VA users initially admitted to Medicare hospitals versus VAMCs at 30 days (15.7% vs. 16.8%, $P < 0.05$) and at 1 year (28.4% vs. 32.0%, $P < 0.001$). These differences, however, were not statistically significant after adjusting for patient characteristics and the type of hospital to which patients were initially admitted. The differences found in the unadjusted mortality rates were attenuated by a higher burden of comorbid diseases and a higher frequency of prior hospitalizations among VA users initially admitted to the VA. Therefore, it is impossible to conclude that the additional procedures made available to Medicare versus VA svstem led to better outcomes. It is possible that the current rates of procedure use in the VA are at a level that is sufficient to confer the benefit of procedural intervention after AMI. This does not address the issue of whether there are other differences in care in the VA and Medicare systems that could augment or diminish the benefits from procedures.

Differences in Cardiac Procedures Use Among Systems of Care

Population-based studies that contrast variation in the use of cardiac procedure and outcomes of patient with AMI in the United States and Canada have generated intense health policy debate in the 1990s.[52] The two countries have different health care financing systems. Canadian expenditures are more centrally controlled than in the U.S. health care system. Substantial differences exist between the two countries in the availability of the technology necessary to perform cardiac procedures. California, for example, has more than 3 times as many cardiac surgery hospitals per capita than 3 provinces in Canada.[53]

Results using patients of all ages enrolled in the Survival and Ventricular Enlargement (SAVE) and the Global Utilization of Streptokinase and Tissue Plasminogen Activator for Occluded Coronary Arteries (GUSTO) trials indicate a different threshold for the use of invasive diagnostic and therapeutic interventions in Canada than in the United States. In the SAVE trial, the United States had higher rates for coronary angiography (68% vs. 35%), coronary angioplasty (22% vs. 8%), and coronary bypass surgery (10% vs. 5%) than Canada.[54] In the GUSTO trial, the United States also had higher rates for coronary angiography (72% vs. 25%), coronary angioplasty (29% vs. 11%), and coronary bypass surgery (14% vs. 3%) than Canada.[55] The procedure rates for patients with AMI were derived from these clinical studies based on selective patient populations, providers, and institutions that volunteered to participate in the studies. Thus, caution should be used in inferring their findings to the population of all elderly patients with AMI.

There are larger population studies, however, that use administrative data to contrast rates of cardiac procedure use between the systems of care for elderly patients hospitalized with AMI. How do cardiac procedure rates for elderly patients differ in the Canadian, VA and Medicare health programs? We examined previously published unadjusted cardiac procedures rates for elderly patients who were hospitalized with AMI between in 1991, the most recent years when data were available from all three health care systems.[56] We calculated procedure rates for the VA for veterans hospitalized during the same time period and list the comparisons in Table 1. Rates for all 3 cardiac procedures were substantially lower in Canada compared to Medicare and the VA. The Medicare and VA have similar rates of coronary angiography (34.9% and 33.1%, respectively), but Medicare has higher rates than the VA for coronary angioplasty (11.7% vs. 5.4%) and coronary bypass surgery

Table 1
Comparison of Cardiac Procedure Rates Among Medicare, Veteran, and Canadian Patients Hospitalized with AMI in 1991 (age ≥ 65)

Procedures	Medicare	VA	Canada
Coronary angiography	34.9	33.1	6.7
Coronary angioplasty	11.7	5.4	1.5
Coronary bypass surgery	10.6	4.8	1.4
Any Revascularization	21.8	9.9	2.8

Note: Cardiac procedures within 30 days of initial admission for AMI. Medicare and Canadian rates previously published by Tu JV, et al. *N Engl J Med,* 336;1500–1505, 1997

(10.6% vs. 9.9%). Caution should be used in interpreting these comparisons, however, due to potential differences in populations observed. adjustment for patient case mix, and other delivery system characteristics.

The observational study of elderly patients with AMI that revealed substantial differences in procedure use did not find survival differences among Medicare, VA, and Canadian patients. Although unadjusted 30-day rates were slightly lower in Medicare, there were no differences in the 1-year mortality rate (34.3% vs. 34.4%).[56] By comparison, the unadjusted 1-year rate for elderly AMI patients hospitalized in the VA was 32.5%. Clinical trial data of AMI patients of all ages suggest, however, that quality of life may be better in U.S. versus Canadian patients. The SAVE trial showed no association between higher procedure use and survival after 2 years, but did find an association between greater procedure use and a lower risk of having activity limiting angina.[54] The GUSTO trial showed that the prevalence of chest pain and dyspnea at 1 year after AMI was higher among the Canadians patients (34% vs. 21% and 45% vs. 29%, respectively).[55] The combined results from the abovementioned clinical studies strongly suggests that there is no survival advantage associated with undergoing coronary angiography, coronary angioplasty, and coronary bypass surgery, but that these procedures may improve patient functional status and quality of life.

Outcomes and Association with Procedure Use

Our observational analyses of the use of cardiac procedures and associated outcomes suggest mixed findings regarding an association between rates of cardiac procedure use and outcomes. The trend in data revealed increased utilization of cardiac procedures and improving survival in elderly veterans hospitalized with AMI in the VA system suggesting a positive association between procedure use and outcomes. In our examination of veterans using VA and nonfederal hospitals there was no apparent association. Veterans who were admitted to nonfederal hospitals (ie, Medicare) had greater procedure use than veterans admitted to VAMCs, but there were no differences in survival. The lack of association was also evident in comparisons among systems of care. They indicate substantially greater procedure use in VA and Medicare than Canada, but no meaningful differences in survival. Clinical trial data on patients of all ages indicate that U.S. patients had less angina and better functional status 1-year after AMI than the Canadians. We do not have comparable measures of cardiac symptoms for veterans using the VA.

Differences in patterns of cardiac procedure use that are not clearly related to differences in outcomes have been observed in other observational studies examining nonclinical characteristics of elderly AMI patients. Using Medicare administrative data, the AMI Patient Outcome Research Team (PORT) reported variation in the use of cardiac procedures by gender and race with no differences in mortality.[57] Additional geographical analyses with clinical data from two states (Texas and New York) showed substantial variation in procedure use, but no differences in mortality or health-related quality of life.[58] Higher procedure rates in hospitals that have onsite availability of cardiac technology have been correlated with lower mortality in the VA[37] and in staff model health maintenance organizations.[59]

Despite the many studies examining variation in care after AMI, it is still not known whether higher rates for diagnostic or revascularization procedures are associated with improvements in mortality. Some have argued that wide variations in procedure use are markers for problems in the appropriateness and quality of care and that they represent opportunities for cost savings if high user areas can be reduced to the utilization of the average, or even the lowest, utilization areas without influencing the health status of patients. Others have argued that these variations are not necessarily "bad" and that it would be a mistake to force convergence on the same rates of use, particularly if the "ideal" rate is not known. From this perspective, these variations may represent differences in patient preferences for health care treatment and/or may represent opportunities to study different practice styles and innovations in care.

Conclusion

Using outcomes research to examine population-based rates of cardiac procedure use and associated outcomes raise important questions about effectiveness of care in the elderly. The results of the most recent observational studies in the VA suggest that more elderly veterans with AMI are receiving cardiac procedures and that patient survival is improving. Alternatively, comparisons across systems of care indicate that greater use of cardiac procedures by elderly patients with AMI is not harmful to patients and that they may be beneficial depending on whether outcomes other than mortality are evaluated. Finding definitive answers about the independent effects of procedures on outcomes will require studies that collect information on detailed clinical characteristics of patients that represent the general AMI population.

References

1. American Heart Association, Cardiovascular Disease Statistics. 1998.
2. Pedersen TR, and the Norwegian Multicenter Study Group. Timolol-induced reduction in mortality and reinfarction in patients surviving acute myocardial infarction. N Engl J Med 34:801–807, 1981.

3. Herlitz J, Elmfeldt D, Holmberg S, et al: The Goteborg metoprolol trial: Mortality and causes of death. *Am J Cardiol* 53:9D, 1984.
4. Beta-blocker Heart Attack Study Group. A randomized trial of propranolol in patients with acute myocardial infarction. *JAMA* 246:2073–2074, 1981.
5. Chadda K, Goldstein S, Byington R, et al: Effect of propranolol after acute myocardial infarction in patients with congestive heart failure. *Circulation* 73:503–510, 1987.
6. Stevenson R, Ranjadayalan K, Wilkinson P, et al: Short and long term prognosis of acute myocardial infarction since introduction of thrombolysis. *BMJ* 307:349–353, 1993.
7. SWIFT Trial Study Group: SWIFT trial of delayed intervention elective intervention versus conservative treatment after thrombolysis with antistreptelase in acute myocardial infarction. *BMJ* 302:555–560, 1991.
8. Williams DO, Braunwald E, Knatterud G, et al: One year results of the thrombolysis in myocardial infarction investigation (TIMI) phase II trial. *Circulation* 85:533–542, 1992.
9. Antiplatelet Triallists' Collaboration: Collaborative overview of randomized trials of antiplatelet therapy. I: Prevention of death, myocardial infarction. and stroke by prolonged antiplatelet therapy in various categories of patients. *BMJ* 308:81–106, 1994.
10. Smith P, Arnesen H, Holme I: The effect of warfarin on mortality and reinfarction after myocardial infarction. *N Engl J Med* 323:147–152, 1990.
11. Anticoagulants in the Secondary Prevention of Events in Coronary Thrombosis Research Group (ASPECT): Effect of long term oral anticoagulant treatment on mortality and cardiovascular morbidity after myocardial infarction. *Lancet* 343:499–503, 1994.
12. Breddin K, Loew D, Lechner K, et al: The German-Austrian aspirin trial: A comparison of acetylsalicylic acid, placebo and phenprocoumon in secondary prevention of myocardial infarction. *Circulation* 62(suppl V):V63-V72, 1980.
13. The EPSIM Research Group. A controlled comparison of aspirin and oral anticoagulants in prevention of death after myocardial infarction. *N Engl J Med* 307:701–708, 1982.
14. Cairns JA: Oral anticoagulants or aspirin after myocardial infarction? *Lancet* 343:497–498, 1994.
15. The Acute Infarction Ramipiril Efficacy Study Investigators: Effect of ramipiril on mortality and morbidity of survivors of acute myocardial infarction with clinical evidence of heart failure. *Lancet* 342:821–828, 1993.
16. Results of the Survival and Ventricular Enlargement trial: Effect of captopril on mortality and morbidity in patients with left ventricular dysfunction after myocardial infarction. *N Engl J Med* 327:669–677, 1992.
17. Swedberg K on behalf of the CONSENSUS II Study Group: Effects of the early administration of enalapril on mortality in patients with acute myocardial infarction. *N Engl J Med* 327:678–684, 1992.
18. Kirklin JW, Naftel CD, Blackstone EH, et al: Summary of a consensus concerning death and ischemic events after coronary artery bypass grafting. *Circulation* 79(suppl I):I81-I191, 1989.
19. Peterson ED, Jollis JG, Bebchuk JD, et al: Changes in mortality after revascularization in the elderly. *Ann Intern Med* 121(12):919–927, 1994.
20. Gillum RF. Trends in acute myocardial infarction and coronary heart disease death in the United States. *J Am Coll Cardiol* 23:1273–1237, 1994.
21. Wennberg JE, Gittelsohn A: Small area variations in health care delivery. *Science* 18:1102, 1973.

22. Wennberg JE, Barnes BA, Zubkoff M: Professional uncertainty and the problem of supplier-induced demand. *Soc Sci Med* 16:811, 1982.
23. Wennberg JE: Future directions for small area variations. *Med Care* 31: YS75-YS80, 1993.
24. Farrow DC, Hunt WC, Samet JM: Geographic variation in the treatment of localized breast cancer. *N Engl J Med* 326:1097–1101, 1992.
25. Roos NP, Roos LL Jr, Henteleff PD: Elective surgical rates: Do high rates mean lower standards? Tonsillectomy and adenoidectomy in Manitoba. *N Engl J Med* 297:360, 1977.
26. Wennberg JE, Mulley AG, Hanley D, et al: Assessment of prostatectomy for benign urinary tract obstruction. Geographic variations and the evaluation of medical outcome. *JAMA* 259:3027–3030, 1988.
27. Luft HS, Bunker JP, Einthoven AC. Should operations be regionalized: The empirical relationship between surgical volume and mortality. *N Engl J Med* 301:1364–1369, 1979.
28. Luft HS, Hunt SS, Maerki SC: The volume-outcome relationship: Practice makes perfect or selective referral patterns. *Health Serv Res* 22(2): 157–181, 1987.
29. Wennberg JE, Freeman JL, Culp WJ: Are hospital services rationed in New Haven or overutilized in Boston? *Lancet* i:1185–1189, 1987.
30. McPherson K, Strong PM, Epstein A, et al: Regional variations in the use of common surgical procedures: Within and between England and Wales, Canada, and the United States of America. *Soc Sci Med* 15A:273–288, 1981.
31. Fisher ES, Welch HG. The future of the Department of Veterans Affairs health care system. *JAMA* 10(4):869–878, 1995.
32. Fonseca M, Smith ME, Klein, RE, et al: The Department of Veterans Affairs Medical Care System and the People it serves. *Med Care* 34(3 suppl):MS9-MS19, 1996.
33. Department of Veterans Affairs: Annual report of the Secretary of Veterans Affairs, FY I 994. Washington, DC, 1995 : DVA.
34. Wright SM, Daley J, Petersen LA: Availability of cardiac technology: Trends in procedure use and outcomes for patient with AMI. Med Care Res Rev 55(2):239- 254, 1998.
35. Pashos CL, Normand ST. Garfinkle JB, et al: Trends in the use of drug therapies in patients with acute myocardial infarction: 1988 to 1998. *J Am Coll Cardiol* 23(5):1023–1030, 1994.
36. Blustein J: High-technology cardiac procedures: The impact of service availability on service use in New York State. *JAMA* 270:344–349, 1993.
37. Wright SM, Peterson ED, Daley J, et al: Outcomes of acute myocardial infarction in the DVA: Does regionalization of healthcare work? *Med Care* 35(2):128–139, 1997.
38. Every NR, Larson EB, Litwin PE, et al: The association between on-site cardiac catheterization facilities and the use of coronary angiography after acute myocardial infarction. *N Engl J Med* 329:546–551, 1993.
39. Barbash GI, White HD, Modan M, et al: Outcome of thrombolytic therapy in relation to hospital size and invasive cardiac services. *Arch Intern Med* 154:2237–2242, 1994.
40. Shortell SM, Gilles RR, Anderson DA: The new world of managed care: Creating organized delivery systems. *Health Affairs* (Winter):45–65, 1994.
41. Gilles RR, Shortell SM, Anderson DA, et al: Conceptualizing and measuring integration: Findings from the health systems integration study. *Hosp Health Serv Admin* 38(4):467–490, 1993.

42. McGovern PG, Pankow JS, Shahar E, et al: Recent trends in acute coronary heart disease. *N Engl J Med* 334(14):884–890, 1996.
43. Naylor DC, Chen E: Population-wide mortality trends among patients hospitalized for acute myocardial infarction: The Ontario experience, 1981 through 1991. *J Am Coll Cardiol* 24:1431–1438, 1994.
44. Pashos CL, Newhouse JP, McNeil BJ: Temporal changes in the care and outcomes of elderly patients with acute myocardial infarction, 1987 through 1990. *JAMA* 270(15):1832–1836, 1993.
45. Hunick MG, Goldman L, Tosteson AN, et al: The recent decline in mortality from coronary heart disease, 1980–1990. *JAMA* 277:535–542, 1997.
46. Gillum RF: Trends in acute myocardial infarction and coronary heart disease death in the United States. *J Am Coll Cardiol* 23:1273–1277. 1994.
47. Gurwitz JH, Goldberg RJ, Chen Z, et al: Recent trends in hospital mortality of acute myocardial infarction: The Worcester Heart Attack Study. *Arch Intern Med* 145:2202–2208, 1994.
48. Gurwitz JH, Osganian V, Goldberg RJ, et al: Diagnostic testing in acute myocardial infarction: Does patient age influence utilization patterns? The Worcester Heart Attack Study. *Am J Epidemiol* 134:948–957, 1991.
49. Gurwitz JH, Goldberg RJ, Chen Z, et al: Beta-blocker therapy in acute myocardial infarction: Evidence for underutilization in the elderly. *Am J Med* 93:605–610, 1992.
50. Weaver WD, Litwin PE, Martin JS, et al: Effect of age on use of thrombolytic therapy and mortality in acute myocardial infarction. *J Am Coll Cardiol* 18:657–662, 1992.
51. Wright SM, Petersen LA, Lamkin RP, et al: Medicare use by veterans with acute myocardial infarction. Poster presentation at 15th Annual Association for Health Services Research Conference, Washington, DC, 1998.
52. Krumholz HM: Cardiac procedures, outcomes, and accountability. *N Engl J Med* 21:1524–1523, 1997.
53. Grumback K, Anderson GM, Luit HS, et al: Regionalization of cardiac surgery in the United States and Canada. *JAMA* 274(16):1282–1288, 1995.
54. Rouleau JL, Moye LA, Pfeffer MA, et al: A comparison of management patterns after acute myocardial infarction in Canada and the United States. *N Engl J Med* 328(11):779–784, 1993.
55. Mark DB, Naylor DC, Hlatky MA, et al: Use of medical resources and quality of life after acute myocardial infarction in Canada and the United States. *N Engl J Med* 331:1130–1135, 1994.
56. Tu JV, Pashos CL, Naylor CD, et al: Use of cardiac procedures and outcomes in elderly patients with myocardial infarction in the United States and Canada. *N Engl J Med* 336:1500–1505, 1997.
57. Udvarhelvi S, Gatsonis C, Epstein AM, et al: Acute myocardial infarction in the Medical population: Process of care and clinical outcomes. *JAMA* 268(18):2530–2536, 1992.
58. Guadagnoli E, Hauptman PJ, Ayanian JZ, et al: Variation in the use of cardiac procedures after acute myocardial infarctn. *JAMA* 333(9):573–578, 1995.
59. Selby JV, Fireman BH, Lundstrom RJ, et al: Variation among hospitals in coronary angiography practices and outcomes after myocardial infarction in a large health maintenance organization. *N Engl J Med* 335: 1888–1896, 1996.

Chapter 12

Medical Management of Stable Angina Pectoris

Gordon L. Pierpont

The term "chronic stable angina" is somewhat of a misnomer. Exertional angina is often fairly predictable, with onset of symptoms tending to recur at the same cardiac workload (heart rate-blood pressure product) on repeated exercise tests.[1] However, during routine daily activities, angina can be quite variable,[2] and influenced by factors such as emotional state,[3] environmental temperature and humidity,[4,5] or circadian hormonal changes.[6] This natural variability in patterns of angina must be considered when adjusting therapy. It is all too easy to increase the dosage of an antianginal, choose alternate therapy, or add a new medication, based on an episode of chest pain that is part of normal variation rather than clear progression of the underlying disease. In the elderly, overmedication with consequent untoward side effects, as well as increased expense and inconvenience, often negate any long-term benefit. Great care must be exercised each time a medication is added or increased in dosage.

Despite this cautionary note, physicians are faced with a growing population of elderly patients with chronic ischemic heart disease requiring medical attention. Medical therapy is often preferred in the elderly because the risk of invasive procedures increases with age. Unfortunately, susceptibility to untoward side effects of medication also increases with age. Therapy for angina is complicated in the elderly by common problems such as resting bradycardia, atrioventricular (AV) nodal conduction delay and susceptibility to heart block, orthostatic or postprandial hypotension, or unexplained syncope or near syncope. Moreover, multiple drugs are often in use in the elderly, and drug inter-

From *Clinical Cardiology in the Elderly. Second Edition,* edited by Elliot Chesler. © 1999, Futura Publishing Company, Armonk, NY.

actions become particularly problematic. For these reasons, this chapter emphasizes the physiological actions of antianginal drugs, and their potential adverse side effects. Particular attention will be given to combination therapy and its role in the elderly.

When choosing medication for angina in an elderly patient, it is helpful to set therapeutic goals that are practical, attainable, and consistent with the patients overall health status. Setting reasonable therapeutic goals for chronic ischemic heart disease (IHD) is complicated by the fact that cardiac ischemia can frequently occur without symptoms. Proper evaluation and therapy for "silent ischemia" has been the subject of much debate in recent years. It is clear that silent ischemia is not always an all-or-none phenomenon. Although some patients may completely deny symptoms during episodes of ischemia[7] or infarction,[8] others may have episodes of ischemia that are symptomatic as well as others that are asymptomatic.[9] It is not unusual when performing exercise tests, for example, to note diagnostic electrocardiographic (ECG) changes[10] or regional wall motion abnormalities[11,12] occurring before symptoms. Should therapeutic goals in the elderly focus only on control of symptoms, or also include attempts to eliminate or minimize all evidence of cardiac ischemia, whether or not symptomatic?

Treatment for an asymptomatic condition is justifiable only when therapy can prolong life or prevent disease from progressing to a symptomatic or debilitating stage. In stable IHD it is not always clear to what extent occasional episodes of intermittent ischemia are detrimental to the myocardium. If the ischemia is prolonged and causes myocardial injury, or if the ischemia produces life-threatening arrhythmias, the adverse effects are readily evident. Alternatively, it is possible that intermittent ischemic episodes promote the development of collateral circulation to jeopardized areas of myocardium, and could thus indirectly be beneficial. Or perhaps metabolic changes occur with "preconditioning" that can blunt the severity of subsequent infarction. Several studies[13-17] suggest that ischemic events on ambulatory electrocardiographic monitoring during daily activity can predict outcome in patients with stable IHD. However, the Total Ischemic Burden European Trial (TIBET),[18] which was specifically designed to determine if the frequency and duration of ischemia in daily life would predict clinical outcome, found that neither presence, frequency, or total duration of ischemic events could predict subsequent cardiac events (cardiac death, myocardial infarction [MI], unstable angina, coronary artery bypass surgery, coronary angioplasty, or treatment failure) in patients with chronic stable angina. Uncertainty as to the long-term outcome of intermittent ischemia suggests that ischemia should not necessarily be treated just because it exists, much as occasional premature ventricular beats should not necessarily be treated simply because they exist. The decision to intervene in silent ischemia thus requires identifying those patients at increased risk for adverse outcome, and choosing therapy for which there is good evidence of either life-prolonging potential or other benefits that could outweigh the risk and cost of intervention.

The decision whether or not to treat silent ischemia in the elderly, and how to treat, cannot be made without a thorough evaluation of the patient. This includes complete definition of all medical problems, a summary of current medication, and knowledge of the patients activities and expectations. It is not unusual to find problems that make treatment decisions easier. For example, if the patient is found to have hypertension, an antihypertensive agent can be chosen that is also efficacious for treating myocardial ischemia. Similarly, if the patient has evidence of previous MI, therapy to prolong life after MI (such as β-adrenergic blockers) can be utilized as discussed in Chapter 9. Alternatively, problems may arise that present relative contraindications to specific therapy, thus limiting the therapeutic choices.

The final, and sometimes most important, information needed to decide when to intervene in silent ischemia is the amount of myocardium at risk, and the status of myocardial function. These assessments are made by exercise testing, provocative drug testing, and cardiac catheterization as discussed elsewhere in this book. Those patients identified as high risk can be considered for coronary artery bypass surgery or coronary angioplasty (Chapter 12). If invasive measures are not warranted, high- risk patients can be treated medically with many of the same considerations in choosing therapy as for symptomatic patients. The remainder of this chapter focuses on medical therapy for stable angina pectoris, where symptoms assist in determining the response to therapy and thus help guide titration of dose and choice of additional or alternate agents. Most of the information is also applicable to patients with silent ischemia, but alternate end points, such as performance on repeat exercise testing must be used.

Aspirin

As noted in Chapter 9, aspirin can prolong life for patients with stable or unstable angina pectoris, and after acute myocardial infarction (AMI). This benefit has recently been shown to include patients with silent ischemia.[19] Aspirin cannot be expected to relieve symptoms of angina. However, unless there are specific contraindications, aspirin should be used in a dose of 81 to 325 mg daily to help prevent future adverse cardiac events.

β-Adrenergic blockers

The studies cited in Chapter 9 demonstrated that β-blocker therapy improves survival after MI, with most of the beneficial evident in the first 6 months. However, it is not clear whether or not β-blockers should be continued permanently, or could be safely stopped after 1 or 2 years. No specific study has adequately addressed this question, but

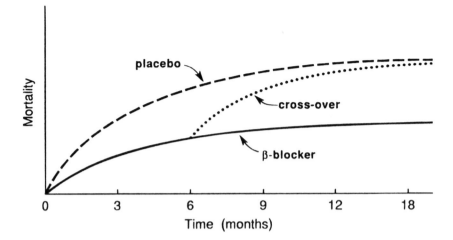

Figure 1: *Possible outcome of a trial to ascertain the need for lifetime use of β-blockers post-myocardial infarction (MI). At 6 months, survival benefit of β-blockade should be evident compared to placebo. If the β-blocker is then stopped, protective effects may be lost (crossover line) compared to continued use. Alternatively, patients receiving the β-blocker may have been protected through a vulnerable period, and continue to do better, even if the β-blocker is stopped at 6 months.*

Figure 1 presents two possible outcomes of a study designed to answer this question. Six months after AMI, patients given a β-blocker would be expected to demonstrate better survival than those on placebo. If the β-blocker were then stopped, the mortality rate could very well increase toward that of the placebo group due to loss of its protective effect. Alternatively, it is possible that the β-blocker succeeded in protecting patients through a more vulnerable period, and is thus no longer needed. In this case, the mortality would stay less than that of the placebo group even after the drug is stopped. Which of these alternatives is more likely remains unclear, but arguments projected from previous studies suggest it is most reasonable to continue the β-blocker long term.[20]

Whereas the data demonstrating life-prolonging effects of β-blockers post-MI are convincing, similar effects on prognosis in patient with IHD who have not had MI are lacking. An uncontrolled review of patients hospitalized for acute cardiac ischemia, but in whom MI was ruled out, suggests that those discharged on β-blockers have a lower 1-year mortality than those not so treated. Fortunately, β-blockers are quite efficacious in helping control symptoms of angina pectoris, and thus are a logical choice as first line therapy for chronic IHD. If hypertension is also present, additional benefit can be obtained because of the antihypertensive effects of β-blockers.

Numerous β-blockers are available for use in treating angina pectoris, making the choice of a specific agent appear confusing. It is therefore important to realize that they all act through the same basic mechanism, namely, competitive inhibition of β-adrenergic receptors. Thadani et al[21] demonstrated that when used at equipotent doses, 5 different β-blockers were equally efficacious in controlling exercise induced angina pectoris. It is likely that no specific agent is better than any other for treating angina pectoris. This allows a specific β-blocker to be chosen by considering such factors as cost and potential side effects, both of which can be important in elderly patients. Significant pulmonary disease is often present, making β_1-selective blockers attractive. It is also common for older patients to have an element of sinus node dysfunction, even though it may be subclinical. As a result, inducing symptomatic bradycardia must be a concern when initiating β-blocker therapy. If the dose of β-blocker required to control exercise heart rate causes severe bradycardia, an agent that possesses intrinsic sympathomimetic activity may alleviate the problem. Sleep disturbances can occasionally be attributed to a β-blocker so that choosing a less lipophilic drug that has limited ability to cross the blood brain barrier might be helpful. Some of the other potential side effects of β-blockers, such as sexual dysfunction or exacerbation of claudication, may be more difficult to remedy by choosing an alternate agent. Table 1 summarizes some of the more important properties of β-blockers to consider in selecting an appropriate agent for an individual patient. Sotalol has not been included in the table because it is used primarily as an antiarrhythmic agent, and esmolol because it is only available for intravenous use.

Table 1
Oral β-Adrenergic Blockers

Generic Name	Trade Name	β-1 Selective	Intrinsic Sympatho-mimetic Activity	Lipophilic	Total Daily Dose (mg)	Cost
Propranolol	Inderal generic	−	−	+	80–640	
Metoprolol	Lopressor Toprol	+	−	+	100–450	
Atenolol	Tenormin	+	−	−	50–200	
Timolol	Blockadren	−	−	−	20–60	
Pindolol	Viskin	−	+	+	10–60	
Labetalol*@	Normodyne	−	−	−	200–1200	
Acebutolol*	Sectral	+	+	−	400–1200	
Carteolol*	Cartrol	−	+	−	2.5–10	
Penbutolol*	Levatol	−	+	+	20–40	
Betaxolol*	Kerlone	+	−	−	10–40	
Carvedilol*@	Corgard	−	−	+	6.5–50	
Bisoprolol*	Zebeta	+	−	+	2.5–20	

* Not FDA approved for angina pectoris; @ Also have α-adrenergic blocking effects.
Propranolol and metoprolol are available in sustained release preparations.

Because left ventricular dysfunction is frequently present in elderly patients with chronic IHD, the use of any negative inotropic agent requires careful consideration. In the previous chapter it was emphasized that β-blockers improved survival following AMI even if mild or moderate heart failure was present. Moreover, placebo was just as likely to induce subsequent episodes of heart failure as was β-blocker in the post—MI studies. Previous ischemic damage is the most common etiology of left ventricular dysfunction in chronic IHD, and it is logical to exclude β-blockers only when congestive heart failure is severe. This outlook is supported by studies that suggest that a β-blocker may even extend life when used carefully in patients with dilated cardiomyopathy.[22,23]

Cost was mentioned as an important consideration in choosing a specific drug. Presence of concomitant medical problems may justify use of a more expensive agent in some patients in an attempt to avoid side effects. However, drug kinetics is a minor issue in this regard. The pharmacological effects of β-blockers last longer than would be predicted based on plasma half-life. As plasma levels fall, release from receptor binding sites lags behind, and some drug effect persists. For example, the plasma half life of propranolol (4 to 6 hours), would suggest an optimal dosing schedule of 4 times daily. However, propranolol has been shown to be equally effective in controlling angina when the same total daily dose is given in a twice daily regimen as when it is divided into 4 equal doses per day.[24] Furthermore, propranolol can adequately control blood pressure in hypertension when given only once a day.[25] This knowledge allows flexibility when considering a dosing schedule for β-blocker use. A convenient once or twice a day regimen can often be used. If other medicine is being taken 3 or 4 times a day, the β-blocker dose can be adjusted to fit the same schedule. For this reason, information on specific drug kinetics is not included in Table 1. Finally, the cost of β-blockers can vary considerably depending not only on the specific drug, but also the source of supply to the patient. As such, a blank column is left in Table 1 to allow entry of local drug prices by the reader. Awareness of these factors can help physicians be of greater service to their patients.

Nitrates

Nitrates have been of known benefit in the treatment of chronic IHD since Brunton[26] reported relief of angina with amyl nitrate in 1867, and Murrell[27] demonstrated similar effects with a 1% solution of nitroglycerin in 1879. Currently, 4 basic nitrate compounds are available for treating angina: nitroglycerin, isosorbide mononitrate, isosorbide dinitrate, and erythrityl or pentaerythritol tetranitrate. These compounds all act via the same mechanism. Nitrates cause direct relaxation of vascular smooth muscle after being converted to nitric oxide within the cells. There is now convincing evidence that nitric oxide is

Table 2
Nitrates

Nitroglycerin	Isosorbide Dinitrate
Sublingual	Oral
Tablet	Oral Sustained Release
Spray	Chewable
Oral Sustained Release	Submucosal
Submucosal	Erythrityl Tetranitrate*
Transdermal	Pentaerythrityl Tetranitrate
Paste	Oral
Patch	Oral sustained release
Isosorbide Mononitrate*	

* oral form only.

the identical compound as endothelium- derived relaxing factor (EDRF), which is endogenous to endothelial cells. Conversion of nitrates to nitric oxide requires reduced sulphhydryl groups. Tolerance to nitrates is felt to be due to progressive depletion of these necessary sulphydryl groups.[28] Changes in neurohormones in response to the drugs, such as an increase in circulating norepinephrine and/or activation of the renin-angiotensin system with consequent fluid retention, may also contribute to nitrate tolerance.[29] This tolerance develops within 24 hours of constant exposure,[30,31] and there is significant cross-tolerance between different nitrate compounds.[32] Providing a nitrate free interval of 8 to 12 hours every day allows for regeneration of sulphhydryl groups and helps avoid tolerance.[33]

Because of tolerance, it becomes critical to understand the kinetics of various nitrate preparations in order to use them properly. Table 2 lists available nitrate preparations, and Figure 2 depicts the relative

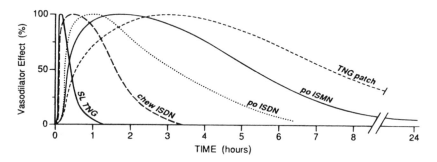

Figure 2: *Relative duration of effect of several commonly used nitrate preparations. SL TNG, sublingual nitroglycerin; chew ISDN, chewable isosorbide dinitrate; po ISDN, oral isosorbide dinitrate; po ISMN, oral isosorbide mononitrate; TNG patch, transdermal nitroglycerin patch.*

duration of effect of several commonly used forms. The rapid onset of sublingual forms of nitroglycerin (tablets or spray) is the reason for their common use to relieve episodes of angina pectoris. Because of this rapid onset of action, they can also be used prophylactically immediately prior to exercise. Chewable isosorbide dinitrate is particularly efficacious for prophylaxis because in addition to an extremely rapid onset of action, it has a longer duration of effect than sublingual nitroglycerin.

For more long-term prophylaxis, the longer acting preparations are needed. Thadani et al[34] provided excellent data applicable to proper use of oral isosorbide dinitrate that can be generalized to other forms as well. They studied effects of isosorbide dinitrate on exercise tolerance in patients with angina in doses ranging from 15 to 120 mg given both acutely, and after chronic therapy 4 times daily. The 15 mg dose was effective acutely, with minimal additional improvement at 30 mg, without additional benefit at higher doses. However, the chronic 4 times daily regimen resulted in significant tolerance. Thus, there appears little reason to use oral isosorbide dinitrate in doses much greater than 20 or 30 mg given 3 times daily. Furthermore, patients should be instructed to take the medication during portions of the day when they are active, rather than just prior to sleep. This will allow a nitrate-free interval overnight, and help avoid tolerance. Breakfast, lunch, and again in the late afternoon work well as appropriate times for many patients to take their isosorbide dinitrate. Similar considerations should be made if longer acting preparations are used. Alternatively, if a nitrate is used to treat nocturnal angina, it should not be given at regular intervals during the day.

Nitrates have an added benefit in patients with angina pectoris and left ventricular dysfunction. In the V-HeFT study of vasodilators in congetive heart failure (CHF),[35] isosorbide dinitrate combined with hydralazine prolonged life. It is not possible to ascertain which of these 2 drugs had the predominant effect, but certainly the results suggest that nitrates alone may have the potential to prolong life in patients with left ventricular dysfunction.

The only 2 significant side effects of nitrates are headaches and hypotension. Tolerance to headaches can develop with long-term use, but this may reflect some concomitant tolerance to the beneficial effects of the drug. Orthostatic hypotension is of particular concern in the elderly, and patients should be warned about the possibility of light-headedness or fainting upon arising. In particularly susceptible individuals, a test dose while under observation is indicated.

In summary, nitrates continue to be very useful in therapy of chronic IHD, but unlike β-blockers, drug kinetics are a major consideration in choosing a particular drug and dosing schedule.

Calcium Channel Antagonists

Intracellular calcium metabolism is very complex, with multiple organelles affecting calcium flux and concentration from the plasma membrane to the myofibrils. The calcium antagonists used to treat angina pectoris are a heterogeneous group of compounds, many of which are structurally quite unrelated. Consequently, although they all exhibit physiological effects by altering cellular calcium, they do not share a common receptor like beta blockers, or a common metabolic pathway equivalent to nitric oxide formation from nitrates. The potency of effect on vascular smooth muscle relative to effects on cardiac myocyte contractile or conduction properties varies considerably among the calcium antagonists. As a result these drugs have differing physiological effects, and it is much more difficult to consider them as a uniform class. Moreover, new entrants into the class continue to appear, making any review incomplete soon after it is published. Table 3 lists calcium antagonists available in the United States at the time of this writing, and Table 4 describes some of their more important properties. Rather than attempt a detailed review of each agent, only those drug effects most pertinent to use in the elderly are highlighted.

Although nifedipine, nicardipine, amlodipine, felodipine, and isradipine each have some unique properties, they can be conveniently discussed together because they are dihydropyridines and share many common effects. The dihydropyridines have vascular effects that predominate more than their myocardial activity. A decrease in blood pressure is predictable, with either no change or a slight reflex increase in heart rate. Felodipine and isradipine are Food and Drug Administration (FDA) approved for use in treating hypertension only, whereas the other dihydropyridines include angina as an indication. In isolated

Table 3
Oral Calcium Antognists

Generic Name	Trade Names	Dihydropyridine	Angina Indication	Daily Dose*
Nifedipine	Procardia, Adalat	yes	yes	30–90 mg
Nicardipine	Cardene	yes	yes	30–120 mg
Amlodipine	Norvasc	yes	yes	5–10 mg
Felodipine	Plendil	yes	no	5–20
Isradipine	DynaCirc	yes	no	2.5–10 mg
Nimodipine	Nimotop	yes	no	240 mg
Nisoldipine	Sular	yes	no	20–60 mg
Verapamil	Calan, Isoptin, Covera, Verelan	no	yes	120–480 mg
Diltiazem	Cardizem, Dilacor, Tiazac	no	yes	60–480 mg
Bepridil	Vascor	no	yes	20–400 mg

* Dose range is given as total daily dose. Depending on the preparation, divided doses are indicated. Nifedipine, nicardipine, verapamil, and diltiazem are available in sustained release type preparations.

Table 4
Comparative Effects of Calcium Antagonists

	Dihydropyridines*	Verapamil	Diltiazem	Bepridil
Heart Rate	↑	↓	↓	0 to ↓
AV Conduction	0	↓	↓	0 to ↓
Contractility	0**	↓	↓	0 to ↓
Blood Pressure	↓↓	↓	↓	0 to ↓
Notable Adverse Effects	Edema, flushing, lightheadedness	Constipation, bradycardia, worsen CHF	Bradycardia, worsen CHF	Proarrhythmic

0: no significant effect; ↑: increase; ↓: decrease; *: all dihydropyridines considered as a class for convenience; and **: reflex increase in contractility counteracts direct negative inotropic effect.

cardiac preparations, these agents have a direct negative inotropic effect. However, the negative inotropic effect is usually not clinically evident when therapy is initiated with these drugs. Single-dose hemodynamic effects may appear beneficial,[36–39] but trials specifically examining use of these agents as vasodilators for patients with symptomatic heart failure have generally failed to show benefit,[40–42] and they may even be dangerous.[43] If a calcium antagonist is needed to help control angina in a patient with left ventricular dysfunction, amlodipine appears to be the agent of choice, as it has been shown to be safe in a large controlled clinical trial of patients with heart failure.[44] Felodipine has also been studied in heart failure patients,[45] but the study was not powered adequately to ensure that adverse effects might be missed due to an inadequate number of patients enrolled. Because of vasodilator activity, side effects most likely to be of concern in the elderly treated with dihydropyridines include light headedness and orthostatic hypotension. Peripheral edema unrelated to heart failure, and gastrointestinal distress are not unusual.

Diltiazem has electrophysiological effects not shared by the dihydropyridines. Diltiazem tends to decrease heart rate and slow conduction through the AV node. As a result it must be used with caution in patients with AV conduction defects or sinus node dysfunction. Aside from the potential electrophysiological problems in susceptible individuals, the drug is usually well tolerated. However, as discussed in the previous chapter, this agent should be used with caution, if at all, in patients with significant left ventricular dysfunction. The Multicenter Diltiazem Postinfarction Trial[46] showed no overall difference in survival or reinfarction in post-MI patients given diltiazem compared to placebo. However, when analyzed prospectively by subgroups according to presence or absence of heart failure, patients with CHF receiving diltiazem had higher mortality than similar patients receiving placebo. Alternatively, patients without CHF tended to do better with diltiazem.

Verapamil also slows heart rate and AV nodal conduction. It has the most potent negative inotropic effect of the calcium antagonists at clinical doses. Caution is therefore needed when there is heart failure. The Danish Verapamil Trial[47,48] provided results in some ways analagous to the Diltiazem Postinfarction Trial.[46] Patients suffering MI treated with verapamil as secondary prevention fared better than those on placebo, but no benefit was evident in the subgroup with evidence of heart failure. In the elderly, constipation can occasionally be a problem with this drug. However, if patients with heart failure, or sinus nodal, or AV node dysfunction are avoided, verapamil can be an effective antianginal agent. It is available generically, and the cost/benefit ratio is often very favorable as a result. Bepridil has electrophysiological effects distinct from those of verapamil or diltiazem. Bepridil prolongs the atrial as well as ventricular refractory periods.[49] This makes the drug of potential use for treating atrial and ventricular tachyarrhythmias, but it is not FDA approved for treatment of any rhythm disturbance. Most notably, bepridil has properties similar to class I antiarrhythmic agents, and can prolong the Q-T interval.[50] This effect can be proarrhythmic, and may cause torsades de pointes type of ventricular tachycardia, especially in elderly patients with diuretic induced hypokalemia.[51] Because of these properties, bepridil should be reserved for use in patients for whom other antianginal drugs have failed to provide adequate relief of symptoms.

In summary, the calcium antagonists have many very important and often distinctive individual characteristics that make generalizations within the class difficult. Great care should be exercised when using any of these agents in the presence of significant heart failure, but a thorough knowledge of each drug and its side effects will otherwise allow appropriate choices to be made in optimizing therapy.

Combination Therapy

All the agents described above can help relieve angina pectoris. However, it is quite common to find that resolution of symptoms is not complete with a single agent, and adding additional drugs are frequently tried to improve the problem. The large variety of drugs available can make combination therapy for angina pectoris quite complicated. This is particularly true in the elderly, among whom side effects are more common than in younger patients.

In treating angina, combining two drugs from the same class of antianginal agents should generally be avoided. Patients are usually given sublingual nitroglycerin for treating acute episodes of angina, independent of whatever long-term prophylactic therapy they are receiving. This is appropriate even when long acting nitrate preparations are used because the high drug concentrations attained for a short duration of time can still be effective. In contrast, combining two different β-blockers is clearly inappropriate as they all act via the same receptors.

Because calcium antagonists have such varying clinical effects, it appears somewhat more logical to try them together in selective combinations. However, using verapamil and diltiazem together is potentially dangerous due to cumulative negative inotropic effects, and additive electrophysiological effects which could lead to symptomatic bradycardia or excess slowing of AV nodal conduction. Using bepridil in combination with most any other calcium antagonist is equally unattractive. Alternatively, because the dihydropyridines have minimal electrophysiological activity, it is reasonable to consider them in combination with other calcium antagonists. Nifedipine has been studied in combination with diltiazem in at least 3 studies.[52–54] This combination tended to improve exercise time compared to either alone, although Frishman et al[52] also noted an increase in troublesome side effects when the 2 drugs were used together. The effect of age on results in these studies was not specifically reported, and the maximum age of participants was 68 to 70 years. Although these studies demonstrate that diltiazem and nifedipine can be used together in the treatment of angina, combining 2 agents from different classes of drugs remains more attractive.

β-Blocker–Nitrate Combination

The addition of a long-acting nitrate to chronic β-blocker therapy has provided the most experience with combination therapy for angina pectoris. A study more than 2 decades ago described a propranolol and isosorbide dinitrate synergism in angina pectoris.[55] Since then, multiple studies with various β-blockers and nitrate preparations have confirmed the clinical experience that this is a reasonable combination. The β-blocker prevents reflex tachycardia usually seen with nitrates and the nitrate helps prevent the initial decrease in cardiac output usually seen with initiation of β-blocker therapy. Also, the side effect profiles of the 2 types of drugs differ, thus avoiding additive adverse reactions.

β-Blocker–Calcium Antagonist Combination

Because calcium antagonists have a different mechanism of action from β-blockers, it appears natural that calcium antagonists would be tried in combination with β-blockers. β-blocker-calcium antagonist combinations are now commonly used, and have been the subject of critical review.[56,57] Adding a dihydropyridine calcium antagonist to a β-blocker is particularly attractive. The systemic vasodilator effects of a drug like nifedipine, for example, could help decrease myocardial workload, while the β-blocker would prevent the reflex increase in heart rate caused by nifedipine.

Several types of studies have examined nifedipine and other dihydropyridines in combination with a β-blocker, but the most appropriate study design to allow valid clinical conclusions is one that is randomized, double-blind, placebo-controlled, and uses exercise tolerance as an end point. Using this type of study design, Lai et al[58] examined atenolol and nifedipine alone and in combination in 10 patients with chronic stable angina on effort. Both were effective in improving exercise workload, and the combination was better than either drug alone. More recently the TIBET study failed to support these results, as no greater improvement in exercise or reduction in ischemia during daily activities were found when atenolol was combined with sustained release nifedipine than with either drug alone.[59] In contrast, the IMAGE (International Multicenter Angina Exercise) study did find added antiischemic benefit from combining nifedipine with metoprolol.[60] They attributed the benefit of combination therapy more to recruitment by the second drug of patients poorly responding to monotherapy than to additive effects in individual patients.

Beneficial effects of combining a dihydropyridine calcium antagonist with a β-blocker for treating angina pectoris is further supported by studies using alternate, less scientifically vigorous, protocols. Uusitalo et al,[61] for example, found that combined treatment with metropolol and nifedipine increased efficacy compared with monotherapy, but there was no baseline using placebo alone. Tweddel et al[62] and Tolins et al[63] found nifedipine to be of additional benefit compared to placebo in patients already taking a β-blocker, and amlodipine also improves exercise tolerance when combined with a β-blocker.[64] Eklund and Oro[65] found nifedipine-β-blocker combination better than single therapy, but in their protocol the combination was always given last, so that there was possible benefit from the training effect of serial exercise testing.

Other studies examined the effects of drugs, singly and in combination, on ST-segment changes recorded by ambulatory monitoring, or during exercise to a fixed maximum workload.[66-68] These studies also reported beneficial effects of the nifedipine-β-blocker combination. In a direct comparison of nifedipine and nicardipine at fixed doses to placebo, Douard et al[69] found exercise duration improved with both drugs when combined with atenolol. Nifedipine has also been compared to isosorbide dinitrate in patients taking propranolol.[70] In this study both combinations were found to be effective, with the nifedipine-propranolol combination more beneficial than isosorbide dinitrate-propranolol. In summary, multiple studies of varying design support use of a β-blocker with a dihydropyridine calcium antagonist as a reasonable combination when monotherapy fails, as long as careful observation is made for potential side effects.

Diltiazem has also been studied in combination with β-blockers in a double-blind, randomized, placebo-controlled trial. Hung et al[71] found diltiazem, propranolol, and the 2 drugs combined, improved exercise duration in 12 patients with stable angina, but the combination was no better than either drug alone. Moreover, adverse side effects required dose reduction in 4 patients on combination therapy. Because both diltiazem and β-blockers slow heart rate and conduction through the AV node, are negatively inotropic, and reduce blood pressure, there must be concern that this combination may cause severe bradycardia, heart block, heart failure, or symptomatic hypotension. There are additional data that diltiazem can be combined with a β-blocker for additional relief of symptoms if used carefully. Studies by Miller et al,[72] and Humen et al[73] used protocols that did not have baseline comparison with placebo, but did demonstrate some additional benefit of diltiazem combined with either nadolol[72] or propranolol[73] compared to monotherapy. Studies by Strauss et al[74] and O'Hara et al[75] found diltiazem-propranolol combination of benefit, but the combination was always tried last in their protocols, thus possibly benefiting from training effect. O'Hara et al[75] emphasized caution because bradycardia can be a serious problem.

Verapamil, like diltiazem, when used in combination with β-blockers raises concern about summation of adverse electrophysiologic effects, potential exacerbation of heart failure, or potentiation of hypotension.[76] However, when used cautiously, Winniford et al[77] and Leon et al[78] have demonstrated that verapamil combined with propranolol can provide additional improvement over either drug alone.

Calcium Antagonist–Nitrate Combination

Using a nitrate with a dihydropyridine calcium antagonist is not a particularily attractive combination. Both types of drugs decrease blood pressure by direct peripheral vasodilation, albeit via different cellular mechanisms. As a result, this combination can readily produce symptomatic hypotension and aggravate orthostatic hypotension. Moreover, both types of drugs tend to reflexively increase heart rate, and this can be additive when the drugs are combined. It is not surprising that only 1 of 12 patients studied by Erlemeier et al[79] preferred the combination of nifedipine with isosorbide mononitrate rather than either drug alone for treatment of chronic angina. Although this combination may be potentially effective in angina presumed due to coronary spasm,[80] it is clearly a poor choice for therapy of elderly patients with exercise induced angina.

It is more logical to combine nitrates with calcium antagonists that have negative chronotropic effects. Such calcium antagonists would counteract the reflex tachycardia induced by nitrates, and the nitrates would not exacerbate slowing of conduction through the AV node caused by the negatively chronotropic calcium antagonists.

Verapamil was combined with isosorbide dinitrate by Silber et al,[81] and this reduced maximal ST segment depression on repeated bicycle exercise tests more than nitrate alone. Like the nifedipine-nitrate combination, a verapamil-nitrate combination has potential efficacy for treatment of coronary spasm.[82] Unfortunately, there are no data showing that a verapamil-nitrate combination improves exercises duration with tolerable side effects.

It is likewise reasonable to consider diltiazem combined with long-acting nitrates but relatively few studies have been performed to assess the efficacy of this combination. Bruce et al[83] studied the exercise response to sustained release nitroglycerin, diltiazem, and both combined in 9 patients with stable angina. Overall results suggested a beneficial effect for those that completed the protocol, but the study was stopped prematurely because 3 patients experienced symptomatic hypotension. Emanuelsson et al[84] failed to show any benefit of isosorbide mononitrate combined with diltiazem in a double-blind cross over study of 25 patients. In this study, diltiazem alone but not nitrate alone, was effective. It is likely that the dose and scheduling used for the nitrate was such that tolerance developed. Additional data would clearly be desirable in order to better define the proper role of diltiazem-nitrate combination therapy for angina pectoris.

It is evident from the discussion above, that several combinations of double therapy may be beneficial in patients whose angina pectoris is inadequately controlled with an optimal dose of a single agent. Choosing the most appropriate combination, however, can be problematic. It is essential to consider all potential side effects of each agent, and the expected result to be achieved in the individual patient. Specific attention must be directed toward evidence of left ventricular, AV nodal and sinus node dysfunction. Studies comparing various combinations of double therapy to each other are relatively few. Morse et al[85] compared nifedipine-propranolol to isosorbide dinitrate-propranolol and concluded that both were better than propranolol alone, and that the former combination was better than the latter. Similar data suggesting better results combining nifedipine rather than a nitrate with a β-blocker was reported by Tolins et al.[63] Nifedipine-propranolol has also been compared to diltiazem-propranolol,[85,86] and while both combinations were effective, it cannot be stated that one was clearly superior. The sustained release form of nifedipine was also compared to diltiazem in patients receiving β-blockers by Siu et al.[87] Both drugs improved exercise tolerance and relieved angina to an equivalent degree. Johnston et al[88] included the combination of verapamil-propranolol in a study that also used nifedipine-verapamil and diltiazem-verapamil. The 3 combinations reduced the incidence of angina and decreased ST-segment depression to an equivalent degree. In summary, they recommended choosing a combination for an initial trial based primarily on expected side effects, a consideration which cannot be overemphasized in the elderly.

Triple Therapy

There is substantial evidence that selected combinations of 2 agents can be beneficial. However, it must be realized that many pertinent studies excluded elderly subjects. Extrapolating study results to older patients may be reasonable if their multiple additional medical problems are carefully considered, adjustments to dosage made when necessary, and close follow-up provided to ensure safety. However, triple therapy is even more complex, and hence more risky than combinations of 2 drugs. More convincing data proving efficacy in the elderly should therefore be required before using triple therapy. Such data are sorely lacking, despite the fact that many forms of triple therapy are used in many practices.

As was the case with double therapy, nitrates and β-blockers can conveniently be considered as relatively homogenous groups, but calcium antagonists must be given special consideration for their very differing physiological effects. Nifedipine was used in triple therapy with a β-blocker and long acting nitrate by Tolins et al[63] who performed serial exercise tests in 19 patients taking a stable effective dose of propranolol. Patients were then randomly given either placebo, isosorbide dinitrate (20 mg), nifedipine (20 mg), or both nifedipine and isosorbide. Both isosorbide and nifedipine improved exercise tolerance compared to placebo in these β-blocked patients. However, when the drugs were combined (triple therapy), results were no better than with double therapy. Figure 3 shows individual responses of patients in that study comparing exercise ability on triple therapy to the best combination of dou-

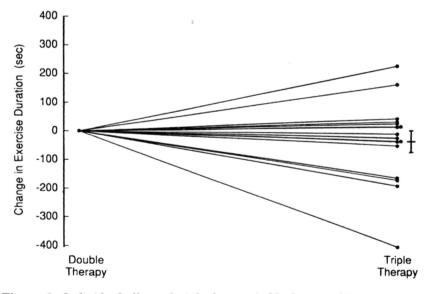

Figure 3: *Individual effects of triple therapy (β-blocker + calcium antagonist + nitrate) compared to double therapy (β-blocker + calcium antagonist) in the study by Tolins et al.[60] Only 2 of 19 patients had significant improvement in exercise duration with triple therapy.*

ble therapy. Only 2 patients showed additional improvement, while 2 additional patients do not appear on the graph because they could not tolerate triple therapy. It was concluded that "maximal therapy is not always optimal therapy" in angina pectoris.

Nesto et al[89] also studied this triple combination by giving nifedipine to 16 patients already taking long term β-blocker and nitrate therapy. After 7 days of triple therapy, bicycle exercise was compared to that done prior to nifedipine. Exercise duration was improved with the addition of nifedipine, but interpretation of the results is clouded by the fact that the study was neither blinded nor randomized. Any training effects of repeated exercise would therefore tend to unfairly provide an advantage favoring addition of nifedipine.

Verapamil was studied in combination with a nitrate and β-blocker by Silber et al.[81] Patients received a constant dose of long acting nitrate, and performed bicycle exercise to a fixed work load determined prior to study. Exercise was repeated with addition of either propranolol or verapamil, then again with the alternate of these 2 drugs (crossver), and finally with both combined (ie, triple therapy, as isosorbide dinitrate was continued during all phases). Maximum ST-segment depression at peak exercise was reduced by both verapamil and propranolol, with further reduction when they were combined. Unfortunately, since exercise duration was fixed in this study, it is difficult to determine if this particular combination of triple therapy would indeed improve exercise tolerance and relieve symptoms. Moreover, the triple therapy was always given last, thus favoring this regimen to the extent that any training or conditioning developed with repeated testing. The clinical value of this particular triple combination must still be considered unproven.

At least 2 studies have examined diltiazem in triple therapy. Boden et al[90] compared diltiazem to placebo in a double-blind randomized fashion in 12 patients who still had exercise induced angina on maximally tolerated doses of propranolol and isosorbide dinitrate. Diltiazem improved exercise duration and reduced maximal ST segment depression. However, by using a maximally tolerated dose of nitrates, which was given in 4 divided doses daily, it is likely that many of the patients were studied under conditions where they would have become tolerant to the nitrates. El-Tamimi et al[91] added a 10-mg dose of isosorbide dinitrate acutely to patients previously given diltiazem alone, and then diltiazem plus atenolol. The addition of nitrate in this study failed to further improve exercise tolerance despite the fact that triple therapy was always given last.

In summary, triple therapy remains of unproved benefit. When used in the elderly as a last resort, potential side effects must be carefully considered, and patients monitored closely to assess results. Moreover, if adding more medication fails to provide additional relief of symptoms, it is important to stop the additional drug(s) to prevent future untoward effects and avoid unnecessary cost and inconvenience.

Risk Factor Intervention

Any discussion of IHD in the young must include a treatise on risk factor identification and intervention. However, in the elderly it is important to put each intervention in proper perspective, because it is fairly easy to do something *to* the patient, but more difficult to do something *for* the patient. Risk factor intervention is generally perceived by patients as having a negative impact on their quality of life, and many elderly patients are more concerned with quality than quantity. A brief review of those major risk factors that can potentially be altered will provide insight into some therapeutic problems worthy of special consideration in the elderly.

Blood pressure is a major determinant of myocardial work load, and hypertension can exacerbate angina. Good control of blood pressure can thus improve angina pectoris, and as noted, anti-anginal drugs are generally also good antihypertensives. It is logical to treat hypertension aggressively in the elderly with chronic IHD, choosing drugs that achieve therapeutic goals with as few side effects as possible. Similarly, close attention to controlling diabetes mellitus is warranted to prevent future complications in other organs as well as the heart.

A common rationale used by older patients addicted to tobacco is that quitting late in life will not make any difference. Epidemiological evidence that stopping the use of tobacco reduces the likelihood of subsequent coronary events is strong enough to warrant aggressive attempts to prevent and reduce smoking. However, it will likely have a greater impact on older patients if data are quoted that demonstrate the benefits of quitting smoking cessation in people who have already developed ischemic heart disease. The most pertinent data comes from the CASS study[92] where effects of smoking cessation were specifically examined in older patients with coronary artery disease. Among 1893 patients 55 years of age or older in the CASS registry with angiographically proven coronary artery disease, 807 patients quit smoking and abstained throughout the study. Those who continued smoking had a relative risk of dying 1.7 times higher than those who quit, and the benefit of stopping did not diminish with advanced age. These data are supported by the Norwegian Multicenter Group Study,[93] where mortality after MI was decreased by 26% and re-infarction by 45%. Similarly, in a report by Hallstrom et al,[92] recurrent cardiac arrest in survivors of out-of-hospital cardiac arrest was lower in those who stopped smoking (19%) than those who continued to smoke (27%). There are, therefore, excellent reasons to stop smoking at any age.

A complete review of the role of dyslipidemia in the pathogenesis of atherosclerosis, as well as various methods of intervention in specific types of lipid disorders, is beyond the scope of this chapter. Important considerations in management of lipid disorders in the elderly are discussed in Chapter 14.

References

1. Smokler P, MacAlpin R, Alvaro A, et al: Reproducibility of a multi-stage near maximal treadmill test for exercise tolerance in angina pectoris. *Circulation* 48:346–351, 1973.
2. Deanfield J, Maseri A, Selwyn A, et al: Myocardial ischaemia during daily life in patients with stable angina: Its relation to symptoms and heart rate changes. *Lancet* ii:753–758, 1983.
3. Taggart P, Gibbons D, Somerville W: Some effects of motor-car driving on the normal and abnormal heart. *Br Med J* 4:130–134, 1969.
4. Taggart P, Parkinson P, Carruthers M: Cardiac responses to thermal, physical, and emotional stress. *Br Med J* 3:71–76, 1972.
5. Epstein S, Stampfer M, Beiser D, et al: Effects of a reduction in environmental temperature on the circulatory response to exercise in man: Implications concerning angina patients. *N Engl J Med* 280:7–11, 1969.
6. Rocco M, Barry J, Campbell S, et al: Circadian variation of transient myocardial ischemia in patients with coronary artery disease. *Circulation* 75:395–400, 1987.
7. Froelicher V, Yanowitz F, Thompson A, et al: The correlation of coronary angiography and the electrocardiographic response to maximal treadmill testing in 76 asymptomatic men. *Circulation* 48:597–604, 1973.
8. Roseman M: Painless myocardial infarction: A review of the literature and analysis of 220 cases. *Ann Intern Med* 41:1–8, 1954.
9. Stern S, Tzivoni D: Early detection of silent ischaemic heart disease by 24-hour electrocardiographic monitoring of active subjects. *Br Heart J* 36:481–486, 1974.
10. Amsterdam E, Martschinske R, Laslett L, et al: Symptomatic and silent myocardial ischemia during exercise testing in coronary artery disease. *Am J Cardiol* 58:43B-46B, 1986.
11. Upton M, Rerych S, Newman G, et al: Detecting abnormalities in left ventricular function during exercise before angina and ST-segment depression. *Circulation* 62:341–349, 1980.
12. Sugishita Y, Koseki S, Matsuda M, et al: Dissociation between regional myocardial dysfunction and ECG changes during myocardial ischemia induced by exercise in patients with angina pectoris. *Am Heart J* 106:1–8, 1983.
13. Rocco, M, Nabel E, Campbell S, et al: Prognostic importance of myocardial ischemia detected by ambulatory monitoring in patients with stable coronary disease. *Circulation* 78:877–884, 1988.
14. Tzivoni D, Weisz G, Gavish A, et al: Comparison of mortality and myocardial infarction rates in stable angina pectoris with and without ischemic episodes during daily activities. *Am Heart J* 63:273–276, 1989.
15. Deedwania P, Carbajal E: Silent ischemia during daily life is an independent predictor of mortality in stable angina pectoris. *Circulation* 81:748–756, 1990.
16. Young A, Barry J, Orav J, et al: Effects of asymptomatic ischemia on long-term prognosis in chronic stable coronary disease. *Circulation* 83:1598–1604, 1991.
17. von Arnim T, for the TIBBS Investigators: Prognostic significance of transient ischemic episodes: Response to treatment shows improved prognosis. *J Am Coll Cardiol* 28:20–24, 1996.
18. Dargie H, Ford I, Fox K, on behalf of the TIBET study group: Total Ischae-

mic Burden European Trial (TIBET): Effects of ischaemia and treatment with atenolol, nifedipine SR and their combination on outcome in patients with chronic stable angina. *Eur Heart J* 17:104–112, 1996.

19. Nyman I, Larsson H, Wallentin L, et al: Prevention of serious cardiac events by low-dose aspirin in patients with silent myocardial ischaemia. *Lancet* 340:497–501, 1992.

20. Olsson G: How long should post-MI β-blocker therapy be continued? *Primary Cardiol* 17:44–49, 1991.

21. Thadani U, Davidson C, Singleton W, et al: Comparison of the immediate effects of five β-adrenoreceptor-blocking drugs with different ancillary properties in angina pectoris. *N Engl J Med* 300:750–755, 1979.

22. Swedberg K, Hjalmarson A, Waagstein F, et al: Beneficial effects of long-term beta-blockade in congestive cardiomyopathy. *Br Heart J* 44:117–133, 1980.

23. Colucci W, Packer M, Bristow, et al: Carvedilol inhibits clinical progression in patients with mild symptoms of heart failure. *Circulation* 94:2800–2806, 1996.

24. Thadani U, Parker J: Propranolol in angina pectoris: Comparison of therapy given two and four times daily. *Am J Cardiol* 46:117–123, 1980.

25. van den Brink G, Boer P, van Asten P, et al: One and three doses of propranolol a day in hypertension. *Clin Pharmacol Ther* 27:9–15, 1980.

26. Brunton T: Use of nitrite of amyl in angina pectoris. *Lancet* ii:97–98, 1867.

27. Murrell W: Nitroglycerin as a remedy for angina pectoris. *Lancet* i:80–81, 1879.

28. Ignarro L, Lippton H, Edwards J, et al: Mechanism of vascular smooth muscle relaxation by organic nitrates, nitrites, nitroprusside and nitric oxide: Evidence for the involvement of s-nitrosothiols as active intermediates. *J Pharmacol Exp Ther* 218:739–749, 1981.

29. Parker J, Farrell B, Fenton T, et al: Counter-regulatory responses to continuous and intermittent therapy with nitroglycerin. *Circulation* 84:2336–2345, 1991.

30. Zimrin D, Reichek N, Bogin K, et al: Antianginal effects of intravenous nitroglycerin over 24 hours. *Circulation* 77:1376–1384, 1988.

31. Steering Committee Transdermal Nitroglycerin Cooperative Study: Acute and chronic antianginal efficacy of continuous twenty-four-hour application of transdermal nitroglycerin. *Am J Cardiol* 68:1263–1272, 1991.

32. Crandall L, Leake C, Loevenhart A, et al: Acquired tolerance to and cross tolerance between the nitrous and nitric acid esters and sodium nitrate in man. *J Pharmacol Exp Ther* 41:103–120, 1931.

33. Parker J, Farrell B, Lahey K, et al: Effect of intervals between doses on the development of tolerance to isosorbide dinitrate. *N Engl J Med* 316:1440–1444, 1987.

34. Thadani U, Fung H, Darke A, et al: Oral isosorbide dinitrate in angina pectoris: Comparison of duration of action and dose-response relation during acute and sustained therapy. *Am J Cardiol* 49:411–419, 1982.

35. Cohn J, Archibald D, Ziesche S, et al: Effect of vasodilator therapy on mortality in chronic congestive heart failure. *N Engl J Med* 314:1547–1552, 1986.

36. Klugmann S, Salvi A, Camerini F: Haemodynamic effects of nifedipine in heart failure. *Br Heart J* 43: 440–446, 1980.

37. Cantelli I, Pavesi P, Naccarella F, et al: Comparison of acute haemodynamic effects of nifedipine and isosorbide dinitrate in patients with heart

failure following acute myocardial infarction. *Int J Cardiol* 1:151–163, 1981.

38. Ludbrook P, Tiefenbrunn A, Sobel B: Influence of nifedipine on left ventricular systolic and diastolic function. *Am J Med* 71:683–692, 1981.

39. Ryman K, Kubo S, Lystash J, et al: Effect of nicardipine on rest and exercise hemodynamics in chronic congestive heart failure. *Am J Cardiol* 58: 583–588, 1986.

40. Elkayam U, Weber L, McKay C, et al: Differences in hemodynamic response to vasodilation due to calcium channel antagonism with nifedipine and direct-acting agonism with hydralazine in chronic refractory congestive heart failure. *Am J Cardiol* 54:126–131, 1984.

41. Agostoni P, De Cesare N, Doria E, et al: Afterload reduction: A comparison of captopril and nifedipine in dilated cardiomyopathy. *Br Heart J* 55: 391–399, 1986.

42. Tan L, Murray R, Littler W: Felodipine in patients with chronic heart failure: Discrepant haemodynamic and clinical effects. *Br Heart J* 58: 122–128, 1987.

43. Elkayam U, Amin J, Mehra A, et al: A prospective randomized, double-blind, crossover study to compare the efficacy and safety of chronic nifedipine therapy with that of isosorbide dinitrate and their combination in the treatment of chronic congestive heart failure. *Circulation* 82:1954–1961, 1990.

44. Packer M, O'Connor C, Ghali J, et al: Effect of amlodipine on morbidity in severe chronic heart failure. *N Engl J Med* 335:1107–1114, 1996.

45. Cohn J, Zeische S, Smith R, et al: Effect of the calcium antagonist felodipine as supplementary vasodilator therapy in patients with chronic heart failure treated with enalapril: V-HeFT III. *Circulation* 96:856–863, 1997.

46. Multicenter Diltiazem Postinfarction Trial Research Group. The effect of diltiazem on mortality and reinfarction after myocardial infarction. *N Engl J Med* 319:385–392, 1988.

47. Danish Study Group on Verapamil in Myocardial Infarction. Secondary prevention with verapamil after myocardial infarction. *Am J Cardiol* 66: 33I-40I, 1990.

48. Danish Study Group on Verapamil in Myocardial Infarction. Effect of verapamil on mortality and major events after acute myocardial infarction (the Danish Verapamil Infarction Trial II - DAVIT II). *Am J Cardiol* 66: 779–785, 1990.

49. Singh B, Nademanee K, Feld G, et al: Comparative electrophysiologic profiles of calcium antagonists with particular reference to bepridil. *Am J Cardiol* 55:14C-19C, 1985.

50. Duchene-Marullaz P, Kantelip J, Trolese J: Effects of bepridil, a new antianginal agent, on ambulatory electrocardiography in human volunteers. *J Cardiovasc Pharmacol* 5:506–510, 1983.

51. Leclercq J, Kural S, Valere P: Bepridil et torsades de pointes. *Arch Mal Coeur* 76:341–348, 1983.

52. Frishman W, Charlap S, Kimmel B, et al: Diltiazem, nifedipine, and their combination in patients with stable angina pectoris: Effects on angina, exercise tolerance, and the ambulatory electrocardiographic ST segment. *Circulation* 77:774–786, 1988.

53. Toyosaki N, Toyo-oka T, Natsume T, et al: Combination therapy with diltiazem and nifedipine in patients with effort angina pectoris. *Circulation* 77: 1370–1375, 1988.

54. Goldberger J, Frishman W: Clinical utility of nifedipine and diltiazem plasma levels in patients with angina pectoris receiving monotherapy and combination treatment. *J Clin Pharmacol* 29:628–634, 1989.
55. Russek H: Propranolol and isosorbide dinitrate synergism in angina pectoris. *Am J Cardiol* 21:44–54, 1968.
56. Strauss W, Parisi A: Combined use of calcium-channel and beta-adrenergic blockers for the treatment of chronic stable angina. *Ann Intern Med* 109: 570–581, 1988.
57. Packer M: Combined beta-adrenergic and calcium-entry blockade in angina pectoris. *N Engl J Med* 320:709–718, 1989.
58. Lai C, Onnis E, Pirisi R, et al: Anti-ischaemic and anti-anginal activity of atenolol, nifedipine and their combination in stable, chronic effort angina. Drugs Exp Clin Res 14:699–705, 1988.
59. Fox K, Mulcahy D, Findlay I, et al: The Total Ischaemic Burden European Trial (TIBET): Effects of atenolol, nifedipine SR and their combination on the exercise test and the total ischaemic burden in 608 patients with stable angina. *Eur Heart J* 17:96–103, 1996.
60. Savonitto S, Ardissino D, Egstrup K, et al: Combination therapy with metoprolol and nifedipine versus monotherapy in patients with stable angina pectoris. *J Am Coll Cardiol* 27:311–316, 1966.
61. Uusitalo A, Arstila M, Bae E, et al: Metoprolol, nifedipine, and the combination in stable effort angina pectoris. *Am J Cardiol* 57:733–737, 1986.
62. Tweddel A, Beattie J, Hutton L, et al: Effects of nifedipine on physical performance in patients with angina pectoris on β-blockers. In P Puech, R Krebs (eds): *Proceedings of the 4th International Adalat Symposium*. Amsterdam, Excerpta Medica, 1980, pp 143–146.
63. Tolins M, Weir E, Chesler E, et al: "Maximal" drug therapy is not necessarily optimal in chronic angina pectoris. *J Am Coll Cardiol* 3:1051–1057, 1984.
64. DiBianco R, Schoomaker F, Singh J, et al: Amlodipine combined with beta blockade for chronic angina: Results of a multicenter, placebo-controlled, randomized double-blind study. *Clin Cardiol* 15:519–524, 1992.
65. Ekelund LG, Oro L: Antianginal efficiency of nifedipine with and without a beta-blocker, studied with exercise test. A double-blind, randomized subacute study. *Clin Cardiol* 2:203–211, 1979.
66. Lynch P, Dargie H, Krikler S, et al: Objective assessment of antianginal treatment: A double-blind comparison of propranolol, nifedipine, and their combination. *Br Med J* 281:184–187, 1980.
67. Dargie H, Lynch P, Krikler, D, et al: Nifedipine and propranolol: A beneficial drug interaction. *Am J Med* 71:676–682, 1981.
68. Egstrup K: Randomized double-blind comparison of metoprolol, nifedipine, and their combination in chronic stable angina: Effects on total ischemic activity and heart rate at onset of ischemia. *Am Heart J* 116:971–978, 1988.
69. Douard H, Mora B, Broustet J: Comparison of the anti-anginal efficacy of nicardipine and nifedipine in patients receiving atenolol: A randomized, double-blind, crossover study. *Int J Cardiol* 22:357–363, 1989.
70. Morse J, Nesto R: Double-blind crossover comparison of the antianginal effects of nifedipine and isosorbide dinitrate in patients with exertional angina receiving propranolol. *J Am Coll Cardiol* 6:1395–1401, 1985.
71. Hung J, Lamb I, Connolly S, et al: The effect of diltiazem and propranolol, alone and in combination, on exercise performance and left ventricular

function in patients with stable effort angina: A double-blind, randomized, and placebo-controlled study. *Circulation* 68:560–567, 1983.

72. Miller W, Vittitoe J, O'Rourke R, et al: Nadolol versus diltiazem and combination for preventing exercise-induced ischemia in severe angina pectoris. *Am J Cardiol* 62:372–376, 1988.

73. Humen D, O'Brien P, Purves P, et al: Effort angina with adequate beta-receptor blockade: Comparison with diltiazem alone and in combination *J Am Coll Cardiol* 7:329–335, 1986.

74. Strauss W, Parisi A: Superiority of combined diltiazem and propranolol therapy for angina pectoris. *Circulation* 71:951–957, 1985.

75. O'Hara M, Khurmi N, Bowles M, et al: Diltiazem and propranolol combination for the treatment of chronic stable angina pectoris. *Clin Cardiol* 10:115–123, 1987.

76. Packer M, Meller J, Medina N, et al: Hemodynamic consequences of combined beta-adrenergic and slow calcium channel blockade in man. *Circulation* 65:660–668, 1982.

77. Winniford M, Huxley R, Hillis L: Randomized, double-blind comparison of propranolol alone and a propranolol-verapamil combination in patients with severe angina of effort. *J Am Coll Cardiol* 1:492–498, 1983.

78. Leon M, Rosing D, Bonow R, et al: Clinical efficacy of verapamil alone and combined with propranolol in treating patients with chronic stable angina pectoris. *Am J Cardiol* 48:131–139, 1981.

79. Erlemeier H, Kupper W, Lange S, et al: Uberprufung der antianginosen wirkung und vertraglichkeit von isosorbid-5-mononitrat oder nifedipin in retardierter form. *Zeitschrift fur Kardiologie* 75:112–114, 1986.

80. Winniford M, Gabliani G, Johnson S, et al: Concomitant calcium antagonist plus isosorbide dinitrate therapy for markedly active variant angina. *Am Heart J* 108:1269–1273, 1984.

81. Silber S, Vogler A, Theisen K: Equal anti-ischemic properties of isosorbide dinitrate plus verapamil and isosorbide dinitrate plus propranolol. A randomized, double-blind and crossover study. *Z Kardiol* 75:100–105, 1986.

82. Freedman S, Richmond D, Kelly D: Long-term follow-up of verapamil and nitrate treatment for coronary artery spasm. *Am J Cardiol* 50:711–715, 1982.

83. Bruce R, Hossack K, Kusumi F, et al: Excessive reduction in peripheral resistance during exercise and risk of orthostatic symptoms with sustained-release nitroglycerin and diltiazem treatment of angina. *Am Heart J* 109:1020–1026, 1985.

84. Emanuelsson H, Ake H, Kristi M, et al: Effects of diltiazem and isosorbide-5-mononitrate, alone and in combination, on patients with stable angina pectoris. *Eur J Clin Pharmacol* 36:561–566, 1989.

85. Morse J: Comparison of combination nifedipine-propranolol and diltiazem-propranolol with high dose diltiazem monotherapy for stable angina pectoris. *Am J Cardiol* 62:1028–1032, 1988.

86. Robinson K, Krikler S, Krikler D: Comparative study of the effect of nifedipine versus diltiazem on exercise performance, serum propranolol levels, and ST-segment abnormalities in patients with chronic stable angina taking propranolol. *Am J Cardiol* 64:27F–30F, 1989.

87. Siu S, Jacoby R, Phillips R, et al: Comparative efficacy of nifedipine gastrointestinal therapeutic system versus diltiazem when added to beta blockers in stable angina pectoris. *Am J Cardiol* 71:887–892, 1993.

88. Johnston D, Lesoway R, Humen D, et al: Clinical and hemodynamic evalua-

tion of propranolol in combination with verapamil, nifedipine and diltiazem in exertional angina pectoris: A placebo-controlled, double-blind, randomized, crossover study. *Am J Cardiol* 55:680–687, 1985.

89. Nesto R, White H, Ganz P, et al: Addition of nifedipine to maximal beta-blocker-nitrate therapy: Effects on exercise capacity and global left ventricular performance at rest and during exercise. *Am J Cardiol* 55:3E-8E, 1985.

90. Boden W, Bough E, Reichman M, et al: Beneficial effects of high dose diltiazem in patients with persistent effort angina on β-blockers and nitrates: A randomized, double-blind, placebo-controlled cross-over study. *Circulation* 71:1197–1205, 1985.

91. El-Tamimi H, Davies G, Kaski J, et al: Effects of diltiazem alone or with isosorbide dinitrate or with atenolol both acutely and chronically for stable angina pectoris. *Am J Cardiol* 64:717–724, 1989.

92. Hermanson B, Omenn G, Kronmal R, et al: Beneficial six-year outcome of smoking cessation in older men and women with coronary artery disease. *N Engl J Med* 319:1365–1369, 1988.

93. Ronnevik P, Gundersen T, Abrahamsen A: Effect of smoking habits and timolol treatment on mortality and reinfarction in patients surviving acute myocardial infarction. *Br Heart J* 54:134–139, 1985.

94. Hallstrom A, Cobb L, Ray R: Smoking as a risk factor for recurrence of sudden cardiac arrest. *N Engl J Med* 314:271–275, 1986.

Chapter 13

Percutaneous Transluminal Coronary Revascularization and Coronary Artery Bypass Surgery in the Elderly

Randall C. Thompson, Bernard J. Gersh

The number of elderly patients with symptomatic coronary artery disease (CAD) is steadily increasing, and it is estimated that over 50% of coronary revascularization procedures in the United States are now performed in individuals older than 65 years.[1-2] This increase has been particularly striking in the very elderly, those over age 80 years. Despite this fact, there has been no direct randomized trial comparison of medical therapy, percutaneous transluminal coronary angioplasty (PTCA), and coronary bypass surgery in older patients. The elderly were generally excluded from older trials of bypass surgery versus medical therapy and have rarely been included in large numbers in recent randomized trials of PTCA versus bypass surgery. Nevertheless, careful review of the rapidly expanding body of data on the results of therapy for cardiovascular disease in the elderly provides a rational approach to choosing the most suitable form of treatment. In considering the reported experience with heart disease in older patients, the distinction between "young-old" (usually considered to be 65 to 75 years) and "old-old" (older than 75 or 80 years) is important to make. In many circumstances, the effect of age on outcome of cardiovascular treatment becomes much more important in the oldest subsets of patients.

From *Clinical Cardiology in the Elderly. Second Edition,* edited by Elliot Chesler. © 1999, Futura Publishing Company, Armonk, NY.

Coronary Artery Bypass Surgery

The increased mortality of coronary bypass graft surgery with age is well established.[3-12] Investigators in the Coronary Artery Surgery Study (CASS) found that the operative mortality was double for patients over age 65 and was higher still as age advanced (Fig. 1).[3] Although cardiac surgical results are quite different now than at the time of the CASS study, contemporary authors such as Hannan and Burke have similarly described a linear relationship between age and bypass surgery operative mortality. In Hannan and Burke's study of 30, 972 patients who underwent coronary surgery in New York State from 1991–1992, the operation mortality was less than 1.5% in patients less than 60 years old but 5.28% in those 75–79 years and 8.31% in those over age 80.[13] (Fig. 1).

Others have reported operative mortality rates of 0%–15.2% for bypass surgery in patients older than 80,[1,14-19] and the larger recent series have reported hospital mortality rates of 5.4%–11.5%.[13,14,19,20] There is other strong evidence that the perioperative survival rates are continuing to improve in older bypass patients. The bypass surgery 30-day mortality in octogenarians was 10.6% from 1987–1990, based on the U.S. national medicare experience.[21] This mortality rate improved over the 4 years involved in the study and very recent data from the Society of Thoracic Surgeons show an overall bypass operation mortal-

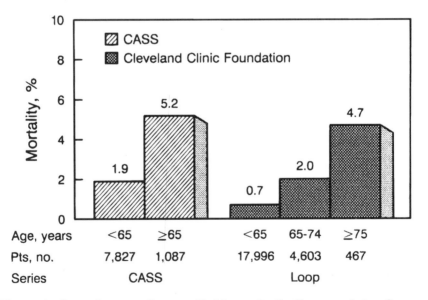

Figure 1: *Operative mortality stratified by age for the Coronary Artery Surgery Study (CASS)*[4] *and a more recent surgical series (Loop, Cleveland Clinic Foundation).*[5] *Operative mortality increases with advancing age.*

ity rate of 5.4% in octogenarians having surgery from 1993–1996 with an elective operation mortality rate of 1.2%.[20]

The frequency of nonfatal morbid complications is also increased in older patients. Stroke is more common in the elderly; the incidence varies from 0%–9.0%,[4,7,15,16,21–23] with the largest surgical series reporting a rate of 2.5% in the group of patients over 65 years old compared with 1% in younger patients.[4] Even very recent series of bypass surgery in octogenarians report stroke rates of up to 5%. This increased risk is perhaps one of the strongest points toward consideration of percutaneous revascularization (PTCR) as an alternative. Also strongly favoring the use of PTCR are the changes in cognitive function[24,25] that prolong hospital stay and represent a major contribution to the greater morbidity of bypass surgery in the elderly, particularly in those older than 75 years.[26–33] Length of stay and hospital costs are understandably greater in the elderly, although both have been substantially reduced in recent years, even in older patients, and many elderly patients are candidates for rapid hospital discharge strategies.[19,20,23,34–36] Also, atrial fibrillation following bypass surgery is a major contribution to increased duration of hospitalization and increased hospital cost and is much more common in elderly patients.[3,4,10,23,37]

Outcomes

Despite these limitations of coronary bypass surgery, relief of angina in the elderly is excellent,[4,14,24] even in the very old,[7,16,38,39] and appears to be at least as good as relief in younger patients (Fig. 2).[40]

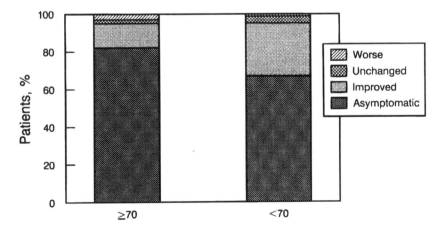

Figure 2: *Symptomatic status of patients 70 years old and older and patients younger than 70 after coronary bypass surgery. Reproduced with permission from Knapp WS, Douglas JS Jr, Craver JM, et al: Efficacy of coronary artery bypass grafting in elderly patients with coronary artery disease. Am J Cardiol 47:923–930, 1981.*

Some series have reported better angina relief than that in younger patients, although noncardiac limitations to physical activity in the elderly may be a factor. Typically, patients over age 70 have an average improvement in angina of about 1.5 NYHA classes, from NYHA classes III-IV to I-II. Also, health related quality of life measurements such as disability and distress are improved in older patients having bypass surgery as are other measurements of functional status and patient reported outcomes. Also, older patients who undergo bypass surgery are more satisfied with the results of their operation than are younger ones, although depression and lack of energy are more common in older patients[12,41–43] and cognitive dysfunction post bypass, sometimes lasting months, is more common in the elderly.[10,18,40,29] Guadagnoli et. al. reported that not only did quality-of-life outcomes 6 months after coronary artery bypass grafting (CABG) not differ between older and younger patients, but also mental health functioning was even better in patients 65 years old or older than in those younger than 65[25] (Fig. 3).

In addition to effective relief of angina, bypass surgery appears to improve survival in some patients older than 65. For patients dismissed from the hospital, long-term survival is excellent[14,23] and is consistently over 80% at 5 years. In some series, overall survival is better than that in the general age-matched population.[4,9,38] Although this finding is perhaps to be expected, since surgical series appropriately exclude pa-

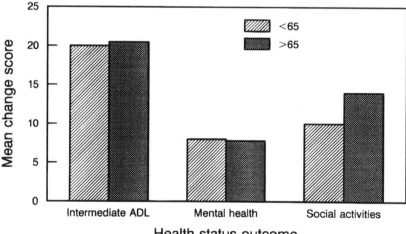

Health status outcome

Figure 3: *Unadjusted health status change score by age group in patients younger than and older than 65 years of age undergoing bypass surgery. ADL: activities of daily living. Reproduced with permission from Guadagnoli E, Ayanian JZ, Cleary PD: Comparison of patient-reported outcomes after elective coronary artery bypass grafting in patients aged ≥ and ≤65 years. Am J Cardiol 70:60–64, 1992.*

tients with other life-threatening co- morbid illnesses, this is not reported in younger patients. Survival in elderly patients is improved with use of the internal mammary artery conduit, as is the case in younger patients.[20,30] The impact of associated noncoronary heart disease on early and late outcomes in the elderly bears emphasis.

Maximal medical management of angina in the elderly is more difficult to achieve. The elderly are more vulnerable to adverse drug reactions for many reasons, including altered pharmacokinetics, comorbid conditions, and interactions between drugs and the physiological changes that accompany aging.[31,32] The attraction of a less invasive approach to management of angina in the elderly is self-evident, but the difficulties in the use of drugs are compounded by more severe symptoms, more extensive anatomical coronary obstructive disease, and left ventricular dysfunction in the elderly. Moreover, randomized trials comparing coronary bypass surgery with medical therapy excluded patients older than 66 years, and elderly patients are frequently excluded from other cardiovascular treatment trials.[33] Management decisions, therefore, need to be based on extrapolation from trials in younger patients and, whereas these data can be reasonably applied to the "young-old," other factors in patients of advanced age are more difficult to take into account.

Despite these caveats, subsets of elderly patients, such as those with three-vessel CAD and poor left ventricular (LV) function[22] or left main equivalent coronary disease, who undergo bypass surgery still appear to have better survival than those treated medically, as do younger patients (Fig. 4).

Determinants of Outcome

A significant component of the increased risk in older people undergoing bypass surgery is related to age itself or other unmeasured or less tangible factors associated with older age. Nonetheless, the bulk of the increased hazard appears to be a function of the increased frequency of co-morbid conditions and more advanced heart disease. Elderly patients who undergo CABG surgery tend to be a sicker group than the younger surgical population. Left main CAD is more frequently encountered, as is, to a lesser extent, three-vessel coronary disease.[3,4,6,13,19,24,26,44–46] Symptoms, including severe angina[6,26,24,38] and congestive heart failure (CHF),[6] are more frequently encountered in the elderly surgical population, as is the frequency of LV dysfunction (Table 1). The increased presence of associated cardiovascular and noncardiovascular comorbid conditions is a major distinction between older and younger patients; for example, peripheral vascular disease, diabetes, hypertension, chronic lung disease, and renal disease are particularly frequent in the oldest subset of patients.

A number of factors have been shown to predict poor outcome with bypass surgery in the elderly. For example, emergency surgery,

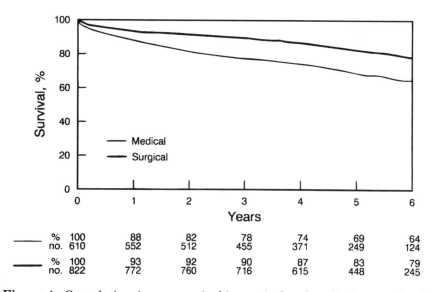

Figure 4: *Cumulative six-year survival in surgical and medical groups for the Coronary Artery Surgery Study (CASS) series, adjusted for LV wall motion score, CHF score, number of diseased vessels, number of associated medical diseases, and age at baseline angiography. Reprinted, by permission of The New England Journal of Medicine, from Gersh BJ, Kronmal RA, Schaff HV, et al: Comparison of coronary artery bypass surgery and medical therapy in patients 65 years of age or older: A nonrandomized study from the Coronary Artery Surgery Study (CASS) Registry. N Engl J Med 313:217–224, 1985.*

cachexia, prior myocardial infarction (MI), Class IV symptoms, cigarette smoking, hypertension, small body size, previous bypass surgery, depressed ejection fraction (<50%), and other indices of poor LV function have all been identified as predictors of increased hospital mortality.[4,6,8,15,39] Based on a large contemporary series of patients undergoing bypass surgery from 1991–1996, the most powerful predictors of mortality in elderly patients appear to be severe LV dysfunction and previous bypass surgery.[47] Female sex has been found to predict operative mortality in some[4,6,11,30,48] series of elderly patients. The impact of co-morbid conditions on early and late outcomes is a pivotal aspect of the preoperative assessment that must be recognized. In a series from the Mayo Clinic, the presence of one or more associated diseases increased perioperative mortality more than threefold among octogenarians undergoing bypass surgery (Fig. 5).[14] Also, in this study and others, the presence of peripheral vascular disease was shown to have a huge impact on the risk of mortality and stroke.[14,49] The explanation for this strong association is believed to be the increased risk of atheroembolism, from the aorta with diffuse involvement of the brain, heart, bowel, and kidneys in patients who have markers for diffuse atheroscle-

Table 1
Baseline Characteristics of Younger and Older Patients Undergoing Coronary Artery Bypass Surgery in Four Large Series

Study	Age, Years	No.	Women, %	Left Main, %	Three-Vessel CAD, %	CHF, %	Unstable Angina, %	PVD, %	HTN, %	Diabetes, %	Prior MI, %	Prior CVD, %
CASS[4]	<65	7,827	—	0.6†	46	3	42	9	35	11	—	2
	≥65	1,087	26	1.7†	61	8	55	10	37	15	—	3
Weintraub et al.[10]	<70	11,295	18.2	11.4	41.0	5.2	61.3*	—	47.6	18.0	50.9	—
	≥70	2,330	33.7	16.9	47.6	8.5	71.7*	—	49.9	20.4	52.0	—
Loop et al.[5]	<65	17,996	13	11	—	—	65‡	13	65	9	—	2
	≥75	467	29	22	—	—	71‡	36	71	13	—	7
Acinapura et al.[26]	<70	3,142	30	16	71	10	42	—	38	4	59	—
	≥70	685	32	35	90	17	60	—	34	60	61	—

The older surgical population tends to have a higher proportion of women, more severe coronary artery disease, and several other medical problems. CAD: coronary artery disease; CASS: Coronary Artery Surgery Study; CHF: history of previous congestive heart failure; CVD: cerebrovascular disease; HTN: history of systemic arterial hypertension; Left Main: significant left main coronary artery stenosis; MI: myocardial infarction; PVD: peripheral vascular disease; *: Class III or IV angina; †: patients with left main artery stenosis were excluded from randomization; and ‡: moderate to severe angina.

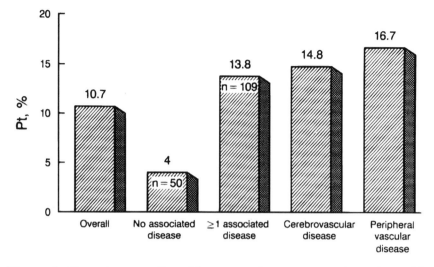

Figure 5: *Operative mortality with coronary bypass surgery in patients older than 80 as stratified by the presence of other medical diseases. Data from Mullaney et al.*[14]

rosis. As the age of the cardiac surgical population has increased, the incidence of atheroembolism has also increased.[50]

Lahey et al.[51] reported the importance of even modest degrees of renal failure in predicting prolonged hospitalization in persons older than 60 undergoing bypass surgery. The number of associated medical diseases has also been found to be an important predictor of long-term survival in the elderly surgical population.[3,4,19,22,45] Left ventricular function and peripheral vascular disease have also been shown to predict late survival.[3,4,19,22,38]

Preoperative assessment needs to take into account not only objective indicators of co-morbid disease but also psychosocial aspects of the patient and his or her way of life. For example, quality of life, functional independence, motivation of the individual and, above all, the expectations of surgery and whether they are realistic all need to be considered.

The key to the most effective use of coronary bypass surgery in the elderly is careful patient selection, and if meticulous attention is paid to the overall status of the patient excellent results (both in terms of morbidity and quality of life) can be ascertained. Mandatory attention to the effects of symptoms on life-style, the coronary anatomy and the degree of LV dysfunction, tolerance of medical therapy, the presence and number of associated medical conditions, and the patient's expectations and desires is the cornerstone of appropriate patient selection. The patient is a key part of the decision and a realistic approach of the potential but limited benefits as well as the potential for death, stroke, and other morbid events is essential and the physician has to know the entire patient and not just the anatomy. That coronary bypass surgery is appropriate treatment for selected patients of advanced age is not in dispute; careful selection and the avoidance of over-utilization are paramount.

Percutaneous Transluminal Coronary Revascularization

The preceding discussion drew attention to the greater morbidity and mortality of CABG surgery in the elderly but also to the potential of bypass surgery to improve survival and quality of life, given the severe symptoms and anatomy of the elderly patient undergoing angiography.

The attractions of a less invasive procedure such as PTCR as an alternative form of revascularization are intuitively obvious. Nonetheless, it must be accepted that the morbidity and mortality associated with PTCR are also increased in the elderly. The frequency of multivessel disease and LV dysfunction in the elderly technically limits the ability of percutaneous approaches to provide complete revascularization in some patients and raises appropriate doubts about the ratio of risk to benefit that is as effective as that of the more definitive cardiac surgery, which is often riskier and has more formidable consequences.

There have been several randomized trials comparing PTCA with coronary bypass surgery in patients with multi-vessel disease. These trials have not included large numbers of very elderly patients, but it does appear that the general results of these randomized studies can be extrapolated to the "young-old" patient population. There are little randomized trial data to guide the clinician in very elderly patients but there is a large published experience of PTCA in older patients and a critical review of these data provide for an educated decision for the individual patient.

Interventional cardiology also continues to rapidly evolve. Numerous devices are now available for coronary revascularization, and intracoronary stents and glycoprotein IIb/IIIa platelet antagonists in particular improve outcome in coronary interventions.[52-56] Numerous advances have steadily lowered the rate of acute complications after percutaneous revascularization[57] particularly in elderly patients[22,58] and, as a result, these procedures are now performed in older, sicker patients than even a few years ago. Studies which evaluate new devices for coronary intervention have typically not included large numbers of older patients. Thus, although the experience with percutaneous revascularization in the elderly is large, this experience is changing with new advances and both critical reevaluation and broad overall perspective remain important for rational decision making in the elderly.

Characteristics of the Elderly Population

As with the surgical population, elderly patients undergoing PTCR are sicker than younger subjects. They have more extensive CAD[1,59-62] and more symptoms, characterized by a more frequent proportion of Class III and IV angina and a higher frequency of unstable angina.[1,61-65] In one series for example, 63% of patients older than 65 undergoing PTCA compared with about 50% in the younger population had unstable angina.[64] In another large series, the incidence of unstable angina was 75% in subjects older than 70 and more than 80% in those older than 75 (Table 2).[1]

Other medical problems are also more common in the elderly undergoing PTCR. Diabetes and hypertension are more frequent,[64] and a history of CHF is more than twice as common in elderly patients as in younger patients. In the National Heart, Lung, and Blood Institute

---

Table 2
Baseline Data for 752 Patients 65 Years Old or Older Undergoing Coronary Angioplasty

	Group A (65–69 years)	Group B (70–74 years)	Group C (≥75 years)	P
Total Number of Patients	326	233	193	
Male, %	66.8	58.8	55.7	0.055
Mean Age, years	67	72	79	
Angina Class, %				
CCS I–II	16.6	13.3	5.7	
CCS III–IV	58.3	63.1	64.9	0.001
V*	17.2	13.3	21.1	
Cardiac and Medical History, %				
Unstable Angina	70.2	75.5	80.4	0.025
Prior CHF	8.9	9.4	24.4	<0.0001
Current CHF	5.8	5.6	18.6	<0.0001
Single Prior MI	36.8	38.6	38.1	0.16
Multiple Prior MI	8.0	9.4	13.9	0.039
Prior CABG	13.5	19.3	11.9	NS
Prior HTN	52.8	55.4	57.9	NS
Prior Active Lifestyle, %	84.4	81.1	66.0	<0.0001

CABG: coronary artery bypass grafting; CCS: Canadian Cardiovascular Society; CHF: congestive heart failure; HTN: systemic arterial hypertension; MI: myocardial infarction; and V*: defined as spontaneous ischemic pain at rest. Reprinted with permission from the American College of Cardiology (Journal of the American College of Cardiology) from Thompson RC, Holmes DR Jr, Gersh BJ, et al: Percutaneous transluminal coronary angioplasty in the elderly: Early and long-term results. J Am Coll Cardiol 1991, 17, 1245–1250.

(NHLBI) PTCA Registry, the incidence of previous CHF was 4% in subjects younger than 65 years and more than 9% in those older than 65.[61] In another series, the incidence of previous CHF was 24% in subjects older than 75 years (Table 3).[1]

Periprocedural Outcome

The distinction between the "old-old" and the "young-old" is particularly cogent to the subject of PTCR in the elderly. Although the technical success rate of PTCR is high in very elderly patients,[1,39,29–33,44,45,48,66,67] several published experiences show that patients in the eldest subgroup not only have more symptoms, but also have the most striking increase in procedural mortality after PTCR (Table 4).[21,61,65,68,69] For example, Thompson et. al., reported that the procedure success rates were similar across age groups within the subgroups of the elderly undergoing PTCA from 1990–1992 (92%–95% success rate)[58] and Nasser et al., found that the procedure success rate was similarly high (95.1%–98.8%) across the elderly subgroups undergoing coronary stent implantation.[70] Increased procedure mortality and fewer bypass operations post-PTCA was consistently reported in the oldest patients in the pre-stent era.[60,70] Physicians treat a number of very old, sick patients with a "salvage PTCR" with the understanding that PTCR complications will be treated medically. The hospital mortality rate for patients over age 75 undergoing PTCR has fallen to about 2%–4% in the more recently published results.[58,69–73] While acute outcomes with coronary interventions will likely continue to improve with further advances, the oldest patients tolerate complications poorly and will understandably continue to have much higher mortality rates than younger patients.

Age per se within the subgroup of patients older than 65 is an independent predictor of procedural mortality. However, it is not the most powerful predictor of short- and long-term outcomes. The most powerful predictor of perioperative PTCA mortality has been reported to be diffuse CAD as defined by the number of coronary segments with significant stenosis.[74] For elderly patients undergoing multivessel PTCA, Bedotto et al.[60] found that an ejection fraction of $< 40\%$, female sex, and three-vessel coronary disease were independent predictors of mortality.

Poor LV function and multi-vessel coronary artery disease are still predictors of procedural mortality in the current stent era.[72] Some elderly patients have heavily calcified coronary arteries which limits the utility of several coronary devices. Calcification may be associated with worsened procedural outcome in the eldest patients undergoing stent implantation, as it was in the past with PTCA. Arterial vascular complications and increased need for blood transfusions occur much more frequently post-PTCR in the elderly,[62,69,70] compared with younger patients.

Table 3
Baseline Characteristics of Younger and Older Patients Undergoing Percutaneous Transluminal Coronary Angioplasty in Four Series

Study	Patients Age, Years	Patients No.	Women, %	Left Main, %	Multivessel CAD, %	CHF, %	Unstable Angina, %	Prior MI, %	Diabetes, %
Kelsey et al.[51]	<65	1,315	21	2	49	4	48	37	12
	65–74	394	39	2	58	9	54	40	18
	≥75	92	46	2	63	17	58	28	11
Thompson et al.[1]	65–74	559	36.5	1.9	44	9.1	72.4	46	—
	≥75	193	44.3	6.7	63	24.4	80.4	52	—
Forman et al.[56]	60–69	570	33	—	30	10	60	49	17
	≥70	337	51	—	41	22	68	52.5	14
Macaya et al.[54]	<65	355	8	—	—	—	50	40	14
	≥65	145	33	—	—	—	63	41	26

The older angioplasty population has a greater proportion of women and a greater incidence of multivessel coronary artery disease, prior heart failure, and unstable angina pectoris. CAD: coronary artery disease; CHF: prior congestive heart failure; Left Main: significant stenosis in the left main coronary artery; and MI: myocardial infarction.

Table 4
Success and Complication Rates in Several Series of Percutaneous Transluminal Coronary Angioplasty (PTCA) in Elderly Patients

| Study | Patients | | Angiographic Success, % | Clinical Success, % | Death, % | MI, % | Emergency CABG, % |
	Age, Years	No.					
Thompson et al.[1]	65–69	326	—	82	1.2	2.7	10.7[#]
Bedotto et al.[50]	65–69	717	†	—	0.8	1.2	0.9
Forman et al.[56]	60–69	570	—	88	2	6	5
Thompson et al.[1]	70–74	233	—	82	2.2	4.3	9[#]
Bedotto et al.[50]	70–74	517	†	—	1.7	1.7	0.9
Kelsey et al.[51]	65–74	394	81	76	3.0	4.6	5.3
Forman et al.[56]	70–79	270	—	88	2	5	4
Thompson et al.[1]	≥75	193	—	92.8	6.2	6.7	4[#]
Kelsey et al.[51]	≥75	92	80	72	3.3	8.7	5.4
Imburgia et al.[56]	≥75	43	68	57	6	12	8
Bedotto et al.[50]	75–79	295	†	—	1.6	1.0	0.6
Kern et al.[67]	≥80	21	78	67	19	—	14
Bedotto et al.[50]	≥80	111	†	—	6.3	2.7	0
Rich et al.[62]	≥80	22	—	93	0	13.6	0
Forman et al.[56]	≥80	67	—	84	6	5	2

The success rate is high in the very elderly. However, PTCA mortality increases with age, and emergency bypass surgery is performed less frequently in the very old. CABG: coronary artery bypass grafting; MI: myocardial infarction; *: includes all bypass surgery within 24 hours of PTCA; and †: overall angiographic success rate is 96%.

Long-Term Survival and Other Long-Term Outcomes

Overall, long-term survival has been found to be quite good in even very old patients undergoing PTCR.[1,22,47,73] For example, a series from the Mayo Clinic found a 4-year survival rate of 86% after PTCA in patients older than 75 years.[1,58] The rates of long-term survival were quite similar between those older than 75 and those 65–75 years old (Fig. 6). Baseline variables found to be predictors of long-term survival free of MI after PTCA in the elderly are the number of the concomitant medical problems and the state of LV function,[74] both of which also predict long-term survival after bypass surgery. Not surprisingly, the extent of CAD strongly influences long-term survival after PTCA.[32,73,74]

In the evaluation of event-free survival after PTCA in the elderly (survival free of MI, bypass surgery, and repeat angioplasty or severe angina pectoris), the number of comorbid medical conditions and LV dysfunction are independent predictors of outcome.[74] However, the extent of CAD, as assessed by either the number of diseased coronary vessels[12] or the number of diseased coronary segments,[74] appears to be the strongest independent predictor of adverse late outcome in older patients, as is the case in younger patients with multivessel disease.[75] For example, a Mayo Clinic series found that at 3 years, a low-risk subset of elderly patients with a single coronary segment stenosis, stable angina, and no or one other medical problem had an event-free

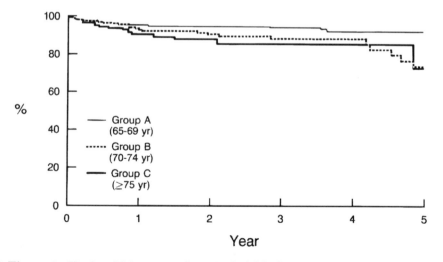

Figure 6: *Kaplan-Meier curve of survival of elderly patients undergoing PTCA. The long-term survival for elderly patients is good. Reprinted with permission from the American College of Cardiology (Journal of the American College of Cardiology) from Thompson RC, Holmes DR Jr, Gersh BJ, et al: Percutaneous transluminal coronary angioplasty in the elderly: Early and long-term results. J Am Coll Cardiol 1991, 17, 1245–1250.*

survival of 72%, whereas the rate was only 37% for a high-risk group of elderly patients with three or four coronary stenoses, two other medical problems, and unstable angina.[74]

Relief of Angina

After coronary bypass graft surgery, relief of angina appears similar in patients above and below the age of 65. The similarity may be due, in part, to less physical activity in older patients limited by noncardiac conditions. In contrast, the relief of angina after PTCR appears to be less with increasing age.[1,58,76]

A complete explanation for this finding is not available, but a higher instance of restenosis is unlikely, since a higher rate of restenosis does not appear to be present in the elderly.[64,77,78] Nonetheless, factors that predispose to restenosis, such as unstable angina,[1,63] multivessel or multilesion PTCR, treatment of the proximal anterior descending artery,[62] and diabetes,[79] may be more frequent in the elderly undergoing PTCR. Restenosis occurs in 30%–50% and repeat revascularization is required in about 20%–50% of successful PTCA cases.[46,78] Randomized, controlled trial data suggest that intracoronary stents reduce the rate of restenosis by about 10 absolute percentage points.[52,53]

The greater incidence of recurrent angina in the "old-old" is likely the result of less complete revascularization among an elderly population with diffuse multivessel disease. More extensive CAD is certainly present in the older patients undergoing angioplasty. Thompson et al.'s[74] review of the Mayo Clinic experience and Bourassa and associates' analysis[66] of the NHLBI Registry found that in many cases, physicians could have performed more extensive revascularization but appeared to have chosen to perform a more limited procedure in this population. For example, the strategy of performing "culprit lesion" PTCA for symptoms of unstable angina has frequently been used in the oldest subgroups. This strategy will likely change somewhat with new devices.

The issue of complete or incomplete revascularization is complex and has a direct bearing on the results of bypass surgery and PTCR in all age groups. Complete revascularization is a desirable objective, particularly in patients with LV dysfunction,[67,80,81] but this must be balanced by the risk of restenosis and of more complex, lengthy procedures in frail elderly patients. Complete as opposed to adequate revascularization is not essential for a satisfactory long-term outcome in all patients with multivessel disease undergoing PTCR.[73,76,82–84] From a practical standpoint, the objective is to provide adequate functional revascularization rather than complete revascularization. The former term implies treatment of all obstructive lesions supplying viable, jeopardized myocardium, and this accomplishment is particularly important in patients with underlying LV dysfunction.

Percutaneous Transluminal Coronary Revascularization for Acute Myocardial Infarction in the Elderly

The mortality rate of elderly patients treated with conventional therapy for acute MI is quite high. For example, in patients over age 80 years old, mortality for acute MI is over 30%.[79,85,86] Thrombolytic therapy benefits older patients but the mortality rate remains high, the risk of intracranial and other major hemorrhage is increased with age, and only a minority of elderly patients are actually treated with thrombolytic therapy.[87-89] Direct PTCR for acute MI has advantages over thrombolytic therapy including, in some studies, lower in-hospital mortality, fewer recurrent events, and lower incidence of stroke.[90-93] While there is not a large published experience with direct PTCR in elderly patients, the reported results are quite encouraging. For example, in the subgroup of patients over age 65 in The Primary Angioplasty in Myocardial Infarction (PAMI) trial, those treated with PTCA had a marked reduction in the endpoint of death or reinfarction (8.6% vs. 20.0%) compared with the thrombolytic group.[87] Also, Laster et al. described the Mid America Heart Institute experience with direct angioplasty for acute MI in octogenarians. Thirty-day mortality was 16%, but was only 10% in patients who were not in cardiogenic shock at presentation. Also, there were no strokes in these patients.[93] These results were better than the reported results of thrombolysis for acute MI in very elderly patients. For example, in the GUSTO Study, the mortality rate in the subgroup of patients over age 75 treated with tissue plasminogen activator was 19.3% and there was a 3.9% stroke rate.[87] Data from the Cooperative Cardiovascular project of 224,377 medicare patients also suggests that PTCA may offer slightly better results than thrombolytic therapy in older patients. This study included 5,131 patients treated with primary PTCA and 16,992 treated with thrombolytic therapy for acute MI from 1994–1995. Hospital mortality rates were similar for the two groups (10.8% vs. 11.4%) but 30-day mortality was lower with primary PTCA (11.8% vs. 14.3%, p < 0.001).

Both thrombolytic and interventional therapies continue to evolve. The use of intracoronary stents appears to improve the short-term outcome compared with PTCA alone for treatment of acute MI.[94] Direct PTCR, when feasible, is an excellent therapy in the elderly, as well as younger patients, who are in the process of having an acute myocardial infarction.

PTCR versus Bypass Surgery in the Elderly

Frequently, the decision about which revascularization strategy to employ is based largely on technical criteria. PTCR is not always technically feasible in elderly patients, but a less invasive approach other than bypass surgery has obvious attraction when it is possible. Older patients who have left main or extensive three vessel disease, especially with poor LV function, are usually better served with bypass surgery, unless their medical problems are severe, as are patients in whom PTCR is technically very difficult. But in older patients who have more limited coronary occlusive disease, a percutaneous approach to revascularization is usually preferred. In many older patients who have multivessel disease and preserved LV function, however, both PTCR and bypass surgery are feasible and the patient and physician have a more difficult decision. Randomized trials of bypass surgery and multivessel PTCA have primarily included younger patients. For example, the average age of combined randomized patients in the EAST,[95] BARI,[96] CABRI,[97] and RITA[98] studies was 60.1 years. However, the consistent results of these trials provide some guidance for treatment decisions in older patients, at least in the "young-old." For randomized patients with multivessel coronary disease there was generally no difference in in-hospital or intermediate-term mortality between the bypass surgery and PTCA groups and overall survival tended to be excellent. For example, 3-year survival was over 93% for both treatment groups in the EAST study.[95] Repeat coronary revascularization was more frequent in the angioplasty groups and relief of angina was less complete. The BARI Study showed improved 5-year survival in the non-prespecified subgroup of diabetic patients who were randomized to bypass surgery.[96]

Indirect comparisons of elderly patients undergoing PTCA or bypass surgery show results which are similar to findings of the randomized trials in younger patients. For example, O'Keefe and colleagues[99] and Thompson et al.[100] found that older patients undergoing PTCA for multivessel disease had similar intermediate term mortality rates versus comparable patients who had undergone bypass surgery. As is the case in younger patients, more of the older angioplasty patients required repeat revascularization procedures than did the surgical patients. As expected, the procedural and subsequent mortality rates tended to be higher in older patients undergoing PTCA or surgery compared with the mortality rates in trials in younger patients.[99,100] Trials of intracoronary stent implantation versus bypass surgery are ongoing.

Approach to Elderly Patients With Angina

The elderly population is a heterogeneous group, and treatment for CAD must be individualized. Age itself should not be the sole deciding factor, but the decision to revascularize and the choice of the procedure should be based on a realistic appraisal of the likelihood of immediate success and long-term benefit. Alternative strategies should be weighed. Careful attention should be paid to modifiable risk factors. The benefit of cigarette smoking cessation in elderly patients with coronary disease is as significant as it is in younger patients.[101] In addition, hypertension is a risk factor for late postoperative bypass mortality in patients older than 65,[40] as it is for all patients in this age group. Thus, elderly smokers should be strongly encouraged to quit, and hypertensive elderly patients with coronary disease should receive careful treatment and follow-up for high blood pressure.

Often, the issue is quality of life rather than long-term survival in elderly patients. For example, an 80-year-old has a life expectancy of approximately eight years.[102] However, independent living and relief of symptoms are important goals, as they are with younger patients. PTCR and surgery can be performed in older persons with a reasonable rate of success and can enhance the quality of life and independence of properly selected older patients. The key is proper patient selection.

For the physician deciding on PTCR or bypass surgery for relief of anginal symptoms in an elderly patient, the following criteria should be considered:

1. The chronologic and physiological ages of the patient;
2. The attitude of the patient, including expectations about surgery and postoperative convalescence;
3. The current activity level of the patient; and expected level to which they would return.
4. The ability of the patient to tolerate medical therapy;
5. The presence of associated medical diseases and their influence on the operative success rate and long-term survival; and
6. The extent of CAD and the potential for technical success in obtaining adequate revascularization.

Our society is faced with a rapidly expanding elderly population that requires a large proportion of total health care expenditures. The feasibility and efficacy of aggressive cardiovascular intervention in this age group are not in dispute, but the proportion of the health care budget that should be devoted to the elderly is a societal issue that will have to be addressed in the current era. The risk and benefits of invasive cardiovascular interventions in the elderly need to focus on the heterogeneity of the chronologically and physiologically elderly populations and take into account the needs and aspirations of our society in this full context.

References

1. Thompson RC, Holmes DR Jr, Gersh BJ, et al: Percutaneous transluminal coronary angioplasty in the elderly: Early and long-term results. *J Am Coll Cardiol* 17:1245–1250, 1991.
2. Feinleib M, Havlik LW, Gillum RF, et al: Coronary heart disease and

related procedures: National Hospital Discharge Survey data. *Circulation* 79(suppl D):I-3-I-18, 1989.

3. Gersh BJ, Kronmal RA, Frye RL, et al: Coronary arteriography and coronary artery bypass surgery: Morbidity and mortality in patients ages 65 years or older: A report from the Coronary Artery Surgery Study. *Circulation* 67:483–491, 1983.

4. Loop FD, Lytle BW, Cosgrove DM, et al: Coronary artery bypass graft surgery in the elderly: Indications and outcome. *Clev Clin J Med* 55: 23–34, 1988.

5. Edmunds LH Jr, Stephenson LW, Edie RN, et al: Open-heart surgery in octogenarians. *N Engl J Med* 319:131–136, 1988.

6. Weintraub WS, Craver JM, Cohen CL, et al: Influence of age on results of coronary artery surgery. *Circulation* 84(suppl 3):III-226-III-235, 1991.

7. Salomon NW, Page US, Bigelow JC, et al: Coronary artery bypass grafting in elderly patients: Comparative results in a consecutive series of 469 patients older than 75 years. *J Thorac Cardiovasc Surg* 101:209–218, 1991.

8. Horvath KA, DiSesa VJ, Peigh PS, et al: Favorable results of coronary artery bypass grafting in patients older than 75 years. *J Thorac Cardiovasc Surg* 99:92–96, 1990.

9. Canber CC, Nichols RD, Cooler SD, et al: Influence of increasing age on long term survival after coronary artery bypass grafting. *Ann Vasc Surg* 62:1123–7, 1996.

10. Carey JS, Cukingham RA, Singer LKM: Quality of life after myocardial revascularization. Effect of increasing age. *J Thorac Cardiovas Surg* 108–115, 1992.

11. Curtis JJ, Walls JT, Bolley TM, et al: Coronary revascularization in the elderly: Determinants of operative mortality. *Ann Thorac Surg* 58: 1069–72, 1994.

12. Kallis P, Unsworth-White J, Munsch C, et al: Disability and distress following cardiac surgery in patients over 70 years of age. *Euro J Cardio-Thorac Surg* 7:306–312, 1993.

13. Hannan EL, Burke J: Effect of age on mortality in coronary artery bypass surgery in New York, 1991–1992. *Am Heart J* 128:1184–9, 1994.

14. Mullany CJ, Darling GE, Pluth JR, et al: Early and late results after isolated coronary artery bypass surgery in 159 patients aged 80 years and older *Circulation* 82(suppl 4):IV-229 IV-236, 1990.

15. Frye RL, Kronmal R, Schaff HV, et al: Stroke in coronary artery bypass graft surgery: An analysis of the CASS experience. *Int J Cardiol* 36: 213–221, 1992.

16. Glower DD, Christopher TD, Milano CA, et al: Performance status and outcome after coronary artery bypass grafting in persons aged 80 to 93 years. *Am J Cardiol* 70:567–571, 1992.

17. Tsai TPT, Chaux A, Matloff JM, et al: Ten year experience of cardiac surgery in patients aged 80 years and older. *Ann Thorac Surg* 58:445–51, 1994.

18. Saher G, Raanani E, Sagia A, et al: Surgical results in cardiac surgical patients over the age of 80 years. *Isr J Med* 32:1322–25, 1996.

19. Peterson ED, Cowper PA, Jollis JG, et al: Outcomes of coronary artery bypass graft surgery in 24,461 patients ages 80 years or older. *Circulation* 92:Suppl II:II-85-II-91, 1995.

20. Pliam MB, Bronstein MH, Zapolanski A, et al: Recent improvement in

result of coronary bypass surgery in octogenarians (Abstract) *Circulation* 96:I-61, 1997.

21. Peterson ED, Jollis JG, Bedchuk JD, et al: Changes in mortality after myocardial revascularization in the elderly, the National Medicare experience. *Ann Intern Med* 121:919–927, .

22. Gersh BJ, Kronmal RA, Schaff HV, et al: Comparison of coronary artery bypass surgery and medical therapy in patients 65 years of age or older: A nonrandomized study from the Coronary Artery Surgery Study (CASS) Registry. *N Engl J Med* 313:217–224, 1985.

23. Paone G, Higgins RSD, Havstad SL: Does age limit the effectiveness of clinical pathways following coronary bypass surgery? (Abstract) *Circulation* 96:I-58, 1997.

24. Knapp WS, Douglas JS Jr, Craver JM, et al: Efficacy of coronary artery bypass grafting in elderly patients with coronary artery disease. *Am J Cardiol* 47:923–930, 1981.

25. Lipowski ZJ: Delirium in the elderly patient. *N Engl J Med* 320:578–582, 1989.

26. Kowalchuk GJ, Siu SC, Lewis SM: Coronary artery disease in the octogenarian: Angiographic spectrum and suitability for revascularization. *Am J Cardiol* 66:1319–1323, 1990.

27. Fuller JA, Adams GG, Buxton B: Atrial fibrillation after coronary artery bypass grafting: Is it a disorder of the elderly? *J Thorac Cardiovasc Surg* 97:821–825, 1989.

28. Gold S, Wong WF, Schatz IJ, et al: Invasive treatment for coronary artery disease in the elderly. *Arch Intern Med* 151:1085–1088, 1991.

29. Guadagnoli E, Ayanian JZ, Cleary PD: Comparison of patient-reported outcomes after elective coronary artery bypass grafting in patients aged > and <65 years. *Am J Cardiol* 70:60–64, 1992.

30. Key EW, Acuff TE, Ryan WH, et al: Determinants of operative mortality in elderly patients undergoing coronary artery bypass grafting, emphasis on the influence of internal mammary artery grafting on mortality and morbidity. *Cardiovasc Surg* 108:73–81, 1994.

31. Nolan L, O'Malley K: Prescribing for the elderly. Part I: Sensitivity of the elderly to adverse drug reactions. *J Am Geriatr Soc* 36:142–149, 1988.

32. Backes RJ, Gersh BJ: The treatment of coronary artery disease in the elderly. *Cardiovasc Drugs Ther* 5:449–455, 1991.

33. Gurwitz JH, Col NF, Avorn J: The exclusion of the elderly and women from clinical trials in acute myocardial infarction. *JAMA* 268:1417–1422, 1992.

34. Ott RA, Gutfinger DE, Miller MP, et al: Rapid recovery after coronary artery bypass grafting: Is the elderly patient eligible? *Ann Thorac Surg* 63:634–9, 1997.

35. Peigh PS, Swartz MT, Vacu KJ, et al: Effect of advancing age on cost and outcome of coronary artery bypass grafting. *Ann Thorac Surg* 58:1362–7, 1994.

36. Weintraub WS, Craver JM, Gott JP, et al: Have coronary surgical services been optimized? (Abstract). *Circulation* 96:I-62, 1997.

37. Aranki SF, Shaw DP, Adams DH, et al: Predictors of atrial fibrillation after coronary artery surgery, current trends and impact on hospital resources. *Circulation* 94:390–397, 1996.

38. Ko W, Gold JP, Lazzaro R, et al: Survival analysis of octogenarian patients with coronary artery disease managed by elective coronary artery bypass

surgery versus conventional medical therapy. *Circulation* 86(suppl 2):II-191II-197, 1992.

39. Tsai T-P, Nessim S, Kass RM, et al: Morbidity and mortality after coronary artery bypass in octogenarians. *Ann Thorac Surg* 51:983–986, 1991.

40. Carey JS, Cukinghan RA, Singer LKM: Quality of life after myocardial revascularization: Effect of increasing age. *J Thorac Cardiovasc Surg* 103: 108–115, 1992.

41. Page SA, Berhoff MS, Emes C: Quality of life, bypass surgery, and the elderly. *Can J Cardiol* 11(9) 777–782, 1995.

42. Walter PJ, Mohan R: Coronary bypass surgery in the elderly - A multidisciplinary opinion: Summary of proceedings of an international symposium held at Antwerp, Belgium, March 9–11 1994. *Quality of Life Research* 4:279–287, 1995.

43. Lazar J, Vanhooser T, Schubach S, et al: Self-rated quality of life of octogenarians after cardiac surgery. (Abstract) *Circulation* 96:I-60, 1997.

44. Christenson JT, Simonet F, Schmazider M: The influence of age on the results of operative coronary artery bypass grafting. *Coronary artery disease* 8:91–95, 1997.

45. Alexander KP, Peterson ED, Muhlbaier LH, et al: Cardiac surgery outcomes in 3,220 octogenarians: Results from the National Cardiovascular Network (Abstract) *Circulation* 96:I-59, 1997.

46. Hirshfeld JW Jr, Schwartz JS, Jugo R, et al: Restenosis after coronary angioplasty: A multivariate statistical model to relate lesion and procedure variables to restenosis. *J Am Coll Cardiol* 18:647–656, 1991.

47. Ellis SG, Cowley MJ, DiSciascio G, et al: Determinants of 2-year outcome after coronary angioplasty in patients with multivessel disease on the basis of comprehensive preprocedural evaluation: Implications for patient selection. *Circulation* 83:1905–1914, 1991.

48. Kitamura M, Endo M, Yamaki F, et al: Long-term results of coronary artery bypass grafting in elderly Japanese patients. *Ann Thorac Surg* 60: 576–9, 1995.

49. Ivanov J, Weisel RD, David TE, et al: Fifteen year trends in risk severity and operative mortality in elderly patients undergoing coronary artery bypass graft surgery. *Circulation* 97:673–680, 1998.

50. Blauth CI, Cosgrove DM, Webb BW, et al: Atheroembolism from the ascending aorta. An emergency problem in cardiac surgery. *J Thorac Cardiovasc Surg* 103:1104–11, 1992.

51. Lahey SJ, Borlase BC, Lavin PT, et al: Preoperative risk factors that predict hospital length of stay in coronary artery bypass patients >60 years old. *Circulation* 86(suppl 2):II-181-II-185, 1992.

52. Fischman DL, Leon MB, Baim DS, et al: A randomized comparison of coronary stent placement and balloon angioplasty and the treatment of coronary artery disease. *N Eng J Med* 331:496–501, 1994.

53. Serruys TW, De Jaeger P, Kiemenei F, et al: Comparison of balloon expandable stent implantation with balloon angioplasty in patients with coronary artery disease. *N Eng J Med* 331:489–95, 1994.

54. Savage MP, Douglas JS, Fischman DL, et al: Stent placement compared with balloon angioplasty for obstructed coronary bypass grafts. *N Eng J Med* 337:740–7, 1997.

55. EPIC Investigators: Use of monoclonal antibody directed against the platelet glycoprotein IIb/IIIa receptor in high risk coronary angioplasty. *N Eng J Med* 330:965–61, 1994.

56. EPILOG Investigators: Platelet glycoprotein IIb/IIIa receptor blockade and low-dose heparin during percutaneous coronary revascularization. *N Eng J Med* 336:1689–96, 1997.
57. Altmann DB, Racz M, Battleman DS, et al: Reduction in angioplasty complications after the introduction of coronary stents; Results from a consecutive series of 2242 patients. *Am Heart J* 132:503–7, 1996.
58. Thompson RC, Holmes DR, Grill DE, et al: Changing outcome of angioplasty in the elderly. *J Am Coll Cardiol* 27:8–14, 1996.
59. Mock MB, Holmes DR Jr, Vlietstra RE, et al: Percutaneous transluminal coronary angioplasty (PTCA) in the elderly patient: Experience in the National Heart, Lung, and Blood Institute PTCA Registry. *Am J Cardiol* 53:89C–9lC, 1984.
60. Bedotto JB, Rutherford BD, McConahay DR, et al: Results of multivessel percutaneous transluminal coronary angioplasty in persons age 65 years and older. *Am J Cardiol* 67:1051–1055, 1991.
61. Kelsey SF, Miller DP, Holubkov R, et al: Results of percutaneous transluminal coronary angioplasty in patients > 65 years of age (from the 1985 to 1986 National Heart, Lung, and Blood Institute's Coronary Angioplasty Registry). *Am J Cardiol* 66:1033–1038, 1990.
62. Lindsay J, Reddy VM, Pinnon EE, et al: Morbidity and mortality rates in elderly patients undergoing percutaneous transluminal coronary angioplasty. *Am Heart J* 128:697–702, 1994.
63. Simpfendorfer C, Raymond R, Schraider J, et al: Early and long-term results of percutaneous transluminal coronary angioplasty in patients 70 years of age and older with angina pectoris. *Am J Cardiol* 62:959–961, 1988.
64. Macaya C, Alfonso F, Iniguez A, et al: Long-term clinical and angiographic follow-up of percutaneous transluminal coronary angioplasty in patients > 65 years of age. *Am J Cardiol* 66:1513–1515, 1990.
65. Forman DE, Berman AD, McCabe CH, et al: PTCA in the elderly: The "young-old" versus the "old-old." *J Am Geriatr Soc* 40:19–22, 1992.
66. Bourassa MG, Holubkov R, Yeh W, et al: Strategy of complete revascularization in patients with multivessel coronary artery disease (a report from the 1985–1986 NHLBI PTCA Registry). *Am J Cardiol* 70:174–178, 1992.
67. Bell MR, Gersh BJ, Schaff HV, et al: Effect of completeness of revascularization on long-term outcome of patients with three-vessel disease undergoing coronary artery bypass surgery: A report from the Coronary Artery Surgery Study (CASS) Registry. *Circulation* 86:446–457, 1992.
68. O'Keefe JH Jr, Rutherford BR, McConahay DR, et al: Multivessel coronary angioplasty from 1980–1989: Procedural results and long-term outcome. *J Am Coll Cardiol* 16:1097–1102, 1990.
69. Fishman RF, Kuntz RE, Carrozza JT, et al: Acute and long-term results of coronary stents and atherectomy in women and the elderly. *Coronary artery disease* 6:159–68, 1995.
70. Nasser TK, Fry ETA, Annan K, et al: Comparison of six month outcome of coronary artery stenting in patients < 65, 65–75, and > 75 years of age. *Am J Cardiol* 80:998–1001, 1997.
71. Jollis JG, Peterson AD, Nelson CL, et al: Relationship between physician and hospital coronary angioplasty volume and outcome in elderly patients. *Circulation* 1995:2485–2491, 1977.
72. De Gregorio J, Kobagashi Y, Albiero R, et al: Coronary artery stenting in the elderly: Short-term outcome and long-term angiographic and clinical follow-up. *J Am Coll Cardiol* 32:577–83, 1998.

73. de Jaegere P, de Feyter P, van Domburg R, et al: Immediate and long term results of percutaneous coronary angioplasty in patients aged 70 and over. *Br Heart J* 67:138–143, 1992.
74. Thompson RC, Holmes DR Jr, Gersh BJ, et al: Predicting outcome of PTCA in the elderly. *Circulation* 88:1577–87, 1993.
75. Vandormael M, Deligonul U, Taussig S, et al: Predictors of long-term cardiac survival in patients with multivessel coronary artery disease undergoing percutaneous transluminal coronary angioplasty. *Am J Cardiol* 67:1–6, 1991.
76. Berg JM, Voors AA, Suttorp MJ, et al: Long-term results after successful percutaneous transluminal coronary angioplasty in patients over 75 years of age. *Am J Cardiol* 77:690–695, 1996.
77. Jackman JD Jr, Navetta Fl, Smith JE, et al: Percutaneous transluminal coronary angioplasty in octogenarians as an effective therapy for angina pectoris. *Am J Cardiol* 68:116–119, 1991.
78. McBride W, Lange RA, Hillis LD: Restenosis after successful coronary angioplasty: Pathology and prevention. *N Engl J Med* 318:1734–1737, 1988.
79. Naylor D, Chen E: Population-wide mortality trends among patients hospitalized for acute myocardial infarction: The Ontario experience, 1981 to 1991. *J Am Coll Cardiol* 24:1431–1438, 1994.
80. Jones EL, Craver JM, Guyton RA, et al: Importance of complete revascularization in performance of the coronary bypass operation. *Am J Cardiol* 51:7–12, 1983.
81. Lavee J, Rath S, Tran-Quang-Hoa, et al: Does complete revascularization by the conventional method truly provide the best possible results? Analysis of results and comparison with revascularization of infarct prone segments (systematic segment myocardial revascularization): The Sheba study. *J Thorac Cardiovasc Surg* 92:279–290, 1986.
82. O'Keefe JH, Allan JJ, McCallister BD, et al: Angioplasty versus bypass surgery for multivessel coronary artery disease with left ventricular ejection fraction < or, > 40%. *Am J Cardiol* 71:897–901, 1993.
83. Reeder GS, Holmes DR Jr, Detre K, et al: Degree of revascularization in patients with multivessel coronary disease: A report from the National Heart, Lung, and Blood Institute Percutaneous Transluminal Coronary Angioplasty registry. *Circulation* 77:638–644, 1988.
84. Bell MR, Bailey KR, Reeder GS, et al: Percutaneous transluminal angioplasty in patients with multivessel coronary disease: How important is complete revascularization for cardiac event-free survival? *J Am Coll Cardiol* 16:553–562, 1990.
85. Goldberg RJ, Gore JM, Gurwitz JH, et al: The impact of age on the incidence and prognosis of initial acute myocardial infarction: The Worchester Heart Attack Study. *Am Heart J* 117:543–549, 1989.
86. Latting CA, Thorberman ME: Acute myocardial infarction in hospitalized patients over age 80. *Am Heart J* 100:311–318, 1980.
87. GUSTO Investigators: International randomized trial comparing 4 thrombolytic strategies for acute myocardial infarction. *N Engl J Med* 329:673–682, 1993.
88. Lew AS, Hanoch H, Cercek B, et al: Mortality and morbidity rates of patients older and younger than 75 years with acute myocardial infarction treated with intravenous streptokinase. *Am J Cardiol* 59:1–5, 1987.
89. Grines CL, Browne KF, Marco J, et al: Comparison of immediate angio-

plasty with thrombolytic therapy for acute myocardial infarction. *N Engl J Med* 328:673–679, 1993.

90. Zijlstra F, VandeBoer M, Hoorntje JCA, et al: A comparison of immediate coronary angioplasty with intravenous streptokinase in acute myocardial infarction. *N Engl J Med* 328:680–684, 1993.

91. Gibbons RJ, Holmes DR, Reeder GS, et al: For the Mayo Coronary Care Unit and Catheterization Laboratory Group. *N Engl J Med* 328:685–691, 1993.

92. de Boer MJ, Hourntse JCA, Ottervanger JP, et al: Immediate angioplasty compared with the administration of a thrombolytic agent followed by conservative treatment for myocardial infarction. *J Am Coll Cardiol* 23: 1004–1008, 1994.

93. Laster SB, Rutherford BD, Giorgi LV, et al: Results of direct percutaneous transluminal coronary angioplasty in octogenarians. *Am J Cardiol* 77: 10–13, 1996.

94. Antoniucci D, Santoro GM, Bolognese L, et al: A clinical trial comparing primary stenting of the infarct-related artery with optimal primary angioplasty for acute myocardial infarction: results from the Florence Randomized Elective Stenting in Acute Coronary Occlusion (FRESCO) trial. *J Am Coll Cardiol* 31(6):1234–9, 1998 May.

95. King SB III, Lembo NJ, Weintraub WF, et al: A randomized trial comparing coronary angioplasty with coronary bypass surgery. *N Engl J Med* 331:1044–50, 1994.

96. The Bypass Angioplasty Revascularization (BARI) Investigators: Comparison of coronary bypass surgery with angioplasty in patients with multivessel disease. *N Engl J Med* 335:217–25, 1996.

97. CABRI Trial Participants: First year results of CABRI (Coronary Angioplasty versus Bypass Revascularization Investigation) *Lancet* 346: 1179–84, 1995.

98. RITA Trial Participants: Coronary angioplasty versus coronary artery bypass surgery: The Randomized Intervention Treatment of Angina (RITA) Trial. *Lancet* 343:573–80, 1993.

99. O'Keefe JH, Sutton MB, McCallister BD, et al: Coronary angioplasty versus bypass surgery in patients greater than 70 years old matched for ventricular function. *J Am Coll Cardiol* 24:425–30, 1994.

100. Thompson RC, Kopecky SL, Mullany CJ, et al: Comparison of percutaneous transluminal angioplasty and coronary artery bypass graft surgery in the elderly resident of Olmsted County, Minnesota. (Abstract) *Circulation* Suppl I, 94:3140, 1996.

101. Hermanson B, Omenn GS, Kronmal RA, et al: Beneficial six-year outcome of smoking cessation in older men and women with coronary artery disease: Results from the CASS registry. *N Engl J Med* 319:1365–1369, 1988.

102. National Center for Health Statistics: U.S. Decennial Life Tables for 1979–81. Washington, DC: United States Department of Health and Human Services; 1985. DHHS Publication No. LPHS] 85–1150–1, Vol 1, No. 1.

Chapter 14

Management of Lipid Disorders

Hanna Bloomfield Rubins

> Take nothing on its looks; take everything on evidence. There
> is no better rule.
>
> Charles Dickens

Coronary heart disease (CHD) is the leading cause of death among
the elderly in the United States and many western countries. In 1992,
for example, 38% of deaths in men and 41% of deaths in women over
age 75 were attributable to heart disease, mostly CHD.[1] The annual
risk for CHD death in men and women age 75 to 79 is 1% to 2%; for
those over age 85 it is as high as 4% to 5%.[2] In addition to mortality,
CHD in the elderly results in substantial morbidity and economic cost.[3]

In middle-aged populations, high levels of serum total cholesterol,
low density lipoprotein cholesterol (LDL-C), and low levels of high density lipoprotein cholesterol (HDL-C) have been clearly implicated as
important risk factors for CHD in observational epidemiological studies. Furthermore, clinical trials in middle-aged individuals have demonstrated that cholesterol lowering therapy reduces the incidence of
first myocardial infarction or CHD death[4] and of recurrent ischemic
events among those with established CHD.[5,6]

For elderly populations, there is less data and more controversy
about the importance of cholesterol as a risk factor for CHD and the
value of screening and treatment. This is an important clinical issue
since there is both a high prevalence of hypercholesterolemia among
the elderly and an increasingly large population of elderly persons in
this country. In this chapter I discuss the evidence pertaining to these
clinically important questions: Are serum lipids and lipoproteins important risk factors for CHD among the elderly? Which elderly persons

From *Clinical Cardiology in the Elderly. Second Edition*, edited by Elliot Chesler. ©
1999, Futura Publishing Company, Armonk, NY.

are appropriate candidates for lipid screening? Under what circumstances and with what modalities should elderly patients be treated for dyslipidemia?

Pathophysiology of Acute Ischemic Events

Although the development of atherosclerotic lesions may take decades, the pathogenesis of acute ischemic events such as myocardial infarction, unstable angina, and sudden death appears to involve processes that can be altered over much shorter periods of time.[7] Angiographic and pathological data suggest that acute ischemic events are precipitated by sudden rupture or erosion and subsequent thrombosis of previously quiescent atherosclerotic plaques.[8] If an occlusive thrombus develops at the rupture site the clinical sequel is usually myocardial infarction; in contrast, nonocclusive thrombi are usually associated with unstable angina or sudden death.[9] The clinical manifestations will depend on the extent, location, and duration of the thrombus and the presence or absence of collateral circulation.

What causes a plaque to rupture? Rupture is related both to the intrinsic properties of the plaque itself and to extrinsic, or "triggering" factors.[9] Intrinsic characteristics that predispose a plaque to rupture include a thin fibrous cap, a large lipid core (>40% of overall plaque volume), and a dense infiltrate of inflammatory cells (in particular, macrophages). Such plaques are typically associated with only modest to moderate luminal obstruction (eg, 30% to 50% stenosis). In contrast to these "vulnerable" plaques, stable lesions have thick fibrous caps, small lipid cores, and moderately to severely obstructed lumens.[8] Triggering factors that can cause disruption of a vulnerable plaque include hemodynamic and mechanical stresses that may be precipitated by increases in sympathetic activity and abnormal vasoconstrictor responses.

There is growing evidence linking hypercholesterolemia to several of the pathogenetic mechanisms underlying acute ischemic events. First, cholesterol in the core of the atherosclerotic plaque is probably derived from circulating oxidized LDL. The level of serum LDL-C is directly related to the size of the lipid core of the atherosclerotic lesion. A large lipid core enhances plaque susceptibility to acute rupture by increasing the circumferential stress and by causing degradative changes in the fibrous cap through activation of inflammatory cells.[10] By preventing further accumulation of lipids in the atherosclerotic plaque and depleting the existing plaque lipid pool, lipid lowering therapy may thus help to stabilize previously vulnerable lesions.[11] Second, oxidized LDL have been implicated in the abnormal endothelial vasomotor response characteristic of atherosclerotic arteries. Specifically, affected arteries show an abnormal, heightened vasoconstrictor response to stimuli such as stress or exercise.[12] Vasoconstriction at the site of a vulnerable plaque may, through increased shear stress, trigger plaque disruption and an acute ischemic event. Several recent clinical studies have shown that lipid lowering therapy improves these abnormal vasoconstrictor responses.[12,13] Third, hypercholesterolemia appears to increase thrombogenic potential by increasing platelet reactivity, an effect that can be reversed by cholesterol lowering therapy.[14] These and other mechanisms may underlie the observation that lipid lowering therapy can reduce acute cardiac ischemic events over relatively short periods of time, (ie, 2 years), even in the absence of marked regression of severely stenotic atherosclerotic lesions.[15]

Role of High-Density Lipoprotein and Triglycerides

While it is generally agreed that HDL is an antiatherogenic lipoprotein, the mechanisms responsible for this effect are still being vigorously investigated.[16] The most widely accepted hypothesis suggests that HDL acts to facilitate removal of cholesterol from the arterial wall and to transport it back to the liver for excretion from the body.[17] Supporting this theory is experimental evidence showing that HDL can remove cholesterol from lipid-laden macrophages in tissue culture.[18] HDL may also play a role in the clearance of atherogenic, triglyceride rich postprandial particles from the circulation and in the prevention of LDL oxidation within the vessel wall.[19]

There are many mechanisms by which triglycerides may contribute to the development of clinically apparent ischemic vascular disease.[20] While triglycerides do not accumulate in the wall of the vessel the way cholesterol does, triglyceride rich lipoproteins, including very low density lipoprotein (VLDL) and chylomicron and VLDL remnants, are known to enter the vessel wall where the cholesterol they carry may contribute to foam cell development.[21] Furthermore, elevated levels of triglycerides are associated with smaller, denser LDL particles which are more susceptible to oxidation and are thought to be more atherogenic than larger LDL particles.[22,23] Finally, high levels of triglycerides may contribute to a hypercoagulable state.[23]

Prevalence of Lipid Abnormalities in the Elderly

Total Cholesterol and LDL-C

Hypercholesterolemia is highly prevalent among the elderly in this country. In the Cardiovascular Health Study, for example, 46% of nearly 5000 community-living persons over the age of 65 had a high LDL-C (>160 mg/dL).[24]

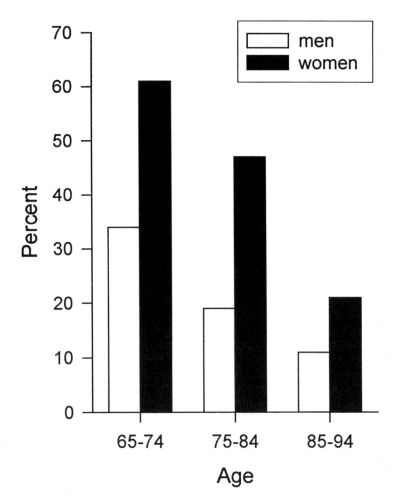

Figure 1: *Prevalence of hypercholesterolemia in elderly men and women. Data from Framingham Heart Study.*[25]

Hypercholesterolemia is more common in elderly women than in men. In the Framingham Heart Study (Figure 1), 34% of men and 61% of women age 65 to 74 had hypercholesterolemia (defined as total cholesterol ≥ 240 mg/dL). This gender difference persists through very old age, although in both men and women the prevalence of hypercholesterolemia declines with extreme old age. Thus, in Framingham, only 11% of men and 21% of women age 85 to 94 had high cholesterol, as defined above.[25] This decline probably represents a "survivor effect"; those with the highest levels of cholesterol die at earlier ages, leaving the oldest age group enriched with people with lower cholesterol levels.

Using cholesterol values and clinical information from the National Health and Nutrition Examination Survey, Sempos and colleagues have estimated that if the 1993 National Cholesterol Education Program Guidelines for treatment were followed, 40% to 50% of men and 50% to 60% of women over age 65 would be candidates for dietary intervention to lower their cholesterol.[26] These authors further estimate that drug treatment to lower cholesterol would be indicated in over 5 million Americans over the age of 65. A similar analysis of the Cardiovascular Health Study population yielded similar findings.[27] It is clear, therefore, that there is a large and growing population of elderly people in whom cholesterol management may be required.

HDL–C and Triglycerides

The National Cholesterol Education Program and the NIH Consensus Conference define low HDL-C as less than 35 mg/dL and triglycerides as normal ($<$200 mg/dL); borderline high (200 to 400 mg/dL); high (400 to 1000 mg/dL); and very high ($>$1000 mg/dL). Using these definitions, approximately 15% of elderly men and fewer than 5% of elderly women have low HDL-C; and fewer than 15% of either men or women have borderline high or higher triglycerides.[24,25] In men but not women, there is a significant decline in triglycerides and increase in HDL-C with increasing age (from mean levels of 145 mg/dL and 48 mg/dL in those aged 65 to 69 to 115 mg/dL and 51 mg/dL, in those over 85 years, respectively).[24] In contrast to total cholesterol and LDL-C, which are not significantly different among those with and without CHD, triglycerides are significantly higher and HDL-C significantly lower in elderly men and women with CHD.[24]

Observational Data: Is Cholesterol a Risk Factor for CHD in the Elderly?

Total Cholesterol and LDL–C as Risk Factors for CHD

The relation between cholesterol level and CHD in the elderly has been highly controversial. Numerous prospective cohort studies have reported variable findings. Several have found no association between cholesterol levels and risk of CHD events in the elderly[28,29]; others have found a positive association[30,31]; and some have reported an inverse or J-shaped association, in which lower cholesterol levels confer increased risk of CHD.[32] However, more recent studies using meta-analysis to combine data from many cohorts,[33] or have adjusted more completely for important confounding variables such as poor general health,[34] appear to support the hypothesis that high levels of cholesterol do indeed predict CHD risk in the elderly.

In 1992, Manolio and colleagues[33] published a pooled analysis of 22 observational epidemiological studies which included over 15,000 women and 49,000 men older than 65. As can be seen from Table 1, the risk of CHD death among older men was 32% higher for those with cholesterol greater than 240 mg/dL than for those with cholesterol less than 200 mg/dL (ie, relative risk of 1.32). The comparable relative risk for younger men was 1.73. The difference in relative risk between younger and older women was even more striking than for men: relative risk of 2.44 in those less than 65 years compared to relative risk of 1.12 for older women. Nevertheless, the increased risk of CHD associated with high cholesterol in the elderly, while of smaller magnitude than in middle aged people, was still significant for both men and women.

In a re-analysis of the data from the Established Populations for Epidemiologic Studies in the Elderly (EPESE), which had originally reported no association between cholesterol and CHD in a community-based cohort of elderly patients (average age 79),[28] a significant association was found when adjustments were made for "frailty," as measured by serum iron and albumin.[34] The rationale behind this approach is that frail patients develop lower cholesterol levels because of their poor general health. Because these patients are the most likely to die during follow-up, often with a cardiac event being the terminal event superimposed on other chronic illnesses, it then appears that a low cholesterol is associated with increased risk of CHD death. If this "spurious" association is accounted for, a positive, linear association between cholesterol levels and CHD death, similar to that seen for middle-aged persons, becomes apparent (Figure 2), with an adjusted relative risk of 1.57 for those with the highest cholesterol (>240 mg/dL) compared to the reference category (161 to 199 mg/dL). No separate analyses by gender

---

Table 1
Relative Risk of Coronary Heart Disease by Total and HDL Cholesterol

	Men		Women	
	<65 years	≥65 years	<65 years	≥65 years
Total cholesterol (≥240 mg/dL vs. <200 mg/dL)	1.73	1.32	2.44	1.12
HDL cholesterol (<50 mg/dL vs. ≥60 mg/dL)	2.31	1.09‡	2.13	1.75

‡ All relative risks are significantly elevated, except 1.09 at P < 09. Sample sizes are: 475,203 for men < 65; 49,078 for men ≥ 65; 70,830 for women < 65; 15,404 for women ≥ 65.

Reproduced with permission from Manolio TA, Pearson TA, Wenger NK, et al: Cholesterol and heart disease in older persons and women: Review of an NHLBI Workshop. *Ann Epidemiol* 2: 161–176, 1992.

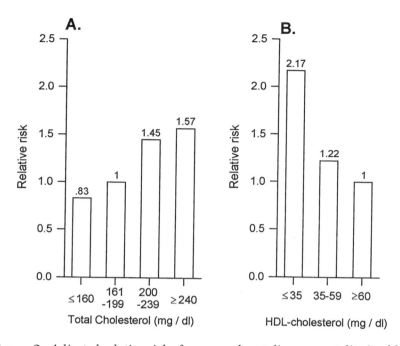

Figure 2: *Adjusted relative risk of coronary heart disease mortality in elderly men and women by cholesterol and HDL-C level. Data from the Established Populations for Epidemiologic Studies in the Elderly. All participants were aged 71 years and older. Relative risks were adjusted for age, sex, coronary heart disease risk factors, serum iron and albumin levels, and excluding first-year deaths. Reproduced with permission from Cori M, Guralnik JM, Salive ME, et al: Clarifying the direct relation between total cholesterol levels and death from coronary heart disease in older persons.* Ann Intern Med *126:753–760, 1997.*

were reported. These authors conclude that in the healthy elderly, cholesterol is indeed a significant risk factor for CHD.

Importance of Excess Risk

It is fair to conclude from the prospective cohort studies that cholesterol remains a significant, although possibly somewhat weaker risk factor for CHD in the elderly than in middle aged people. Nevertheless, since CHD is so much more common among elderly people, even a small increase in relative risk conferred by an elevated cholesterol can have important clinical and public health implications. To understand this point requires an understanding of the difference between relative and excess (also known as attributable) risk.[35] Relative risk, defined as the ratio of disease incidence in those with the risk factor to disease incidence in those without the risk factor, is the best measure for assessing

Table 2
Comparison of Relative and Excess Risk of Coronary Heart Disease Death by Serum Cholesterol and Age*

Age	Relative Risk‡	Excess Risk‡ (per 1000 person-years)
65–69	1.6	5.2
70–74	1.7	7.9
75–79	1.7	11.3

* Adapted from Rubin et al based on data from 2746 white men, reference 103.

‡ Relative risk and excess risk were calculated using mortality in the highest quartile of serum cholesterol compared to the lower three quartiles.

* Adapted with permission from Rubin SM, Sidney S, Black DM, et al: High blood cholesterol in elderly men and the excess risk for coronary heart disease. *Ann Intern Med* 113:916–920, 1990.

the causal association between risk factor and disease. The higher the relative risk the more likely that the risk factor actually causes or contributes to the pathogenesis of the disease. The excess risk, however, which is the difference between rates in 2 different risk groups, takes into account the underlying prevalence of disease in the population, and is a better estimate of how much disease could be prevented in a given population by eliminating or treating the risk factor. Because CHD is much more common in elderly patients than in younger patients, the excess risk of CHD associated with high compared to low levels of cholesterol is actually much greater for older than for younger patients, as demonstrated in the example in Table 2. This implies that more CHD events could be prevented by treating elevated cholesterol in an elderly than in a younger population, although definitive proof of this hypothesis requires clinical trial confirmation.

HDL-C as a Risk Factor for CHD

Many cohort studies have demonstrated that HDL-C is a strong, independent, inverse risk factor for CHD in all age groups and both genders, especially in elderly women. In the EPESE study of over 2500 men and 1300 women all over age 70, the relative risk of cardiac death in those with HDL-C less than 35 mg/dL compared to those with HDL-C of greater than 60 mg/dL, was 2.5 (95% confidence interval, 1.6 to 4.0).[34,36] This association held for both men and women in both age groups (71 to 80 and over 80 years) and persisted after adjustment for other risk factors, including total cholesterol (Figure 2). Other observational studies have reported similar findings (Table 1).[33] In the Framingham population, low HDL-C was associated with increased risk of CHD death for all age groups between 50 and 80 years, although the magnitude of the association declined with advancing age.[29] In the large pooled analysis published in 1992, low HDL-C was a significant risk factor in elderly women and was trending towards significance in elderly men (P = .09).[33]

Triglyceride as a Risk Factor for CHD

The importance of triglycerides as an independent risk factor for CHD is controversial even for middle aged populations. Although triglycerides almost always show a strong positive association with CHD by univariate analyses, the association tends to disappear when multivariate methods are used to control for other lipid fractions, especially HDL-C. This was interpreted as suggesting that triglycerides are not important. The more recent view is that it is not useful to attempt to "disentangle" complex and highly interrelated metabolic processes involving multiple lipid and lipoprotein fractions by statistical techniques, especially because such techniques are known to be unreliable when 2 or more predictor variables are highly correlated.[21] Recent epidemiological studies have attempted, instead, to consider the joint effects of triglycerides with other lipids and lipoprotein fractions rather than to try to isolate the "independent" role of triglycerides. These studies suggest that hypertriglyceridemia is an important risk factor for CHD especially when accompanied by low HDL-C[37]; by a high LDL-C:HDL-C ratio[22,38]; or in conjunction with other metabolic abnormalities, such as obesity, hypertension, and abnormal glucose metabolism, often referred to as the insulin resistance syndrome.[37]

Most of the epidemiological data examining the triglyceride-CHD relation in the elderly are from older studies using the old analytic approach of trying to isolate the role of triglycerides. In Manolio's pooled analysis, in which unadjusted relative risks were included from 10 studies, triglycerides ≥ 130 mg/dL compared to a level of less than 100 mg/dL conferred for men a 24% and for women a 39% increased risk of CHD death (P < .05 for both).[33] However, other studies have not confirmed this relationship,[39,40] and there continues to be uncertainty regarding the significance of triglycerides at any age. The triglyceride question will probably never be satisfactorily resolved by observational epidemiological data. Two trials currently underway using triglyceride lowering agents in patients up to age 75 with established CHD will likely provide valuable insight into this perplexing clinical dilemma.[41,42]

Clinical Trial Data: Does Lipid Intervention Prevent Clinical Events in Older Patients?

Although the pathophysiology and the observational data suggest that dyslipidemia is an important reversible cause of CHD in the el-

Table 3
Major Recent Clinical Trials of Cholesterol Lowering for the Prevention of Coronary Heart Disease

| | Age | n | Cumulative CHD Incidence at 5 years | | RRR‡ | ARR | NNT:5 |
			Placebo	Statin			
Secondary Prevention							
4S	<60	3318	27.6%	17.6%	39%	10%	10
	60–70	1126	28.3%	21%	29%	7.3%	14
CARE	<60	2030	26%	21%	20%	5%	20
	60–75	2129	27%	20%	27%	7%	14
Primary Prevention							
WOSCOPS	<55	3225	6.1%	3.5%	40%	2.6%	38
	55–64	3370	9.8%	7.3%	27%	2.5%	40

CHD, coronary heart disease death or nonfatal myocardial infarction; RRR, relative risk reduction; ARR, absolute risk reduction; NNT:5, number needed to treat for 5 years to prevent 1 event; 4S, Scandinavian Simvastatin Survival Study[5]; CARE, Cholesterol and Recurrent Events Study[6]; WOSCOPS, West of Scotland Coronary Prevention Study.[4]
‡ for all RRR, $P \leq .02$

derly, only clinical trial data can definitively demonstrate the efficacy of treatment. Traditionally, trials have enrolled either patients with or without known CHD at baseline (secondary or primary prevention studies, respectively). Results from the major recent trials are summarized in Table 3.

Secondary Prevention Trials

There are 2 main categories of secondary prevention trials: those which assess the effects of lipid lowering diets or drugs on the angiographic appearance of coronary artery lesions ("regression studies") and those in which clinical events such as myocardial infarction and CHD death are the primary outcome measures. Because regression studies have focused almost exclusively on middle-aged patients, I will not discuss these studies.

Until recently, major secondary prevention trials either did not include patients over age 65, or had too few patients to evaluate the results separately by age. In the recently published Scandinavian Simvastatin Survival Study (4S)[5] and the Cholesterol and Recurrent Events trial (CARE),[6] there were sufficient numbers of older patients to allow for separate analyses of the oldest age groups.

The 4S enrolled 4444 men and women age 35 to 70 with documented CHD and average LDL-C of 189 mg/dL. Subjects received either simvastatin, at a dose of 20 or 40 mg/day, or placebo, and were followed for about 5 years. All-cause mortality, CHD death, nonfatal myocardial infarction, and other clinical events such as hospitalization for angina, revascularization procedures, and stroke, were recorded. The relative risk of death from any cause in the treated compared to the placebo group was 0.70 (95% confidence interval, 0.58 to 0.85, $P = 0.0003$). A significant reduction in all-cause mortality was also seen in the subgroup of patients 60 to 70 years old.[5]

The CARE trial extends the results of the 4S to patients up to age 75 and to those with more moderate levels of LDL-C. In this trial, 4159 CHD patients age 21 to 75, with a mean level of total cholesterol of 209 mg/dL and LDL-C of 139 mg/dL, received either pravastatin 40 mg/day or placebo and were followed for 5 years for the occurrence of atherosclerotic events. There was no significant difference in all-cause mortality between the two treatment groups. However, there was a 24% reduction in the primary endpoint (fatal coronary disease and nonfatal myocardial infarction) in the pravastatin group (95% confidence interval, 9% to 36%, $P = 0.003$). Among the patients over age 60 (n = 2129), the relative risk reduction was 27% (95% confidence interval, 12% to 38%, $P < 0.001$) (Table 3). Patients whose LDL-C was below 125 mg/dL at baseline did not benefit from pravastatin.[6]

In both these trials, patients assigned to the statin had a lower incidence of revascularization procedures, unstable angina, and stroke. In neither study was there an increased risk of cancer in the treated patients; however, in CARE, 12 women assigned to pravastatin and only 1 woman assigned to placebo developed breast cancer ($P = 0.002$).

Based on these 2 secondary prevention trials it may be concluded that cholesterol-lowering therapy with statins safely reduces the 5-year risk of CHD morbidity and mortality in elderly patients up to age 70 to 75, with a documented history of CHD and LDL-C above 125 mg/dL. Aside from their CHD, patients entered into these trials were generally healthy; any severe chronic or life threatening disease, with the exception of well-controlled diabetes, excluded a patient from entry. Similarly, good functional status and ability to comply with a medical regimen and study visits were required for entry. Thus it would be inappropriate to extrapolate the results of these trials to frail, sick elderly patients.

Primary Prevention Trials

None of the major primary prevention trials of cholesterol treatment have enrolled elderly patients. Maximum age in these studies ranged from 55 to 64. The West of Scotland Trial, which included 6595 men with a mean LDL-C of 192 mg/dL did have sufficient numbers of patients to perform a subgroup analysis based on age (comparing < 55 with 55 to 64). In this trial, patients received either pravastatin or placebo and were followed for 5 years. As can be seen in Table 3, there was a significant reduction in the combined end point (nonfatal myocardial infarction and CHD death) in both younger and older age groups.[4]

Data from this trial demonstrate the relationship between baseline risk, relative risk reduction, and absolute risk reduction. Baseline risk is represented by the event rate in the control group. Relative risk reduction, analagous to relative risk for observational studies (see above), is defined as the difference between event rates in the two treatment groups divided by the event rate in the control group. The absolute risk reduction, analagous to the excess or attributable risk for observational studies, is defined simply as the difference in the event rates between the 2 treatment groups. Thus, for the older population (Table 3) the baseline 5-year risk was 9.8%, the relative risk reduction with pravastatin was 27% ([9.8% - 7.3%]/7.3%) and the absolute risk reduction was 2.5% (9.8% to 7.3%).

The absolute risk reduction indicates the number of events that will be prevented with treatment. Thus, in a similar cohort of patients pravastatin can be expected to prevent 2.5 CHD deaths or nonfatal MIs for every 100 patients treated for 5 years. Or, put another way, it would be necessary to treat 40 patients with pravastatin for 5 years to prevent one event. This latter formulation (the reciprocal of the absolute risk reduction) has been termed "number needed to treat."

Inspection of the data in Table 3 reveals some useful insights about the importance of baseline risk. For example, in West of Scotland, even though the younger group had a much more pronounced relative risk reduction with pravastatin than the older group (40% compared to 27%), the absolute risk reduction was nearly identical (2.6% vs. 2.5%). This is because the baseline risk was higher in the older group (control group event rate of 9.8% in the older group compared to 6.1% in the younger) and is consistent with the observational data: lower relative risk in the elderly but, because of higher disease incidence, equivalent or even higher absolute risk. Similarly, if one compares the older age groups in CARE and in West of Scotland, it is noteworthy that the relative risk reduction is identical at 27% but the absolute risk reduction in CARE is almost three times as high as for West of Scotland (7% vs. 2.5%), again because of the higher baseline risk for events in the CARE population, all of whom had established heart disease (27% in CARE vs. 9.8% in West of Scotland). Thus the potential benefit to be derived from cholesterol lowering is highly dependent on the baseline risk, and this risk is an important factor for individual treatment decisions.

Extrapolating from Clinical Trial Data in Primary Prevention

In the absence of clinical trial data for elderly persons without CHD, how can we best decide who should be screened and treated?

Table 4
Framingham Risk Equation

A. Identify risk points for each of the following 5 categories:

1. Age

male	points	female	points
65–67	16	61–67	10
68–70	17	68–74	11
71–73	18		
74	19		

2. HDL-cholesterol (mg/dL)

25–26	7	47–50	0
27–29	6	51–55	−1
30–32	5	56–60	−2
33–35	4	61–66	−3
36–38	3	67–73	−4
39–42	2	74–80	−5
43–46	1	81–87	−6
		88–96	−7

3. Total cholesterol (mg/dL)

139–151	−3	220–239	2
152–166	−2	240–262	3
167–182	−1	263–288	4
183–199	0	289–315	5
200–219	1	316–330	6

4. Systolic blood pressure (mm Hg)

98–104	−2	130–139	2
105–112	−1	140–149	3
113–120	0	150–160	4
121–129	1	161–172	5
		173–185	6

5. Other factors

cigarette smoking	4
diabetes	
male	3
female	6
ECG-LVH	9

B. Add up points from sections 1–5
C. Find probability of CHD over 5 years based on point total

Points	Probability (%)	Points	Probability (%)
0–7	1	23	12
8–10	2	24	13
11–13	3	25	14
14	4	26	16
15–16	5	27	17
17	6	28	19
18	7	29	20
19–20	8	30	22
21	9	31	24
22	11	32	25

ECG-LVH, electrocardiographic left ventricular hypertrophy.

Reproduced with permission from Anderson KM, Wilson PWF, Odell PM, et al: An updated coronary risk profile: A statement for health professionals. *Circulation* 83:356–362, 1991.

One recommended approach is to use the available observational and clinical trial data to quantitatively estimate the potential benefits and harm for a given patient, as illustrated in the following example.

Example: A 75-year-old asymptomatic man with a total cholesterol of 240 mg/dL, an HDL-C of 45 mg/dL, systolic blood pressure of 135 mm Hg, who does not smoke and is not diabetic, with a normal electrocardiogram.

Step #1: Estimate this patient's 5-year risk of developing a CHD event. Using the Framingham multivariate risk function which has been conveniently formatted for easy use[43] (Table 4), the estimated risk of a major CHD event over the next 5 years is about 12%.

Step #2: Estimate the expected relative risk reduction. Relative risk reductions for the combined endpoint of fatal CHD and nonfatal myocardial infarction have been remarkably similar in the oldest age groups in the three recent trials of statins: 27% in West of Scotland, 29% in 4S, and 27% in CARE (Table 3). However, because the observational data suggest a lower relative risk in older persons, we will conservatively estimate a relative risk reduction of only 20% for this 75-year-old man.

Step #3: Apply the relative risk reduction to the baseline risk. A 20% risk reduction applied to a 12%–5-year risk yields an absolute risk reduction of 0.024 (0.20 × 0.12). In other words, treating this patient would reduce his 5-year risk of major CHD events from 12% to 9.6% (0.12 - 0.024). Put another way, you would need to treat 42 similar people for 5 years with a statin to prevent 1 event ("number needed to

---

Table 5
Number Needed to Treat for 5 years (NNT:5) to Prevent 1 Event for Various Clinical Scenarios

Patient Profile	Intervention	Event Prevented	NNT:5	Reference
CHD patients age 60–70 with very high cholesterol	simvastatin	CHD death/nonfatal MI	10	5
CHD patients age 60–75 with moderate cholesterol	pravastatin	CHD death/nonfatal MI	14	6
Patients without CHD age 55–64 with very high cholesterol	pravastatin	CHD death/nonfatal MI	40	4
Males age 65 with systolic and diastolic hypertension	diuretic	CHD death/nonfatal MI	35	104
Healthy men over 40 years	aspirin	Myocardial infarction	110	105
Unstable angina	aspirin	Death/myocardial infarction	2	105
Annual fecal occult blood tests		Colon cancer death	1000	105

CHD, coronary heart disease; MI, myocardial infarction.

treat" = 1/absolute risk reduction = 1/0.024). For comparison, for a 75-year-old female diabetic smoker, with systolic hypertension, and a total cholesterol of 240 mg/dL with an HDL-C of 34 mg/dL, whose 5-year CHD risk is around 25%, the "number needed to treat" is 20.

Step #4: Factor in possible harm from therapy.The net benefit of treatment equals the benefit minus the harm. The risk of a serious side effect from a statin that would be equivalent to a myocardial infarction or CHD death is less than 1 in 1000, a risk too small to change the result in Step 3.

At what "number neededed to treat" is treatment indicated? There is no definite answer to this and many other factors must be weighed, including patient preference, cost, inconvenience and other quality of life considerations. It is useful, however, to compare the "numbers needed to treat" for cholesterol treatment for elderly patients and for other commonly used therapeutic interventions (Table 5).

Screening Recommendations

Patients with Established Vascular Disease

Although the secondary prevention trials have focused specifically on patients with established CHD, most authorities apply the same screening and treatment recommendations to those with a history of symptomatic cerebrovascular or peripheral vascular disease because these patients are at an equally high risk of cardiovascular morbidity and mortality.[44,45] Patients of any age with clinically evident atherosclerotic vascular disease who have a life expectancy of 5 or more years, an interest in modifying their lipids, and an acceptable functional status should be screened with a full fasting lipid profile (total cholesterol, triglycerides, LDL-C, and HDL-C).

If screening reveals dyslipidemia that requires treatment, the frequency of further lipid determinations will be guided by the treatment plan, as detailed below. For patients with initially acceptable values, the National Cholesterol Education Program recommends yearly repeat screening.[46] However, it is acceptable to extend this period to several years if the initial screening values are well below treatment thresholds (see below).

Patients without Established Vascular Disease

This is an area of controversy, because, as discussed above, there are no clinical trial data for elderly people without CHD. The National Cholesterol Evaluation Program (NCEP) recommends screening for all people over the age of 20 (no upper age limit).[46] The American College of Physicians, adopting a more conservative, evidence-based approach, considers such screening optional in those aged 65 to 75 years of age and does not recommend screening for those over age 75.[44,47] Given the lack of clear-cut data, decisions for screening and treatment should be based on an assessment of the individual's patient's overall or "baseline" CHD risk and his/her preferences. It is reasonable to screen patients at "high" overall risk for CHD who express an interest in complying with a lipid modifying program. High risk often refers to an annual risk of more than 3% per year.[48] Risk can be estimated either quantitatively through use of the Framingham risk equation (as illustrated above and Table 4) or qualitatively (for example, an elderly patient with at least one of the other risk factors in Table 6 is considered high risk).

If screening is chosen, the NCEP recommends the following approach, which is summarized in Figure 3. Initial screen consists of a nonfasting total cholesterol and HDL-C, with a full lipid profile reserved for those who have either: (1) HDL-C <35 mg/dL; (2) total cholesterol > 240 mg/dL; or (3) total cholesterol 200 to 239 mg/dL and one or more other cardiac risk factors (Table 6). If the LDL-C is more than 130 mg/dL, intervention is indicated and the frequency of repeat testing is determined by the treatment plan. If the LDL-C is less than 130 mg/ dL, treatment is not indicated and repeat screening with a nonfasting

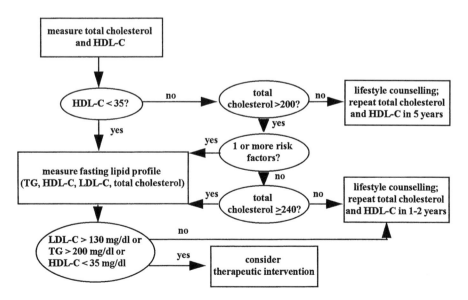

Figure 3: *Screening algorithm for elderly persons without established vascular disease.*

Table 6
National Cholesterol Education Program Cardiac Risk Factors

Positive Risk Factors
- Age:
    Male: ≥45 years
    Female: ≥55 years or premature menopause without estrogen replacement
        therapy
- Family history of premature CHD (definite myocardial infarction or sudden death
  before 55 years of age in father or other male first-degree relative, or before 65
  years of age in mother or other female first-degree relative)
- Current cigarette smoking
- Hypertension (≥140/90 mm Hg, or on antihypertensive medication)
- Low HDL-cholesterol (<35 mg/dL)
- Diabetes mellitus
Negative Risk Factor
- High HDL-cholesterol (≥60 mg/dL)

See National Cholesterol Education Program.[45]

total cholesterol and HDL-C should be repeated in 1 to 2 years. For patients who do not meet criteria for a full lipid profile based on initial screen, repeat screening with a nonfasting total cholesterol and HDL-C should be performed again in 5 years for those with total cholesterol lower than 200, and after 1 to 2 years for those with total cholesterol 200 to 239 mg/dL.

General Treatment Approach

The general approach to diagnosing and treating lipid disorders is described below.

Establishing Baseline Lipid Levels

Because there are many factors, both biological and analytic, contributing to variability in lipid measurements, treatment decisions should be based on a minimum of 2 lipid profiles obtained several weeks apart.[49,50] If values differ by more than 20% on the first 2 profiles, a third should be obtained. This is analagous to the recommended practice of measuring blood pressure at least 3 times over several weeks before either labeling a patient hypertensive or initiating antihypertensive treatment. Lipid profiles should be obtained while patients are in their usual state of health; those obtained during periods of stress, including hospitalization, are often inaccurate.[51]

Secondary Dyslipidemias

If an abnormal lipid profile is obtained and confirmed on repeat testing, secondary causes of hyperlipidemia (Table 7), especially obesity, hypothyroidism, diabetes and excess alcohol intake, should be considered. Although the yield is probably low,[52] it could be argued that it is worth screening for hypothyroidism in elderly patients with an elevated LDL-C, because it is often occult in older individuals and is easily treatable.[45] Diabetes should be considered in anyone with hypertriglyceridemia and low HDL-C, the classic diabetic dyslipidemia. Diabetics are not more likely to have an elevated LDL-C than the general population.[53] In patients with hypertriglyceridemia, inquiry about alcohol intake is indicated. Excess alcohol intake is one of the few circumstances in which hypertriglyceridemia is usually accompanied by elevated levels of HDL-C (estrogen therapy is another). Renal and obstructive liver disease severe enough to affect lipids are rarely occult and thus do not need to be screened for with laboratory testing if the clinical history is negative.

Initial Therapeutic Approach

As the initial therapeutic approach, dietary modification should be encouraged for a minimum of 3 to 6 months. In patients with CHD whose LDL-C is very high, diet and medications may be initiated simultaneously. Other preventive measures, including smoking cessation,

---

Table 7
Secondary Causes of Dyslipidemia

Causes of High LDL-C
    Hypothyroidism
    Nephrotic syndrome
    Obstructive liver disease
Causes of Low HDL-C
    Diabetes
    Smoking
    Overweight
    Chronic renal failure
    Thiazides, loop diuretics, β-blockers, androgens
Causes of High Triglycerides
    Diabetes
    Alcohol
    Excess carbohydrates
    Overweight
    Chronic renal failure

low-dose aspirin, exercise, treatment of hypertension, and, for women, hormone replacement therapy should be addressed, as appropriate.

LDL-C in Patients with Established Vascular Disease

Treatment is indicated for patients up to the age of 75 years with CHD and LDL-C greater than 130 mg/dL. Older patients who are interested and have a reasonable life expectancy (at least 5 years) may also be offered treatment. If LDL-C remains greater than 130 mg/dL after diet, treatment with either a statin, niacin, or a bile acid binding resin should be instituted. Because statins are well tolerated and safe (at least in short term studies) and have been the agents used in the most persuasive clinical trials[5,6] they should be the first choice. However, if cost considerations are important or in patients with very low levels of HDL-C or very high levels of triglycerides, niacin is a reasonable alternative. In an older secondary prevention trial, niacin reduced CHD events and, in a 15-year follow-up study, total mortality.[54,55] Bile acid binding resins should be considered second-line agents because they are not cheaper than statins and are poorly tolerated and difficult to combine with other medications. Fibrates are not currently indicated for the treatment of patients with CHD.

The NCEP sets the goal LDL-C for CHD patients at less than 100 mg/dL and the drug initiation level at 130 mg/dL. If the LDL-C is between 100 and 130 mg/dL either initially or following institution of lipid lowering therapy, it is controversial whether to initiate or intensify drug therapy in an attempt to achieve an LDL-C lower than 100 mg/dL.[56-58] Direct clinical trial data are lacking. In the CARE study there was no benefit from pravastatin in the subgroup of 800 patients with baseline LDL-C lower than 125 mg/dL.[6] This was admittedly a *post hoc* subgroup analysis; however it may be the most relevant data available at this time.

Other data relevant to this issue come from a recent clinical trial of aggressive cholesterol lowering in 1351 patients age 21 to 74 (mean: 61.5 years) recruited 1 to 11 years after coronary artery bypass graft surgery.[59] The mean baseline LDL-C was around 155 mg/dL (range 130 to 175 mg/dL). Patients were randomly assigned to either 2.5 mg/day of lovastatin (which could be increased to 5 mg if LDL-C remained above 140 mg/dL) or 40 mg/day (which could be increased to 80 mg if LDL-C remained above 85 mg/dL). The mean LDL-C in the aggressively treated group was 93 mg/dL, a 40% decrease, compared to 136 mg/dL in the moderate treatment group, a 12% decrease. In the aggressively treated group, the mean percentage of grafts with progression of atherosclerosis, as determined by angiography was 27% compared to 39% for the moderate treatment group ($P < 0.001$). The study was not large enough to detect any difference in clinical end points. Unfortunately this study does not answer the question of whether achieving an LDL-C below 100 mg/dL is better than achieving an LDL-C < 130 mg/dL, because it was not designed to detect differences in clinically meaning-ful end points, such as deaths and myocardial infarctions, and also because it compared a very aggressive lipid regimen to a suboptimal regimen. A dose of 2.5 mg of lovastatin is about a tenth of the usual starting dose of 20 mg and, not unexpectedly, resulted in only a 12% decrease in LDL-C to a level above 130 mg/dL.

It is clear from CARE that some cholesterol lowering is beneficial in CHD patients whose initial LDL-C is above 125–130 mg/dL, but what defines optimal LDL-C is currently unknown. At least 1 meta-analysis of cholesterol-lowering trials for prevention of death in CHD patients suggested that a reduction of total cholesterol of at least 10% to 20% represents a threshold that must be achieved for benefit but that greater reductions are not necessarily associated with more bene-fit.[57] For elderly patients, I do not advise overly aggressive therapy with medications and would consider a reasonable goal for LDL-C to be less than 130 mg/dL.

Patients without CHD who have cerebral or peripheral manifesta-tions of atherosclerotic vascular disease are often treated with the same intensity as those with CHD, although clinical trial data justifying such an approach are lacking.

LDL-C in Patients without Established Vascular Disease

It should be remembered that there are no clinical trial data to support the treatment of hyperlipidemia in elderly patients without CHD. For this reason, healthy, elderly patients should be considered candidates for cholesterol lowering medication only if their CHD risk is high. Even for these patients, it is important to consider cost, safety, inconvenience, side effects, and patient preference for diet or drugs.

If treatment of cholesterol is deemed necessary and desirable by the patient-provider team for individuals 65 to 75 years old, the goal LDL-C should be established based on overall CHD risk. The NCEP guidelines recommend a goal LDL-C of less than 130 mg/dL for patients with 2 or more risk factors (because age is one risk factor, for elderly patients this means 1 additional risk factor, see Table 6).[46] Medications are reserved for patients who cannot achieve an LDL-C below 160 mg/dL with diet. For elderly patients without other risk factors for CHD, treatment should be considered strictly optional at any cholesterol level. Diet may be considered at an LDL-C of 160 mg/dL with drugs reserved for LDL-C above 190 mg/dL.

Bile acid binding resins, gemfibrozil, and statins have all been shown to be beneficial in primary prevention studies in middle aged men. Choice of drug must be individualized based on anticipated side effects, costs, and consideration of HDL-C and triglyceride levels.

Most authorities would not recommend treatment of any level of cholesterol for patients over the age of 75 who do not have CHD. Many are also reluctant to treat women of any age with drugs because their baseline risk of CHD and the relative risk associated with high cholesterol is lower than for men.[60] Furthermore, no primary prevention trial of lipid-lowering drugs has included women of any age.

Low HDL-C and High Triglycerides

The primary approach to low HDL-C and high triglycerides is nonpharmacological. Secondary causes should first be considered and treated if indicated (Table 7). For low HDL-C, weight loss, smoking cessation, moderate alcohol intake, and exercise are useful.[45] Generally, patients who do not drink alcohol should not be advised to start, because of concerns about abuse and dependence. However, patients who inquire may be reassured that alcohol intake not to exceed two drinks a day may raise HDL-C. For high triglycerides, weight loss, exercise, abstention from alcohol, and avoidance of excess carbohydrates are recommended. Carbohydrate intake should not be replaced with excess dietary fat, which can raise total cholesterol and LDL-C. Perhaps most important is adequate glycemic control for diabetics. Hypertriglyceridemia is often highly refractory to treatment in the presence of poorly controlled diabetes.

Low levels of HDL-C and high levels of triglycerides should not be treated with medications in the elderly, although it is appropriate to take into consideration the level of HDL-C and triglycerides in patients for whom medication is indicated for a high LDL-C. Ongoing trials that include patients up to age 75 are examining the benefits of fibric acids, which primarily raise HDL-C and lower triglycerides, for the subset of CHD patients with low levels of HDL-C.[41,42] These trials, scheduled to report results in 1998, will help clarify the role of HDL-C and triglyceride modification for CHD patients.

Dietary Treatment

American Heart Association Step I and Step II Diet

Despite discouraging evidence on the efficacy of diet in the treatment of hyperlipidemia,[61–63] diet is the first-line treatment for patients with lipid disorders. The primary goals of the NCEP and American Heart Association Step I diet are to: (1) achieve ideal body weight; (2) decrease total fat intake to no more than 30% of total calories; (3) decrease saturated fat to no more than 10% of total calories; and (4) reduce daily cholesterol intake to less than 300 mg. The Step II diet further restricts saturated fat intake to 7% of total calories and cholesterol ingestion to no more than 200 mg/day. Fish should be encouraged as a low-fat, protein-rich substitute for red meat. High levels of fish intake have been associated in epidemiological studies with reduced cardiovascular mortality and morbidity.[64] Furthermore, patients should be advised to ingest adequate fiber and incorporate a reasonable exercise regimen into their daily lives (eg, 30 minutes per day of brisk walking). Finally, although alcohol raises HDL-C and has been linked to reduced cardiovascular mortality,[65,66] it should not be actively promoted for obvious reasons. Nevertheless, if a patient is already ingesting up to two alcoholic drinks a day without evidence of medical or social problems, he or she may be reassured that this habit is acceptable.

The least controversial of these dietary recommendations is achieving ideal body weight. Weight loss favorably affects all components of the lipid profile, in particular HDL-C and triglycerides.[67–69] Moreover, obesity has been identified as a risk factor for cardiovascular disease and all-cause mortality in the elderly independent of known risk factors such as lipids and hypertension.[70,71] However, when prescribing diets for the elderly the importance of maintaining adequate nutrition must be emphasized and drastic weight loss efforts should be avoided. The recommendation to decrease intake of saturated fat is also well accepted. However, controversy continues to center around the issue of whether the saturated fat should be preferentially replaced by carbohydrates or by unsaturated fats, such as monounsaurates or polyunsaturates.[72,73] In any case, elderly patients adopting a low saturated fat diet need to be cautioned to maintain adequate calcium intake (from skim dairy products or other sources such as green leafy vegetables and broccoli).

Vitamin Supplementation

The role of vitamin therapy for the prevention of CHD has received a lot of attention in recent years. Interest has focused primarily on folic acid to treat hyperhomocysteinemia and on antioxidants such as vitamin C, vitamin E, and beta-carotene. Strong epidemiological data indicate that hyperhomocysteinemia is an important risk factor for cardiovascular events[74,75] and folate supplementation of 1 to 2 mg/day can normalize homocysteine levels.[76] Because no clinical trials have yet documented the efficacy of supplemental folate for prevention of cardiovascular events, such therapy is not recommended; however, it is certainly appropriate to encourage patients to maintain adequate dietary intake of folate.

Epidemiological data also suggest an association between high intake of supplemental or dietary antioxidant vitamins, especially beta carotene and vitamin E, and reduced risk of atherosclerotic vascular disease in both young and older populations.[77,78]

Results from clinical trials reported in the last few years, however, have failed to confirm these findings. These trials make it quite clear that supplemental beta- carotene is not protective against either cancer or cardiovascular disease and may in fact be harmful in smokers.[79,80] Thus, patients should be actively discouraged from using over-the-counter beta-carotene supplements. The usefulness of vitamin E, however, remains controversial. One large trial found no benefit; however the dose of vitamin E may have been suboptimal.[79] A second randomized controlled trial in patients of all ages (mean: 61 years) with established CHD demonstrated a statistically and clinically significant 47% reduction in myocardial infarction and CHD deaths in patients receiving vitamin E (at a higher dose). Total mortality was slightly but not significantly increased in the vitamin E group.[81] Thus, vitamin E supplementation appears to be a promising but as yet unproven modality.

When counseling elderly patients wishing to reduce their risk for CHD, it is important for the provider to help the patient appreciate the difference between therapies of proven and those of uncertain value. The elderly may be particularly susceptible to exaggerated media or commercial claims and may waste money, often from limited incomes, on useless or even potentially harmful products. Supplemental vitamin E, for example, even in relatively low doses may not be harmless; a nonsignificant excess of fatal hemorrhagic stroke was noted in one large clinical trial.[79]

Hormone Replacement Therapy

Epidemiological data strongly suggest that postmenopausal women who use hormone replacement therapy, either estrogen alone or in combination with a progestin, have about half the CHD risk as those who do not.[82] Whether elderly women are also protected is less clear, because most of the available studies have not included many women over the age of 65. However, in the recent 16-year follow-up report from the Nurses Health Study, the risk of CHD among women age 60 to 71 years old was 34% lower among hormone users compared to nonusers.[82] A similar beneficial effect in elderly women was noted in at least one other large observational study.[83] The Women's Health Initiative, a large clinical trial funded by the National Institutes of Health, is expected to provide more definitive information on the risks and benefits of hormone replacement therapy.

Estrogen-only and combined estrogen-progestin regimens reduce LDL-C by about 10% to 15%. HDL-C increases by 10%–15% with unopposed estrogen and somewhat less with combined regimens. All regimens tend to raise triglycerides by 15% to 25%,[84] which may be problematic in women with a history of high triglycerides. Ultimately, decisions about hormone replacement therapy must be based on an overall assessment of an individual patient's risk for osteoporosis and breast cancer, as well as cardiovascular disease. If a choice is made to use hormone replacement therapy, assessment of lipids should not be made until the patient has been on the chosen regimen for at least 3 to 6 months and triglycerides should be monitored in women with high baseline levels.

Medications

The major categories of lipid altering medications include bile acid binding resins, niacin, HMG co-A reductase inhibitors, also known as "statins," and fibrates (Table 8). Excellent reviews of lipid-lowering medications are available[85]; the comments that follow focus primarily on issues relevant to prescribing these medications in the elderly.

Patients started on lipid-lowering agents should have repeat lipids and liver function tests checked within the first 6 to 8 weeks of starting therapy and then every 3 to 6 months for the first year and once or twice a year thereafter. Closer monitoring may be advisable for patients with hepatic dysfunction, renal insufficiency, and in frail patients on multiple medications.

Niacin

The advantages of niacin are that it is cheap and that, in addition to lowering LDL-C (by 20% to 30%), it also lowers triglycerides (by 20% to 40%) and raises HDL-C (by 10% to 30%). Niacin has not been extensively studied in older patients. In one randomized controlled trial of wax-matrix sustained release niacin, subjects were analyzed by age (20 to 50 vs. 50 to 70 years). Compared to younger patients assigned to niacin, older patients had significantly greater reductions in total cholesterol, LDL-C and triglycerides. HDL-C was increased significantly in the niacin treated groups, with no differences between older

Table 8
Commonly Used Lipid-lowering Medications

Drug	*Usual Dose Range (total daily dose)*	*Lipid Effect** *LDL-C*	*HDL-C*	*TG*
Statins				
Atorvastatin	10–80 mg	↓ 20%–40%	↑ 2%–8%	↓ 20%–40%
Fluvastatin	10–40 mg	↓ 15%–25%	↑ 2%–8%	↓ 10%–15%
Lovastatin	10–80 mg	↓ 20%–30%	↑ 2%–8%	↓ 10%–15%
Pravastatin	10–40 mg	↓ 20%–30%	↑ 2%–8%	↓ 10%–15%
Simvastatin	5–40 mg	↓ 25%–40%	↑ 2%–8%	↓ 10%–15%
Gemfibrozil	1200 mg	↓ 5%–15%	↑ 5%–20%	↓ 30%–40%
Resins				
Colestipol	10–20 gm	↓ 15%–25%	↑ 3%–5%	↑ 0%–10%
Cholestyramine	8–16 gm	↓ 15%–25%	↑ 3%–5%	↑ 0%–10%
Niacin	1.5–4.5 gm	↓ 20%–30%	↑ 10%–30%	↓ 20%–40%

* Lipid effects are for a mid-range dose

and younger patients. Furthermore, there were fewer side effects reported by the older compared to the younger patients and compliance was equally good. However, there was a higher incidence of elevation in liver function tests among older patients; nevertheless, in the majority of these patients the liver function tests remained within the normal range.[86]

In a retrospective cohort study of 969 predominantly older men (mean age 61.7 years), controlled-release niacin was effective but was discontinued by close to half of all patients because of adverse effects, including worsening of glycemic control in over 40% of diabetics. Probable or possible niacin-induced hepatotoxicity was documented in fewer than 5% of patients. There was no association between age and hepatic dysfunction.[87]

In summary, niacin can be used in older patients, with proper monitoring of liver function. It should probably be avoided in elderly diabetics. Peptic ulcer disease and gout may occasionally be exacerbated by this agent. Overall, one can expect that about 50% to 70% of elderly patients will be able to stay on this medication long-term.[88] In order to maximize compliance, patient education is critical. Specifically, patients need to be informed that flushing is a very common but harmless side effect that generally wanes with time. To minimize this reaction, niacin should be titrated up very slowly over several weeks and it should be ingested with meals but not with hot liquids. Pretreatment with one aspirin may minimize the flushing reaction.[89] Finally, patients must be cautioned against substituting a controlled-release niacin preparation, available over-the-counter, for regular, crystalline niacin. Controlled-release niacin, in daily doses over 1.5 g has been associated with a high incidence of hepatotoxicity.[90]

Bile Acid Binding Resins

Resins such as cholestyramine and colestipol typically reduce LDL-C by 15% to 25%. HDL-C and triglycerides tend to increase modestly. Cholestyramine was the intervention used in the Lipid Research Clinics Coronary Primary Prevention Trial, the first major clinical trial to demonstrate reductions in CHD morbidity and mortality with cholesterol-lowering.[91] While these nonsystemic drugs are generally safe, they can be difficult to use in the elderly for 2 reasons. First, they can cause distressing gastrointestinal side effects such as bloating and constipation.[92] Adequate intake of fiber, fluids and exercise can often ameliorate these problems but clinical experience suggests that many elderly patients do not tolerate these agents well. Second, other medications must be taken either 1 hour before or 3 to 4 hours after the ingestion of resins, in order to avoid binding in the intestinal tract. This constraint is a nuisance and often interferes with patient compliance. In fact, the discontinuance rate of resins among patients aged 71 to 80 has been shown to be close to 60%.[88]

Resins are particularly useful as second line drugs for lowering LDL-C both for patients who cannot tolerate or do not respond to other agents or in conjunction with other agents to maximize the cholesterol-lowering effect. Hypertriglyceridemia may be precipitated by these agents; they should be avoided in those with initially high levels of triglycerides.

HMG Co–A Reductase Inhibitors (Statins)

Statins are the best tolerated and most potent cholesterol-lowering medications currently available. Currently there are 5 available agents (fluvastatin, pravastatin, lovastatin, simvastatin, and atorvastatin) with varying potency. Lovastatin and pravastatin are considered equipotent; within the ususal dose range of 20 to 40 mg/day, they lower LDL-C by 20% to 30%. Simvastatin is about twice as potent, lowering LDL-C by about 40% at a dose of 40 mg/day. Fluvastatin tends to be roughly half as potent as lovastatin and pravastatin. All statins tend to have minimal HDL-C-raising and triglyceride-lowering effects, with the exception of atorvastatin that can lower triglycerides by 20% to 40%.[93,94] Otherwise there do not appear to be major differences among the statins in either efficacy or tolerability.

The best information on the efficacy, side effects, and safety of statins in the elderly comes from the Cholesterol Reduction in Senior Persons trial that enrolled 431 patient over the age of 65 (mean age 71) with baseline LDL-C between 160 and 220 mg/dL. Patients were randomly assigned to either placebo or lovastatin 20 or 40 mg/day and followed for 1 year. Reductions in total cholesterol (17% to 20%) and LDL-C (24% to 28%) were observed in both the lovastatin groups; the higher dose of lovastatin did not result in significantly greater reductions than the lower dose. In this elderly population, self-report of both abdominal pain and changes in visual acuity were more common in the drug-treated group. Nevertheless, prevalence of side effects was low and overall adherence was high.[63] The safety and efficacy of lovastatin and other statins in the elderly has been confirmed in other trials.[95,96]

In summary, statins are highly effective and well tolerated in the elderly. Muscle aches and pains without creatine kinase elevations and nonspecific GI complaints are occasionally seen. Hepatoxicity, severe myopathy, or rhabdomyolysis are rare complications. There has been speculation but currently no substantial cause for concern about the potential long-term carcinogenic effects of these agents.[97]

Fibrates

The only fibrate currently available in the United States is gemfibrozil. In the Helsinki Heart Study this medication was found to decrease the incidence of CHD morbidity and mortality in hypercholesterolemic middle aged men without prior evidence of CHD.[98] However, the finding of a nonsignificant excess of fatal intracranial hemorrhage and of accidental and violent deaths in the gemfibrozil treated group raised concerns about the safety of this drug. A large-scale secondary prevention trial scheduled to report results at the end of 1998, is evaluating whether gemfibrozil prevents nonfatal myocardial infarction and CHD death in men with low levels of HDL-C (mean of 32 mg/dL) and normal levels of LDL-C (mean of 111 mg/dL). In this study, 72% of patients are over the age of 60.[99] Gemfibrozil reliably lowers triglycerides by 30% to 40%; raises HDL-C by 15% to 20%; and lowers LDL-C by 5% to 15%. This drug is especially useful for patients with high triglycerides. It is now available in an inexpensive generic form and is generally well tolerated. Nonspecific gastrointestinal complaints are the most common side effects. Development of gallstones and potentiation of the effect of warfarin may also be noted.

Combination Therapy

Combination therapy may be required for patients with severe elevations in LDL-C unresponsive to maximal doses of a single agent or for patients with combined hyperlipidemia in whom both cholesterol and triglyceride lowering is required. A statin combined with a resin is a particularly useful combination for lowering LDL-C that cannot be effectively treated with one drug.[100] For patients with combined hyperlipidemia, atorvastatin may effectively lower both LDL-C and triglycerides.[93] Alternatively, statins may be combined with either gemfibrozil or with niacin, although patients must be carefully monitored for the occurrence of myopathy.[101] Because combination therapy may increase the risk of side effects and toxicity, it is rarely indicated in the elderly.

Conclusions

The value of lowering LDL-C in patients with known CHD has been established and should be offered to patients of any age who are in reasonable health and have an interest in lowering their cholesterol. For elderly patients without CHD, decisions about screening and treatment must be individualized, based on an overall assessment of CHD risk, other health issues, and patient interest. The federally sponsored ALLHAT study which is investigating the value of cholesterol intervention in several thousand high risk older patients will likely yield important new insights into the relative benefits and harms of this therapy in the elderly. Other ongoing trials which include elderly patients will also be available over the next several years to help inform clinical decision-making.[102]

References

1. Parker SL, Tong T, Bolden S, et al: Cancer statistics, 1996. *CA Cancer J Clin* 46:5–7, 1996.
2. Walsh JME, Grady D: Treatment of hyperlipidemia in women. *JAMA* 274:1152–1158, 1995.
3. American Heart Association. *Heart and Stroke Facts: 1996 Statistical Supplement.* 1995.
4. Shepherd J, Cobbe SM, Ford I, et al: Prevention of coronary heart disease with pravastatin in men with hypercholesterolemia. *N Engl J Med* 333: 1301–1307, 1995.
5. Scandinavian Simvastatin Survivial Study Group: Randomised trial of cholesterol lowering in 4444 patients with coronary heart disease: The Scandinavian Simvastatin Survival Study (4S). *Lancet* 344:1383–1389, 1994.
6. Sacks FM, Pfeffer MA, Moye LA, et al: The effect of pravastatin on coronary events after myocardial infarction in patients with average cholesterol levels. *N Engl J Med* 335:1001–1009, 1996.
7. Levine GN, Keaney JF, Vita JA: Cholesterol reduction in cardiovascular disease: Clinical benefits and possible mechanisms. *N Engl J Med* 332: 512–521, 1995.
8. Libby P: Molecular bases of the acute coronary syndromes. *Circulation* 91:2844–2850, 1995.
9. Falk E, Shah PK, Fuster V: Coronary plaque disruption. *Circulation* 92: 657–671, 1995.
10. Davies MJ: The composition of coronary-artery plaques. *N Engl J Med* 336:1312–1314, 1997.
11. Burke AP, Farb A, Malcom GT, et al: Coronary risk factors and plaque morphology in men with coronary disease who died suddenly. *N Engl J Med* 336:1276–1282, 1997.
12. Anderson TJ, Meredith IT, Yeung AC, et al: The effect of cholesterol-lowering and antioxidant therapy on endothelium-dependent coronary vasomotion. *N Engl J Med* 332:488–493, 1995.
13. Leung W, Lau C, Wong C: Beneficial effect of cholesterol-lowering therapy on coronary endothelium-dependent relaxation in hypercholesterolaemic patients. *Lancet* 341:1496–1500, 1993.
14. Lacoste L, Lam JYT, Hung J, et al: Hyperlipidemia and coronary disease: Correction of the increased thrombogenic potential with cholesterol reduction. *Circulation* 92:3172–3177, 1995.
15. Brown BG, Zhao X, Sacco DE, et al: Lipid lowering and plaque regression: New insights into prevention of plaque disruption and clinical events in coronary disease. *Circulation* 87:1781–1791, 1993.
16. Lacko AG, Miller NE: International Symposium on the Role of HDL in Disease Prevention: Report on a Meeting. *J Lipid Res* 38:1267–1273, 1997.
17. Gwynne JT: HDL and atherosclerosis: An update. *Clin Cardiol* 14:I-17-I-24, 1991.
18. Brown MS, Goldstein JL: Lipoprotein metabolism in the macrophage: Implications for cholesterol deposition in atherosclerosis. *Ann Rev Biochem* 52:223–261, 1983.
19. Mackness MI, Abbott CA, Arrol S, et al: The role of high density lipopro-

tein and lipid-soluble antioxidant vitamins in inhibiting low-density lipoprotein oxidation. *Biochem J* 294:829–835, 1993.

20. Austin MA: Plasma triglyceride and coronary heart disease. *Arterioscl Thromb* 11:2–14, 1991.

21. Ginsberg HN: Is hypertriglyceridemia a risk factor for atherosclerotic cardiovascular disease? A simple question with a complicated answer. *Ann Intern Med* 126:912–914, 1997.

22. Stampfer JJ, Krauss RM, Ma J, et al: A prospective study of triglyceride level, low- density lipoprotein particle diameter, and risk of myocardial infarction. *JAMA* 276:882–888, 1996.

23. LaRosa JC: Triglycerides and coronary risk in women and the elderly. *Arch Intern Med* 157:961–968, 1997.

24. Ettinger WH, Wahl PW, Kuller LH, et al: Lipoprotein lipids in older people: Results from the Cardiovascular Health Study. *Circulation* 86:858–869, 1992.

25. Kannel WB: Range of serum cholesterol values in the population developing coronary artery disease. *Am J Cardiol* 76:69C–77C, 1995.

26. Sempos CT, Cleeman JI, Carroll MD, et al: Prevalence of high blood cholesterol among US adults. *JAMA* 269:3009–3014, 1993.

27. Manolio TA, Furberg CD, Wahl PW, et al: Eligibility for cholesterol referral in community-dwelling older adults. *Ann Intern Med* 116:641–649, 1992.

28. Krumholz HM, Seeman RE, Merrill SS, et al: Lack of association between cholesterol and coronary heart disease mortality and morbidity and all-cause mortality in persons older than 70 years. *JAMA* 272:1335–1340, 1994.

29. Kronmal RA, Cain KC, Zhan Y, et al: Total serum cholesterol levels and mortality risk as a function of age: A report based on the Framingham data. *Arch Intern Med* 153:1065–1073, 1993.

30. Benfante R, Reed D: Is elevated serum cholesterol level a risk factor for coronary heart disease in the elderly? *JAMA* 263:393–396, 1990.

31. Sorkin JD, Andres R, Muller DC, et al: Cholesterol as a risk factor for coronary heart disease in elderly men: The Baltimore Longitudinal Study of Aging. *Ann Epidemiol* 2:59–67, 1992.

32. Anderson KM, Castelli WP, Levy D: Cholesterol and mortality: 30 years of follow-up from the Framingham study. *JAMA* 257:2176–2180, 1987.

33. Manolio TA, Pearson TA, Wenger NK, et al: Cholesterol and heart disease in older persons and women: Review of an NHLBI Workshop. *Ann Epidemiol* 2:161–176, 1992.

34. Cori M, Guralnik JM, Salive ME, et al: Clarifying the direct relation between total cholesterol levels and death from coronary heart disease in older persons. *Ann Intern Med* 126:753–760, 1997.

35. Malenka DJ, Baron JA: Cholesterol and coronary heart disease: The importance of patient-specific attributable risk. *Arch Intern Med* 148:2247–2252, 1988.

36. Corti M, Gurainik JM, Salive ME, et al: HDL cholesterol predicts coronary heart disease mortality in older persons. *JAMA* 274:539–544, 1995.

37. Tenkanen L, Pietila K, Manninen V, et al: The triglyceride issue revisited: Findings from the Helsinki Heart Study. *Arch Intern Med* 154:2714–2720, 1994.

38. Manninen V, Tenkanen L, Koskinen P, et al: Joint effects of serum triglyceride and LDL cholesterol and HDL cholesterol concentrations on coro-

nary heart disease risk in the Helsinki Heart Study: Implications for treatment. *Circulation* 85:37–45, 1992.

39. Benfante RJ, Reed CM, MacLean CJ, et al: Risk factors in middle age that predict early and late onset of coronary heart disease. *J Clin Epidemiol* 42: 95–104, 1989.

40. Criqui MH, Heiss G, Cohn R, et al: Plasma triglyceride level and mortality from coronary heart disease. *N Engl J Med* 328:1220–1225, 1993.

41. Rubins HB, Robins SJ, Iwane MK, et al: Rationale and design of the Department of Veterans Affairs High-Density Lipoprotein Cholesterol Intervention Trial (HIT) for secondary prevention of coronary artery disease in men with low high-density lipoprotein cholesterol and desirable low-density lipoprotein cholesterol. *Am J Cardiol* 71:45–52, 1993.

42. Goldbourt U, Behar S, Reiss-Reicher H, et al: Rationale and design of a secondary prevention trial of increasing serum high-density lipoprotein cholesterol and reducing triglycerides in patients with clinically manifest atherosclerotic heart disease (the Bezafibrate Infarction Prevention Trial). *Am J Cardiol* 71:909–915, 1993.

43. Anderson KM, Wilson PWF, Odell PM, et al: An updated coronary risk profile: A statement for health professionals. *Circulation* 83:356–362, 1991.

44. American College of Physicians: Guidelines for using serum cholesterol, high- density lipoprotein cholesterol, and triglyceride levels as screening tests for preventing coronary heart disease in adults. *Ann Intern Med* 124:515–517, 1996.

45. National Cholesterol Education Program. Second Report of the Expert Panel on Detection, Evaluation, and Treatment of High Blood Cholesterol in Adults (Adult Treatment Panel II). NIH Publication No. 93–3095, 1993.

46. Expert Panel on Detection, Evaluation, and Treatment of High Blood Cholesterol in Adults: Summary of the second report of the National Cholesterol Education Program (NCEP) Expert Panel on Detection, Evaluation, and Treatment of High Blood Cholesterol in Adults (Adult Treatment Panel II). *JAMA* 269:3015–3023, 1993.

47. Garber AM, Browner WS, Hulley SB: Cholesterol screening in asymptomatic adults, revisited. *Ann Intern Med* 124:518–531, 1996.

48. Ramsy LE, Haq IU, Jackson PR, et al: Targeting lipid-lowering drug therapy for primary prevention of coronary disease: An updated Sheffield table. *Lancet* 348:387–388, 1996.

49. Cooper GR, Myers GL, Smith J, et al: Blood lipid measurements: Variations and practical utility. *JAMA* 267:1652–1660, 1992.

50. Wilson PWF: Cholesterol screening: Once is not enough. *Arch Intern Med* 155:2146–2147, 1995.

51. Leidig GA, Pasternak RC, Horowitz G, et al: Effects of heparin and cardiac catheterization on serum lipoprotein and triglyceride levels. *Am J Cardiol* 74:47–52, 1994.

52. Evans P, Gray DP: Value of screening for secondary causes of hyperlipidaemia in general practice. *BMJ* 309:509–510, 1994.

53. Laakso M, Ronnemaa T, Lehto S, et al: Does NIDDM increase the risk for coronary heart disease similarly in both low- and high-risk populations? *Diabetologia* 38:487–493, 1995.

54. The Coronary Drug Project Research Group: Clofibrate and niacin in coronary heart disease. *JAMA* 231:360–381, 1975.

55. Canner PL, Berge KG, Wenger NK, et al: Fifteen year mortality in Coro-

nary Drug Project patients: Long-term benefit with niacin. *J Am Coll Cardiol* 8:1245–1255, 1986.

56. Rubins HB: Cholesterol in patients with coronary heart disease: How low should we go? *JGIM* 10:464–471, 1995.
57. Marchioli R, Marfisi R, Carinci F, et al: Meta-analysis, clinical trials, and transferability of research results into practice: the case of cholesterol-lowering interventions in the secondary prevention of coronary heart disease. *Arch Intern Med* 156:1158–1172, 1996.
58. Kreisberg RA: Cholesterol-lowering and coronary atherosclerosis: Good news and bad news. *Am J Med* 101:455–458, 1996.
59. The Post Coronary Artery Bypass Graft Trial Investigators: The effect of aggressive lowering of low-density lipoprotein cholesterol levels and low-dose anticoagulation on obstructive changes in saphenous-vein coronary-artery bypass grafts. *N Engl J Med* 336:153–162, 1997.
60. Hulley SB, Newman TB: Cholesterol in the elderly: Is it important? *JAMA* 272:1372–1374, 1994.
61. Hunninghake DB, Stein EA, Dujovne CA, et al: The efficacy of intensive dietary therapy alone or combined with lovastatin in outpatients with hypercholesterolemia. *N Engl J Med* 328:1213–1219, 1993.
62. Ives DG, Kuller LH, Traven ND: Use and outcomes of a cholesterol-lowering intervention for rural elderly subjects. *Am J Prev Med* 9:274–281, 1993.
63. LaRosa JC, Applegate W, Crouse III JR, et al: Cholesterol lowering in the elderly: results of the Cholesterol Reduction in Seniors Program (CRISP) pilot study. *Arch Intern Med* 154:529–539, 1994.
64. Daviglus ML, Stamler J, Orencia AJ, et al: Fish consumption and the 30-year risk of fatal myocardial infarction. *N Engl J Med* 336:1046–1053, 1997.
65. Suh I, Shaten J, Cutler JA, et al: Alcohol use and mortality from coronary heart disease: The role of high-density lipoprotein cholesterol. *Ann Intern Med* 116:881–887, 1992.
66. Stampfer MJ, Colditz GA, Willett WC, et al: A prospective study of moderate alcohol consumption and the risk of coronary disease and stroke in women. *N Engl J Med* 319:267–273, 1988.
67. Wood PD, Stefanick ML, Dreon DM, et al: Changes in plasma lipids and lipoproteins in overweight men during weight loss through dieting as compared with exercise. *N Engl J Med* 319:1173–1179, 1988.
68. Wood PD, Stefanick ML, Williams PT, et al: The effects on plasma lipoproteins of a prudent weight-reducing diet, with or without exercise, in overweight men and women. *N Engl J Med* 325:461–466, 1991.
69. Schaefer EJ, Lichtenstein AH, Lamon-Fava S, et al: Body weight and low-density lipoprotein cholesterol changes after consumption of a low-fat ad libitum diet. *JAMA* 274:1450–1455, 1995.
70. Harris T, Cook EF, Garrison R, et al: Body mass index and mortality among nonsmoking older persons. *JAMA* 259:1520–1524, 1988.
71. Cornoni-Huntley JC, Harris TB, Everett DF, et al: An overview of body weight of older persons, including the impact on mortality: The National Health and Nutrition Examination Survey I—Epidemiologic Follow-up Study. *J Clin Epidemiol* 44:743–753, 1991.
72. Connor WE, Connor SL: Should a low-fat, high-carbohydrate diet be recommended for everyone? *N Engl J Med* 337:562–563, 1997.
73. Katan MB, Grundy SM, Willett SC: Beyond low-fat diets. *N Engl J Med* 337:563–566, 1997.

74. Nygard O, Nordrehaug JE, Refsum H, et al: Plasma homocysteine levels and mortality in patients with coronary artery disease. *N Engl J Med* 337:230–236, 1997.
75. Stampfer MJ, Malinow MR, Willett WC, et al: A prospective study of plasma homocyst(e)ine and risk of myocardial infarction in US physicians. *JAMA* 268:877–881, 1992.
76. Stampfer MJ, Malinow MR: Can lowering homocysteine levels reduce cardiovascular risk? *N Engl J Med* 332:328–329, 1995.
77. Kushi LH, Folsom AR, Prineas RJ, et al: Dietary antioxidant vitamins and death from coronary heart disease in postmenopausal women. *N Engl J Med* 334:1156–1162, 1996.
78. Jha P, Flather M, Lonn E, et al: The antioxidant vitamins and cardiovascular disease: A critical review of epidemiologic and clinical trial data. *Ann Intern Med* 123:860–872, 1995.
79. The Alpha-Tocopherol Beta Carotene Cancer Prevention Study Group: The effect of vitamin E and beta carotene on the incidence of lung cancer and other cancers in male smokers. *N Engl J Med* 330:1029–1035, 1994.
80. Hennekens CH, Buring JE, Manson JE, et al: Lack of effect of long-term supplementation with beta carotene on the incidence of malignant neoplasms and cardiovascular disease. *N Engl J Med* 334:1145–1149, 1996.
81. Stephens NG, Schofield PM, Kelly F, et al: Randomized controlled trial of vitamin E in patients with coronary disease: Cambridge Heart Antioxidant Study (CHAOS). *Lancet* 347:781–786, 1996.
82. Grodstein F, Stampfer MJ, Manson JE, et al: Postmenopausal estrogen and progestin use and the risk of cardiovascular disease. *N Engl J Med* 335:453–461, 1996.
83. Henderson BE, Paganini-Hill A, Ross RK: Decreased mortality in users of estrogen replacement therapy. *Arch Intern Med* 151:75–78, 1991.
84. The Writing Group for the PEPI Trial: Effects of estrogen or estrogen/progestin regimens on heart disease risk factors in postmenopausal women: The Postmenopausal Estrogen/Progestin Interventions (PEPI) Trial. *JAMA* 273:199–208, 1996.
85. Larsen ML, Illingworth DR: Drug treatment of dyslipoproteinemia. *Med Clin North Am* 78:225–245, 1994.
86. Keenan JM, Bae C, Fontaine PL, et al: Treatment of hypercholesterolemia: Comparison of younger versus older patients using wax-matrix sustained-release niacin. *J Am Geriatr Soc* 40:12–18, 1992.
87. Gray DR, Morgan T, Chretien SD, et al: Efficacy and safety of controlled-release niacin in dyslipoproteinemic veterans. *Ann Intern Med* 121:252–258, 1994.
88. Schectman G, Hiatt J, Hartz A: Evaluation of the effectiveness of lipid-lowering therapy (bile acid sequestrants, niacin, psyllium and lovastatin) for treating hypercholesterolemia in veterans. *Am J Cardiol* 71:759–765, 1993.
89. Jungnickel PW, Maloley PA, Vander Tuin EL, et al: Effect of two aspirin pretreatment regimens on niacin-induced cutaneous reactions. *J Gen Intern Med* 12:591–596, 1997.
90. McKenney JM, Proctor JD, Harris S, et al: A comparison of the efficacy and toxic effects of sustained- vs immediate-release niacin in hypercholesterolemic patients. *JAMA* 271:672–677, 1994.
91. The Lipid Research Clinics Coronary Primary Prevention Trial Results. II.The relationship of reduction in incidence of coronary heart disease to cholesterol lowering. *JAMA* 251:365–374, 1984.

92. Garg A, Grundy SM: Cholestyramine therapy for dyslipidemia in non-insulin- dependent diabetes mellitus. *Ann Intern Med* 121:416–422, 1994.
93. Bakker-Arkema RG, Davidson MH, Goldstein RJ, et al: Efficacy and safety of a new HMG-CoA reductase inhibitor, Atorvastatin, in patients with hypertriglyceridemia. *JAMA* 275:128–133, 1996.
94. Hsu I, Spinler SA, Johnson NE: Comparative evaluation of the safety and efficacy of HMG-CoA reductase inhibitor monotherapy in the treatment of primary hypercholesterolemia. *Ann Pharmacother* 29:743–759, 1995.
95. Glasser SP, DiBianco R, Effron BA, et al: The efficacy and safety of pravastatin in patients aged 60 to 85 years with low-density lipoprotein cholesterol >160 mg/dL. *Am J Cardiol* 77:83–85, 1996.
96. Shear CL, Franklin FA, Stinnett S, et al: [(EXCEL)] study results: Effect of patient characteristics on lovastatin-induced changes in plasma concentrations of lipids and lipoproteins. *Circulation* 85:1293–1303, 1992.
97. Newman TB, Hulley SB: Carcinogenicity of lipid-lowering drugs. *JAMA* 275:55–60, 1996.
98. Frick MH, Elo O, Haapa K, et al: Helsinki Heart Study: Primary prevention trial with gemfibrozil in middle-aged men with dyslipidemia. *N Engl J Med* 317:1237–1245, 1987.
99. Rubins HB, Robins SJ, Collins D: The Veterans Affairs High-Density Lipoprotein Intervention Trial: Baseline characteristics of normocholesterolemic men with coronary artery disease and low levels of high-density lipoprotein cholesterol. *Am J Cardiol* 78:572–575, 1996.
100. Brown G, Albers JJ, Fisher LD, et al: Regression of coronary artery disease as a result of intensive lipid-lowering therapy in men with high levels of apolipoprotein B. *N Engl J Med* 323:1289–1298, 1990.
101. Wiklund O, Bergman M, Bondjers G, et al: Pravastatin and gemfibrozil alone and in combination for the treatment of hypercholesterolemia. *Am J Med* 94:13–20, 1993.
102. Cholesterol Treatment Trialists' (CTT) Collaboration: Protocol for a prospective collaborative overview of all current and planned randomized trials of cholesterol treatment regimens. *Am J Cardiol* 75:1130–1134, 1995.
103. Rubin SM, Sidney S, Black DM, et al: High blood cholesterol in elderly men and the excess risk for coronary heart disease. *Ann Intern Med* 113:916–920, 1990.
104. MRC Working Party: Medical Research Council trial of treatment of hypertension in older adults: Principal results. *BMJ* 304:405–412, 1992.
105. Rajkumar SV, Sampathkumar P, Gustafson AB: Number needed to treat is a simple measure of treatment efficacy for clinicians. *JGIM* 11:357–359, 1996.

Chapter 15

Arrhythmias

Charles C. Gornick, Arthur H. L. From

Among older patients, the diagnosis and treatment of cardiac arrhythmias must take into consideration the severity of any concomitant heart and, or lung disease. These diseases are frequently causally related to the arrhythmia and, even if not, may worsen symptomatology when an arrhythmia occurs. Clinical presentation is quite variable. In some patients, there is a history of arrhythmias complicating long-established heart disease, whereas in others a new arrhythmia may develop without clinically evident heart disease. Furthermore, significant symptoms may only develop when an acute illness such as pneumonia or acute myocardial infarction is superimposed upon a previously well-tolerated arrhythmia. It is important that the physician look carefully for these precipitating factors as well as others including congestive heart failure, acid/base and electrolyte abnormalities, and adverse drug effects.

Age-associated alterations in the conduction system may result in conduction delays that facilitate the development of reentrant arrhythmias. Additionally, if an appropriate arrhythmia substrate is present, an age or disease associated increase in the frequency of premature atrial or ventricular beats can trigger supraventricular or ventricular arrhythmias. Lastly, although the frequency and distribution of cardiac arrhythmias changes with age, it is not uncommon to have older individuals present with atrioventricular (AV) nodal or AV reentry tachycardia, arrhythmias that are more often encountered among the young. The importance of recognizing such arrhythmias is that specific treatment options including catheter ablation may be applied equally well to the elderly patient.

From *Clinical Cardiology in the Elderly. Second Edition,* edited by Elliot Chesler. © 1999, Futura Publishing Company, Armonk, NY.

Bradyarrhythmias

Sinus Node Dysfunction

Sinus node dysfunction is the most common bradyarrhythmia encountered among the elderly (Figure 1).[1-4] It may manifest as isolated bradycardia with symptoms such as fatigue, exercise intolerance, dizziness or syncope.[5] It may also present as the so called "tachycardia-bradycardia syndrome."[6] In the latter, symptoms relating to either bradycardia or tachycardia may predominate. The usual tachyarrhythmias are atrial fibrillation or flutter but other primary atrial tachycardias may also occur. With spontaneous or therapeutic interruption of the tachyarrhythmia, severe symptomatic bradycardia may supervene because of "overdrive" suppression of sinus node function. Also, pharmacological treatment aimed at controlling the tachyarrhythmia, by further depressing sinus node function, may precipitate or accentuate bradycardia.

Various invasive pacing tests that measure sinus node recovery time and sino-atrial conduction time have been devised to assess sinus node function. Unfortunately, while these tests are fairly specific (90%), they are insensitive and normal in up to 30% of individuals ultimately proven to have symptomatic sinus node dysfunction.[5] Thus, the clinical utility of invasive testing is limited, and the diagnosis is generally made by a suggestive history supported by electrocardiographic documentation.[7] Ambulatory 24 hour electrocardiography is useful, particularly if symptoms occur during the monitoring period. Electrocardiographic (ECG) event recorders enable prolonged monitoring when symptoms are infrequent.[8] Among patients in whom the major manifestation of sinus node dysfunction is exertional fatigue, exercise testing may document failure of heart rate to increase appropriately with exercise.[5] It must be emphasized, however, that heart rate response to exercise is blunted in the elderly and this should be taken into account before ascribing any symptoms to chronotropic incompetence. [9]

Pathophysiology

The mechanisms underlying sinus node dysfunction are not well defined but abnormalities have been classified as *intrinsic* when there is apparent abnormality of the sinoatrial (SA) node or SA nodal exit block, or *extrinsic* when there is abnormal neural input to the node.[5] A technique that may be used to separate intrinsic from extrinsic dysfunction is measurement of the "intrinsic heart rate" (corrected for age) that is defined as the heart rate after complete autonomic blockade with atropine and propranolol.[10] The intrinsic heart rate is normal in patients with autonomically mediated sinus dysfunction. However, be-

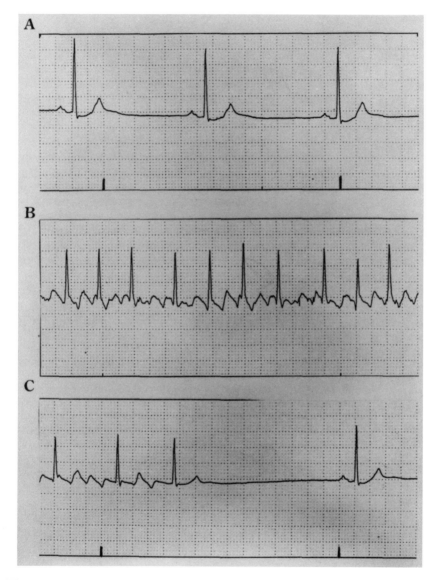

Figure 1: *ECG findings in a patient with sinus node dysfunction and tachy-brady syndrome. (A) demonstrates significant sinus bradycardia (36 beats per minute), (B), episodes of atrial fibrillation and (C), termination of tachycardia with a 2.5-second pause.*

cause therapy is not usually influenced by this distinction, such testing is rarely performed except for research purposes.

Treatment

Patients presenting with symptoms of sinus node dysfunction require careful scrutiny of their medications. β-adrenergic blockers, calcium channel blockers, digoxin, sympatholytic antihypertensive agents, and antiarrhythmic agents have been implicated in sinus node dysfunction and symptoms may abate when treatment is stopped. A sometimes overlooked route of administration of β-blocking agents is eye drops used for treatment of glaucoma. Drugs less commonly associated with sinus node dysfunction include lithium carbonate, cimetidine, antidepressants such as amitriptyline, and phenothiazines.[11]

In patients with symptomatic sinus node dysfunction without an otherwise correctable cause, electrical pacing is standard therapy.[12-14] Pacing is effective because in patients with symptoms resulting from bradycardia the resting heart rate is increased and chronotropic incompetence can be corrected. In patients with predominant tachycardia-related symptoms, pacing may prevent recurrence or permit the use of drug suppressive therapy that would otherwise be limited by the underlying sinus node dysfunction. It cannot be overemphasized that pacing should be reserved for symptomatic patients because there is no evidence that pacing improves longevity in asymptomatic patients.[15-17] If symptoms are not clearly attributable to sinus node dysfunction, it is reasonable to seek additional documentation using ambulatory electrocardiography before implanting a pacemaker. Occasionally, when sinus node dysfunction is attributable to extrinsic neural factors, anticholinergic drugs such as propantheline bromide and scopolamine, and agents such as theophylline[18] (which enhances sympathetic activity) have been advocated as alternatives to pacing in selected patients. However, in elderly patients, these pharmacological approaches rarely control the bradycardia at tolerable dosages.[19]

Lastly, chronotropic incompetence, and especially, that occurring in the context of significant left ventricular systolic dysfunction may contribute to decreased exercise tolerance and fatigue. In such patients the ability to increase stroke volume in response to exercise may be quite limited and cardiac output can only increase with tachycardia. Hence, increasing the basal heart rate and restoring the capacity to increase heart rate with exercise (with rate responsive pacing) may significantly increase exercise capacity and reduce exercise associated symptoms. Detailed discussion of appropriate pacemaker selection will be presented subsequently.

Abnormalities of AV Conduction

Diagnostic Features

When there is intermittent or established complete heart block, the severity of symptoms depends on the rate of the subsidiary pacemaker. An adequate heart rate is often maintained by a junctional rhythm with a QRS configuration similar to that seen previously in sinus rhythm (Figure 2). Under these circumstances, symptoms may be mild or nonspecific, such as fatigue. A lower, slower (and less reliable) ventricular escape rhythm, characterized by wide and aberrant QRS configuration, often results in severe weakness, symptoms of congestive heart failure and, or dizziness or syncope. Syncope occurs as a result of transient asystole or bursts of ventricular tachycardia associated with the severe bradycardia (Stokes-Adams attacks).[20] Clinically significant AV conduction disturbances are usually readily diagnosed by ECG. However, when symptoms are intermittent or occur only with exercise, ambulatory electrocardiography, patient activated ECG "event" recorder studies or exercise electrocardiography may be necessary for diagnosis.

Pathophysiology

Among the elderly, ischemic heart disease is frequently thought to be the cause of AV conduction abnormalities. In fact, only about 20% of cases can be directly attributed to this cause by pathologic examination. Primary degeneration of the conduction system (Lev-Lenegre's disease) is felt to be the usual cause.[21] The latter diagnosis may be inferred when a careful history and physical examination appear to exclude other causes. Acute myocardial infarction is complicated by AV block in 5% to 8% of patients. With inferior infarction partial (usually

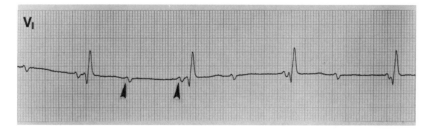

Figure 2: *ECG lead V_1 demonstrating complete AV dissociation. P waves are marked with arrows. QRS morphology is the same as was seen previously in sinus rhythm.*

Möbitz type I) or complete heart block may occur. Temporary pacing may be required if there is hemodynamic instability due to severe bradycardia, marked left ventricular dysfunction, or associated clinically significant right ventricular infarction. In many patients pacing is not required as symptoms resulting from the heart block (which is usually associated with a stable junctional escape rhythm of 40 to 55 beats per minute) are minimal and the prognosis for complete recovery of AV nodal function is excellent. Permanent pacing should be reserved for those with significant block persisting for at least 7 to 10 days.[22] In contrast, AV block associated with anteroseptal myocardial infarction is usually a result of extensive myocardial damage and the short- and long-term prognosis with or without pacing is poor.[22-26] Temporary transvenous or transcutaneous pacing should be instituted or be available in all patients with second degree AV block or complete AV block associated with acute anteroseptal infarction and in those with new bundle branch block since heart block may develop acutely in 20% to 30% of these patients.[27] Valvular heart disease, particularly calcific aortic stenosis, may be associated with impaired AV conduction.[28] This results from extension of valvular calcification into the bundle of His or proximal bundle branches that traverse the ventricular septum. Additionally, surgical replacement of the aortic and, or mitral valves may result in heart block when sutures are placed too deeply in the ventricular septum. Rheumatoid arthritis, ankylosing spondylitis and mycotic aneurysms of the aortic root may also involve the AV node or bundle of His by direct extension.[28] Lyme myocarditis may be associated with heart block (generally occurring above the bundle of His) that usually resolves with antibiotic therapy.[28] Temporary pacing is sometimes required if the escape rhythm is excessively slow and the patient symptomatic.

Treatment Strategies

Temporary Pacing. When heart block is likely to be temporary and is not symptomatic (as in acute inferior myocardial infarction), treatment is not required. If the patient is symptomatic, treatment with atropine or isoproterenol may occasionally be successful. However, these drugs are less desirable than temporary pacing because of their side effects. In asymptomatic patients our practice is to place temporary transcutaneous pacing patches,[29] ensure that they function properly and leave them in standby mode. If transcutaneous pacing is subsequently required for more than a brief period, temporary transvenous ventricular pacing is instituted since prolonged transcutaneous stimulation can be uncomfortable. In some patients with complete heart block, such as those with associated, severe right ventricular infarction, temporary dual chamber pacing may afford an additional hemodynamic advantage because the atrial contribution to ventricular filling may be considerable.[30]

Although patients with AV block associated with acute anterior infarction may be temporarily stabilized with drugs and, or transcutaneous pacing, temporary transvenous pacing is the most reliable therapeutic modality. In the setting of acute anterior infarction, an apparently reliable or pharmacologically supported ventricular escape rhythm may rapidly deteriorate. A transcutaneous pacemaker can be used to support the patient while preparations are made for placing a temporary transvenous pacing system. Similarly, a standby transcutaneous pacing system should be placed in patients with new bundle branch block while preparing for transvenous pacing.

In patients without acute myocardial infarction, it must be established that AV block is irreversible before placing a permanent pacemaker. In the setting of drug induced or aggravated AV block, adequate time must be allowed for medications to "wash out" It should be recognized that some elderly patients may not know what medications they are receiving or be confused about dosage. Hence, the physician should always be alert to the possibility of drug induced AV block, especially in the context of atrial fibrillation where an excessively slow rate may be caused by unrecognized overmedication.

Permanent Pacing. Progressive advances in technology have made a wide variety of reliable pacing systems available. Thus, once a patient has a definite indication for pacemaker implantation, the next important decision is the type of pacing system to use.

Pacemaker Codes. Agreed on symbols or codes to describe pacemakers are an indispensable means of communication. In 1974, The Inter-Society Commission on Heart Disease Resources (ICHD) recommended a 3-position letter code to provide a simple way of describing pacing systems.[31] This system has been modified as pacemakers have become more complicated with additional letter positions added.[32] Table 1 summarizes the widely used 3-position pacemaker coding system. Addition of an R to the 3-position code indicates the pacemaker is able to increase rate in response to exercise with an additional sensor.

Table 1
Three-Position ICHD Code

I. Chamber(s) paced	II. Chamber(s) sensed	III. Mode of response(s)
V-Ventricle	V-Ventricle	V-Ventricle
A-Atrium	A-Atrium	I-Inhibited
D-Double	D-Double	D-Double
	O-None	O-None

General Considerations. Pacemakers that utilize atrial sensing, AV synchrony and or rate responsiveness often improve exercise capacity considerably. Among younger patients with normal ventricular function, the increase in heart rate associated with exercise is probably the most important determinant of increased cardiac output and, consequently, exercise performance, especially at high levels of exercise. In the elderly, AV-synchrony may be more important since less time is spent at high exertional levels with high heart rates. AV synchrony with appropriately timed atrial contraction, augments left ventricular filling when systolic or diastolic abnormalities are present. Among the elderly, decreased ventricular compliance is common although often not recognized.[33] This diastolic abnormality is more likely if there is a history of hypertension with associated left ventricular hypertrophy.[34]

Retrospective and a recent prospective studies have demonstrated increased morbidity and possibly mortality among patients treated with single lead ventricular pacemakers compared to those that include an atrial lead. This appears to be a result of a higher incidence of atrial fibrillation and stroke.[35-37] Retrospective data suggest that there is a 5-fold increase in the incidence of atrial fibrillation in patients with VVI pacing as compared to those paced with systems that include atrial sensing and pacing.[36,38] In a prospective trial of atrial versus ventricular pacing, 7% of atrially paced patients versus 13% of ventricular paced patients developed chronic atrial fibrillation.[37] Moreover, in many patients with "sick sinus syndrome", AV conduction is intact. In such patients, VVI pacing can induce retrograde atrial activation during ventricular contraction resulting in the "pacemaker syndrome."[39] This syndrome is characterized by symptoms induced by hypotension and a sensation of pulsation and fullness in the neck that occurs during periods of intermittent ventricular pacing.

Among patients with sick sinus syndrome, the decision to pace the atrium alone versus both atrium and ventricle depends on the possibility of later development of atrial fibrillation or clinically significant AV block. The incidence of new atrial fibrillation after pacing is reported to be 3.9% to 7% and for development of new AV block 2% to 8.4%.[37-40] On the basis of these data, an atrial pacemaker can probably be used successfully in many patients with isolated "sick sinus syndrome." Other factors to be considered in selecting a pacemaker are anticipated life span and functional capacity. Without specific indications, complex pacing systems that include AV synchrony and or rate responsiveness are not useful in patients with poor prognosis or markedly diminished functional capability. However, it should be recognized that while single chamber ventricular pacemakers are less complex and costly, these should not be the only considerations. Such a choice may represent false economy since symptoms such as the "pacemaker syndrome" may necessitate conversion to dual chamber pacing. Also, there may be long-term sequelae such as atrial fibrillation and systemic embolism with ventricular pacing alone.[37,38,40]

Appropriate Pacemaker Selection. In most patients, dual chamber pacing is desirable and the first step is to determine whether the atrium can be reliably sensed and paced. Among patients with chronic atrial fibrillation or a large "silent" right atrium unresponsive to stimulation, an atrial lead is clearly contraindicated. Episodic atrial arrhythmias also make the decision more difficult. However, it should also be appreciated that in some instances, atrial pacing decreases the frequency of atrial arrhythmias. If a standard dual chamber pacemaker programmed in the DDD mode is in place and an atrial arrhythmia such as atrial fibrillation supervenes, the pacemaker will attempt to track the atrium resulting in ventricular pacing at a rate near the pacemakers programmed upper rate limit (Figure 3). In this situation, the pacemaker can be programmed to the VVI mode so that the atrium is not sensed. Alternatively, the upper rate limit can be reduced to limit the upper tracking rate of the pacemaker but still preserving AV synchrony should there be return to sinus rhythm. Either of these options obviously limits pacemaker function if and when the patient reverts to sinus rhythm. Pacemakers are available with additional features such as DDI, DDIR, and automatic mode switching that can be programmed to alter the way in which the atrium is tracked to prevent rapid ventricular pacing rates. With the DDI mode, atrial rate tracking with exercise is lost, with the DDIR mode rate increase with exercise is provided by an activity sensor, and with automatic mode switching when an atrial tachyarrhythmia is detected the pacemaker reverts to a DDI or DDIR mode. In the latter modes, the pacemaker continues to track the atrium (pacing the ventricle at the activity sensor determined rate) until the atrial arrhythmia terminates allowing the pacemaker to return to either a DDD or DDDR mode automatically. Such devices have advantages and disadvantages but all attempt to maintain the benefits of dual chamber pacing, despite the occurrence of episodic atrial arrhyth-

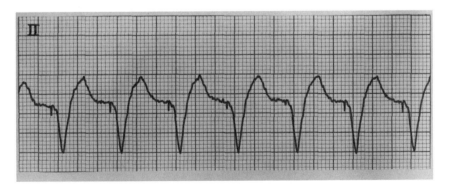

Figure 3: *ECG demonstrating atrial tracking of atrial fibrillation with ventricular pacing at the programmed upper rate limit of 100 beats per minute in a DDD pacemaker.*

mias. These devices should be considered for use in patients with a prior history of atrial arrhythmias.

In patients in whom (single chamber) atrial pacing is being considered, the second step is to test AV conduction. If AV conduction is normal at the time of pacemaker implantation, the risk of subsequent AV block has been reported to have an annual incidence of 1.2%.[39] It is important to recognize however, that AV conduction can be affected by pharmacological therapy or episodic neural influences. An example of the latter would include use of a dual chamber rather than an atrial pacemaker to control bradycardia associated with carotid hypersensitivity syndrome. Even though AV conduction is normal at baseline, associated neural influences can precipitate AV block just at a time when pacing is required for treatment of sinus bradycardia or sinus arrest.

Heart rate response to exercise is an important consideration in selected patients. If a patient has chronotropic competence of the SA node, tracking the atrial response during exercise yields the most physiologic ventricular pacing rate. In approximately 25% of patients with complete AV block, the SA node does not respond with an appropriate rate increase with exercise. In such patients, a rate responsive pacing system, using a sensor incorporated into the pacing system, can improve exercise performance. If patients are temporarily unable to exercise during an acute illness, heart rate response to atropine or isoproterenol can be helpful in assessing chronotropic competence of the SA node.

Finally, there should be an assessment of left ventricular function. Clearly, it is important to maintain AV synchrony when there is decreased left ventricular compliance and, or ejection fraction. Dual chamber pacing with a short AV interval has been advocated to improve the hemodynamic performance in patients with severe left ventricular dysfunction.[40] The eventual role of pacing in the treatment of congestive heart failure continues to evolve.[41]

In summary, when the atrium can be reliably paced and, or sensed, a pacemaker that includes an atrial lead should be used unless there are extenuating circumstances. The decision to include an exercise rate response feature must be determined on an individual basis.

Tachyarrhythmias

Primary Atrial Arrhythmias

Atrial Fibrillation

Etiology. Premature atrial contractions are the most frequent intermittent arrhythmia in the elderly, but atrial fibrillation is the most frequent chronic tachyarrhythmia. The incidence is reported to be 3.8%

Table 2
Conditions Associated with Atrial Fibrillation

Cardiac	Systemic
Ischemic heart disease, acute or chronic	Age
	Chronic pulmonary disease
Pericarditis	Alcohol
Cardiac Surgery	Thyrotoxicosis
Cardiomyopathy	Cerebrovascular accident
Valvular heart disease	Fever
Cardioversion	Electrolyte abnormalities
Tachybradycardia syndrome	(eg, decreased K^+, decreased Mg^{++})
Tumors, lipomatous hypertrophy	Trauma
Pre-excitation syndromes	Hypovolemia
Hypertension/ventricular	Hypothermia
hypertrophy	Electrocution
Ventricular pacing	

in men in their sixth decade but lower in women.[42] Among individuals over age 70 years, the incidence increases to 9% in the general population.[42]

Among the elderly, atrial fibrillation is usually associated with underlying cardiac disease. Although the list of associated cardiac diseases is long (Table 2), atrial fibrillation is most frequently associated with ischemic, hypertensive, valvular heart disease or cardiomyopathy. Systemic disorders such as hyperthyroidism or amyloidosis are less frequent causes.

The history and physical examination taken together with the electrocardiogram and chest roentgenogram will often reveal the nature of the underlying cardiac disease. An echocardiogram provides more precise definition of chamber size and performance and valvular function. Hyperthyroidism should be excluded by laboratory studies since its clinical features are often cryptic in older individuals; effective treatment with restoration to a euthyroid state is often associated with reversion to sinus rhythm.

Clinical Presentation. In 30% to 50% of elderly patients with atrial fibrillation, there may be no symptoms or merely a sensation of irregular heart beat even when a rapid ventricular response is induced by exercise.[43] Patients with moderately severe heart disease often present with exertional fatigue and dyspnea. Those with significant left ventricular dysfunction, severe coronary artery disease or severe left ventricular hypertrophy may present with symptoms and signs of congestive heart failure and, or angina. Patients with severe aortic and mitral stenosis, hypertrophic cardiomyopathy, or restrictive myocardial disease are especially vulnerable to rapid development of heart failure. The loss of the atrial "kick" and rate related shortening of the diastolic filling period can result in marked elevation of left atrial and left ventricular filling pressures.

In some patients with or without underlying cardiac disease, the arrhythmia only manifests during the stress of surgery, sepsis, alcohol withdrawal, exacerbation of heart failure, or bronchospasm. Following resolution of the primary problem, reversion to sinus rhythm often occurs. The incidence of atrial fibrillation post cardiac surgery (either coronary artery bypass surgery and/or valve surgery) is as high as 30% to 50% and increases with the age of the patient.[44,45] Atrial fibrillation may present as a paroxysmal arrhythmia whose frequency varies from once a day to once a year. This arrhythmia may occur in the presence or absence of evident underlying heart disease although recent data suggest that even in patients without obvious heart disease atrial histology may be abnormal.[46] In some patients with paroxysmal atrial fibrillation, chronic atrial fibrillation eventually ensues.[47] In many patients with paroxysmal atrial fibrillation, the arrhythmia is associated with disturbing symptoms.

Unfortunately, embolic stroke may be the initial presentation of patients with otherwise asymptomatic atrial fibrillation. In the Framingham study, the prevalence of atrial fibrillation in patients presenting with stroke increased from 6.7% among those aged 50 to 59 years to 36.2% among those aged 80 to 89 years.[48]

Electrocardiographic Features. Atrial fibrillation is easily diagnosed by ECG features that include absence of regular atrial activity, a fine or coarse undulating baseline, and irregularly irregular R-R intervals (Figure 4). Occasionally, a coarse undulating baseline with so called "fibrillatory" waves may be confused with other atrial arrhythmias such as atrial flutter or paroxysmal atrial tachycardia which may also be associated with variable AV conduction. This confusion often occurs when the ventricular response is not very irregular.

When the resting ventricular response without drug therapy is less than 80 beats per minute and there is only a modest increase in response to exercise stress, there is associated disease of the AV node. In contrast, a resting ventricular response of 120 to 160 beats per minute suggests that AV nodal function is normal. If the resting ventricular response is more than 150 beats per minute, the sympathetic nervous system is activated either by the underlying illness or the stress of the altered hemodynamic state created by atrial fibrillation. Resting ventricular rates of more than 200 beats per minute suggest the presence of enhanced AV nodal conduction or the presence of an accessory AV connection. Under the latter circumstance, the QRS morphology is aberrant and the rhythm may be confused with ventricular tachycardia (Figure 5).

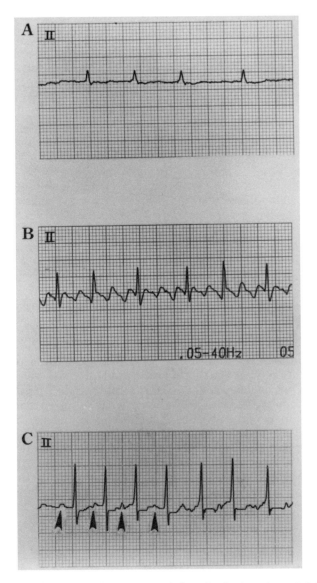

Figure 4: *ECG examples of primary atrial arrhythmias. A: atrial fibrillation; B: atrial flutter; C: multifocal atrial tachycardia with arrows marking P waves of multiple morphologies.*

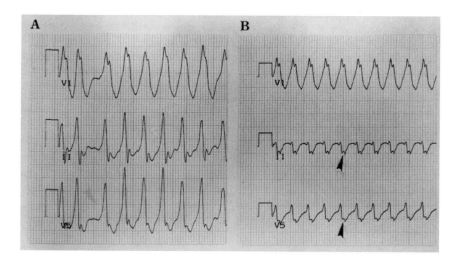

Figure 5: *ECG examples of (A) atrial fibrillation in a patient with a left-sided accessory AV connection resulting in an irregular rate with wide bizarre QRS complexes. (B) Antidromic reciprocating tachycardia utilizing a left-sided accessory AV connection in the antegrade direction resulting in wide bizarre QRS pattern. P waves are marked with arrows.*

Complications. In addition to its effect on cardiac performance, atrial fibrillation is a marker for a 5-fold increase in incidence of stroke[49] and increased cardiac mortality compared to subjects in sinus rhythm.[42] Of interest, younger patients with so called "lone" atrial fibrillation, defined by the absence of evident heart disease, hypertension or diabetes, have an extremely low risk for embolism.[50] In the elderly with "lone atrial fibrillation," sufficient long-term follow-up data in large populations is not available. On the basis of available information, the incidence of stroke appears to be low. Atrial fibrillation occurring following cardiac surgery prolongs hospitalization and increases costs.[44]

Therapeutic Approach. Optimally, patients presenting with atrial fibrillation should be converted to, and maintained in permanent sinus rhythm. Unfortunately, this goal is impossible in many patients. Even with aggressive pharmacological therapy, long-term maintenance of sinus rhythm is achieved in only 60% of patients.[51] Therefore, a therapeutic strategy that carefully evaluates risks and benefits of a specific intervention in the individual patient is warranted. Overzealous treatment may lead to side effects of medication including the potential for proarrhythmia.[52] In some patients with atrial fibrillation, with underlying sinus node disease conversion to sinus rhythm may result in symptoms secondary to bradycardia. An ongoing National Institutes of Health (NIH) sponsored trial, Atrial Fibrillation Follow-up Investigation of Rhythm Management (AFFIRM) may provide evidence on whether rate vs rhythm control is more appropriate in asymptomatic patients with atrial fibrillation.[53]

The ventricular response to atrial fibrillation can usually be controlled with drugs. Alternatively, radiofrequency modification of AV nodal conduction or ablation, and ventricular pacing can be used in drug refractory cases.[54,55] Adequate rate control both at rest and during exercise is important since chronic tachycardia has been associated with further deterioration of cardiac function (so called tachycardic myocardiopathy).[56] In certain patients presenting after an episode of atrial fibrillation with rapid ventricular response and left ventricular (LV) dysfunction, conversion to sinus rhythm or adequate rate control of atrial fibrillation has resulted in improvement of LV systolic function.[56]

Immediate Therapy. Four subgroups of clinical presentations may be defined:

1. Acute hemodynamic failure and, or unstable angina;
2. Hemodynamically stable with mild to moderate heart failure;
3. Few symptoms;
4. Extremely rapid heart rate.

When elderly patients, including immediately postoperative patients, present with acute onset of atrial fibrillation and severe hemodynamic failure (hypotension and, or pulmonary edema) and, or persisting angina, the arrhythmia must be rapidly controlled or corrected. The most efficacious treatment is electrical cardioversion under sedation, preferably with an anesthesiologist in attendance. Synchronized DC cardioversion using 100 J or more will be required.[57] If this fails, the energy level may be doubled and then increased to 300 to 360 J. If cardioversion fails, intravenous β-blocking drugs such as esmolol,[58] or calcium channel antagonists such as diltiazem,[59] can be used to slow the ventricular rate response. Both drug types must be used with caution because of the risk of severe hypotension or worsening of congestive heart failure in patients with significant left ventricular dysfunction.

Adjunctive therapy to control congestive failure, hypotension, and angina must also be used to stabilize the patient. Drug dosages should be adjusted in relation to diminished renal and hepatic function because elderly patients often have altered drug pharmacokinetics.

Preoperative and postoperative use of β-blockers has been effective in reducing the incidence of atrial fibrillation complicating cardiac surgery. Recently, pretreatment with amiodarone for 1 week prior to cardiac surgery, continued during the immediate post operative period, has been shown to reduce the incidence of atrial fibrillation from 53% to 25%.[45]

In patients presenting with atrial fibrillation and rapid ventricular response but without hypotension, severe cardiac failure, hypoxemia or significant angina, the initial goal is to control ventricular rate. Rate control can often be achieved with intravenous digoxin. The total loading dose should be adjusted for body weight and the maintenance dosage determined depending on renal function and clinical response. In patients with severe heart failure who are relatively stable, the success of pharmacological or electrical cardioversion is greatest after therapy for failure has been optimized and heart failure controlled.[60] Hence, delayed cardioversion after a period of treatment and anticoagulation may be advantageous because it not only facilitates the success rate of cardioversion but also decreases risk of embolism.

In many patients with atrial fibrillation precipitated by stress, particularly in the perioperative period, adrenergic activity is elevated and digoxin may not be adequate to control heart rate. Increased sympathetic nervous system activity limits the effectiveness of digoxin on the AV node and perpetuates the arrhythmia. If there are no specific contraindications to β-blocking drugs, an intravenous preparation with a short half-life, such as esmolol, is probably the initial drug of choice in most postoperative patients because of its short half-life.[61,62] In situations in which β-blocking drugs are relatively contraindicated, we use intravenous diltiazem. Examples include patients with severe left ventricular dysfunction and catecholamine support required to maintain hemodynamic stability, or significant lung disease, particularly with bronchospasm.[50] Intravenous diltiazem can be initiated with gradual increases in dosage to control ventricular rate without precipitating severe hypotension or worsening of congestive heart failure in many patients. If pharmacological strategy fails and/or the patient becomes unstable, cardioversion should be performed promptly.

Many elderly patients with atrial fibrillation present with few or no symptoms. Some have ventricular rates that range from 50 to 80 beats per minute at rest and this increases only modestly with activity. Others will have more rapid heart rates at rest, particularly during stress. The former require no treatment for rate control and indeed, the use of digoxin or other drugs may cause severe bradycardia. Among patients with unusually slow ventricular response to atrial fibrillation, the possibility of a drug impairing AV nodal conduction should be excluded before considering implantation of a pacemaker. This consideration is especially true in the elderly patient with early dementia who may be confused about medications and dosages.

In elderly patients requiring treatment for control of ventricular rate, optimal resting and exercise heart rates can often be achieved with oral digoxin alone because AV nodal function is somewhat depressed. However, in many patients with normal AV nodal function, oral β-blockers[63] or calcium blockers such as verapamil[64] or diltiazem[65] must be added to, or used instead of digoxin, to control exercise tachycardia.

In some patients, medication may control exercise-induced tachycardia, but symptomatic bradycardia may occur at rest and VVI pacing may be required. If drug therapy fails to control ventricular rate, AV conduction can be slowed or completely interrupted by radiofrequency catheter ablation.[54,55] Catheter ablation has proven to be safe and effective even in elderly patients with significant underlying heart and lung disease. The use of radiofrequency ablation to modify and slow AV nodal conduction has a reported success rate of 60% to 70%.[54] Permanent pacer implantation is required in about 30% of patients because of development of significant, or complete AV block. The potential advantage of successful AV junction modification is that permanent pacing is not required. Unfortunately AV modification does not always control ventricular response rate.[66] In contrast, catheter ablation of the AV junction and subsequent VVI or VVIR (R = activity sensing mode) pacing is highly effective in dealing with this problem and this latter approach has the most certain outcome of controlling rate and regularizing rhythm.[55]

Certain patients with atrial fibrillation have ventricular response greater than 200 beats per minute. If the QRS complexes are wide and bizarre (normal QRS complexes may be interspersed), conduction through an accessory AV connection such as seen with the Wolff-Parkinson-White syndrome (WPW) should be considered. In treating atrial fibrillation with a very rapid response due to antegrade conduction though an accessory pathway, digoxin and verapamil are contraindicated since they may further accelerate conduction through the accessory connection and induce ventricular fibrillation. Indeed, rapid rate induced ventricular fibrillation is thought to be the mechanism for those rare instances of sudden death in patients with WPW. The most appropriate initial therapy in these patients is cardioversion followed by treatment with a type I antiarrhythmic drug and a β-blocking drug. Both drugs can decrease conduction through the accessory connection. If immediate cardioversion is not possible, intravenous procainamide, given slowly to avoid hypotension, will often slow conduction in the accessory connection, thereby reducing ventricular rate to tolerable levels. However, this is a temporary expedient and if the atrial fibrillation is not converted by the procainamide, DC cardioversion is still required.

Long-term Therapy. Electrical cardioversion of patients with atrial fibrillation has an initial success rate of up to 90%.[67] Factors associated with a higher initial cardioversion rate include younger age and shorter duration of arrhythmia.[68] The major problem in treating atrial fibrillation is maintenance of sinus rhythm after cardioversion. Unless the arrhythmia is related to an acute illness or stress, such as cardiac surgery, a recurrence rate of 80% at 1 year should be expected following cardioversion.[43] Thus, in many patients antiarrhythmic drugs are used in an attempt to maintain sinus rhythm. The choice of drug is largely empiric but individual drug toxicity, side effects and proarrhythmia as

Table 3
Commonly Used Antiarrhythmic Drugs

Drug	Oral Dose (mg)	Therapeutic Level (mg/mL)	Major Elimination Route	Primary Side Effects
Quinidine	300–600 q6h	3–6	Liver	Diarrhea G.I. upset Cinchonism Proarrhythmia
Procainamide	750–1250 q6h	4–10	Kidneys	Lupus syndrome G.I. upset
Disopyramide	100–400 q6–8h	2–5	Kidneys	Urinary retention Dry mouth Congestive failure
Flecainide	100–200 q12h	0.2–1.0	Liver	Pro-arrhythmia CNS symptoms
Propafenone	150–300 q8–12h	0.2–3.0	Liver	Unusual taste G.I. upset Conduction disturbances CNS symptoms
Amiodarone	200–400 qd	0.5–1.5	Kidneys	Photosensitivity Liver/lung toxicity Thyroid abnormalities
Moricizine	200–300 q8h	—	Liver	CNS symptoms G.I. upset Conduction disturbances
Mexilitine	150–300 q8h	0.75–2	Liver	CNS symptoms GI upset
Sotalol	80–160 q12h	—	Liver	CNS symptoms Conduction disturbances Proarrhythmia

well as the nature and severity of the underlying heart disease should be taken into account. Table 3 summarizes the commonly used antiarrhythmic medications (with the exception of mexilitene) which have been used in attempts to control recurrences.

If possible, patients should be hospitalized and monitored during initial treatment with antiarrhythmic drugs to detect pro-arrhythmia (marked QT prolongation and, or arrhythmia) and to ensure medication is otherwise well tolerated. An initial period of hospital observation when initiating antiarrhythmic therapy is especially important in most elderly patients among whom underlying heart and other diseases are the rule rather than the exception. It is important to correct electrolyte abnormalities before drug therapy and to consider potential adverse interactions of the antiarrhythmic agent with other drugs such as digoxin, warfarin, and cimetidine.

Long-term maintenance of sinus rhythm with quinidine has been reported in up to 60% of patients.[69] The class IC agent propafenone[70,71] and sotalol, a combined β-blocking-type III agent,[72,73] have been reported as successful in 40% to 67% of cases. Amiodarone, a class III agent has been successful in restoring and maintaining sinus rhythm in up to 79% of cases in whose other antiarrhythmic agents have failed.[74] Other class I agents such as procainamide and moricizine, have also been used successfully to prevent recurrent atrial fibrillation.

Results from current ongoing trials including the NIH sponsored AFFIRM trial should prove helpful in assessing not only the wisdom of rhythm control as opposed to rate control but also assist in the choice of antiarrhythmic drug.[53] In the AFFIRM trial, the initial choice of selecting an antiarrhythmic for treatment of atrial fibrillation is being tested in a major substudy. Patients are being randomized to receive amiodarone, sotalol, or class I agents as the first choice at attempted rhythm control.[53]

Our current practice is to begin with procainamide, quinidine, or sotalol and if unsuccessful, other drugs including amiodarone may be tried. In general, we avoid class IC agents if there is any evidence of heart disease because of excess deaths reported in the CAST trial.[75] When procainamide and quinidine are used alone they may accelerate ventricular response to atrial fibrillation should the arrhythmia recur. The proposed mechanisms are neurally mediated enhancement of AV nodal conduction and slowing of the fibrillatory rate allowing faster conduction through the AV node.[76] Generally, digitalis (or alternatively β-blockers or calcium channel antagonists) are given in conjunction with procainamide or quinidine to provide AV slowing should atrial fibrillation recur.

If the need to maintain the patient in sinus rhythm is pressing and other drugs have failed or if the patient has severe underlying heart disease which increases the likelihood of recurrence, we use amiodarone.[74] Amiodarone has the additional beneficial effect of slowing conduction through the AV node which is useful should atrial fibrillation recur. After loading with amiodarone, doses as low as 200 mg/day may be effective.[77] Proarrhythmia seems less of a problem than with other antiarrhythmic medications and LV function is not significantly depressed by orally administered amiodarone. Amiodarone might well be the most efficacious drug but it's potential for other organ system toxicity, especially thyroid, hepatic and pulmonary, is always a concern. However, since many elderly patients with underlying cardiac or other diseases have quite limited life expectancy, the long-term risk of toxicity may be less concerning. It must be stressed that the use of long-term amiodarone therapy commits the physician to an organized follow-up plan to detect toxic effect on the thyroid, lung and liver. This surveillance is superimposed on the routine clinical follow-up plan and this is best accomplished by including a flowsheet in the patients chart so that liver, thyroid and pulmonary function tests and chest x-ray results are regularly recorded.

In patients with stress-induced atrial fibrillation following coronary artery bypass or other surgery, or an acute medical illness, long-term treatment is often unnecessary. Therapy may be terminated after resolution of the precipitating event and re-instituted only if atrial fibrillation recurs. In practice, most patients in this category have their antiarrhythmic medication discontinued at their first follow-up visit (2–4 weeks). It is disturbing to note that many elderly patients are still taking digoxin, quinidine and other antiarrhythmic agents unnecessarily many months, and sometimes years, after a short episode of stress induced atrial fibrillation.

Prediction of long-term maintenance of sinus rhythm has been correlated with younger age, shorter duration of atrial fibrillation, a low New York Heart Association functional class and absence of rheumatic heart disease.[68] Large left atrial size has been implicated in the past as predicting long-term cardioversion failure.[78–80] Other large studies, however have not demonstrated left atrial size to be a useful tool in predicting long-term maintenance of sinus rhythm.[68] In a group of 50 patients, Dethy et al[81] has described return of atrial contraction when assessed by Doppler echocardiography, as a useful indicator of persistence of sinus rhythm at 6 months following cardioversion.

More recently, the atrial maze operation has been proposed as a potential "cure" for selected patients with atrial fibrillation.[82] In this procedure, multiple incisions are made in both atria to limit the amount of myocardium that could potentially participate in sustaining the multiple reentry loops considered to be the basis of the arrhythmia. Reported results indicate that postoperative left atrial transport function returns in many patients. However, some patients need long-term pacing to maintain heart rate, probably a result of coexisting intrinsic sinus node dysfunction. At present we do not believe there is a major role for this procedure among the elderly in whom underlying heart disease and other diseases increase surgical risk and in whom the contribution to overall quality of life compared to conventional therapy would be modest at best. More recently, attempts have been made to duplicate the maze procedure using catheter based selective radiofrequency induced lesions in the atria.[83] Reports of the results of this methodology are too preliminary to permit recommendations. However, when acceptable risk and efficacy are demonstrated in elderly patients, this may prove to be useful in these patients severely limited functionally by atrial fibrillation.

Long-term atrial pacing has been demonstrated to reduce the occurrence rate of atrial fibrillation in patients with sinus node dysfunction.[37] More recently dual site atrial pacing (simultaneous pacing of high and low right atrium)[84] and Bachmann's bundle pacing[85] have demonstrated some success in reducing the incidence of recurrent atrial fibrillation. However, experience with the technique is too limited to justify recommendation at this time.

In elderly patients with short-duration atrial fibrillation (less than 6 months) who have minimal or no symptoms and mild or no underlying heart disease, cardioversion and a period of several months of antiarrhythmic therapy may be a reasonable approach. Such patients may have a decreased likelihood of recurrence and long-term antiarrhythmic therapy and anticoagulation can be avoided if this strategy works. In asymptomatic patients with rate controlled chronic atrial fibrillation (6 months to 1 year's duration), previous logic for attempting conversion to sinus rhythm was aimed at preventing systemic embolism and the possibility that a reasonable number of such patients would maintain sinus rhythm with antiarrhythmic therapy. Recent studies in patients with nonrheumatic atrial fibrillation have demonstrated that low intensity warfarin therapy (international normalized ratio [INR] 2–3) decreases the risk for stroke to rates close to that of age matched controls and is safe even in elderly patients.[86–89] There is also some evidence that aspirin may reduce the risk of stroke.[87] Our current practice is to treat all older patients with chronic atrial fibrillation with low intensity warfarin unless there are contraindications in which case we consider aspirin. Hence, repeated attempts to maintain sinus rhythm in otherwise asymptomatic elderly patients may no longer be appropriate because with substantial reduction of risk of embolization by anticoagulation, the risk of proarrhythmia may outweigh the benefits of sinus rhythm. As noted earlier, the AFFIRM trial should determine whether rate control or a vigorous effort to obtain and maintain sinus rhythm will yield a better long-term outcome in patients with atrial fibrillation.[53] The results of this study are expected to serve as a basis for evidence based decision making in this controversial area in which there are currently few relevant data.

Lastly, the role of warfarin in preventing stroke may be more than just prevention of embolization from left atrial thrombi. A recent echocardiographic study suggests that other mechanisms including mitral valve disease, patent foramen ovale, regional ventricular wall motion abnormalities, and atrial septal aneurysm may also be responsible.[90] Others have cited the low incidence of embolism in patients with "lone atrial fibrillation" and suggested that embolism associated with atrial fibrillation results from coexisting myocardial infarction, mitral valve disease, or aortic and carotid atherosclerosis.[91]

Cardioversion. There are several considerations that apply to elective cardioversion. A major one is the possibility of embolism associated with the procedure. Although the risk for stroke is low,[92] it is has become standard, practice in patients, in whom atrial fibrillation has been present for more than 48 hours, to anticoagulate with warfarin for 3 to 4 weeks before, and 3 to 4 weeks after cardioversion. The rationale for continuing anticoagulation after successful cardioversion is the known delay in return of atrial mechanical function in some patients.[93] Prior to cardioversion, patients are monitored and placed on a suppressive antiarrhythmic drug for the period of time required to achieve a therapeutic blood level for the specific agent chosen. Digoxin need not be stopped but if quinidine or other drugs that elevate digoxin levels are selected, then the dose of digoxin should be reduced. Approximately 10% to 20% of patients will convert with type I antiarrhythmic therapy alone.[94] Additionally, about one third of patients with atrial fibrillation can be pharmacologically converted with ibutilide an intravenous class III agent.[95,96] The drug is most effective when atrial fibrillation or flutter is of recent onset (ie, < 30 days). We have occasionally used ibutilide in attempts at cardioversion when there is a strong reason to avoid the brief general anesthesia required for electrical cardioversion. If ibutilide is used, the patient must be carefully monitored for a few hours after drug administration since the incidence of polymorphous ventricular tachycardia has been reported to be 8.3%.[95] Postconversion warfarin is recommended for 1 month if the atrial fibrillation is of more than 48 hours in duration.

Recently, transesophageal echocardiography has been proposed as a technique to rule out the presence of left atrial thrombus prior to cardioversion thereby eliminating the need for anticoagulation prior to cardioversion.[97] Lastly, the role of anticoagulation with warfarin after cardioversion is unclear in patients with atrial fibrillation of short duration (ie, <48 hours). We recommend initial heparinization on admission if cardioversion is to be delayed. It may be prudent to anticoagulate patients with atrial fibrillation of 4 to 6 weeks duration until it is clear that there is not an early recurrence.

Atrial Flutter

Etiology. In the acute setting, atrial flutter may complicate myocardial infarction, pneumonia, or a variety of surgical procedures particularly cardiothoracic operations. Chronic atrial flutter is much less common than atrial fibrillation, but tends to be associated with the same diseases. However, atrial flutter is more frequent among elderly than younger patients. Acute or chronic atrial flutter are uncommon in the absence of underlying heart or advanced pulmonary disease.

Clinical Presentation. The onset of atrial flutter may be associated with angina or congestive heart failure. Uncommonly, it is an unexpected finding at routine examination. The ventricular response is characteristically approximately 150 beats per minute. In the absence of ventricular ectopy or varying degrees of AV block, the rhythm is regular. As is the case with atrial fibrillation, patients with severe aortic and mitral valvular stenosis, hypertrophic myocardiopathy, or restrictive myocardial diseases are especially vulnerable to severe symptoms following loss of effective atrial contraction and rate related shortening of the diastolic filling period. In patients with less severe myocardial disease, atrial flutter may decrease exercise tolerance and induce mild heart failure.

Electrocardiographic Features. The typical appearance is a "saw tooth" pattern intervening between QRST complexes in inferior leads II, III, and AVF (Figure 4). This pattern may be obscured by the QRST complex. Occasionally, flutter waves are best seen in lead V_1. The atrial flutter rate of 250 to 340 per minute is typically twice that of the ventricular rate response. Generally, some degree of AV block (usually 2:1) is present. Rarely, 1:1 conduction may occur when there is accelerated AV nodal conduction or an accessory AV connection or if the flutter rate is relatively slow (~200 per minute) and AV conduction is rapid.

Among patients with primary abnormalities of AV nodal function or those receiving drugs that depress AV nodal conduction, AV block may be greater than 2:1 but it is always in multiples of the atrial flutter rate. As the flutter rate is usually near 300 beats per minute, atrial flutter should be suspected in every regular supraventricular tachycardia with a ventricular rate in the range of 150 beats per minute even if flutter waves are not readily visible on ECG. If the patient is stable, maneuvers that transiently increase AV block such as carotid massage, or adenosine 6 to 12 mg intravenously, can be used to unmask flutter waves. If conversion to sinus rhythm occurs, then AV nodal or AV reentrant rhythm rather than atrial flutter is the likely diagnosis. If these maneuvers fail to unmask flutter waves, an atrial electrogram using an esophageal or intra-atrial electrode is helpful. In postoperative cardiac patients, surgically attached temporary atrial pacing electrodes facilitate diagnosis and can be used to overdrive pace the arrhythmia.[98]

Atrial flutter is differentiated from other atrial tachycardias primarily by rate. With flutter, the atrial rate is generally more than 250 beats per minute, whereas the rate in primary atrial tachycardia is less. An exception is atrial flutter in the elderly patient with abnormal intra-atrial conduction receiving an antiarrhythmic agent in whom the flutter rate may fall below 200 beats per minute.

Complications

The hemodynamic consequences are similar to those seen with atrial fibrillation. Unlike atrial fibrillation, the reported incidence of systemic embolism has been low and cardioversion has not been considered an increased risk. This may be because mechanical activity of the atria during flutter is more coordinated than during fibrillation so that there is less stagnation of blood in the left atrium. Recently, however, echocardiographic studies of patients with atrial flutter have demonstrated a surprisingly high incidence of thrombus in the left atrial appendage and/or blood stasis ("smoke").[99] Hence, although the embolic risk with flutter is undoubtedly lower than with atrial fibrillation, it may be prudent to anticoagulate patients with chronic atrial flutter because embolism may rarely occur.[100]

Immediate Therapy. Four subgroups of clinical presentations may be defined:

1. Acute hemodynamic failure and, or unstable angina;

2. Rapid response with minimal symptoms;

3. Slow ventricular response or slow flutter rate with minimal symptoms;

4. Extremely rapid ventricular response.

Patients with atrial flutter and rapid ventricular response of 150 beats per minute or more may present with various combinations of hypotension, congestive failure, and angina. The treatment of choice is QRS synchronized DC cardioversion or atrial overdrive pacing. The latter is particularly useful following cardiac operations when a temporary atrial lead is in place[98] and in patients with severe chronic lung disease in whom even a brief period of general anesthesia may be undesirable. The advantage of DC cardioversion is that it is generally available, highly effective, and can be used in anticoagulated patients. Atrial flutter is usually converted with 50 J or less, but if this fails the energy level can be increased as required. It should also be noted that when the flutter rate is more than 340 beats per minute, atrial overdrive is frequently ineffective and cardioversion is the preferred treatment.[98]

In patients who present with acute atrial flutter with few or no symptoms, the usual ventricular response is 150 beats per minute or less. Early cardioversion by one of the aforementioned techniques is again the most efficient treatment. Initial therapy with digoxin and either quinidine or procainamide results in conversion in a minority of cases (10%–20%), so there is little rationale for prolonged efforts at pharmacological conversion. In up to 50% of cases of *acute* atrial flutter associated with surgery or stress, conversion to sinus rhythm with intravenous esmolol therapy may occur.[61,62] Intravenous ibutilide has been used with fair success (63%). Conversion usually occurs within the first 30 minutes. After ibutilide administration, patients need to be carefully monitored for a few hours because of the risk for polymorphous ventricular tachycardia.[95]

A few patients present with atrial flutter and greater than 2:1 AV block without drug therapy and some of these patients also have a slow flutter rate (between 180 and 220 beats per minute). Such presentation is more common in the elderly and a case can be made for simply controlling ventricular response with drugs that slow AV nodal conduction. If the patient is symptomatic and rate control does not result in marked improvement, standard conversion and suppressive treatment can be used. In patients where both suppression and rate control are unsuccessful, AV nodal ablation and subsequent VVI or VVIR pacing is indicated.

A small number of patients present with a 1:1 AV conduction and a ventricular rate close to 300 beats per minute. As with atrial fibrillation, this suggests that accelerated AV nodal conduction or an accessory AV connection is present. The latter, with atrial fibrillation, is suggested by abnormal QRS morphology compatible with pre-excitation. This ECG pattern may be confused with ventricular tachycardia if there is not variable AV block. In either case the rapid heart rate itself poses a major threat to the patient and urgent cardioversion is indicated.

Long-term Therapy. After acute atrial flutter has been converted, duration of drug therapy is variable and largely determined by the cause. In patients with acute stress-induced atrial flutter after cardiac surgery, therapy may be terminated after a few days to weeks and re-instituted only if flutter recurs.

In patients with chronic atrial flutter, pharmacological control of ventricular rate, particularly during exercise, is often difficult or impossible with normal AV nodal function. Thus, conversion and suppression, rather than rate control is the therapeutic goal. The long-term suppressive strategy is comparable to that described for atrial fibrillation. After cardioversion, patients should receive digoxin and either quinidine or procainamide or another antiarrhythmic drug. The logic in combining digoxin with quinidine or procainamide therapy is to slow AV nodal conduction to prevent acceleration of heart rate should flutter recur because type I drugs slow the flutter rate and also accelerate AV nodal conduction. β-adrenergic and calcium channel blocking drugs can also prevent this complication. As with atrial fibrillation, other antiarrhythmic agents such as propafenone, ethmozine, and sotalol have been used successfully. Amiodarone is also quite effective in preventing recurrence of atrial flutter should other drugs fail. Many of these other agents also depress AV nodal conduction and concomitant therapy with digoxin or other agents may not be required.

Catheter ablation of the flutter "circuit" using radiofrequency energy has been used to treat chronic or recurrent typical atrial flutter.[101] In typical atrial flutter, predominantly negative flutter waves are seen in inferior leads II, III, and AVF on the surface ECG. Ablation of the isthmus between the tricuspid valve and inferior vena cava can be curative in a substantial number of patients. Unfortunately, up to 30% of patients subsequently develop atrial fibrillation, but in some cases this can be suppressed with antiarrhythmic therapy.[102] If drug regimens and ablation fail, catheter ablation of the AV node followed by VVI or VVIR (R = activity sensor) pacemaker implantation is the therapy of choice. Anticoagulation for chronic atrial flutter or for cardioversion of patients with atrial flutter of more than 48 hours has traditionally not been recommended because the frequency of systemic embolic has been considered negligible. However, this recommendation should be tempered with caution especially in light of more recent echocardiographic data indicating a significant incidence of intra-atrial clot and, or blood stasis ("smoke")in such patients.[99] Furthermore, it is uncertain how frequently there are associated paroxysms of atrial fibrillation in patients with atrial flutter and this may account for these echocardiographic observations. Hence, we now consider it prudent to offer anticoagulation to patients with chronic atrial flutter unless there are contraindications.

Multifocal Atrial Tachycardia

Etiology. Multifocal atrial tachycardia (MAT) is a common arrhythmia that is almost never primary.[76] It is most frequently encountered in the intensive care unit complicating severe cardiac or pulmonary disease, particularly exacerbations of chronic obstructive lung disease. It may result from stress precipitated surge in serum catecholamine levels combined with atrial abnormalities such as acute stretch. Patients receiving xanthines, and catecholamine bronchodilatators are particularly susceptible to MAT and the theophylline blood level should be determined in any patient with MAT who receives this drug. It should be noted that MAT is not a manifestation of digitalis toxicity, but toxicity may supervene when this agent is used in a vain attempt to control the ventricular rate response.

Electrocardiographic Features. The characteristic pattern is a rapid, irregular ventricular rhythm with each QRS complex preceded by P waves of varying morphology (Figure 4). Nonconducted premature P waves are also frequent. The typical heart rate is 100 to 130 beats per minute, although faster rates may occur and be complicated by aberrant ventricular conduction.[103] MAT may be associated with intermittent atrial flutter or fibrillation. Usually, 3 or more different P wave morphologies are required for diagnosis.[104] If the electrocardiographic pattern is similar but the atrial rate is 100 beats per minute or less, the term "chaotic atrial rhythm" is sometimes used.

Complications. MAT may worsen the hemodynamic status and/or ischemia in patients who are already quite ill if the ventricular rate is more than ~130 per minute. In clinically stable patients, the rhythm generally poses no threat unless the ventricular response becomes very rapid (~150 per minute).

Therapy. The primary intent of therapy is to stabilize the underlying disease process and to eliminate other precipitating causes of MAT such as xanthine toxicity. The major indication for treating MAT is a ventricular rate not tolerated by the patient. β-adrenergic blocking drugs or calcium channel antagonists may be useful to control the ventricular rate.[105] The role of β-blockers is limited by the frequency of severe lung disease although low dose esmolol therapy is often effective and well tolerated in such patients. If these drugs fail, procainamide can be added in an attempt to slow the atrial rate.[76] Digoxin is usually ineffective, and if vigorously administered may induce toxicity. In a few particularly refractory cases of more chronic MAT we have had some success with amiodarone therapy. The latter not only slows atrial rate, but also slows AV conduction resulting in slower ventricular rates.

Paroxysmal Atrial Tachycardia

Etiology. Sustained paroxysms of atrial tachycardia (PAT) are relatively uncommon among the elderly, although short asymptomatic bursts are often detected by 24-hour Holter monitor recordings; occasionally recurrent symptomatic PAT may be a problem in some patients. PAT has several intra-atrial electrophysiological mechanisms and is usually associated with underlying cardiac disease.[106] A relatively small number of cases of PAT with variable AV nodal block are a result of digitalis toxicity,although this arrhythmia is characteristic of digitalis toxicity.[107]

Clinical Presentation. As in the case of other atrial tachyarrhythmias, the patient may be asymptomatic or present with unstable hemodynamics, or unstable angina. In addition, when PAT is a consequence of digitalis toxicity, patients may have other manifestations such as nausea, vomiting, confusion and rarely, yellow vision.

Electrocardiographic Characteristics. The atrial rate is 160 to 250 beats per minute and P waves are present before each QRS complex unless AV block is present. The P wave may have a normal axis suggesting an origin from the high right atrium. Alternatively, P waves may have a superiorly directed axis with negative P waves in inferior leads suggesting a low atrial origin, so- called "inferior atrial rhythm." Differentiation between atrial flutter and PAT is made primarily on the basis of atrial rate. Carotid massage or intravenous adenosine (6–12 mg intravenous, given rapidly) may induce AV block in PAT with 1:1 conduction. This response identifies the atrium as the source of the arrhythmia. If these interventions terminate the arrhythmia, AV nodal reentry or reentry using an accessory connection should be strongly considered.

Complications. The major complications associated with PAT are worsening hemodynamic status and myocardial ischemia. In patients with digitalis toxicity, there may be associated ventricular arrhythmias and high grade AV block.

Therapy. This is determined by clinical urgency and etiology of the arrhythmia. When digitalis toxicity is suspected because of PAT with AV block, the drug should be withheld and hypomagnesemia and hypokalemia should be corrected when present. Digoxin antibody administration is usually not required unless PAT is rapid and, or the patient is in jeopardy. A substantially elevated serum digoxin level (>3 ng/mL) supports a diagnosis of digoxin toxicity. Unstable patients with frank digitalis toxicity should not be cardioverted because of the substantial danger of postcardioversion ventricular arrhythmias; antibody administration is the preferred treatment. If digoxin is not the cause of PAT and the patient is clinically unstable, cardioversion should be used. In patients with an intra-atrial reentrant tachycardia, conversion to sinus rhythm may occur. Type 1 antiarrhythmic drugs may be effective in suppressing recurrent PAT. If the arrhythmia is automatic in origin, stimulants such as theophylline and caffeine should be avoided and a trial of β-blocker therapy may be warranted. In patients with recurrent drug resistant PAT, an electrophysiological study may be useful in clarifying the nature of the arrhythmia. Surgical or catheter ablation of an atrial focus has been successful in selected cases.[106] AV nodal ablation combined with VVI or VVIR pacing is reserved for refractory cases

Nonparoxysmal Junctional Tachycardia

Etiology. Nonparoxysmal junctional tachycardia (NPJT) is an accelerated junctional rhythm with ventricular rate between 70 and 140 beats per minute.[107] It may be caused by digitalis toxicity[108] or be associated with cardiac surgery, acute myocardial infarction or other severe illnesses that elevate serum catecholamine levels. It should not be confused with a junctional escape rhythm occurring in the presence of physiological or pathological sinus bradycardia where the junctional escape rate is usually less than 50 beats per minute.

Clinical Presentation. The patient may be asymptomatic or have symptoms and signs of the underlying disease. "Cannon A waves" may at times be present in the jugular venous pulse because of AV dissociation; the intensity of the first heart sound varies for the same reason. The ventricular rate is generally somewhat irregular because of intermittent sinus capture beats and periodic resetting of the sinus node by retrograde atrial activation. Loss of atrial contribution to ventricular filling may precipitate or aggravate heart failure.

Electrocardiographic Characteristics. The junctional rate exceeds that of the sinus node. There may be regular or intermittent retrograde atrial activation that resets the sinus node. Sinus capture beats often make the ventricular response irregular. NPJT may occur in the presence of atrial fibrillation or sinus rhythm. At more rapid rates, NPJT may be confused with slow ventricular tachycardia when there is aberrant intra-ventricular conduction.

Therapy. When NPJT is a manifestation of digitalis toxicity and the patient is hemodynamically stable as is usually the case, withholding digoxin and correcting hypomagnesemia and hypokalemia are all that is required. If the patient is unstable and the arrhythmia is thought to be contributory, digitalis antibody can be administered. In the absence of digitalis toxicity, in a stable patient, nothing need be done beyond treating the underlying problem. If lack of atrial "kick" is associated with hemodynamic instability, atrial pacing may be used to overdrive the junctional pacemaker and restore a normal sequence of contraction. If tachycardia aggravates angina, a short acting β-adrenergic blocking drug such as esmolol may be tried cautiously to slow the rate. However, this is unlikely to correct the arrhythmia. There are no long-term therapeutic recommendations since this tachyarrhythmia is transitory in the setting of an acute illness or perioperative stress.

AV Nodal and AV Reentrant Arrhythmias

In the elderly, new presentation of these arrhythmias is less common than in the young but accurate diagnosis is equally important in selecting pharmacological therapy and the availability of potentially curative ablation therapy.[109–112]

AV Nodal Reentry

Etiology

AV nodal reentry tachycardia is usually precipitated by a premature atrial impulse that is conducted slowly through the AV nodal region only to reenter using a fast conduction pathway in the retrograde direction (Figure 6). This pattern of slow antegrade conduction with fast retrograde conduction (slow-fast AV nodal reentry) can continue as a circus movement tachycardia until such time as the circuit is interrupted. A much less common form (fast-slow AV nodal reentry) results from fast antegrade conduction and slow retrograde conduction. In most patients only one form of the tachycardia is observed. However, intermediate forms with variable conduction times in either antegrade or retrograde direction may occur.

Clinical Presentation. Typically, attacks of tachycardia begin and end suddenly. Generally, the heart rate is in the range of 160 to 180 beats per minute but faster rates may occur and occasionally result in syncope (see Figure 8, Chapter 13). Syncope may result, in part, from the hemodynamic consequences of simultaneous contraction of the atria and ventricles, rapid rate, or other neurally mediated causes.[113]

ECG Diagnosis. The ECG during tachycardia generally has a narrow QRS complex, or QRS morphology similar to that of sinus rhythm. Typical right or left bundle branch block conduction pattern may also occur. In the common slow-fast tachycardia, the atria and ventricles are activated nearly simultaneously so that the P wave is buried in the QRS complex (Figure 7). An esophageal electrode can be used at the bedside to document simultaneous activation of the atria and ventricles. In the uncommon form of AV node reentry (fast-slow), the P wave may be visible during tachycardia. Under this circumstance the distance from the preceding R wave to the P is longer than the subsequent PR interval. During sinus rhythm, patients with AV nodal reentry tachycardia do not have delta waves to suggest ventricular pre-excitation. Although a probable diagnosis of AV nodal reentry can often be made based on the presenting clinical and electrocardiographic features, an invasive electrophysiological study is needed to confirm the diagnosis.

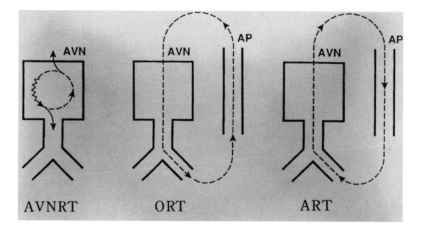

Figure 6: *Schematic representation of AV nodal reentry tachycardia (AVNRT). In this tachycardia reentry occurs in the area of the AV node with secondary activation of the atria and ventricles. Orthodromic reciprocating tachycardia (ORT) utilizes the normal conduction system in an antegrade direction and an accessory AV connection in the retrograde direction to complete the reentry loop. Antidromic reciprocating tachycardia (ART) utilizes an accessory AV connection in the antegrade direction and the normal conduction system in the retrograde direction.*

Immediate Therapy. At the time of presentation, patients may have already discovered that certain maneuvers such as holding their breath, Valsalva maneuver, or carotid massage can interrupt the tachycardia.[114] When these are successful, termination of tachycardia is the rule as opposed to the transient increase in AV block seen in patients with primary atrial tachycardias. If vagal maneuvers fail, intravenous adenosine or a calcium channel blocking drug such as verapamil is usually successful. Adenosine (6–12 mg rapidly intravenously) is preferable because its rapid onset and offset of action limits the duration of any side effects. Intravenous verapamil (5–15 mg intravenously) is also quite effective, but can result in significant hypotension particularly if rapid conversion to sinus rhythm does not occur. Pretreatment with intravenously administered calcium has been shown to prevent or attenuate the hypotension without affecting the AV nodal blocking effect.[105] DC cardioversion is rarely necessary.

Long-term Therapy. Patients with infrequent, brief, well-tolerated episodes that are self terminating may require no therapy. If drug therapy is necessary, β-blockers, calcium channel blockers, and antiarrhythmic drugs have been used with varying degrees of success and the choice of antiarrhythmic agents is empirical, the goal being to select an agent that is well tolerated and effective; in this regard, newer agents such as propafenone are increasingly favored. Catheter ablation has been found to be extremely effective in treating both "slow" and "fast" pathways in over 90% of cases.[109,112] Selective AV nodal modification is occasionally complicated by complete AV block that appears to be more common when the primary attempt is to ablate a "fast" pathway.[112] Catheter ablation has become the primary mode of therapy in many patients with frequent symptomatic episodes of AV nodal reentry tachycardia.

AV Reentry Tachycardia and the WPW syndrome

Etiology. AV reentry tachycardia uses an accessory connection and the normal specialized conduction system as a macro-reentry tachycardia loop (Figure 6).[115] The arrhythmia is precipitated by premature atrial or ventricular impulses that are conducted differently through the normal specialized conduction system compared to the accessory connection.

Clinical Presentation. Like AV nodal reentry, episodes of tachycardia start and end abruptly. Tachycardia rates are similar to that seen with AV nodal reentry. Elderly patients usually give a history of intermittent tachycardia for years. Often, their major complaint is that the tachycardia has recently become much more symptomatic. This is often related to development of other cardiovascular disease, especially coronary artery disease. An increase in frequency and inability to self terminate episodes of tachycardia are also frequent complaints.

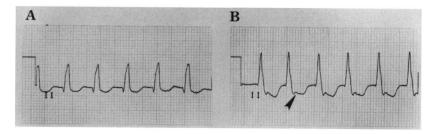

Figure 7: *ECG examples of **A**: AV nodal reentry tachycardia. Note the absence of P waves secondary to their inscription at the same time as the QRS. **B**: Orthodromic reciprocating tachycardia utilizing an accessory AV connection. P waves are marked with arrows.*

ECG Diagnosis. The ECG in sinus rhythm may demonstrate evidence of ventricular pre-excitation in the form of delta waves (Figure 8).[115] The presence of delta waves depends on the location of the connection, its ability to conduct in an antegrade fashion and the conduction properties of the AV node. If the connection does not conduct in an antegrade direction, it is called "concealed." Orthodromic reciprocating tachycardia (ORT) (Figures 6 and 8), the most common form of AV reentrant tachycardia, utilizes the normal AV node and His conduction system in an antegrade direction and the accessory connection in retrograde direction to complete the reentry loop. Hence, delta waves, if present during sinus rhythm, disappear during the tachycardia (Figure 8). The ventricular rate during ORT is frequently in the range of 180 to 200 beats per minute in the older age group, although faster rates (200 to 240 beats per minute) are occasionally encountered. Unlike AV node reentry, careful examination of the ECG during ORT will often reveal P waves (Figure 7). The timing of the P waves is such that the R to P interval is usually less than the subsequent P to R interval. If P waves are not visible, techniques to record atrial electrical activity such as an esophageal lead can be used. During ORT the QRS is typically narrow but right or left bundle branch block may occur. Antidromic reciprocating tachycardia (ART) (Figure 6) is much less common and involves antegrade conduction through the accessory connection with retrograde conduction via the His and AV nodal conduction system.[115] In ART the QRS is wide and bizarre because of abnormal ventricular activation through the accessory connection (Figure 5). Patients with accessory connections may present with severe symptoms and fast ventricular rates in response to atrial fibrillation or flutter. This occurs when the accessory pathway has a rapid antegrade conduction velocity and a short refractory period. Under these circumstances the QRS is wide and bizarre (Figure 5) and very rapid ventricular rates can occur. A more complex situation arises when there is an accessory connection that is not an active participant in the tachycardia. An example is the occurrence of AV nodal reentry tachycardia with a "by-

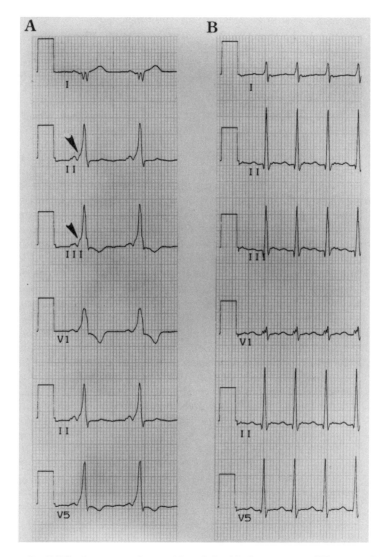

Figure 8: *ECGs from a patient with a left-sided accessory AV connection.* **A:** *In sinus rhythm note delta waves marked with arrows.* **B:** *During orthodromic reciprocating tachycardia the QRS normalizes as antegrade conduction is through the AV node with the reentrant circuit completed by the accessory connection.*

stander" accessory AV connection that does not participate in the reentry loop but does activate the ventricles abnormally producing wide aberrant QRS complexes.[115] This diagnosis is made by careful invasive electrophysiological study. Other accessory AV connections that are variants of pre-excitation also exist but are decidedly less common. Examples are atrio-fasicular connections that arise in the right atrium and insert in the vicinity of the right bundle branch. Similarly, nodo-fasicular and nodoventricular connections may arise in the AV node and insert in the vicinity of the right bundle branch or right ventricle.[116]

Immediate Therapy. As in AV nodal reentry tachycardia, patients may use techniques such as the Valsalva maneuver or carotid massage to interrupt episodes of tachycardia. If vagal maneuvers fail and QRS morphology is normal or has a morphology of typical right or left bundle branch block, then adenosine (6–12 mg rapidly, intravenous) or verapamil (5–15 mg intravenous) can be used to terminate orthodromic tachycardia. Whether vagal maneuvers, adenosine or verapamil are used, termination almost always occurs with inscription of a P wave, because block occurs in the AV node. Synchronized DC cardioversion or procainamide infusion can be used if the aforementioned drugs fail. If DC conversion is performed, an energy level of 50 J synchronized to the R wave is generally adequate.

If antidromic tachycardia (either antegrade conduction through an accessory connection and retrograde conduction through the normal conduction system or atrial fibrillation or flutter with rapid antegrade conduction through an accessory pathway) is suspected, prompt cardioversion is the safest and most expeditious therapy and will likely be successful. If the wide complex tachycardia is well tolerated, slow infusion of intravenous procainamide (10–15 mg/kg) given at a rate of no greater than 25 mg/min, carefully monitoring for hypotension, may be successful. Agents that slow conduction in the AV node such as digoxin and calcium channel blockers should be avoided in treatment of these tachycardias as they may facilitate conduction through the accessory connection and further accelerate heart rate. The differentiation of rapid antegrade AV reentry tachycardia from a regular atrial tachycardia (such as PAT or flutter) with rapid antegrade conduction down an accessory connection may be difficult. This diagnostic problem reinforces our recommendation to use cardioversion as the primary therapy, or slow procainamide infusion, if cardioversion cannot be performed promptly. It must be emphasized that wide complex tachycardia in older patients with known accessory pathways cannot always be assumed to be related to the accessory connection. For example, an elderly patient may have had pre-excitation since childhood but with the development of ischemic heart disease, ventricular tachycardia may occur, making clinical distinction difficult. Electrophysiological study can identify inducible ventricular tachycardia and also map the accessory pathway.

Long-term Therapy. As in AV nodal reentry, no treatment may be necessary in patients with infrequent, well tolerated, self terminating episodes of orthodromic AV reentry tachycardia. In patients with ORT requiring treatment, drugs that slow AV nodal conduction such as digoxin and calcium channel blockers may be effective. However, these drugs could potentially increase the frequency of tachycardia by providing the critical AV nodal delay required for impulses to reenter the accessory connection. Drugs that slow accessory pathway conduction such as β-blockers and most type 1 antiarrhythmic drugs can be used successfully.[117] In patients with antidromic tachycardia or rapid ventricular response to atrial fibrillation, the latter drugs are especially important. Amiodarone has been found to be particularly effective in the management of some refractory tachycardias. However, as discussed subsequently, radiofrequency catheter ablation of the accessory pathway may be the best approach in these patients.

Catheter ablation is a relatively safe and effective curative therapy (>90%) for patients with accessory connections and frequent and, or life threatening ORT or ART.[110,111] Previously, surgical techniques to interrupt pathways tended to be used in younger, and only highly symptomatic older patients. We have used radiofrequency catheter ablation successfully in a number of older patients including several with significant coexisting diseases, especially severe pulmonary disease. In many such patients, this is a better and perhaps safer option than lifelong complex pharmacological therapy.

Ventricular Arrhythmias

Premature Ventricular Contractions and Nonsustained Ventricular Tachycardia

Etiology

Premature ventricular contractions (PVCs), and even runs of nonsustained ventricular tachycardia (VT) are common in elderly patients and their frequency increases with age. They may be encountered in the absence of clinically evident heart disease, but usually complicate ischemic or hypertensive heart disease or cardiomyopathy.

Clinical Presentation

Many patients are unaware of the arrhythmia. Palpitation or a sensation of throbbing in the neck are presumably caused by "cannon

A waves." Anxiety may result from awareness of an irregular heart beat. Weakness and presyncope are rare and may result from ventricular bigeminy with a slow effective heart rate. Ambulatory ECG recordings and clinical observation indicate that most PVCs are asymptomatic. Perception of PVCs is more likely to occur when the patient is at rest, especially before sleep when external stimuli are minimal.

Electrocardiographic Features

PVCs are usually easily recognized by their patterns of atypical left bundle branch block or right bundle branch block, or greater degrees of aberration. A full compensatory pause usually occurs because of block of the next sinus beat following retrograde conduction and penetration of the AV node. Usually, the coupling interval between the PVC and the preceding normal QRS complex is fixed and a reentrant mechanism is likely. If retrograde conduction is absent as with closely coupled PVCs, the subsequent sinus P wave will be conducted and the PVC is then said to be *interpolated*. When the coupling interval is variable but the interval between PVCs is constant, or a multiple of a constant interval, *ventricular parasystole* is present. Ventricular parasystole reflects abnormal automaticity and has no more clinical significance than re-entrant PVCs. However, parasystole is more resistant to drug therapy than reentrant extrasystoles. Nonsustained VT has electrocardiographic features comparable to those described below for sustained ventricular tachycardia.

Therapy

There is evidence that frequent PVCs, including PVCs in pairs, or short runs of less than 5 beats, and nonsustained VT of less than 20 to 30 seconds duration, are independent markers for sudden death in the presence of significant underlying heart disease.[118–120] However, there are no data to indicate that treatment with antiarrhythmic drugs improves prognosis except for possibly amiodarone.[121] The latter drug has demonstrated mixed results when used in patients at high risk after myocardial infarction, or with congestive heart failure. The lesson of the Cardiac Arrhythmia Suppression Study (CAST) study is that certain antiarrhythmic drugs may actually increase mortality after myocardial infarction despite controlling ventricular ectopy.[75] Whether these data apply to other antiarrhythmic drugs or other cardiac diseases remains to be determined.

Symptomatic patients should be reassured that PVCs are not dangerous. This will often reduce anxiety and make sensed PVCs more tolerable. When the frequency of PVCs is increased by caffeine, alcohol, smoking, or excessive fatigue, their frequency may be markedly reduced by changes in life style. β-adrenergic blockers may be used for their anxiolytic effect, when symptoms are intolerable, provided there are no contraindications. However, control of PVCs themselves is infrequent with β- blockers alone.

Therapy with antiarrhythmic drugs should be reserved for the very few patients with intractable and distressing symptoms willing to accept risks inherent in such therapy. Treatment should usually be instituted in hospital to monitor for early proarrhythmia and inappropriate prolongation of the QT or other conduction intervals. The choice of drug should consider the potential for proarrhythmia, side effect profiles, and special problems of older patients. For example, disopyramide has marked negative inotropic and anticholinergic properties and should not be used in men with poor left ventricular function and, or obstructive uropathy. Because the main benefit of therapy is relief of symptoms and not prolongation of life, the minimal dose that will achieve this effect should be used. Given the uncertain risk/benefit ratio of treating PVCs with antiarrhythmic drugs, it cannot be overemphasized that treatment is the last resort reserved for patients with poorly tolerated symptoms. Table 3 summarizes the drugs commonly used in the treatment of ventricular arrhythmias.

Similar considerations apply to nonsustained ventricular tachycardia in asymptomatic patients who have relatively well preserved left ventricular function. In patients with an ejection fraction of less than 30% to 35%, complex ventricular ectopy identifies a group of patients at high risk for sudden death.[118-120] The MADITT trial using ambulatory monitoring evaluated post-myocardial infarction patients with ejection fractions ≤35% and nonsustained ventricular tachycardia (≥3 beats).[122] Patients were subjected to electrophysiological testing and if found to be inducible and not suppressible with antiarrhythmic drugs were randomly assigned to receive conventional therapy versus an implantable defibrillator. Improved survival was demonstrated in the ICD group with significant reduction in arrhythmic death. In contrast, in a group of patients referred for coronary artery bypass with ejection fractions ≤35% and an abnormal signal averaged ECG, implantation of a defibrillator at the time of surgery did not have a survival benefit.[123] Thus, the use of prophylactic implanted cardioverter-defibrillators appears promising in selected post-myocardial infarction patients with significantly decreased ejection fractions and nonsustained ventricular tachycardia. The current high cost of this procedure and numbers of potential patients may limit their widespread use but, this may change with advances in technology and improved ability to identify the highest risk patients. Among the elderly, the presence and severity of cardiac, and other underlying diseases, must be considered before applying the results of the MADITT trial to this population.

Sustained Ventricular Tachycardia and Ventricular Fibrillation

Etiology. Chronic ischemic heart disease with myocardial scarring and left ventricular dysfunction is by far the most common substrate

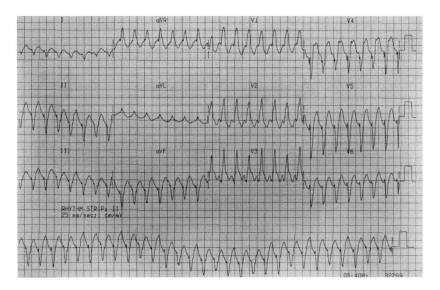

Figure 9: *Twelve-lead ECG during ventricular tachycardia from a patient with ischemic heart disease. Note the atypical right bundle branch appearance with very wide QRS complexes. In the frontal plane the QRS axis is superiorly directed.*

for recurrent ventricular tachycardia (Figure 9), ventricular fibrillation, and sudden death. Evidence of abnormalities of myocardial excitation can frequently be detected by signal averaged ECG, a technique that can detect late potentials in an extended terminal portion of the QRS.[124]

The next most common cause of ventricular arrhythmias is nonischemic myocardiopathy with left ventricular dysfunction. In the older age group, common causes of left ventricular dysfunction include those related to valvular disease, long-standing hypertension, idiopathic cardiomyopathy and, long-term alcohol abuse. Drug-induced ventricular arrhythmias including those associated with QT prolongation (torsades de pointes)[125] (Figure 10) and digitalis toxicity[107] must also be considered. Drugs associated with QT prolongation and torsades de pointes include most standard antiarrhythmic drugs such as quinidine, procainamide, disopyramide, propafenone, sotalol, etc; in contrast, amiodarone is an uncommon cause of this arrhythmia despite the fact that QT prolongation is generally present.[125] The calcium channel blocker, bepridil, which also has sodium channel opening properties, and psychotropic drugs such as amitryptyline and phenothiazines may also result in QT prolongation and torsade.[125] Antibiotics such as intravenous erythromycin have also been implicated.[125] Other abnormalities associated with the long QT syndrome include hypokalemia, hypomagnesemia, lithium therapy, hypophosphatemia, a liquid protein diet or

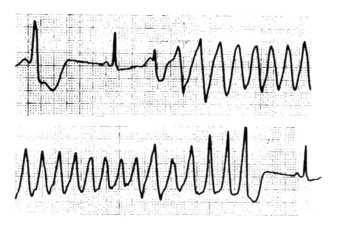

Figure 10: *ECG (continuous strip) example of torsades de pointes which occurred in a patient recently placed on quinidine therapy. Note initiation of tachycardia after a pause and spontaneous termination of the arrhythmia despite the rapid rate.*

starvation and severe bradyarrhythmias such as sinus node dysfunction or complete heart block.[20,125]

Clinical Presentation. Although most patients who present with severe ventricular arrhythmias have a history of significant cardiac disease, in some the arrhythmia may be the first manifestation of the disease. Even among patients with a known history of heart disease, the clinical course may have been quite stable until onset of the arrhythmia. Patients generally present with palpitation, weakness, dizziness, angina, or symptoms of heart failure, or, more dramatically with syncope or cardiac arrest. The presenting symptoms and signs are generally proportional to the rate of tachycardia and severity of cardiac disease. If the ventricular tachycardia rate is slow and underlying heart disease is mild, there may be few symptoms. Physical findings relatively specific for ventricular tachycardia include intermittent cannon A waves in the jugular venous pulse and variation in intensity of the first heart sound, both a result of AV dissociation. If there is retrograde AV conduction, these findings are absent and the jugular venous pulse demonstrates continuous cannon A waves.

The advent of mobile paramedic units has significantly increased the number of patients resuscitated from an episode of out of hospital cardiac arrest. Long-term survival following ventricular fibrillation and sudden death is strongly linked to severity of cardiac and noncardiac disease and the type of long-term therapy used. In the elderly patient, ventricular fibrillation may be the terminal event in a variety of medical illnesses. This in part explains the low success rate in attempts to resuscitate patients already hospitalized for advanced illness whether cardiac or noncardiac. Thus, in an elderly population it is essential to define the resuscitation status of all patients receiving long-term care. This decision should include a detailed evaluation of long-term prognosis and should incorporate the views of the patient and family. Prior determination of resuscitation status generally prevents tragic futile efforts that deny the patient and family the comfort and dignity of a peaceful death.

Electrocardiographic Findings. Ventricular tachycardia is characterized by abnormal QRS morphology and duration and is one of the causes of "wide QRS complex tachycardia." Other causes include: (1) supraventricular tachycardias with right bundle branch block, left bundle branch block, or nonspecific intraventricular conduction delay and (2) tachycardias involving ventricular activation via an accessory pathway such as the WPW syndrome.[126] Physicians are generally eternal optimists and often try to make the most benign diagnosis in the face of a wide QRS complex tachycardia especially if the tachycardia is well tolerated. It should be emphasized that, in an older population and especially in those with underlying heart disease, the most common wide QRS complex tachycardia is ventricular tachycardia.[126] A number of criteria have been proposed for analysis of wide complex QRS tachycardias[127]:

(1) AV dissociation is present in about 50% of ventricular tachycardias and should be carefully sought by looking for P waves independent of QRS complexes in the 12 lead ECG.
(2) The presence of fusion beats strongly supports AV dissociation (Figure 11).

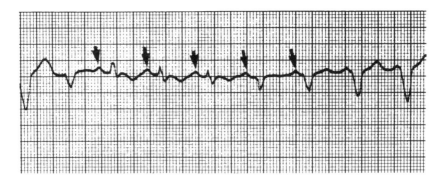

Figure 11: *ECG example of slow ventricular tachycardia with competing sinus rhythm producing fusion beats. From left to right wide complex ventricular beats with fusion resulting from above (P's marked with arrows).*

(3) Unless typical right bundle branch block or left bundle branch block is present, a diagnosis of ventricular tachycardia is strongly favored, provided an earlier ECG with sinus rhythm does not show comparable QRS morphology.

(4) Ventricular tachycardia is usually monomorphic (Figure 9).

(5) QRS duration greater than 140 msec with atypical right bundle branch block (Figure 9) or 160 msec with atypical left bundle branch block favors ventricular tachycardia.

(6) A negative, monomorphic QRS complex in all precordial leads is nearly always ventricular tachycardia.

(7) A markedly leftward frontal plane QRS axis is highly suggestive of ventricular tachycardia (Figure 9).

Even with these useful guidelines and a strong probability that a wide QRS tachycardia in an elderly patient is ventricular tachycardia, it should be appreciated that in some patients only electrophysiological study can define the true nature of a tachycardia.

Torsades de pointes (Figure 10) is the type of ventricular tachycardia most often associated with QT prolongation, although monomorphic ventricular tachycardia may also occur with QT prolongation. Torsades de pointes is characterized by rapid rate and marked variations of QRS morphology (ie, rapid changes of the QRS from positive to negative) over short periods of time. Persistent torsades may result in cardiovascular collapse and deteriorate into ventricular fibrillation. Torsades is often initiated by a long-short sequence of R-R intervals (Figure 10). For example, a sinus beat followed by a PVC generates a compensatory pause and the next sinus beat has marked prolongation of the QT interval with a significant after potential that triggers the arrhythmia.[125]

Digitalis associated ventricular tachycardia or fibrillation may occur in the patient with severe heart disease even if digoxin levels are not markedly elevated, and especially if hypokalemia or hypomagnesemia are present.[107] In patients with less severe disease, ventricular arrhythmia may occur with very high digoxin levels. The classic, but uncommon, digitalis induced bidirectional ventricular tachycardia is felt to result from alternation of intraventricular conduction.[107]

Ventricular fibrillation is characterized by chaotic variations in the electrocardiographic baseline that may be coarse in amplitude or quite fine. The term ventricular flutter has been used to designate regular sinusoidal oscillations of moderate amplitude with the rate varying from 175 to 300 cycles per minute.

Immediate Therapeutic Approach. This is dictated by the clinical presentation. If the patient with ventricular tachycardia is stable enough to tolerate a brief delay in cardioversion, a 12-lead ECG should be obtained. This will aid initial diagnosis and, most importantly, will be useful for reference in those patients undergoing subsequent electrophysiological study. In the unstable patient with ventricular tachycardia, a monitor strip may be all that is obtainable and immediate synchronized DC cardioversion is indicated following adequate sedation. Patients who are stable can be loaded with lidocaine or procainamide. If tachycardia persists, DC cardioversion can be performed under brief general anesthesia. Although bretylium tosylate may slow ventricular tachycardia, it is usually not very effective in terminating or preventing the arrhythmia. The hypotensive effects of bretylium limits its use in patients with marginal hemodynamic status. In patients with acute, recurring ventricular tachycardia or fibrillation, intravenous amiodarone is often effective when other agents have failed.

For patients presenting with ventricular fibrillation, the American Heart Association Advanced Cardiac Life Support (ACLS) guidelines for emergency therapy should be followed. In all patients with ventricular arrhythmias particular attention should be paid to identifying underlying myocardial infarction, ischemia, heart failure, electrolyte, acid-base and arterial blood gas abnormalities and drug toxicity because correction of such abnormalities facilitates resuscitation. Further, definition of a reversible cause of the arrhythmia will markedly influence long-term therapy.

Long-Term Therapeutic Approaches. Long-term therapeutic goals and approach to treatment are determined by severity of arrhythmia and associated cardiac and noncardiac diseases. In the setting of acute transmural myocardial infarction, the risk of late recurrence of early ventricular arrhythmia is relatively low. The primary determinants of subsequent untoward events are the severity of left ventricular dysfunction, the presence of myocardial ischemia, and the presence of persisting ventricular ectopy or nonsustained ventricular tachycardia. These patients should undergo the usual postinfarction risk stratification including, contrast angiography, exercise stress testing, and determination of left ventricular function using echocardiography or nuclear angiography. In elderly patients, particularly those with multiple limiting concomitant problems, risk stratification may not be feasible or particularly useful. If inducible ischemia is present, it should be dealt with as discussed in Chapter 10.

In patients presenting with acute ventricular arrhythmias without myocardial infarction, we perform angiography to assess severity of any underlying coronary disease and also to assess left ventricular function unless age or debility is a contraindication. We recommend revascularization without further evaluation of the arrhythmia when there is severe coronary disease. After optimal management of the coronary artery disease, the patient then undergoes an electrophysiological study to determine whether inducible ventricular arrhythmia is present.

In patients without critical coronary disease, we perform electrophysiological testing following angiography. However, in patients in whom the clinically significant arrhythmia is readily detected by rest or ambulatory monitoring, an alternate approach is serial trials of anti-arrhythmic drugs followed by 24-hour ambulatory ECG monitoring and exercise testing to ensure suppression. In the subpopulation of patients with significant ambulatory arrhythmias, electrophysiological testing or Holter monitoring appear to be equally effective in predicting drug efficacy.[128] Drugs used to treat ventricular arrhythmias are summarized in Table 3. In patients without significant ventricular arrhythmia during monitoring, electrophysiological testing is superior. In the setting of ischemic heart disease, electrophysiological testing results in arrhythmia induction in about 80% to 90% of cases. In nonischemic cardiomyopathy, the yield is only about 50% or less.[129] It is important to recognize that even with serial antiarrhythmic drug testing using many drugs, the likelihood of success measured by provocative electrophysiological testing is only about 45%.[106] In patients with the poorest ventricular function, finding tolerable and effective drug therapy is difficult. Unfortunately, this group is at the highest risk for recurrence of arrhythmia and sudden death. In the ESVEM study when a drug was judged effective either by electrophysiological testing or Holter monitoring, 150 of 296 patients suffered arrhythmia recurrence and there were 34 arrhythmic deaths.[128] Patients presenting with sustained ventricular tachycardia that is hemodynamically tolerable will more frequently benefit from serial drug testing. Even in this group, however, there is a substantial risk of sudden death.

Other modes of therapy include surgical[130] and more recently, catheter[131] and chemical ablation.[132] In patients with 1 or 2 morphologies of ventricular tachycardia and left ventricular aneurysm, surgical plication of the aneurysm coupled with arrhythmia mapping and selective endocardial ablation can be very successful.[130] Catheter ablation using either DC or radiofrequency energy are successful in about 50% of selected cases.[131] Usually, catheter ablation is reserved for cases refractory to drug treatment with frequent recurrence. Instillation of intracoronary alcohol through an angioplasty balloon catheter has been used to ablate arrhythmias in a few selected cases but remains an investigational procedure.[132]

Currently, the most successful therapy used to treat patients with symptomatic life-threatening ventricular arrhythmias is the implantable cardioverter-defibrillator. Mortality rates as low as 7% over the first year after implantation have been reported as has an arrhythmic death rate over 5 years of follow-up of less than 5%.[133] The Antiarrhythmic versus Implantable Defibrillators Trial found a significant benefit using device versus pharmacologic therapy.[134] In our experience, adjunctive drug therapy and also radiofrequency ablation may reduce frequency of cardioverter-defibrillator discharges in patients when they impinge on the quality of life. Fortunately, with modern devices capable of rapid pacing conversion of ventricular tachycardia, the frequency of uncomfortable shocks is often minimal.

Unfortunately, many patients who have suffered significant ventricular arrhythmias are poor candidates for aggressive therapy with implanted devices. Included in this group are patients with severe intractable heart failure and those with significant multisystem diseases. Additionally, some elderly patients are quite averse to this form of treatment. In such patients we have used amiodarone empirically and this has been well tolerated even in the presence of severe left ventricular dysfunction. Concerns about long-term complications, including serious hepatic and pulmonary toxicity, need to be balanced against potential benefit of the drug. We regularly monitor thyroid and liver function and obtain annual pulmonary function tests including diffusing capacity of lung for carbon monoxide (D_{lco}). The latter seems to be helpful only in patients with gradually progressive pulmonary toxicity. Most cases of pulmonary toxicity present subacutely with dry cough and the problem is to rule out other causes.

Sotalol (a type 3 antiarrhythmic agent with β-blocking properties) has also been reported to be effective in treating ventricular tachyarrhythmias and can be used if the ejection fraction is not severely depressed and there are no other contraindications to β-blockade. [73,128]

Therapy for Long QT-Associated Ventricular Tachycardia. Temporary ventricular pacing or acceleration of heart rate with infusion of isoproterenol or dobutamine are frequently successful in shortening the QT interval and abolishing torsades.[125] Drug withdrawal and, or correction of hypokalemia and hypomagnesemia is important when these are thought to be responsible or contributory. Intravenous magnesium infusion is often effective in controlling torsades even in patients without magnesium deficiency and this is now first line therapy.[125]

Therapy for Digitalis Toxic Ventricular Tachycardia. If the patient is not compromised by a relatively slow tachycardia, withholding digitalis, correcting electrolyte deficiencies and careful monitoring is appropriate. If there is evidence of major toxicity, characterized by elevation of serum potassium levels, severe tachyarrhythmia or bradyarrhythmias and hemodynamic instability, digoxin antibody (FAB) is the most effective treatment.

Antitachycardia and Defibrillator Devices

As pointed out earlier, implanted cardioverter-defibrillators (ICDs) are highly effective in treating sudden arrhythmic cardiac death.[133] It must be recognized, however, that such therapy is "after-the -fact," and recurrence of arrhythmia is not prevented. This treatment is a welcome addition to current options, considering the high failure rate of drugs. Previously, ICDs required a thoracotomy for implantation which increased mortality and morbidity. However, the recent availability of transvenous leads and other methods of cardioversion such as overdrive pacing make device therapy even more appealing. The cost of device therapy remains high, but will likely decrease. The success of ICD devices in prolonging life has generated another social issue, ie, when can such patients be permitted to drive their automobiles? Physicians may consult the detailed recommendations included in the AHA/NASPE Medical/Scientific Statement [135] and relevant State regulations. Although currently available ICD's substantially decrease the risk of sudden death, they do not decrease mortality from heart failure.[136,137] The decision to implant a defibrillator in a younger individual with good left ventricular function and an episode of sudden cardiac death is relatively easy, but the decision is more difficult in the elderly patient and particularly those patients with multiple diseases. Severe left ventricular dysfunction is associated with a higher implantation mortality. In patients with progressive heart failure, an ICD may prolong, but not improve the quality of life. It is important, therefore, for physicians to help elderly patients exercise their autonomy and make informed decisions as to whether or not to accept this treatment. As indicated, empiric drug therapy may be a reasonable alternative for some members of this group of patients.

Acknowledgment

The authors wish to thank Dr. Howard B. Burchell for his detailed critique of this chapter and many helpful suggestions, to Karleen Pratt for secretarial assistance and to Peggy Fashingbauer for her help in preparation of the figures.

References

1. Rokseth R, Hatle L: Prospective study on the occurrence and management of chronic sinoatrial disease, with follow-up study. *Am Heart J* 109: 513–522, 1985.
2. Hartel G, Talvensaari T: Treatment of sinoatrial syndrome with permanent cardiac pacing in 90 patients. *Acta Med Scand* 198:341–347, 1975.
3. Jordan J, Yamaguchi I, Mandel M: Function and dysfunction of the sinus node: Clinical studies in the evaluation of sinus node function. In: F Bonke, (ed.) *The Sinus Node: Structure, Function, and Clinical Relevance.* The Hague: Martinus Nijhoff, 1978, pp 3–22.
4. Rickards A, Donaldson R: Rate responsive pacing. *Clin Prog Pacing Electrophysiol* 1:21–29, 1983.
5. Benditt D, Milstein S, Goldstein M, et al: Sinus node dysfunction: Pathophysiology, clinical features, evaluation and treatment. In: D Zipes, J Jalife, (eds.) *Cardiac Electrophysiology: From Cell to Bedside.* Philadelphia, PA: WB Saunders, 1990, pp 708–734.
6. Short D: The syndrome of alternating bradycardia and tachycardia. *Br Heart J* 16:208–214, 1954.

7. Lekieffre J, Libersa C, Caron J, et al: Electrocardiographic aspects of sinus node dysfunction: Use of the holter electrocardiographic recording. In: S Levy, M Scheinman M, (eds.) *Cardiac Arrhythmias: From Diagnosis to Therapy*; Mount Kisco, NY, Futura Publishing Company, 1984, pp 73–105

8. Antman E, Ludmer P, McGowan N, et al: Transtelephonic electrocardiographic transmission for management of cardiac arrhythmias. *Am J Cardiol* 58:1021–1024, 1986.

9. Kostis J, Moreyra A, Amendo M, et al: The effect of age on heart rate in subjects free of heart disease. *Circulation* 65:141–145, 1982.

10. Jose A, Collison D: The normal range and the determinants of the intrinsic heart rate in man. *Cardiovasc Res* 4:160–166, 1970.

11. Benditt D, Sakaguchi S, Goldstein M, et al: Sinus node dysfunction: Pathophysiology, clinical features, evaluation and treatment. In: D Zipes, J Jalife, (eds.) *Cardiac Electrophysiology, From Cell to Bedside*. Second edition. Philadelphia, PA, W.B. Saunders Company, 1995, pp 1215–1247.

12. Skagen K, Hansen J: The long-term prognosis for patients with sinoatrial block treated with permanent pacemaker. *Acta Med Scand* 199:13–15, 1975.

13. Sasaki S, Takeuchi A, Ohzeki M, et al: Long-term follow-up of paced patients with sick sinus syndrome. In: K Steinbach, D Glogar, A Laszkovics, et al: *Cardiac Pacing. Proceedings of the VIIth World Symposium on Cardiac Pacing*. Darmstadt, Steinkopff Verlag, 1983, pp. 85–90.

14. Conde C, Leppo J, Lipski J, et al: Effectiveness of pacemaker treatment in the bradycardia-tachycardia syndrome. *Am J Cardiol* 32:209–214, 1973.

15. Alt E, Volker R, Wirtzfeld A, et al: Survival and follow-up after pacemaker implantation: A comparison of patients with sick sinus syndrome, complete heart block and atrial fibrillation. *PACE* 8:849–855, 1985.

16. Wohl A, Laborde J, Atkins JM, et al: Prognosis of patients permanently paced for sick sinus syndrome. *Arch Intern Med* 136:406–408, 1976.

17. Lichstein E, Aithal H, Jonas S, et al: Natural history of severe sinus bradycardia discovered by 24 hour Holter monitoring. *PACE* 5:185–189, 1982.

18. Benditt D, Benson DJ, Kriett J, et al: Electrophysiologic effects of theophylline in young patients with recurrent symptomatic bradyarrhythmias. *Am J Cardiol* 52:1223–1229, 1983.

19. Benditt D, Benson D Jr, Dunnigan A, et al: Drug therapy in sinus node dysfunction. In: E Rapport, (ed.). *Cardiology Update-1984*. New York, Elsevier, 1984, pp 79–101.

20. Parkinson J, Papp C, Evans W: The electrocardiogram of the Stokes-Adams attack. *Br Heart J* 3:171–199, 1941.

21. Davies M, Anderson R, Becker A: *The Conduction System of the Heart*. London: Butterworth & Co., 1983.

22. Rotman M, Wagner G, Wallace A: Bradyarrhythmias in acute myocardial infarction. *Circulation* 45:703, 1972.

23. Norris R: Heart block in posterior and anterior myocardial infarction. *Br Heart J* 31:352, 1969.

24. Norris R, Mercer C: Significance of idioventricular rhythms in acute myocardial infarction. *Prog Cardiovasc Dis* 16:455, 1974.

25. Mavric Z, Zaputovic L, Matana A, et al: Complete heart block associated with acute myocardial infarction. *Am Heart J* 119:823, 1990.

26. Kostuk W, Beanlands D: Complete heart block associated with acute myocardial infarction. *Am J Cardiol* 26:380, 1970.

27. Lamas G, Muller J, Turi Z, et al: A simplified method to predict occurrence of complete heart block during acute myocardial infarction. *Am J Cardiol* 57:1213–1219, 1986.

28. Waller B: Clinicopathological correlations of the human cardiac conduction system. In: D Zipes, J Jalife J, (eds.) *Cardiac Electrophysiology: From Cell to Bedside.* Philadelphia, PA, WB Saunders, 1990, pp 249–269.

29. Madsen J, Meibom J, Videbach R: Transcutaneous pacing: Experience with the Zoll noninvasive temporary pacemaker. *Am Heart J* 116:7, 1988.

30. Matangi M: Temporary physiologic pacing in inferior wall acute myocardial infarction with right ventricular damage. *Am J Cardiol* 59:1207, 1987.

31. Parsonnet V, Furman S, Smyth N: Implantable cardiac pacemakers: Status report and resource guidelines. *Circulation* 50:A21, 1974.

32. Parsonnet V, Furman S, Smyth N: Revised code for pacemaker identification. *PACE* 4:400, 1981.

33. Lakatta E, Mitchell J, Pomerance A, et al: Human aging: Changes in structure and function. *J Am Coll Cardiol* 10:42A-47A, 1987.

34. Lakatta E: Do hypertension and aging have a similar effect on the myocardium? *Circulation* 75:169–177, 1987.

35. Alpert M, Curtis J, Sanfelippo J, et al: Comparative survival following permanent ventricular and dual-chamber pacing for patients with chronic symptomatic sinus node dysfunction with and without congestive heart failure. *Am Heart J* 113:958–965, 1987.

36. Rosenqvist M: Atrial pacing for sick sinus syndrome. *Clin Cardiol* 13:43–47, 1990.

37. Andersen H, Thuesen L, Bagger J, et al: Prospective randomised trial of atrial versus ventricular pacing in sick-sinus syndrome. *Lancet* 344:1523–1528, 1994.

38. Sutton R, Kenny R: The natural history of sick sinus syndrome. *PACE* 9:1110–1114, 1986.

39. Barold S, Zipes D: Cardiac pacemakers and antiarrhythmic devices. In: E Braunwald, (ed.) *Heart Disease: A Textbook of Cardiovascular Medicine.* Philadelphia, PA, WB Saunders, 1992, pp. 726–755.

40. Hochleitner M, Hortnagl H, Hortnagl H, et al: Long-term efficacy of physiologic dual-chamber pacing in the treatment of end-stage idiopathic dilated cardiomyopathy. *Am J Cardiol* 70:1320–1325, 1992.

41. Brecker S, Gibson D: Clinical perspectives: What is the role of pacing in dilated cardiomyopathy? *Eur Heart J* 17:819–824, 1996.

42. Kannel W, Abbott R, Savage D, et al: Epidemiologic features of chronic atrial fibrillation. *N Engl J Med* 306:1018–1022, 1982.

43. Lundstrom T, Ryden L: Chronic atrial fibrillation: Long term results of direct current conversion. *Acta Med Scand* 223:53–59, 1988.

44. Aranki S, Shaw D, Adams D, et al: Predictors of atrial fibrillation after coronary artery surgery. *Circulation* 94:390–397, 1996.

45. Daoud E, Strickberger S, Man C, et al: Preoperative amiodarone as prophylaxis against atrial fibrillation after heart surgery. *N Engl J Med* 337:1785–1791, 1997.

46. Frustaci A, Chimenti C, Bellocci F, et al: Histological substrate of atrial biopsies in patients with lone atrial fibrillation. *Circulation* 96:1180–1184, 1997.

47. Takahashi N, Seki A, Imataka K: Clinical features of paroxysmal atrial fibrillation. An observation of 94 patients. *Jpn Heart J* 22:143–149, 1981.

48. Wolf P, Abbott R, Kannel W: Atrial fibrillation: A major contributor to stroke in the elderly. *Arch Intern Med* 147:1561–1564, 1987.
49. Wolf P, Dawber T, Emerson T Jr, et al: Epidemiologic assessment of chronic atrial fibrillation and the risk of stroke: The Framingham Study. *Neurology* 28:973–977, 1978.
50. Kopecky S, Gergh B, McGoon M, et al: The natural history of lone atrial fibrillation. *N Engl J Med* 317:669–674, 1987.
51. Crijns H, Van Gelder I, Van Gilst W, et al: Serial antiarrhythmic drug treatment to maintain sinus rhythm after electrical cardioversion for chronic atrial fibrillation or atrial flutter. *Am J Cardiol* 68:335–341, 1991.
52. Coplen S, Antman E, Berlin J, et al: Efficacy and safety of quinidine therapy for maintenance of sinus rhythm after cardioversion. A meta-analysis of randomized control trials. *Circulation* 82:1106–1116, 1990.
53. Investigators TPaSCotASftNA. Atrial fibrillation follow-up Investigation of Rhythm Management: The AFFIRM study design. *Am J Cardiol* 79:1198–1202, 1997.
54. Williamson B, Man K, Daoud E, et al: Radiofrequency catheter modification of atrioventricular conduction to control the ventricular rate during atrial fibrillation. *N Engl J Med* 331:910–917, 1994.
55. Yeung-Lai-Wah J, Alison J, Lonergan L, et al: High success rate of atrioventricular node ablation with radiofrequency energy. *J Am Coll Cardiol* 18:1753–1758, 1991.
56. Grogan M, Smith H, Gersh B, et al: Left ventricular dysfunction due to atrial fibrillation in patients initially believed to have idiopathic dilated cardiomyopathy. *Am J Cardiol* 69:1570–1573, 1992.
57. Kerber R, Jensen S, Grayzel J, et al: Elective cardioversion: Influence of paddle-electrode location and size on success rates and energy requirements. *N Engl J Med* 305:658–662, 1981.
58. The Esmolol vs Placebo Multicenter Study Group: Comparison of the efficacy and safety of esmolol, a short-acting beta blocker, with placebo in the treatment of supraventricular tachyarrhythmias. *Am Heart J* 111:42–48, 1986.
59. Salerno D, Dias V, Kleiger R, et al: Efficacy and safety of intravenous diltiazem for treatment of atrial fibrillation and atrial flutter. *Am J Cardiol* 63:1046–1051, 1989.
60. Crijns H, Van den Berg M, Van Gelder I, et al: Management of atrial fibrillation in the setting of heart failure. *Eur Heart J* 18(suppl C): , 1997.
61. Gray R, Bateman T, Czer L, Conklin C, et al: Esmolol: A new ultrashort-acting beta-adrenergic blocking agent for rapid control of heart rate in postoperative supraventricular tachyarrhythmias. *J Am Coll Cardiol* 5:1451–1456, 1985.
62. Platia E, Michelson E, Porterfield J, et al: Esmolol versus verapamil in the acute treatment of atrial fibrillation or atrial flutter. *Am J Cardiol* 63:925–929, 1989.
63. David D, Di Segni E, Klein H, et al: Inefficacy of digitalis in the control of heart rate in patients with chronic atrial fibrillation: Beneficial effect of an added beta adrenergic blocking agent. *Am J Cardiol* 44:1378–1382, 1979.
64. Panidis I, Morganroth J, Baessler C: Effectiveness and safety of oral verapamil to control exercise-induced tachycardia in patients with atrial fibrillation receiving digitalis. *Am J Cardiol* 52:1197–1201, 1983.
65. Steinberg J, Katz R, Bren G, et al: Efficacy of oral diltiazem to control

ventricular response in chronic atrial fibrillation at rest and during exercise. *J Am Coll Cardiol* 9:405–411, 1987.

66. Kreiner G, Heinz G, Siostrzonek P, et al: Effect of slow pathway ablation on ventricular rate during atrial fibrillation: Dependence on electrophysiological properties of the fast pathway. *Circulation* 93:277–283, 1996.

67. Lown B, Perlroth M, Kaidbey S, et al: Cardioversion of atrial fibrillation. *N Engl J Med* 269:325–331, 1963.

68. Van Gelder I, Crijns H, Van Gilst W, et al: Prediction of uneventful cardioversion and maintenance of sinus rhyhtm from direct-current electrical cardioversion of chronic atrial fibrillation and flutter. *Am J Cardiol* 68: 41–46, 1991.

69. Borgeat A, Goy J, Maendly R, et al: Flecainide versus quinidine for conversion of atrial fibrillation to sinus rhythm. *Am J Cardiol* 58:496–498, 1986.

70. Antman E, Beamer A, Cantillon C, et al: Long-term oral propafenone therapy for suppression of refractory symptomatic atrial fibrillation and atrial flutter. *J Am Coll Cardiol* 12:1005–1011, 1988.

71. Antman E, Beamer A, Cantillon C, et al: Therapy of refractory symptomatic atrial fibrillation and atrial flutter: A staged care approach with new antiarrhythmic drugs. *J Amer Coll Cardiol* 15:698–707, 1990.

72. Juul-Moller S, Edvardsson N, Rehnqvist-Ahlberg N: Sotalol versus quinidine for the maintenance of sinus rhythm after direct current conversion of atrial fibrillation. *Circulation* 82:1932–1939, 1990.

73. Haverkamp W, Martinez-Rubio A, Hief C, et al: Efficacy and safety of d,l-sotalol in patients with ventricular tachycardia and in survivors of cardiac arrest. *J Am Coll Cardiol* 30:487–495, 1997.

74. Gold R, Haffajee C, Charos G, et al: Amiodarone for refractory atrial fibrillation. *Am J Cardiol* 57:124–127, 1986.

75. The Cardiac Arrhythmia Supression Trial (CAST) Investigators: Preliminary report: Effect of encainide and flecainide on mortality in a randomized trial of arrhythmia supression after myocardial infarction. *N Engl J Med* 321:406–412, 1989.

76. Benditt D, Benson D Jr, Dunnigan A, et al: Atrial flutter, atrial fibrillation, and other primary atrial tachycardias. *Med Clin North Am* 68: 895–918, 1984.

77. Middlekauff H, Wiener I, Saxon L, et al: Low-dose amiodarone for atrial fibrillation: time for a prospective study? *Ann Intern Med* 116:1017–1020, 1992.

78. Henry W, Morganroth J, Pearlman A, et al: Relation between echocardiographically determined left atrial size and atrial fibrillation. *Circulation* 53:273–279, 1976.

79. Halpern S, Ellrodt G, Singh B, et al: Efficacy of intravenous procainamide infusion in converting atrial fibrillation to sinus rhythm: Relation to left atrial size. *Br Heart J* 44:589–595, 1980.

80. Ewy G, Ulfers L, Hager W, Rosenfeld A, et al: Response of atrial fibrillation to therapy: role of etiology and left atrial diameter. *J Electrocardiol* 13:119–124, 1980.

81. Dethy M, Chassat C, Roy D, et al: Doppler echocardiographic predictors of recurrence of atrial fibrillation after cardioversion. *Am J Cardiol* 62: 723–726, 1988.

82. Cox J, Boineau J, Shuessler R, et al: Successful surgical treatment of atrial fibrillation. *JAMA* 266:1976–1980, 1991.

83. Swartz J, Pellersels G, Silvers J, et al: A catheter-based curative approach to atrial fibrillation in humans. *Circulation* 90:335A, 1994.

84. Prakash A, Saksena S, Hill M, et al: Acute effects of dual-site right atrial pacing in patients with spontaneous and inducible atrial flutter and fibrillation. *J Am Coll Cardiol* 29:1007–1014, 1997.
85. Bailin S, Johnson W, Hokyt R: A prospective randomized trial of Bachmann's Bundle Pacing for the prevention of atrial fibrillation. *J Am Coll Cardiol* 29:74A, 1997.
86. Ezekowitz M, Bridgers S, James K, et al: Warfarin in the prevention of stroke associated with nonrheumatic atrial fibrillation. *N Engl J Med* 327:1406–1412, 1992.
87. Stroke Prevention in Atrial Fibrillation Investigators: Stroke prevention in atrial fibrillation study: Final results. *Circulation* 84:527–539, 1991.
88. The Boston Area Anticoagulation Trial for Atrial Fibrillation Investigators: The effect of low-dose warfarin on the risk of stroke in patients with non-rheumatic atrial fibrillation. *N Engl J Med* 323:1505–1511, 1990.
89. Petersen P, Boysen G, Godtfredsen J, et al: Placebo-controlled, randomised trial of warfarin and aspirin for prevention of thromboembolic complications in chronic atrial fibrillation: The Copenhagen AFASAK study. *Lancet* 1:538–545, 1989.
90. Archer S, Kvernen L, James K, et al: Detection of left atrial thrombus in chronic nonrheumatic atrial fibrillation by transesophageal echocardiography. *Am Heart J* 130:287–295, 1995.
91. Chesebro J, Fuster V, Halperin J: Atrial fibrillation: Risk marker for stroke. *N Engl J Med* 323:1556–1558, 1990.
92. Arnold A, Mick M, Mazurek R, et al: Role of prophylactic anticoagulation for direct current cardioversion in patients with atrial fibrillation or atrial flutter. *J Am Coll Cardiol* 19:851–855, 1992.
93. Manning W, Leeman D, Gotch P, et al: Pulsed Doppler evaluation of atrial mechanical function after electrical cardioversion of atrial fibrillation. *J Am Coll Cardiol* 13:617–623, 1989.
94. Fenster P, Comess K, Marsh R, et al: Conversion of atrial fibrillation to sinus rhythm by acute intravenous procainamide infusion. *Am Heart J* 106:501–504, 1983.
95. Stambler B, Wood M, Ellenbogen K, et al: Efficacy and safety of repeated intravenous doses of ibutilide for rapid conversion of atrial flutter or fibrillation. *Circulation* 94:1613–1621, 1996.
96. Kowey P, VanderLust J, Luderer J: Analysis of safety and risk/benefit of ibutilide for conversion of atrial fibrillation/flutter. *Am J Cardiol* 78(8A): 46–52, 1996.
97. Manning W, Silverman D, Gordon S, et al: Cardioversion from atrial fibrillation without prolonged anticoagulation with use of transesophageal echocardiography to exclude the presence of atrial thrombi. *N Engl J Med* 328:750–755, 1993.
98. Wells J Jr, MacLean W, James T, et al: Characterization of atrial flutter - studies in man after open heart surgery using fixed atrial electrodes. *Circulation* 60:665–673, 1979.
99. Irani W, Grayburn P, Afridi I: Prevalence of thrombus, spontaneous echo contrast, and atrial stunning in patients undergoing cardioversion of atrial flutter. A prospective study using transesophageal echocardiography. *Circulation* 95:962–966, 1997.
100. Mehta D, Baruch L: Thromboembolism following cardioversion of "common" atrial flutter. Risk factors and limitations of transesophageal echocardiography. *Chest* 110:1001–1003, 1996.

101. Feld G, Fleck R, Chen P, et al: Radiofrequency catheter ablation for the treatment of human type 1 atrial flutter. *Circulation* 86:1233–1240, 1992.
102. Poty H, Saoudi N, Nair M, et al: Radiofrequency catheter ablation of atrial flutter. *Circulation* 94:3204–3213, 1996.
103. Chung E: *Manual of Cardiac Arrhythmias*. Stoneham, MA: Butterworth, 1986.
104. Shine K, Kastor J, Yurchak P: Multifocal atrial tachycardia: Clinical and electrocardiographic features. *N Engl J Med* 279:344–349, 1968.
105. Salerno D, Anderson B, Sharkey P, et al: Intravenous verapamil for treatment of multifocal atrial tachycardia, with and without calcium pretreatment. *Ann Intern Med* 107:623–628, 1987.
106. Swerdlow C, Liem L: Atrial and junctional tachycardias: Clinical presentation, Course, and therapy. In: D Zipes, J Jalife, (eds.) *Cardiac Electrophysiology: From Cell to Bedside*. Philadelphia, PA, WB Saunders, 1990, pp 742–755.
107. Wantanabe Y, Nishimura M, Noda T, et al: Atrioventicular junctionaltachycardias. In: D Zipes, J Jalife, (eds.) *Cardiac Electrophysiology: From Cell to Bedside*. Philadelphia, PA, WB Saunders, 1990, pp 564–570.
108. Fisch C: Digitalis induced tachycardias. In: B Surawicz, C Reddy, E Prystowsky, (eds.) *Tachycardias*. Boston, MA, Martinus Nijhoff, 1984, pp 399–406.
109. Jackman W, Beckman K, McClelland J, et al: Treatment of supraventricular tachycardia due to atrioventricular nodal reentry by radiofrequency catheter ablation of slow-pathway conduction. *N Engl J Med* 327: 313–318, 1992.
110. Schluter M, Geiger M, Siebels J, et al: Catheter ablation using radiofrequency current to cure symptomatic patients with tachyarrhythmias related to an accessory atrioventricular pathway. *Circulation* 84: 1644–1661, 1991.
111. Lesh M, Van Hare G, Schamp D, et al: Curative percutaneous catheter ablation using radiofrequency energy for accessory pathways in all locations: Results in 100 consecutive patients. *J Am Coll Cardiol* 19: 1303–1309, 1992.
112. Lee M, Morady F, Kadish A, et al: Catheter modification of the atrioventricular junction with radiofrequency energy for control of atrioventricular nodal reentry tachycardia. *Circulation* 83:827–835, 1991.
113. Leitch J, Klein G, Yee R, et al: Syncope associated with supraventricular tachycardia: An expression of tachycardia rate or vasomotor response? *Circulation* 85:1064–1071, 1992.
114. Waxman M, Wald R, Sharma A, et al: Vagal techniques for termination of paroxysmal supraventricular tachycardia. *Am J Cardiol* 46:655, 1980.
115. Gornick C, Benson D: Electrocardiographic aspects of the preexcitation syndromes. In: D Benditt, D Benson, (eds.) *Cardiac Preexcitation Syndromes: Origins, Evaluation, and Treatment*. Boston, MA, Martinus Nijhoff, 1986, pp 43–73.
116. Gallagher J, Selle J, Sealy W, et al: Variants of pre-excitation: Update 1989. In: D Zipes, J Jalife, (eds.) *Cardiac Electrophysiology: From Cell to Bedside*. Philadelphia, PA, WB Saunders, 1990, pp 480–502.
117. Wellens H, Brugada P, Penn O, et al: Pre-excitation syndromes. In: D Zipes, J Jalife, (eds.) *Cardiac Electrophysiology: From Cell to Bedside*. Philadelphia, PA, WB Saunders, 1990, pp 691–702.
118. Gradman A, Deedwania P, Cody R, et al: Predictors of total mortality and

sudden death in mild to moderate heart failure. *J Am Coll Cardiol* 14: 564–590, 1989.

119. Mukharji J, Rude P, Poole K, et al: Risk factors and sudden death following acute myocardial infarction: Two year follow-up. *Am J Cardiol* 54: 31–36, 1984.

120. Bigger J, Fleiss J, Kleiger R, et al: The relationship between ventricular arrhythmias, left ventricular dysfunction and mortality in the two years after myocardial infarction. *Circulation* 69:250–258, 1984.

121. Investigators ATM-A: Effect of prophylactic amiodarone on mortality after acute myocardial infarction and in congestive heart failure: Meta-analysis of individual data from 6500 patients in randomised trials. *Lancet* 350:1417–1424, 1997.

122. Moss A, Hall J, Cannom D, et al: Improve survival with an implanted defibrillator in patients with coronary disease at high risk for ventricular arrhythmia. *New Engl J Med* 335:1933–1940, 1996.

123. Bigger J, Investigators CABG: PT: Prophylactic use of implanted cardiac defibrillators in patients at high risk for ventricular arrhythmias after coronary artery bypass graft surgery. *N Engl J Med* 337:1569–1575, 1997.

124. Kuchar D, Thornburn C, Sammel N: Prediction of serious events after myocardial infarction: Signal averaged electrocardiogram. Holter monitoring and radionuclide ventriculography. *J Am Coll Cardiol* 9:531–538, 1987.

125. Jackman W, Friday K, Anderson J, et al: The long QT syndromes: A critical review, new clinical observations and a unifying hypothesis. *Prog Cardiovasc Dis* 31:115–172, 1988.

126. Akhtar M, Shenasa M, Mohammand J, et al: Wide QRS complex tachycardia: Reappraisal of a common clinical problem. *Ann Intern Med* 109: 905–912, 1988.

127. Wellens H, Conover M: *The ECG in Emergency Decision Making*. Philadelphis, PA, WB Saunders, 1992.

128. Mason J, Investigators ESVEM: A comparison of electrophysiologic testing with Holter monitoring to predict antiarrhythmic drug efficacy for ventricular tachyarrhythmias. *N Engl J Med* 329:445–451, 1993.

129. Naccarelli G, Prystowsky E, Jackman W, et al: Role of electrophysiologic testing in managing patients who have ventricular tachycardia unrelated to coronary artery disease. *Am J Cardiol* 50:165–171, 1982.

130. Cox J: Patient selection criteria and results of surgery for refractory ischemic ventricular tachycardia. *Circulation* 79:I-163-I177, 1989.

131. Harvey M, Kalbfleisch S, El-Atassi R, et al: Radiofrequency catheter ablation of ventricular tachycardia in patients with coronary artery disease. *Circulation* 86:519, 1992.

132. Brugada P, de Swart F, Bar W, et al: Transcoronary termination and chemical ablation of arrhythmias. In: D Zipes, J Jalife, (eds.) *Cardiac Electrophysiology: From Cell to Bedside*. Philadelphia, PA, WB Saunders, 1990, pp 1005–1014.

133. Winkle R, Mead R, Ruder M, et al: Long term outcome with the implantable cardioverter-defibrillator. *J Am Coll Cardiol* 13:1353–1361, 1989.

134. Investigators TAvID: A comparison of antiarrhythmic-drug therapy with implantable defibrillators in patients resuscitated from near-fatal ventricular arrhythmias. *N Engl J Med* 337:1576–1583, 1997.

135. Epstein A, Miles W, Benditt D, et al: Personal and public saftey issues related to arrhythmias that may affect conciousness: Implications for reg-

ulation and physician recommendations. A medical/scientific statement from the American Heart Association and the North American Society of Pacing and Electrophysiology. *Circulation* 94:1147–1166, 1996.

136. Tchou P, Kadri N, Anderson J, et al: Automatic implantable cardioverter defibrillators and survival of patients with left ventricular arrhythmias. *Ann Intern Med* 109:529–534, 1988

137. Kjekshus J: Arrhythmias and mortality in congestive heart failure. *Am J Cardiol* 65:42–48, 1990.

Chapter 16

Evaluation and Treatment of the Elderly Patient with Syncope

Charles C. Gornick

Syncope is a sudden temporary loss of consciousness and postural tone usually followed by spontaneous and complete recovery within minutes. Syncope is a common medical problem, particularly among the elderly. In the Framingham study, the prevalence of syncope was 0.7% in men age 35 to 44 years and 5.6% in men age 75 years and older.[1] Syncope recurrence was reported in about 30%. Similarly, an annual incidence of 6% with a recurrence rate of 30% has been described in a group of elderly patients living in long-term care institutions.[2,3] Table 1 summarizes the differential diagnosis of syncope.

The approach to patients with syncope can be frustrating to both patient and physician. The patient is often frightened by a spell and worries about recurrences. The physician often finds little wrong at initial examination and knows from past experience that even extensive evaluation may not result in a firm diagnosis. Uncertainty is compounded by an awareness that isolated episodes of syncope are common and although usually harmless, recurrences are often unpredictable and may result in serious injury and even fatality especially if the cause is a ventricular tachyarrhythmia. The evaluation of syncope in the elderly is complicated by the frequent presence of coexisting illnesses.

Recently, electrophysiological testing and use of autonomic maneuvers such as head up tilt testing have made accurate diagnosis in patients with unexplained syncope much more likely. Such testing can

From *Clinical Cardiology in the Elderly. Second Edition,* edited by Elliot Chesler. © 1999, Futura Publishing Company, Armonk, NY.

Table 1
Differential Diagnosis of Syncope

I. Orthostatic	**II. Neurally-mediated**
A. Drug induced	A. Situational
B. Other	Emotional
Idiopathic	Carotid sinus syndrome
Shy Drager	Cough
diabetic neuropathy	Micturition/defecation
Parkinson's	Swallowing
Other neuropathies	Glossopharyngeal, trigeminal
III. Cardiac	neuralgia
A. Bradyarrythmias	B. Nonsituational
Sick sinus syndrome	**IV. Neurological/psychiatric**
AV block	A. Seizures
Pacemaker malfunction	B. Cerebrovascular disease
B. Tacharrhythmias	Subclavian steel
Ventricular	Vertebral-basilar insufficiency
Supraventricular	C. Psychogenic
C. Obstruction to flow	anxiety
aortic stenosis	depression
hypertrophic cardiomyopathy	panic disorders
atrial myxoma	
mitral stenosis	
Pulmonary	
embolus	
hypertension	
valvular stenosis	

confirm a clinical diagnosis, study the pathophysiology, and aid in the selection of therapy for patients with syncope.

General Considerations

A careful history and physical examination will often identify the cause of syncope or at least suggest some possibilities. A wide variety of tests are available to evaluate such patients, but the goal should be to use them judiciously and selectively. Unfortunately, test results often only indicate a likely cause so that at least two problems may arise. First, in up to 40% of patients none of the test results may be abnormal, leaving the cause undiagnosed.[4] Second, more than one test result may be abnormal, suggesting multiple possible causes for syncope.

On initial examination, it is usually possible to decide whether to pursue a neurological as opposed to a cardiovascular evaluation. Syncope must be differentiated from vertigo, seizures, and sleep disorders;

therefore, evidence obtained from a witness is crucial. Without seizures or specific neurological signs, computed tomography (CT) or magnetic resonance imaging (MRI) scans are of low yield and expensive. If there is no cardiac history or abnormal physical findings, additional cardiovascular evaluation may also have a low yield.

An electrocardiogram (ECG) should be obtained in all older individuals in whom a clear cause for syncope cannot be identified by initial history and physical examination. Although the ECG has low sensitivity for detecting arrhythmias, when abnormalities are found, decision making is accelerated. Conversely, a normal ECG makes a cardiac cause unlikely. When the cause remains obscure after the initial examination and ECG, it is helpful to triage patients into those with, and those without heart disease. As a rule of thumb, when there is structural heart disease, electrophysiological study tends to be the most rewarding procedure. In patients without detectable heart disease, autonomic maneuvers such as carotid sinus massage and head up tilt testing are probably the most cost-effective tests.

Patients with Heart Disease

Aortic valve stenosis, hypertrophic cardiomyopathy, atrial myxoma, severe pulmonary hypertension, and right to left shunts may be responsible for syncope without arrhythmia and are readily detected by routine examination and echocardiography. Acute myocardial infarction, especially inferior in location, may present with dizziness or syncope as a result of hypotension with or without heart block. The clinical presentation usually makes this diagnosis obvious and the ECG is confirmatory. Patients with coronary artery disease, cardiomyopathy, valvular heart disease, and conduction system disease such as bundle branch, or bifasicular blocks have a high likelihood that arrhythmia is the cause of their syncope. Initial ECG monitoring forms the first step in evaluating these patients. If, as often happens, monitoring is not diagnostic, provocative electrophysiological (EP) testing is appropriate for both diagnosis and selecting the most effective therapy. When EP studies are negative, patients tend to have a favorable prognosis and empiric pacing or antiarrhythmic drugs are not warranted. In patients with recurrent syncope where there is a strong suspicion for arrhythmia despite negative EP studies, patient activated event recorders permit longer ECG monitoring that at times may capture a "spell."[5]

Patients without Heart Disease

Patients with a history of syncope younger than age 60 years without heart disease have an excellent prognosis. When the resting ECG is normal, prolonged ECG monitoring and EP studies tend to be of limited use in making a diagnosis. Many of these patients have "neurally mediated" syncope diagnosed by autonomic manuevers such as head-up tilt testing.

Older patients without evident heart disease are probably similar to their younger counterparts in that cardiac arrhythmias are an uncommon cause. However, one must be careful to exclude occult cardiac disease. Thus, there is probably a more important role for prolonged ECG monitoring and EP testing in the elderly. Orthostatic syncope is the most common etiology of syncope in the elderly. Although "neurally mediated" syncope is also common in the elderly, precipitating factors and mechanisms can be different from that in younger individuals. In our experience, emotional faints and psychogenic syncope are uncommon in older patients.

Orthostatic Hypotension

Incidence

Orthostatic hypotension is reported in up to 20% of elderly medical outpatients older than age 65 years[6,7] and up to 30% among those older than age 75 years,[6] whereas in healthy normotensive elderly subjects the prevalence is less than 7%.[8,9] Data from the National Health and Nutrition Examination Survey (1976–1980), confirm an increased prevalence of postural hypotension with advancing age.[10] This increase was found to be related to an increased incidence of supine hypertension.

Orthostatic hypotension is usually defined as a drop in systolic blood pressure of 20 mm Hg or more with assumption of upright posture.[11] However, the high prevalence of this finding, large day to day variability, and frequent lack of associated symptoms raises important questions about the clinical value of this definition in elderly patients. Clinically, symptoms associated with orthostatic fall in blood pressure is clearly significant. Yet even without symptoms, a fall in blood pressure may be a predictor of a poor prognosis. Two separate epidemiological studies have shown that a reduction of 20 mm Hg or more within 3 minutes of standing is a significant risk factor for subsequent falls and syncope.[3,12]

Mechanisms

In normal young individuals, change to the upright position is accompanied by pooling of approximately 500–700 cc of blood in the lower extremities. This leads to a secondary transient reduction in cardiac output, stimulation of the carotid, aortic and cardiopulmonary baroreceptors and increased sympathetic outflow in an attempt to maintain adequate cardiac output.[13] In the elderly, it is well recognized that there is decreased ability to adapt to orthostatic stress.[11] For example, heart rate does not increase in response to orthostatic stress to the magnitude that it does in younger individuals.

Conditions that interfere with diastolic cardiac filling such as reduction in intravascular volume or reduced venous return may result in a significant fall in cardiac output with resultant orthostatic hypotension. A common cause of hypovolemia with associated symptomatic orthostatic hypotension is diuretics such as furosemide and bumetamide. Hypovolemia may also result from general medical conditions such as gastrointestinal hemorrhage, poorly controlled diabetes, chronic diarrhea and Addison's disease. The elderly tolerate volume reduction poorly,[14] probably as a result of impaired cardiac diastolic filling associated with reduced left ventricular compliance.[15] Additionally, alterations in venous compliance in the lower extremities such as occurs with venous insufficiency, can significantly aggravate venous pooling. Several age-related physiological changes make elderly persons vulnerable to dehydration. Changes in renal function may promote salt wasting[16-18] and elderly patients do not experience the same thirst as their younger counterparts during water deprivation.[19] Therefore, orthostatic hypotension may be observed in elderly persons during any acute illness that increases fluid losses or limits access to oral fluids.

With aging there is an increase in stiffness of the vasculature resulting in elevated systolic blood pressure,[20] increased afterload and moderate left ventricular hypertrophy.[15] Systolic hypertension increases in prevalence with aging, so that more than 30% of persons older than age 75 years have resting systolic blood pressures above 160 mm Hg.[21] Systolic hypertension interacts with other effects mentioned above to further impair the normal response to orthostatic stress. Paradoxically therefore, in old age hypertension increases the likelihood of orthostatic hypotension. Hypertension also increases the risk of cerebral ischemia from a sudden drop in blood pressure. Hypertension and aging are both associated with decreased resting cerebral blood flow, close to the threshold for cerebral ischemia.[22] As a result, transitory reductions in blood pressure in hypertensive individuals are more likely to produce symptoms.[23]

Many drugs used to treat hypertension, cardiac, and psychiatric disorders have a vasodilator action that aggravates orthostatic hypotension. So-called "triple therapy" (β-blocker, nifedipine and a long acting nitrate) used for treatment of angina can cause symptomatic hypotension because of summation of the vasodilator effects.[24] β-blockers and calcium channel blockers may also be responsible for syncope by impairing cardiac conduction. An often overlooked source of β-blocker toxicity is the use of eye drops for the treatment of glaucoma. Surreptitious, or overuse of medications by confused elderly patients can lead to drug toxicity. Drugs commonly responsible for syncope are listed in Table 2.

Postprandial hypotension has been described in 15% of elderly patients in an institution, most of whom are asymptomatic.[25] However,

Table 2
Drugs Causing Syncope

I. Antihypertensives
  Vasodilators
  Diuretics
III. Cardiac
  B blockers
  Digitalis
  Nitrates
  Ca^{++} Channel blockers
  Anti arrhythmics
    proarrhythmia
    torsade de pointe (i.e. Quinidine, sotolol)
	II. Psychiatric
	  Antidepressants
	  Phenothiazines
	IV. Recreational
	  Alcohol
	  Marijuana
	  Cocaine

in some, a severe drop in blood pressure may result in syncope and even severe injury.[26] The effect of upright posture and the post prandial state may be additive and the resultant hypotension may be severe.

Impaired baroreceptor responsiveness and a variety of neurological conditions have been associated with failure of autonomic control of blood pressure in response to changes in posture. These have been arbitrarily divided into those that are a result of central nervous system dysfunction, those related to failure of peripheral nervous system regulation and those with features of both. Associated symptoms include visual difficulty, impotence, incontinence, constipation, anhidrosis, heat intolerance, impotence, and fatigue.[27]

In patients with central nervous system autonomic dysfunction (Figure 1), serum norepinephrine fails to rise appropriately with orthostatic stress. Also, there tends to be an exaggerated response to infused

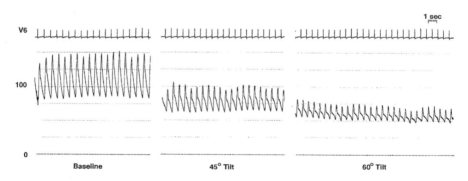

Figure 1: *ECG lead V$_6$ and blood pressure (mm Hg) recordings supine (150/85), 45° (100/65) and 60° (75/50) upright tilt in a 70-year-old man with "progressive autonomic insufficiency." Norepinephrine levels measured in the supine (242 pg/mL) and 60° upright positions (256 pg/mL) and heart rate were unchanged despite the severe fall in blood pressure.*

norepinephrine suggestive of peripheral denervation. In the absence of other neurological symptoms or findings, these syndromes have been called "idiopathic orthostatic hypotension" or "progressive autonomic insufficiency".[28,29] Several central nervous system disorders that have evidence of autonomic insufficiency include Shy-Drager syndrome (multiple-system atrophy), brain stem lesions, Parkinson's disease, myelopathy, and multiple cerebral infarcts.[28-31]

Diabetes is the most common cause of peripheral autonomic insufficiency.[32] Diabetics often have autonomic and peripheral neuropathy with gastroparesis and sensory and motor loss. Less common disorders affecting the peripheral autonomic nervous system include amyloidosis, vitamin deficiencies, and carcinomatous neuropathy.

Diagnosis

Orthostatic hypotension in the elderly may be a nonspecific finding, but development of symptoms with standing implies that it is the probable cause of syncope. Alternatively, if the blood pressure falls to less than 90 mm Hg on standing even without symptoms, orthostatic hypotension is the likely cause of syncope. Some patients will have an immediate decline in blood pressure with standing, but others will have a gradual fall only evident after a few minutes.[11]

Orthostatic blood pressure measurements should be made following a supine period of 10 to 15 minutes. Blood pressure should be measured immediately on standing and repeated over a 2- to 5-minute period.[33] Although rarely necessary, ambulatory blood pressure monitoring may be useful in patients with infrequent episodes. Because medications and eating may cause significant hypotension in the elderly, it is important to measure postural blood pressure changes at the time of peak effect of medication or 30 minutes after eating.

The heart rate response to postural changes can provide helpful information. Minimal cardioacceleration (less than 10 beats per minute) in the face of hypotension suggests impaired baroreceptor-reflexes, whereas tachycardia (greater than 100 beats per minute) suggests volume depletion. Since there can be an age related decrease in sensitivity of the baroreceptors, the absence of cardioacceleration does not exclude volume depletion in the elderly.[11]

The remainder of the evaluation of patients with orthostatic symptoms should focus on other associated autonomic or neurological symptoms and evidence for diseases associated with autonomic dysfunction. On physical examination, significant hypertension and evidence of other cardiovascular or neurological diseases should be pursued.

Treatment

Orthostatic hypotension, even if asymptomatic, is a risk factor for subsequent falls or syncope and patients should be warned of this and instructed to avoid sudden change in posture. When there are significant symptoms, the most important initial consideration is to ensure that medications are not contributory.[34] In patients with hypertension, vasodilator therapy can be replaced with agents such as β-blockers that have a similar effect on blood pressure in both supine and upright positions. In some cases it may be necessary to forgo treatment of mild hypertension because of the side effects of medication. In more severe cases, use of thigh-high support stockings prevent venous pooling when standing and may improve symptoms. Liberalization of salt intake (including supplementation if necessary) and volume expansion with a mineralocorticoid such as fluorohydrocortisone acetate can also be used. Fluorohydrocortisone acetate not only results in volume expansion, but may also sensitize adrenergic receptors to the effects of circulating catecholamine. Mineralocorticoid use requires careful monitoring for severe supine hypertension, congestive heart failure, and hypokalemia.[11] Elevation of the head of the bed 30° can be used to prevent nocturnal diuresis and supine hypertension that result from shifts of interstitial fluid from the legs to the circulation at night. Exercises such as dorsiflexing the feet before standing that promote venous return, accelerate heart rate, and increase blood pressure may be helpful.[11]

When symptoms persist despite attempts at volume expansion, oral midodrine[35,36] or ephedrine can be used to raise blood pressure. Their side effects include tachyphylaxis and exacerbation of supine hypertension. We try to dose these agents most heavily in the early morning when orthostatic symptoms are usually most severe. This allows for low drug levels at night during recumbency and avoids severe supine hypertension. If supine hypertension is severe, treatment with vasodilators such as hydralazine at night along with midodrine or ephedrine during the day may be required.[37] Other agents found to be useful include: (1) Inhibitors of prostaglandin synthesis such as indomethacin and other nonsteroidal antiinflammatory agents that inhibit prostaglandin mediated vasodilatation.[38] (2) The peripheral α_2-agonist clonidine promotes peripheral venoconstriction in patients with reduced central sympathetic outflow.[39] (3) The central α_2-adrenergic antagonist yohimbine increases the activity of the sympathetic nervous system.[40,41] (4) β-blockers that block β_2-vasodilator receptors or have intrinsic sympathomimetic activity.[40,41] (5) Other sympathomimetic agents such as caffeine,[42] phenylpropanolamine,[43] and dihydroergotamine.[44] (6) Subcutaneous somatostatin for treatment of severe postprandial hypotension.[45] (7) Erythropoietin can cause remarkable improvement in orthostatic tolerance when administered to patients with autonomic failure,[46] and finally (8) Serotonin reuptake inhibitors have been used with success.[47]

Neurally Mediated Syncope

Sir Thomas Lewis described fainting attacks as "vasovagal" because they were accompanied by hypotension and bradycardia.[48] He correctly concluded that bradycardia was not the main cause of syncope since the heart rate rarely fell below 50 beats per minute and hypotension was not affected by administration of atropine that prevented bradycardia. Subsequently, many patients have been described with syncope attributed to impaired neurovascular control. In some, bradycardia predominates but in others hypotension is the major finding. In most, there is a combination of hypotension and bradycardia. Uncommonly, tachycardia is associated with severe hypotension. For this reason, we prefer use of the broader term "neurally mediated" syncope that does not imply the presence of both bradycardia and hypotension and can be used to describe a variety of syndromes.

Neurally-mediated syncope can be separated into situational and nonsituational types (Table 1). Situational syncope occurs in response to fear, anxiety, pain, carotid sinus pressure, cough, micturition or defecation, etc. Nonsituational, syncope occurs without clear associated or precipitating factors. In an elderly population, the causes of neurally mediated syncope are similar to those in a younger population, but the distribution frequency is different. For example, carotid sinus hypersensitivity is more frequent in older individuals and emotional faints are more common in the young. Although much is known about the factors predisposing to neurally mediated syncope, the exact mechanisms responsible for sudden bradycardia and vasodilatation remain incompletely understood.

Situational Syncope

The usual sequence of events is typified by the so called emotional or common faint. Emotional stress initially results in an increase in heart rate and blood pressure with little change in total peripheral vascular resistance. This is followed by an abrupt decrease in peripheral vascular resistance, fall in blood pressure and syncope. Heart rate usually decreases, but may remain unchanged and less often may even increase. The hypotension appears to be a result of vasodilatation due to inhibition of sympathetic vasoconstriction[49,50] or other mechanisms.[51] Bradycardia, is relatively unimportant in terms of its hemodynamic consequences unless heart rate is extremely slow or there is asystole.

Carotid sinus syncope occurs primarily in older men, particularly in association with hypertension, or a prior history of head and neck cancer treated with radiation or surgery. Classically, syncope follows direct pressure by a tight collar. This syndrome is the best example of neurally mediated syncope, in that both the afferent and to some extent, the efferent paths of the reflex response have been described. Baroreceptors are located in the internal carotid artery just above the bifurcation of the common carotid artery. Under normal conditions, afferent impulses travel through the glossopharyngeal and perhaps vagus nerves to the sensory nucleus of the vagus and vasomotor centers in the brain stem. An increase in intrasinus pressure leads to activation of efferent nerves (fibers of vagus nerve) that cause cardiac slowing (cardioinhibitory effect). Simultaneous activation of the vasomotor center results in decreased blood pressure probably as a result of sympathetic inhibition(vasodepressor effect). Under abnormal circumstances, the response to changes in carotid sinus pressure can be markedly exaggerated and result in syncope. A rare form of syncope associated with swallowing[52–56] or cold stimulation of the pharynx ("ice cream syncope") likely has afferent and efferent limbs similar to that of carotid sinus syncope.

Syncope immediately before, during, or after micturition is relatively common[57,58] and responsible for 8% to 9% of cases of syncope Figures 2 and 3).[59,60] Several hypotheses have been proposed to account for syncope associated with urination: (1) orthostatic, related to getting up quickly at night; (2) high vagal tone at night; (3) vasodepressor, and or cardioinhibitory reflexes arising from the rapidly emptied bladder, or the Valsalva maneuver required to empty the bladder in men with prostatic hypertrophy. When micturition syncope occurs in the young, men are primarily affected. In older individuals, women are also affected and orthostatic hypotension (both symptomatic and asymptomatic) is present in most cases.[59] Syncope associated with defecation is

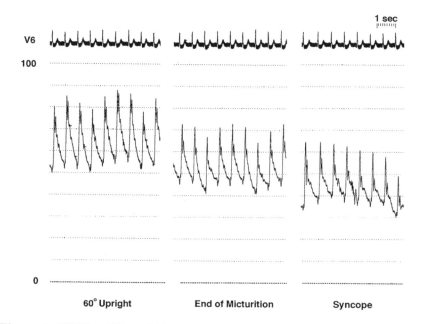

Figure 2: *ECG lead V₆ and blood pressure (mm Hg) recordings measured during an episode of micturation syncope in a 75 year old man positioned at 60° upright tilt. Timing of recordings from left to right were just prior to, immediately after, and when syncope occurred 1½ minutes postvoiding.*

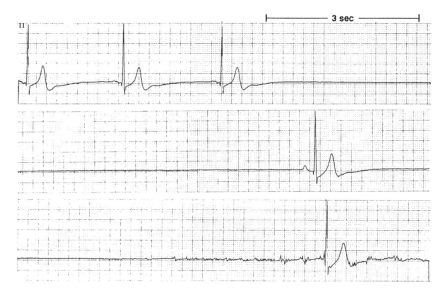

Figure 3: *ECG lead II recording obtained during a syncopal event immediately post voiding in a 75-year-old man with multiple episodes of micturation syncope. Baseline rhythm was sinus at a rate of 60 beats per minute just prior to this recording.*

rare.[61,62] It affects both sexes with equal frequency and is usually associated with concomitant orthostatic hypotension.[61]

Post-tussive syncope occurs predominantly in men with a history of significant chronic lung disease (Figure 4).[63,64] The mechanisms responsible for syncope associated with cough are not well defined. Increased intrathoracic pressure during coughing is transmitted to all intrathoracic structures including the heart and great vessels. Initially, the blood pressure is elevated, but subsequently raised intrathoracic pressure reduces venous return that can induce a cardioinhibitory, or vasodepressor response, or both, in susceptible people.

Severe pain, of any cause, can induce a cardioinhibitory and/or a vasodepressor response resulting in dizziness or syncope. Glossopharyngeal and trigeminal neuralgia can be associated with syncope presumably as a direct result of abnormal nerve activity.[65,66]

Nonsituational Syncope

In many patients ultimately found to have neurally mediated syncope, an association to a "triggering" event cannot be identified despite a careful history. In some, associated gastrointestinal symptoms, sweating, and a cold clammy feeling are suggestive of a neurally me-

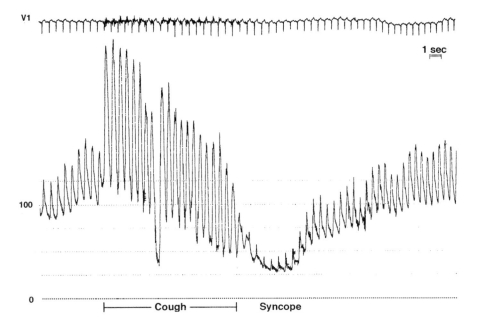

Figure 4: *ECG lead V₁ and blood pressure (mm Hg) recordings during an episode of cough syncope in a 56-year-old man with chronic obstructive pulmonary disease. During cough at 75° upright tilt increased intrathoracic pressure is reflected in the aortic pressure tracing. After cough, syncope occurred lasting several seconds.*

diated cause. The mechanisms responsible for syncope appear to be similar to those of situational syncope except no specific "trigger" can be identified.

Diagnosis

Spontaneous episodes of neurally mediated syncope are infrequently documented since they are unpredictable and their frequency quite variable.. Neurological testing, extensive ECG monitoring, and EP testing have been of low yield. Previously, patients were assumed to have neurally mediated syncope after exclusion of other known causes. Recently more specific clinical tests including autonomic maneuvers such as carotid sinus massage, Valsalva maneuver, cough, and head up tilt testing (HUT), with and without isoproterenol have been used in diagnosis. Unfortunately, these tests are not absolutely specific and may produce symptoms and findings in normal individuals.[67]

Carotid sinus massage is generally performed on either side for 10–12 seconds just lateral to the thyroid cartilage and close to the angle

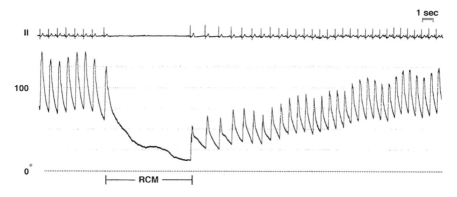

Figure 5: *ECG lead II and blood pressure (mm Hg) recordings during right carotid massage (RCM) performed in the supine position in a 56-year-old man with a history of syncope. After 8 seconds of asystole (cardioinhibitory effect) persistant hypotension remains (vasodepressor effect).*

of the jaw with continuous ECG monitoring (Figure 5).[68] Blood pressure can be monitored continuously with an arterial line, or noninvasively just before massage, at completion of massage, and for 1 to 2 minutes following massage. We perform carotid massage in the supine position first and if a significant vasodepressor component is present, repeat massage with 30°–60° of upright tilt. Three types of abnormal responses to carotid massage have been described: (1) cardioinhibitory type with cardiac asystole of greater than 3 seconds; (2) vasodepressor type with more than a 50 mm Hg fall in blood pressure or a lesser fall associated with reproducible symptoms; and (3) a combination of both 1 and 2.[69] Unfortunately, carotid sinus hypersensitivity using these criteria has been reported in 5%–25% of an asymptomatic population, most often in the elderly and especially in men.[70–74] Hence, an unequivocal diagnosis of carotid sinus syncope can only be made with the above findings and a clinical history of syncope associated with neck pressure. Complications of carotid massage are rare, but prolonged asystole and permanent neurological deficits may result.[75,76] The test should not be performed in patients with suspected cerebrovascular disease, unless the pretest likelihood of carotid sinus syndrome is high.

The Valsalva maneuver is reproducibly performed by having the patient take a deep breath and then expiring forcefully for 10–12 seconds or as long as possible through a tube connected to a sphygmomanometer.[13] Examples of a normal and abnormal response to the Valsalva manuever are presented in Figure 6. Most subjects can maintain a pressure of 40–60 mm Hg. The ECG and blood pressure should be continuously monitored. In normal subjects (Figure 6A), there is an increase in heart rate during the initial expiratory phase, blood pressure falls, but equilibrates at a lower level. After release, there is an overshoot of blood pressure with reflex bradycardia. Under abnormal

A

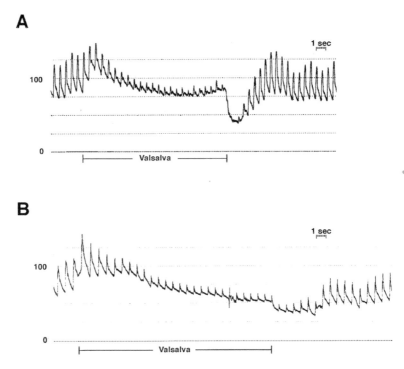

Figure 6: ***Panel A*** *contains blood pressure recording during a normal response to Valsalva to 50 mm Hg performed at 60° of upright tilt in a 69-year-old man (see text).* ***Panel B*** *contains a similar recording during Valsalva to 40 mm Hg at 60° upright tilt in a 75-yearold man with a history of micturation syncope. At the start of the strain phase, blood pressure initially rises then falls. On release, blood pressure only slowly rises and in this case took over 40 seconds to return to baseline.*

circumstances (Figure 6B), blood pressure either fails to rise after release, or falls further, leading to symptoms especially if the patient is upright. We prefer to perform this test at 30°–60° of upright tilt in an attempt to reproduce symptoms.

Patients with a history of post-tussive syncope are asked to cough vigorously for several seconds while positioned at 30°–60° of upright tilt during continuous ECG and blood pressure monitoring. An abnormal response to cough can include either significant bradycardia[77–79] or significant hypotension (Figure 4) .

HUT with and without pharmacological provocation with agents such as isoproterenol, edrophonium, and nitroglycerin has been used in the evaluation of patients with syncope but protocols have not been standardized.[51] Figure 7 demonstrates an abnormal HUT. We use 75°–80° upright tilt for up to 45 minutes. In elderly patients, we do not generally use pharmacological provocation if the baseline tilt study is

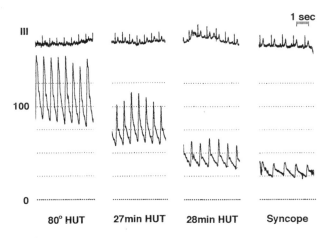

Figure 7: *ECG lead III and blood pressure(mm Hg) recordings during an 80°
head-up tilt in a 73-year-old man with a history of syncope. Tracings from left
to right were obtained immediately following HUT, and at 27 minutes, and at
28 minutes when a sudden fall in blood pressure and mild slowing of heart rate
occurred resulting in syncope.*

negative. A positive HUT is usually defined as induction of syncope
with sudden significant hypotension; heart rate usually slows and
frank asystole can occur. Tachycardia with hypotension is uncommon.
With various HUT protocols approximately 70%–80% of young patients
with suspected neurally mediated syncope will have a positive test.[51]
In elderly patients, similar large series are not yet available but in our
experience they are less likely to have a positive tilt study.[80–82] HUT
appears to be reasonably specific in that only 10%–20% of control subjects without a prior history of syncope have positive studies, in most
series.[51] In one series, the false-positive rate was much higher.[67] Several studies have reported fair reproducibility (70%) of HUT whether
the studies are performed on the same or different days.[51] To improve
reproducibility, it is recommended that studies be performed in as near
as identical circumstances as possible, including factors such as time
of day, hydration status and medications.

Treatment

A decision to treat patients with neurally mediated syncope depends on the frequency and severity of spells and whether potential
"triggers" can be avoided. Treatment can be as simple as having men
sit before, during and after urination, or therapy to prevent cough. It
is important to reemphasize that the elderly often have changes in
regulation of cerebral blood flow that makes them more susceptible to

minor changes in blood pressure induced by neurally mediated reflexes. Efforts to ensure that elderly patients are adequately hydrated including avoidance of diuretics can be helpful. In some patients, volume expansion with mineralocorticoids or use of support stockings may be useful.

If these measures fail, control of significant bradycardia can be achieved with pacing techniques.[83] In patients with neurally mediated syncope, pacing appears to be useful only in patients with a significant bradycardic component.[84] Dual chamber pacemakers used have a form of rapid rate drop hysteresis. When heart rate drops precipitously, pacing begins at a higher rate hopefully to prevent or alleviate symptoms. Eventually, hemodynamic sensors incorporated into pacemakers will further optimize this form of therapy, coupling pacing with blood pressure response.[83] With carotid sinus hypersensitivity, control of significant bradycardia can control or eliminate symptoms in up to 80% or more of patients.[85] Although ventricular pacing has been successfully used, dual chambered pacing is more effective.[86,87] Anticholinergic agents such as probantheline bromide[87] and scopolamine patches may be successful in selected patients.

In many patients bradycardia is either not significant or only partially responsible for symptoms, and treatment must be aimed at the vasodepressor component. β-blockers[88] and disopyramide[89] have been used successfully in some patients and their efficacy appears to be partially related to effects on the "triggering" mechanisms. The second approach is to use sympathomimetics such as ephedrine,[68] phenylpropanolamine,[43] or midodrine.[35,36] Because they may precipitate significant hypertension in the elderly, combined therapy with β-blockers and hydralazine may be required.[37] Other agents which have been used with variable success include: theophylline[90] and serotonin uptake inhibitors such as fluoxetine and sertraline.[47]

Cardiac Syncope

Syncope has significant morbidity and mortality when cardiac related. In a study by Kapoor et al[91] of patients with cardiac syncope older than age 60 years, the 2 year mortality rate was 38%. In this study, even if an initial diagnosis of non cardiac syncope was made, mortality was 21%, with many of the patients dying later as a result of cardiovascular disease. The causes of cardiovascular syncope (Table 1) can be divided into those associated with either brady-or tachyarrhythmias or specific structural abnormalities such as aortic stenosis.

Diagnosis

When structural cardiac abnormalities have been excluded, a stepwise approach to diagnosis should be followed. Diagnosis is often difficult since symptoms have usually resolved by the time of evaluation. Making a causal inference on the basis of arrhythmias detected by ECG monitoring during asymptomatic periods is a major problem since there are no validated criteria. Studies that report the yield of ambulatory ECG monitoring and electrophysiological studies suffer from lack of a definitive diagnostic standard to which they can be compared. These problems will be discussed further with each of the following: (1) ECG and rhythm strips; (2) 24-hour ambulatory ECG monitoring and ECG event recorders; (3) signal averaged ECG, and (4) EP testing.

ECG

The electrocardiogram is abnormal in up to one half of patients with syncope.[92] Findings include bifascicular block, old myocardial infarction, and left ventricular hypertrophy. In various reports, the ECG has been used to assign a cause in 2%–11% of patients.[92,93] Evidence has been derived from monitoring strips obtained by paramedics in the field, rhythm strips in the emergency department or hospital, and 12-lead ECGs. The most common causes include ventricular tachycardia and bradyarrhythmias and occasional examples of acute myocardial infarction.

Exercise treadmill testing has been used in attempts to provoke syncope, or diagnose exercise related tachyarrhythmias or bradyarrhythmias.[94–97] The data on exercise testing consists only of case reports and individual experiences. In one study of 119 patients in which exercise testing was compared to ambulatory monitoring in the diagnosis of syncope, only 3 patients had an abnormality detected with exercise.[98] In general, exercise stress testing is neither sensitive nor cost effective in the diagnosis of arrythmias and syncope unless there is a clear history of exercise provocation of symptoms.

Ambulatory ECG Monitoring and Event Recorders

Most detected arrhythmias are brief and frequent in otherwise normal ambulatory asymptomatic individuals.[99–108] For example, sinus bradycardia (fewer than 40 beats per minute during sleep) was found in 24%, brief runs of supraventricular tachycardia in 50%, premature atrial contractions in 50%, and premature ventricular contractions (PVCs) in up to75% with complex PVCs in 15% of normal individuals.[4] However, sinus pauses greater than 2 seconds are uncommon in asymptomatic individuals and complete AV block and non sustained ventricular tachycardia lasting longer than 5 beats are even less frequent.

Because there are no definitive standards with which to compare the results of ambulatory monitoring, one method of assessing accuracy has been to determine the proportion of patients who had a correlation between recorded arrhythmias and symptoms. Overall correlation with symptoms has been noted in only about 4% of patients. In approximately 17% of patients, symptoms were not associated with arrhythmias and therefore arrhythmias are excluded as a cause for syncope. In more than 80% of patients there were no symptoms, yet arrhythmias were found in many patients.[4] Thus the causal relationship between arrhythmias and syncope as assessed by ambulatory monitoring is difficult to define. Also, the optimal duration of ambulatory ECG monitoring has not been determined. In one study an ECG finding was noted in 15% after 24 hours, 11% after 48 hours, and 4.2% after 72 hours.[109] Only 1 of the arrhythmias detected was in a symptomatic patient. Thus monitoring for 48 hours is generally considered sufficient.

Certain arrhythmias detected by monitoring patients with syncope have been related to subsequent mortality and sudden death. Frequent or repetitive ventricular ectopy, has been found to be an independent predictor of mortality conferring a 3.7 times increase in total mortality and 14.9 times increase of sudden death.[99] No data have been reported to date to indicate that treatment of these arrhythmias alters this risk. Inferences can probably be made however in patients with ischemic heart disease and low ejection fractions (<35%) with nonsustained ventricular tachycardia on monitoring and inducible ventricular tachycardia with EP testing. In this latter group of patients, implantable cardioverter-defibrillators have shown a survival benefit.[110] In the future other high-risk groups may be identified including patients with unexplained syncope that might benefit from this type of therapy.

Patient-activated event recorders with a memory loop can be useful in selected patients. These devices are more likely to capture an event after an episode since several minutes of retrograde ECG recording is possible. In 1 reported study, 14 of 39 patients with frequent syncopal episodes had symptoms during monitoring (average 28 days; range 3–140 days). Only 3 of the patients had arrhythmias, whereas 11 had a "normal" cardiac rhythm.[111] The clear drawback of these devices is that they are only useful in patients with frequent symptoms. In a follow up study by Kapoor et al,[112] only 5% of patients reported recurrent symptoms at 1 month, 11% at 3 months, and 16% at 6 months. Thus, cardiac event monitoring is likely to be useful for capturing a spell in a small subset of patients with frequent recurrence in whom initial evaluation is negative and arrhythmias are not diagnosed by other means such as 24 hour ambulatory ECG monitoring or EP testing. Transtelephonic monitoring is not useful in patients with abrupt loss of consciousness, since the patient is unable to transmit a recording during a spell. This technique is more useful for the evaluation of dizziness, presyncope, and pacemaker malfunction. Implantable loop recorders are now available. Implantation of this pacemaker sized device now allows long term monitoring of patients with syncope of unknown etiology in which other diagnostic modalities have failed.[113] In 24 such patients, Krahn et al[113] was able to identify 10 patients with recurrent infrequent syncope secondary to bradycardia (8 patients) and tachycardia (2 patients). In 9 patients, recordings during a syncopal episode ruled out arrhythmia as a cause.

Signal Averaged ECG

Signal averaging is a computer technique that reduces random noise in the ECG to enhance detection of low amplitude signals in the terminal portion of the QRS complex. Detection of these low amplitude signals, or late potentials, has been reported to have a sensitivity of about 80% and specificity of 90% for prediction of inducible sustained ventricular tachycardia in patients with syncope.[114-116] Unfortunately, QRS widening with bundle branch block or other conduction system disease makes interpretation of the signal averaged ECG difficult.

The usefulness of this test in evaluating patients with syncope is not clear. Some centers have advocated using the signal averaged ECG as a screening before EP testing. However, in patients with heart disease in whom arrhythmias are suspected as a cause, an electrophysiological study (EPS) probably be performed anyway because of lack of sensitivity of the signal averaged ECG. Furthermore, other abnormalities including sinus node dysfunction, AV nodal conduction abnormalities, His-Purkinje conduction abnormalities, and other arrhythmias can only be excluded by EPS.

EPS

The current role of EPS in patients with syncope is not clearly defined. EPS is invasive and costly, but relatively safe. In patients without identifiable heart disease the yield is low. However, in patients with recurrent unexplained syncope and significant organic heart disease, EPS can be very useful in identifying arrhythmias and selecting therapy.

Krol et al[117] reported that predictors of a negative EPS included absence of heart disease by history, ejection fraction greater than 40%, normal ECG and 24 hour ambulatory monitoring, absence of injury, and multiple or prolonged episodes (>5 minutes) of syncope. EPS are also more likely to be abnormal in patients with bundle branch block. In a study involving patients 75 years and older, EPS provides a likely diagnosis in 68% of studies. Abnormal findings included sinus node dysfunction (55%), abnormal His bundle conduction (39%), ventricular tachycardia (14%) and more than one abnormality.[118] In some patients, attempts have been made to correlate syncopal symptoms by upright tilt during the induced arrhythmias.[119]

The sensitivity and specificity of abnormalities identified at EPS need to be addressed when evaluating patients with syncope. The ECG findings of sinus node disease have been well described and diagnosis is generally established by the history and ambulatory electrocardiography. A prolonged sinus node recovery time has low sensitivity for the diagnosis of sinus node dysfunction (18%–69%), but appears to be specific (45%–100%) when compared to ambulatory monitoring.[120] The value of other tests of sinus node function such as the siro atrial conduction time is controversial. Screening tests for AV nodal conduction and refractoriness are difficult to interpret because the sensitivity and specificity of these measurements are not known.[121,122] Ascribing syncope to abnormalities of H-V conduction is often difficult. A markedly prolonged HV interval and block between the H and the V spike during atrial pacing is a marker of conduction system disease that may result in bradycardia and syncope. However, definition of a prolonged HV interval varies widely from greater than 55 ms to 100 ms. Unfortunately, the finding of an HV interval greater than 100 ms is uncommon even in patients with syncope.[121–124]

Induction of supraventricular tachycardia in patients without a prior history of tachycardia is uncommon. Figure 8 demonstrates induction of AV nodal reentry tachycardia in an elderly man with a prior history of arrhythmias and a recent history of syncope. Atrial fibrillation or flutter may also be initiated, but their significance is uncertain

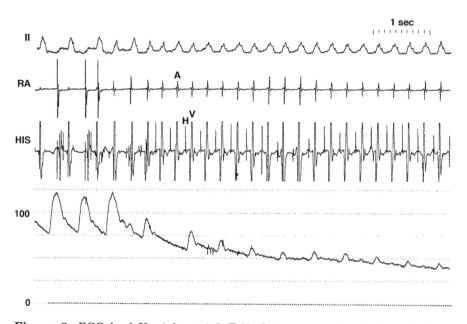

Figure 8: *ECG lead II, right atrial (RA) electrogram (A), His bundle electrogram (H), ventricular electrogram (V), and blood pressure (mm Hg) recorded during induction of AV nodal reentry tachycardia. From left to right, 2 atrial drive train beats followed by a single atrial extrastimulus with induction of tachycardia. Despite being supine, severe hypotension persisted until tachycardia was terminated.*

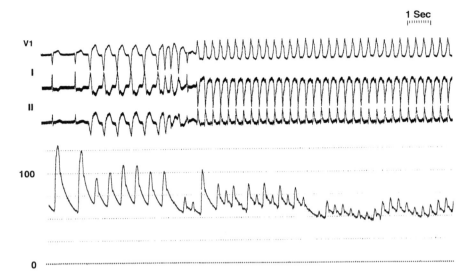

Figure 9: *ECG leads V₁, I, II and blood pressure (mm Hg) recorded during EPS in a 68-year-old man with a history of syncope secondary to ventricular tachycardia. From left to right, 2 sinus beats followed by a 6-beat ventricular drive train and a single extrastimulus with induction of monomorphic ventricular tachycardia. Despite being in the supine position, note the significant hypotension that occurred.*

unless they reproduce spontaneous symptoms.[121,122,124] A higher proportion of patients with heart disease will have inducible ventricular arrhythmias (55%–70%) compared to those without cardiac disease (20%).[4] Figure 9 is an example of ventricular tachycardia induced at EPS in a patient with known ischemic heart disease with syncope secondary to the tachycardia documented by ECG monitoring. Inducible sustained monomorphic ventricular tachycardia has a sensitivity and specificity of 90% or greater for predicting spontaneous ventricular tachycardia when EPS is compared to prolonged ambulatory ECG monitoring.[125] Induction of polymorphic or nonsustained ventricular tachycardia is often a nonspecific response. Based on available data the following EPS findings are important: (1) sustained monomorphic ventricular tachycardia; (2) sinus node recovery time longer than 3 seconds; (3) pacing induced infranodal block or an HV interval of more than 100 ms; (4) supraventricular tachycardia with symptomatic hypotension similar to a spontaneous episode.

Evaluation of the efficacy of EPS in the diagnosis and treatment of syncope depends on the ability to predict recurrence. Many studies report fewer recurrences in patients with positive EPS and subsequent directed therapy compared to recurrence in patients with negative EPS.[4] Since syncope is often sporadic, it is often difficult to assess rates of recurrence unless prior symptoms were frequent, or follow-up is very long. EPS focused on mortality, report markedly higher death rates in patients with positive findings as high as 61%–3-year mortality and 48% sudden death rate in one series.[126] The Antiarrhythmics versus Implantable Defibrillators (AVID) Investigators reported improved survival with device therapy.[127] Included in this study were survivors of sudden death and patients with symptomatic (including syncope) ventricular tachycardia and an ejection fraction of 40% or less. Thus in patients with heart disease and inducibility of significant ventricular arrhythmias at EPS, it can be inferred that there may well be survival benefit with aggressive evaluation and therapy.

Neurological or Psychiatric Syncope

Syncope resulting from cerebral vascular disease is uncommon. Cerebral ischemia or infarction tends to present as a neurological deficit and not syncope. However, cerebrovascular disease can potentiate susceptibility to syncope when there is associated postural hypotension. Syncope associated with neurological symptoms localized to the brainstem suggest vertebro-basilar insufficiency,[128] basilar artery migraine,[129,130] vertebral artery compression by degenerative cervical spine disease, and subclavian steal.[131] Occasionally, transient neurological symptoms that can be mistaken for transient ischemic episodes can be a result of neurally-mediated hypotension.[132]

Seizures may be confused with syncope. Generally, the presence of an aura, typical tonic-clonic movements, and post-ictal state associated with an abnormal EEG make differentiation possible. Unfortunately, myoclonic jerking can be associated with any cause of syncope associated with hypotension which when witnessed by an untrained observer may result in erroneous diagnosis of seizure. HUT was used by Grubb et al[133] to separate these diagnostic possibilities.

Sleep disorders including sleep apnea can generally be differentiated from syncope by history, with sleep studies only occasionally required. Drug ingestion and in particular alcohol abuse need careful evaluation.[134] Several effects of acute and chronic alcohol abuse may cause loss of consciousness including reversible autonomic dysfunction with orthostatic hypotension, chronic postural hypotension related to sympathetic damage, cardiomyopathy with associated arrhythmias, and alcohol withdrawal seizures.[135,136]

Anxiety and panic disorders and major depression have been associated with syncope in younger individuals.[137] In an older population, these conditions are rarely responsible for syncope.

Syncope and Driving

The most frequent question either asked or avoided by syncope patients (and sometimes their physicians) regards the ability to resume driving. For patients, the inability to drive is often viewed as so confining as to be considered a major disability. This is especially true in rural areas where inability to drive renders patients house bound. On the other hand, motor vehicle accidents are one of the leading causes of death and disability in the western world. Thus, it would seem self evident that driving should be restricted in patients with syncope since their risk of loss of consciousness while driving is presumably higher than in the general population. Recently, the American Heart Association and North American Society of Pacing and Electrophysiology released a policy statement regarding recommendations for patients with arrhythmias that may affect consciousness and syncope.[138] This policy statement is not a legal document, but rather provides recommendations from recognized authorities in the field.

In discussing the ability to return to driving in patients who have suffered an episode of syncope, the treating physician must consider 3 major issues. Firstly, there are the patient's wishes, secondly safety issues, and thirdly any legal or regulatory issues.

Most patients will follow their physician's advice in terms of refraining from driving for at least a prescribed period until it becomes clear that resumption of driving is safe. Some patients however continue driving despite their physician's recommendations or may seek another physician with a more favorable opinion. It is important to note that although patients with syncope are at increased risk while driving, so are other groups of patients including those with significant ischemic heart disease and advanced cardiomyopathy. Similary, teenage drivers have a high accident risk. Yet, neither of these latter groups of individuals have been restricted from driving. Thus in all fairness to the syncopal patients, physicians must attempt to address several key issues: (1) What is the likelihood of syncope while driving? (2) How is the latter affected with treatment? (3) What are the circumstances under which syncope is most likely to occur? (4) Does any warning occur prior to loss of consciousness? (5) How often and in what environment does the patient drive? (6) Finally, are there any legal implications to the physician's recommendations?

It is beyond the scope of this chapter to attempt to list what are perceived to be the risks of recurrent syncope or alteration in awareness while driving in different population groups. Rather the reader is referred to several recent publications which provide a more in depth view.[138,139] Several generalizations however can be made. Firstly, if syncope is infrequent and not severe, or the condition is treatable with an expected good response, restriction from driving may be inappropriate. Examples include patients with mild vasovagal or neurally mediated syncope which occurrs infrequently or only in the upright position, or a treatable condition such as complete heart block following pacemaker implantation. On the other hand, patients with frequent recurrence of syncope especially in the seated position, should be warned to not drive. A good example would be a patient with ventricular arrhythmias with repeated syncope terminated by an ICD. Most patients, however, fall between the examples given, and it is the responsibility of the physician to carefully review each patient's circumstances and use the best judgement to make recommendations. We follow the general guidelines of (1) allowing patients to drive immediately if there is no apparent increased risk, (2) restrict driving for 3 months if the risk is felt to be low and a short period of response to treatment is desired, (3) no driving for 6 months if a longer period of observation is required, and (4) permanently restrict driving when the risk of recurrence remains high despite the best medical treatment.

In general the legal medical criteria for driving in the United States are determined by the individual states. Therefore, it is important for physicians to know what the local laws are and what are their responsibilities concerning individual patients. These laws are subject to change and do change. In most states, currently, it is the individual driver's (patient's) responsibility to report an episode of syncope to the appropriate government agency; however, some states require physician reporting. In general the legal risks to physicians regarding driver recommendations appear low provided the issues are discussed with the patient, documented, and if necessary reported to the proper legal authority. With proper diagnosis and treatment, it is hoped that prudent guidelines for driving can be established in most patients using common sense and published guidelines.[138]

Conclusion

Syncope is a common and troubling problem for both physicians and patients. Algorithms developed to evaluate syncope have generally not been very effective partly because there are so many potential causes. Even with extensive evaluation, infrequent episodes will remain undiagnosed. A careful history and physical examination are invaluable in the judicious application of tests used to evaluate these patients. The issue of the need for hospitalization for emergent, as opposed to outpatient evaluation has not been addressed unless a potentially life threatening cardiac cause is suspected. Further directions in the management of patients with syncope include not only improvements in diagnosis, but also identification and assessment of potential successful therapies to prevent recurrence and mortality.

Acknowledgments

Secretarial assistance from JoAnne Underhill and preparation of the figures and tables by Margaret Fashingbauer are gratefully acknowledged.

References

1. Savage D, Corwin L, McGee D, et al: Epidemiologic features of isolated syncope: The Framingham Study. *Stroke* 16:626–629, 1985.
2. Lipsitz L, Wei J, Rowe J: Syncope in an elderly, institutionalized population: Prevalence, incidence and associated risk. *Q J Med* 15:45–55, 1985.
3. Lipsitz L, Pluchino F, Wei J, et al: Syncope in institutionalized elderly: The impact of multiple pathological conditions and situational stress. *J Chronic Dis* 39:619–630, 1986.
4. Kapoor W: Diagnostic evaluation of syncope. *Am J Med* 90:91–106, 1991.
5. Antman E, Ludmer P, McGowan N, et al: Transtelephonic electrocardiographic transmission for management of cardiac arrhythmias. *Am J Cardiol* 58:1021–1024, 1986.
6. Caird F, Andrews G, Kennedy R: Effect of posture on blood pressure in the elderly. *Br Heart J* 35:527–530, 1973.
7. MacLennan W, Hall M, Timothy J: Postural hypotension in old age: Is it a disorder of the nervous system or of blood vessels? *Age Ageing* 12:25–32, 1980.
8. Myers M, Kearns P, Kennedy D, et al: Postural hypotension and diruetic therapy in the elderly. *Can Med Assoc J* 119:581–584, 1978.
9. Mader S, Josephson K, Rubenstein L: Low prevalence of postural hypotension among community-dwelling elderly. *JAMA* 258:1511–1514, 1978.
10. Harris T, Kleinman J, Lipsitz L, et al: Is age or level of systolic blood pressure related to positional blood pressure change? *Gerontologist* 26:59A, 1986.
11. Lipsitz L: Orthostatic hypotension in the elderly. *N Engl J Med* 321:952–957, 1989.
12. Tinetti M, Williams T, Mayewski R: Fall risk index for elderly patients based on number of chronic disabilities. *Am J Med* 80:429–434, 1986.
13. Eckberg D-L: Parasympathetic cardiovascular control in human disease: A critical review of methods and results. *Am J Physiol* 239:H581-H593, 1980.
14. Shannon R, Wei J, Rosa R, et al: The effect of age and sodium depletion on cardiovascular response to orthostasis. *Hypertension* 8:438–443, 1986.
15. Lakatta E, Mitchell J, Pomerance A, et al: Human aging: Changes in structure and function. *J Am Coll Cardiol* 10:42A-47A, 1987.
16. Crane M, Harris J: Effect of aging on renin activity and aldosterone excretion. *J Lab Clin Med* 87:947–959, 1976.
17. Epstein M, Hollenberg N: Age as a determinant of renal sodium conservation in normal man. *J Lab Clin Med* 87:411–417, 1976.
18. Haller B, Zust H, Shar S, et al: Effects of posture and ageing on circulating atrial natriuretic peptide levels in man. *J Hypertens* 5:551–556, 1987.
19. Phillips P, Rolls B, Ledingham J: Reduced thirst after water deprivation in healthy elderly men. *N Engl J Med* 311:753–759, 1984.
20. Wei J: Age and the cardiovascular system. *N Engl J Med* 327:1735–1739, 1992.
21. Kannel W. Hypertension and aging. In: C Finch, E Schneider, (eds.) *Handbook of the Biology of Aging.* 2nd ed. New York: Van Nostrand Reinhold, 1985, pp 00-00.
22. Meyer J, Shaw T: Cerebral blood flow in aging. In: M Albert, (ed.) *Clinical Neurology of Aging.* New York, Oxford University Press, 1984.
23. Strandgaard S: Autoregulation of cerebral blood flow in hypertensive pa-

tients: The modifying influence of prolonged antihypertensive treatment on the tolerance to acute, drug-induced hypotension. *Circulation* 53: 720–727, 1976.

24. Tolins M, Weir E, Chesler E, et al: Maximal drug therapy is not necessarily optimal in chronic angina pectoris. *J Am Coll Cardiol* 3:1051–1057, 1984.
25. Ferrara L, Cicerano U, Marotta T, et al. Postprandial and postural hypotension in the elderly. *Cardiol Elderly* 1:33–37, 1993.
26. Lipsitz L, Pluchino F, Wei J, et al: Cardiovascular and norepinephrine responses following meal consumption in elderly (older than 75 years) persons with post-prandial hypotension and syncope. *Am J Cardiol* 58: 810–815, 1986.
27. Bannister R. Introduction and classification. In: R Bannister, (eds.) *Autonomic Failure: A Textbook of Clinical Disorders of the Autonomic Nervous System*. 2nd ed. London: Oxford, 1988, pp 1–20.
28. Ziegler M, Lake C, Kopin I: The sympathetic-nervous-system defect in primary orthostatic hypotension. *N Engl J Med* 296:293–297, 1977.
29. Polinsky R, Kopin I, Ebert M, et al: Pharmacologic distinction of different orthostatic hypotension syndromes. *Neurology* 31:1–7, 1981.
30. Shy G, Drager G: A neurological syndrome associated with orthostatic hypotension. *Arch Neurol* 2:511–527, 1960.
31. Schatz I: Orthostatic hypotension. I. Function and neurogenic causes. *Arch Intern Med* 144:773–777, 1984.
32. Edmonds M, Watkins P: Clinical presentations of diabetic autonomic failure. In: R Bannister, (eds.) *Autonomic Failure: a Textbook of Clinical Disorders of the Autonomic Nervous System*. 2nd ed. London, Oxford, 1988, pp 632–653.
33. Mader S, Palmer R, Rubenstein L: Effect of timing and number of baseline blood pressure determinations on postural blood pressure response. *J Am Geriatr Soc* 37:444–446, 1989.
34. Lipsitz L, Fluchino F, Wei J, et al: Syncope in institutionalized elderly: The impact of multiple pathological conditions and situational stress. *J Chronic Dis* 39:619–630, 1986.
35. Jankovic J, Gilden J, Hiner B, et al: Neurogenic orthostatic hypotension: A double-blind, placebo-controlled study with midodrine. *Am J Med* 95: 38–48, 1993.
36. Kaufmann H, Brannan T, Krakoff L, et al: Treatment of orthostatic hypotension due to automatic failure with a peripheral alpha-adrenergic agonist (midodrine). *Neurology* 38:951–956, 1988.
37. Fouad F, Bravo E, Onyekwere O, et al: Supine hypertension associated with orthostatic hypotension. *Cardiol Elderly* 1:273–280, 1993.
38. Kochar M, Itskovitz H: Treatment of idiopathic orthostatic hypotension (Shy-Drager syndrome) with indomethacin. *Lancet* 1:1011–1014, 1978.
39. Robertson D, Goldberg M, Hollister A, et al: Clonidine raises blood pressure in severe idiopathic orthostatic hypotension. *Am J Med* 74:193–200, 1993.
40. Schatz I. Orthostatic hypotension. II. Clinical diagnosis, testing, and treatment. *Arch Intern Med* 144:1037–1041, 1984.
41. Onrot J, Goldberg M, Hollister A, et al: Management of chronic orthostatic hypotension. *Am J Med* 80:454–464, 1986.
42. Onrot J, Goldberg M, Biaggioni I, et al: Hemodynamic and humoral effects of caffeine in automatic failure: Therapeutic implications for postprandial hypotension. *N Engl J Med* 313:549–554, 1985.

43. Biaggioni I, Onrot J, Steward C, et al: The potent pressor effect of phenyl-propanolamine in patients with autonomic impairment. *JAMA* 258: 236–239, 1987.
44. Hoeldtke R, Cavanaugh S, Hughes J, et al: Treatment of orthostatic hypotension with dihydroergotamine and caffeine. *Ann Intern Med* 105: 168–173, 1986.
45. Hoeldtke R, Boden G, O'Dorisio T: Treatment of postprandial hypotension with a somatostatin analogue (SMS 201–995). *Am J Med* 81:83–87, 1986.
46. Hoeldtke R, Streeten D: Treatment of orthostatic hypotension with erythropoietin. *N Engl J Med* 329:611–615, 1993.
47. Grubb B, Kosinski D: Serotonin and syncope: An emerging connection? *Eur J Cardiac Pacing Electrophysiol* 5:306–314, 1996.
48. Lewis T: Vasovagal syncope and the carotid sinus mechanism. *Br Med J* 1:873–876, 1932.
49. Wallin B, Sundlof G: Sympathetic outflow in muscles during vasovagal syncope. *J Autonom Nerv Syst* 6:287–291, 1982.
50. Wallin B, Westerberg C-E, Sundlof G: Syncope induced by glossopharyngeal neuralgia: Sympathetic outflow to muscle. *Neurology* 34:522–524, 1984.
51. Benditt D, Lurie K, Adler S, et al: Rationale and methodology of head-up tilt table testing for evaluation of neurally-mediated (cardioneurogenic) syncope. In: D Zipes, J Jalife, (eds.) *Cardiac Electrophysiology: From Cell to Bedside.* 2nd ed. Philadelphia, PA, W. B. Saunders Co., 1995, pp 00-00.
52. Golf S. Swallowing syncope. *Acta Med Scand* 201:585–586, 1977.
53. Wik B, Hillestad L: Deglutition syncope. *Br Med J* 3:747, 1975.
54. Kalloor G, Singh S, Collis J: Cardiac arrhythmias on swallowing. *Am Heart J* 93:235–238, 1977.
55. Kunis R, Garfein O, Pepe A, et al: Deglutition syncope and atrioventricular block selectively induced by hot food and liquid. *Am J Cardiol* 55:613, 1985.
56. Kadish A, Wesler L, Marchlinski F: Swallowing syncope: Observations in the absence of conduction system or esophageal disease. *Am J Med* 81: 1098–2000, 1986.
57. Lukash W, Sawyer G, Davis J. Micturition syncope produced by orthostasis and bladder distension. *N Engl J Med* 270:341–344, 1964.
58. Paulson O, Lund M. Natural history of micturition syncope. *Acta Scand* 52:401–406, 1975.
59. Kapoor W, Peterson J, Karpf M: Micturition syncope. *JAMA* 253:796–798, 1985.
60. Schiavone A, Biasi M, Buonomo C, et al: Micturition syncopes. *Funct Neurol* 6:305–308, 1991.
61. Kapoor W, Peterson J, Karpf M: Defecation syncope. A symptom with multiple etiologies. *Arch Intern Med* 146:2377–2379, 1986.
62. Pathy M: Defecation syncope. *Age Ageing* 7:233–236, 1978.
63. Kerr A, Derbes V: The syndrome of cough syncope. *Ann Intern Med* 39: 1240–1252, 1953.
64. Pedersen A, Sandoe E, Hvidberg E, et al: Studies on the mechanism of tussive syncope. *Acta Med Scand* 179:653–661, 1996.
65. Kapoor W, Janetta P: Trigeminal neuralgia associated with seizure and syncope. *J Neurosurg* 61:594–595, 1984.
66. Hassam A, Abindar E, Goldhammer E, et al: Complete heart block and trigeminal neuralgia. *Neurology* 37:1089–1090, 1987.

67. Kapoor W, Brant N: Evaluation of syncope by upright tilt testing with isoproterenol: A nonspecific test. Ann Intern Med 116:358–363, 1992.
68. Almquist A, Gornick C, Benson W Jr, et al: Carotid sinus hypersensitivity: Evaluation of the vasodepressor component. *Circulation* 71:927–936, 1985.
69. Walter P, Crawley I, Dorney E: Carotid sinus hypersensitivity and syncope. *Am J Cardiol* 42:396–403, 1978.
70. Lown B, Levine S: The carotid sinus: clinical value of its stimulation. *Circulation* 23:766–788, 1961.
71. Tuckman J, Slater S, Mendlowitz M: The carotid sinus reflexes. *Am Heart J* 70:119–134, 1965.
72. Stryjer D, Friedensohn A, Schlesinger Z: Carotid sinus hypersensitivity: Diagnosis of vasodepressor type in the presence of cardioinhibitory type. *PACE* 5:793–800, 1982.
73. Heidorn G, McNamara A: Effect of carotid sinus stimulation on the electrocardiograms of clinically normal individuals. *Circulation* 14: 1104–1113, 1956.
74. Smiddy J, Lewis H, Dunn M: The effect of carotid massage in older men. *J Cardiol* 27:209–211, 1972.
75. Cohen M: Ventricular fibrillation precipitated by carotid sinus pressure report and review of the literature. *Am Heart J* 84:681–686, 1972.
76. Askey J: Hemiplegia following carotid sinus stimulation. *Am Heart J* 31: 131–137, 1946.
77. Hart G, Oldershaw P, Cull R, et al: Syncope caused by cough-induced complete atrioventricular block. *PACE* 5:564–566, 1982.
78. Baron S, Huang S: Cough syncope presenting as Mobitz type II atrioventricular block-an electrophysiologic correlation. *PACE* 10:65–69, 1987.
79. Choi Y, Kim J, Oh BH et al: Cough syncope caused by sinus arrest in a patient with sick sinus syndrome. *PACE* 12:883–886, 1989.
80. Brignole M, Menozzi C, Gianfranchi L, et al: Carotid sinus massage, eyeball compression, and head-up tilt test in patients with syncope of uncertain origin and in healthy control subjects. *Am Heart J* 122:1644–1651, 1991.
81. Grubb B, Wolfe D, Samoil D, et al: Recurrent unexplained syncope in the elderly: The use of head-upright tilt table testing in evaluation and management. *J Am Geriatr Soc* 40:1123–1128, 1992.
82. Lipsitz L, Marks E, Koestner J, et al: Reduced susceptibility to syncope during postural tilt in old age. *Arch Intern Med* 149:2709–2712, 1989.
83. Benditt D, Petersen M, Lurie K, et al: Cardiac pacing for prevention of recurrent vasovagal syncope. *Ann Intern Med* 122:204–209, 1995.
84. Petersen M, Chamberlain-Webber R, Fitzpatrick A, et al: Permanent pacing for cardioinihibitory malignant vasovagal syndrome. *Br Heart J* 71: 274–281, 1994.
85. Thomas J. Diseases of the carotid sinus syncope. In: P Vinken, G Bruyn, (eds.) *Handbook of Clinical Neurology*. Amsterdam, North-Holland, 1972, pp 532–551.
86. Morley C, Perrins E, Grant P, et al: Carotid sinus syncope treated by pacing. *Br Heart J* 47:411–418, 1982.
87. Sugrue D, Gersh B, Holmes DR, et al: Symptomatic isolated carotid sinus hypersensitivity: Natural history and results of treatment with anticholinergic drugs or pacemakers. *J Am Coll Cardiol* 7:158–162, 1986.
88. Goldenberg I, Almquist A, Dunbar D, et al: Prevention of neurally-me-

diated syncope by selective beta-1 adrenoceptor blockade (abstract). *Circulation* 76(Suppl 4):133, 1987.

89. Milstein S, Buetikofer J, Dunnigan A, et al: Usefulness of disopyramide for prevention of upright tilt-induced hypotension-bradycardia. *Am J Cardiol* 65:1339–1344, 1990.

90. Nelson S, Stanley M, Love C, et al: Autonomic and hemodynamic effects of oral theophylline in patients with vasodepressor syncope. *Arch Intern Med* 51:2425–2429, 1991.

91. Kapoor W, Snustad D, Peterson J, et al: Syncope in the elderly. *Am J Med* 80:419–428, 1980.

92. Kapoor W: Evaluation and outcome of patients with syncope. *Medicine* 69:160–175, 1990.

93. Kapoor W, Peterson J, Karpf M: The usefulness of initial electrocardiogram in evaluating patients with syncope (abstract). *Clin Res* 35:762A, 1987.

94. Kapoor W: Syncope with abrupt termination of exercise (brief clinical observation). *Am J Med* 87:597–599, 1989.

95. Eichna L, Horvath S, Bean W. Post-exertional orthostatic hypotension. *Am J Med Sci* 213:641–654, 1947.

96. Schlesinger Z: Life-threatening "vagal reaction" to physical fitness test (letter). *JAMA* 226:1119, 1973.

97. Huycke E, Card H, Sobol S, et al: Postexertional cardiac asystole in a young man without organic heart disease. *Ann Intern Med* 106:844–845, 1987.

98. Boudoulas H, Schaael S, Lewis R, et al: Superiority of 24-hour outpatient monitoring over multi-stage exercise testing for the evaluation of syncope. *J Electrocardiol* 12:103–108, 1979.

99. Kapoor W, Cha R, Peterson J, et al: Prolonged electrocardiographic monitoring in patients with syncope: The importance of frequent or repetitive ventricular ectopy. *Am J Med* 82:20–28, 1987.

100. Clark P, Glasser S, Spoto E: Arrhythmias detected by ambulatory monitoring: Lack of correlation with symptoms of dizziness and syncope. *Chest* 77:722–725, 1980.

101. Gibson T, Heitzman M: Diagnostic efficacy of 24-hour electrocardiographic monitoring for syncope. *Am J Cardiol* 53:1013–1017, 1984.

102. Abdon N, Johansson B, Lessem J: Predictive use of routine 24-hour electrocardiography in suspected Adams-Stokes syndrome. Comparison with cardiac rhythm during symptoms. *Br Heart J* 47:553–558, 1982.

103. Gordon M, Huang M, Gryfe C: An evaluation of falls, syncope, and dizziness in prolonged ambulatory cardiographic monitoring in a geriatric institutional setting. *J Am Geriatr Soc* 30:6–12, 1982.

104. Brodsky M, Wu D, Denes P, et al: Arrhythmias documented by 24-hour continuous electrocardiographic monitoring in 50 male medical students without apparent heart disease. *Am J Cardiol* 39:390–395, 1977.

105. Clarke J, Hamer J, Shelton J, et al:The rhythm of the normal human heart. *Lancet* 2:508–512, 1976.

106. Winkle R, Derrington D, Schroeder J: Characteristics of ventricular tachycardia in ambulatory patients. *Am J Cardiol* 39:487–492, 1977.

107. Glasser S, Clark P, Applebaum H: Occurrence of frequent complex arrhythmias detected by ambulatory monitoring: Findings in an apparently healthy asymptomatic elderly population. *Chest* 75:565–568, 1979.

108. Barrett P, Peter C, Swan H, et al: The frequency and prognostic signifi-

cance of electrocardiographic abnormalities in clinically normal individuals. *Prog Cardiovasc Dis* 23:299–319, 1981.

109. Bass E, Curtiss E, Arena VC, et al: The duration of holter monitoring in patients with syncope: Is 24 hours enough? *Arch Intern Med* 150: 1073–1078, 1990.

110. Moss A, Hall J, Cannom D, et al: Improved survival with an implanted defibrillator in patients with coronary disease at high risk for ventricular arrhythmia. *N Engl J Med* 335:1933–1940, 1996.

111. Linzer M, Pritchett E, Pontinen M, et al: Diagnosing the undiagnosable: Use of continuous loop electrocardiographic recorders in unexplained syncope (abstract). *Circulation* 1989;80:35, 1989.

112. Kapoor W, Peterson J, Wieand H, et al: Diagnostic and prognostic implications of recurrences in patients with syncope. *Am J Med* 83:700–708, 1987.

113. Krahn A, Klein G, Norris C, et al: The etiology of syncope in patients with negative tilt table and electrophysiologic testing. *Circulation* 92: 1819–1824, 1995.

114. Kuchar D, Thorburn C, Sammel N: Signal-averaged electrocardiogram for evaluation of recurrent syncope. *Am J Cardiol* 58:949–953, 1986.

115. Gang E, Peter T, Rosenthal ME, et al: Detection of late potentials on the surface electrocardiogram in unexplained syncope. *Am J Cardiol* (1014–1020), 1986.

116. Winters S, Stewart D, Gomes J: Signal averaging of the surface QRS complex predicts inducibility of ventricular tachycardia in patients with syncope of unknown origin: A prospective study. *J Am Coll Cardiol* 10: 775–781, 1987.

117. Krol R, Morady F, Flaker G, et al: Electrophysiologic testing in patients with unexplained syncope: Clinical and noninvasive predictors of outcome. *J Am Coll Cardiol* 10:358–363, 1987.

118. Sugrue D, Holmes D Jr, Gersh B, et al: Impact of intracardiac electrophysiologic testing on the management of elderly patients with recurrent syncope or near syncope. *J Am Geriatr Soc* 35:1079–1083, 1987.

119. Hammill S, Holmes D, Wood DL, et al: Electrophysiologic testing in the upright position: Improved evaluation of patients with rhythm disturbances using a tilt table. *J Am Coll Cardiol* 4:65–71, 1984.

120. Benditt D, Milstein S, Goldstein M: Sinus node dysfunction: pathophysiology, clinical features, evaluation, and treatment. In: D Zipes, J Jalife, (eds.) *Cardiac Electrophysiology: From Cell to Bedside.* 2nd ed. Philadelphia, PA, W.B. Saunders Co., 1990.

121. DiMarco J: Electrophysiologic studies in patients with unexplained syncope. *Circulation* 75:III 144–145, 1987.

122. McAnulty J: Syncope of unknown origin: The role of electrophysiologic studies. *Circulation* 75:144–145, 1987.

123. Fujimura O, Yee R, Klein GJ, et al: The diagnostic sensitivity of electrophysiologic testing in patients with syncope caused by transient bradycardia. *N Engl J Med* 321:1703–1713, 1989.

124. Morady F, Scheinman M: The role and limitations of electrophysiologic testing in patients with unexplained syncope. *Int J Cardiol* 4:229–234, 1983.

125. Vandepol C, Farshidi A, Spielman SR, et al: Incidence and clinical significance of induced ventricular tachycardia. *Am J Cardiol* 45:725–731, 1980.

126. Bass E, Elson J, Fogoros R, et al. Long-term prognosis of patients undergo-

ing electrophysiologic studies for syncope of unknown origin. *Am J Cardiol* 62:1186–1191, 1988.

127. Investigators TAvID: A comparison of antiarrhythmic-drug therapy with implantable defibrillators in patients resuscitated from near-fatal ventricular arrhythmias. *N Engl J Med* 337:1576–1583, 1997.

128. Goldstein M, Bokis C: *Cerebrovascular Disorders: a Clinical and Research Classification.* Geneva, WHO, 1978. vol 43.

129. Bickerstaff E: Impairment of consciousness in migraine. *Lancet* 2:1057–1059, 1961.

130. Swanson J, Vick N: Basilar artery migraine. *Neurology* 132:278–281, 1978.

131. Fields W, Lemak N: Joint study of extracranial arterial occlusion VII. Subclavian steal-a review of 168 cases. *JAMA* 222:1139–1143, 1972.

132. Grubb B, Samoil D, Temesy-Armos P, et al: Episodic periods of neurally mediated hypotension and bradycardia mimicking transient ischemic attacks in the elderly: Identification with head-up tilt-table testing. *Cardiol Elderly* 1:221–225, 1993.

133. Grubb B, Gerard G, Roush K, et al: Differentiation of convulsive syncope and epilepsy with head-up tilt testing. *Ann Intern Med* 115:871–876, 1991.

134. Kapoor W, Karpf M, Wieand S, et al: A prospective evaluation and follow-up of patients with syncope. *N Engl J Med* 309:197–204, 1983.

135. Johnson R, Eisenhofer G, Lambie D: The effects of acute and chronic ingestion of ethanol on the autonomic nervous system. *Drug Alcohol Depend* 18:319–328, 1986.

136. Johnson R: Autonomic failure in alcoholics. In: Bannister R, (eds.) *Autonomic Failure. A Textbook of Clinical Disorders of the Autonomic Nervous System.* New York, Oxford University Press, 1989.

137. Linzer M, Felder A, Hackel A, et al: Psychiatric syncope. *Psychosomatics* 31:181–188, 1990.

138. Epstein A, Miles W, Benditt D, et al: Personal and public safety issues related to arrhythmias that may affect consciousness: Implications for regulation and physician recommendations. *Circulation* 94:1147–1166, 1996.

139. Grubb B, Olshansky B. *Syncope: Mechanisms and Management.* Armonk, NY, Futura Publishing Company, 1998.

Chapter 17

Hypertension in the Elderly

Geza Simon

Hypertension is frequent in the elderly and is a risk factor for cardiovascular disease.[1-5] Recent large clinical trials have clearly established that pharmacological treatment of both systolic/diastolic and isolated systolic hypertension in the elderly reduces cardiovascular morbidity and mortality.[6,7] The present review summarizes the differences that exist in our diagnostic approach and treatment of elderly compared to otherwise healthy middle-aged hypertensive patients. The emphasis is on stroke prevention as the main benefit of antihypertensive therapy, and on the hazards of overzealous treatment of hypertension with complicating vascular diseases, principally, atherosclerosis.

Prevalence and Risk

The prevalence of hypertension is grossly overestimated when measurement of blood pressure is taken on a single occasion. After repeated examinations in one study, the prevalence of diastolic hypertension (>99 mm Hg) in a middle-aged population fell from 15.6% to 5.5%, and that of systolic hypertension in an elderly population from 13.9% to 2.7%.[5] However, the true prevalence of systolic hypertension in this study may have been underestimated by exclusion from follow-up of those subjects who had systolic and diastolic hypertension during initial examination. It has been suggested that to detect sustained hypertension, any estimate of prevalence based on a single set of casual readings be divided by 3. Similarly, clinicians who make treatment decisions based on a single set of readings may treat many patients unnecessarily, especially when these readings are made during intercurrent illness.[5]

From *Clinical Cardiology in the Elderly. Second Edition,* edited by Elliot Chesler. © 1999, Futura Publishing Company, Armonk, NY.

Dividing by the "rule of 3," the prevalence of sustained diastolic hypertension in subjects older than age 60 years ranges from 12% to 14%. The incidence is higher in men and decreases with age.[5] In the Systolic Hypertension in the Elderly Program (SHEP), using repeated blood pressure measurements on 3 separate occasions, the prevalence of sustained isolated systolic hypertension was 6%, 11%, and 18% between 60–69, 70–79, and above 80 years of age, respectively.[8] It is estimated that at age 70 years, the prevalence of diastolic or systolic hypertension, or both, is between 20% and 25%.

Based on the Framingham data and other studies among the elderly, systolic hypertension is more predictive of future cardiovascular morbidity and mortality than diastolic hypertension.[9] The risk of cardiovascular complications (coronary events, stroke, claudication, congestive heart failure) rises sharply with systolic pressure in elderly men, but not as sharply in elderly women. There are similar risk associations between cardiovascular disease and diastolic pressure in elderly men. For older women, the curve relating the incidence of cardiovascular disease to diastolic pressure is relatively flat. The same relationships hold for blood pressure and specific cardiovascular complications, such as stroke and myocardial infarction, as for cardiovascular complications as an aggregate. Left ventricular hypertrophy (LVH), measured by electrocardiography (ECG) or echocardiography, has emerged as an independent cardiovascular risk factor that may interact with blood pressure.[10,11] LVH is more prevalent in the elderly than in younger age groups and is highly correlated with systolic hypertension. In the very old (older than 80 years), some of the abovementioned relationships may no longer hold. Among the noninstitutionalized very old (aged 84–88 years), mortality rate due principally to coronary events was found to be relatively high, not only in subjects with hypertension, but also in subjects with low blood pressure (<70 mm Hg diastolic). The lowest mortality in this study population was found among subjects with systolic blood pressure between 140–169 mm Hg and diastolic blood pressure between 70–99 mm Hg.[12] These findings were confirmed and extended by others. In men aged 75 and older, diastolic blood pressures less than 75 mm Hg were associated with increased cardiovascular mortality.[13] Coronary risk was increased 5–7-fold in untreated hypertensive men, aged 65–84, who experienced a spontaneous fall in diastolic blood pressure over a 5-year period, compared to that of men whose diastolic blood pressure increased or remained stable.[14]

What is the pathophysiological significance and what are the therapeutic implications of the predominant role of systolic pressure as a cardiovascular risk factor in the elderly? Systolic hypertension is the result of reduced aortic distensibility with aging, although stroke volume, peak left ventricular ejection velocity, and timing of the reflected pulse wave from the periphery may also contribute.[15,16] Systolic hypertension is more common in women than in men. The reason for this may be the shorter stature of women than of men, as a result of which the arrival of the reflected pulse wave from the periphery may coincide with peak systolic pressure generated by the left ventricle in the arch of the aorta, resulting in higher pressure. Whether systolic hypertension itself, without evidence of rigid large arteries, is associated with cardiovascular disease is still being debated. One awaits the application of modern techniques for the measurement of distensibility of large arteries to define the pathophysiological alterations that are responsible for the association between systolic hypertension and cardiovascular risk.

Pathophysiology

The hallmark of hypertension in the elderly as in middle-aged patients is increased peripheral vascular resistance. The aim of antihypertensive therapy is to decrease peripheral vascular resistance and thereby ameliorate hypertension. A number of pathophysiological alterations in the elderly, however, make them vulnerable to sudden or excessive lowering of blood pressure. These include the high incidence of atherosclerosis, decreased baroreceptor responsiveness, and impaired autoregulation of blood flow related to age and hypertension.

Atherosclerosis

The incidence of coronary events and stroke increases with age and is even higher when there is hypertension.[9] The incidence of coronary events in the elderly is about twice that in middle-aged individuals, and there is a 2–3-fold increase in coronary events in hypertensive, compared with normotensive elderly patients. Severe internal carotid artery disease (>75% stenosis) was found by Doppler shifted ultrasound in 14% of elderly hypertensive patients without a history of cardiovascular disease (mean age 75 years, range 65–97) and in 23% of elderly hypertensives with a previous stroke (mean age 75 years, range 65–91).[17] In a matched group of asymptomatic normotensive volunteers (mean age 76, range 68–90 years), there was no evidence of severe internal carotid artery disease.

Some degree of atherosclerosis of the renal arteries is detectable in 45% of normotensive and 76% of hypertensive patients older than age 60 years.[18] The incidence of hemodynamically important renal artery stenoses is more difficult to ascertain because of difficulty in determining what is a flow-limiting lesion. The incidence of renovascular hypertension is 15% in white patients older than age 40 years with poorly controlled hypertension or renal insufficiency or history of analgesic abuse.[18] Renovascular hypertension was diagnosed in only 0.65% of black patients referred for evaluation of severe hypertension, abnormal intravenous pyelography, or abdominal bruits.[18] Renal artery atherosclerosis is a progressive disease; in 4 studies, the rate of progression was 9.5% of patients per year (range 4.5–18.0).[19–22] Surprisingly, control of blood pressure did not correlate with progression of renovascular stenosis.

Baroreceptors

All components of baroreceptor reflexes are dampened in the elderly.[23,24] Increased rigidity of large arteries secondary to aging and atherosclerosis appears to be the main reason for this reduced responsiveness. Hypertension aggravates age-related atherosclerosis and causes further dampening of baroreceptor function. Impaired baroreceptor function in the elderly is manifested by increased moment-to-moment fluctuations in blood pressure and decreased heart rate response after lowering or raising blood pressure. Although healthy old people may appear to be well compensated under optimal conditions, the slightest change in hemodynamic status may cause postural changes. This may be a result of volume depletion by diuretics or vasodilation produced by antihypertensive medications. In one study, 6 healthy old subjects (aged 65–80 years) were able to maintain their blood pressure during a 60° upright tilt during basal conditions, but experienced a 24 mm Hg drop in systolic blood pressure during tilt after 2 days of modest sodium depletion and a daily dosage of 100 mg hydrochlorothiazide; 3 of the subjects described postural symptoms.[25] Other common causes of orthostatic hypotension in the elderly are tricyclic antidepressants and underlying malignancy. Occult malignancy may be the cause of unexplained amelioration of hypertension before the onset of weight loss, presumably, due to the release of vasodilator substances.

Another example of impaired regulation of blood pressure in the elderly is postprandial hypotension.[26] In institutionalized elderly patients with a history of syncope, postprandial hypotension persisted for 60 minutes, with a fall in mean systolic pressure of 25 mm Hg at 35 minutes and without a compensatory rise in heart rate.[27] The degree of postprandial hypotension correlated directly with the level of basal blood pressure before the meal, a finding consistent with the clinical observation that hypertension increases the risk for orthostatic hypotension in the elderly. Postprandial hypotension has also been demonstrated in an unselected population of institutionalized elderly patients (aged 78 ± 9 years, mean ± SD), and was severe enough in some to produce symptoms.[28] The presumed cause of postprandial hypotension is impaired baroreceptor compensation after pooling of blood in the splanchnic circulation during digestion. Several gastrointestinal and pancreatic peptides may play a role in splanchnic vasodilatation. Postprandial hypotension can be prevented by ocreotide, an analogue of somatastatin that inhibits release of intestinal vasodilator peptides.[26]

Autoregulation

Regulation of organ blood flow at tissue level is a phenomenon referred to as autoregulation, and this is impaired in the elderly. Autoregulation has been most extensively investigated in the cerebral circulation because this vascular bed is accessible to external radiotracer counting. In normal people, cerebral blood flow remains constant between mean arterial pressures of about 60 to 120 mm Hg. This constancy is maintained by intrinsic myogenic mechanisms and sympathetic nervous control. In patients with moderate or severe hypertension, cerebral blood flow is the same as in normotensives, but the autoregulatory range shifts to higher mean arterial pressures of about 100 to 180 mm Hg.[29,30] This maintains a normal cerebral blood flow despite higher pressures but makes these patients more vulnerable to cerebral ischemia when the pressure falls to a level well tolerated by normotensives (Figure 1). For example, acute lowering of the blood pressure from 160/110 (mean 127) to 140/85 (mean 102) in a hypertensive patient may induce cerebral hypoperfusion, although hypotension in the conventional sense has not occurred. Impaired cerebral autoregulation is the likely explanation for weakness, faintness and postural dizziness experienced by patients during the first few days after initiating antihypertensive therapy.

Impaired cerebral autoregulation may also occur in the elderly without hypertension. In one study, 7 of 11 elderly patients (aged 65–90 years) with orthostatic hypotension showed bilateral or unilateral failure of cerebral autoregulation during tilt testing, but 4 asymptomatic control patients (1 aged 86 years) did not.[31] Fortunately, impairment of cerebral autoregulation is reversible with effective long-term antihypertensive therapy.[30] Although not as well studied, impaired autoregulation may also be present in the myocardium and kidneys of chronically hypertensive patients. This may explain the development of angina without obstructive coronary artery disease, and the transitory deterioration of renal function that may follow rapid and excessive lowering of blood pressure in these patients.

Implications for Antihypertensive Therapy

The combination of severe atherosclerosis, reduced baroreceptor responsiveness, and impaired vascular autoregulation in the elderly may result in serious complications when there is sudden or excessive lowering of blood pressure. The development of stroke shortly after the initiation of diuretic or antihypertensive therapy is well known. Seven such patients were identified among 100 stroke victims by Jansen and colleagues,[32] 6 of whom had furosemide added to their therapeutic regimen within 3 weeks (10 days mean) of stroke; a significant drop in blood pressure was documented in 4. It has been estimated that 4% of strokes in the elderly may be caused by antihypertensive therapy. The administration of oral or sublingual nifedipine to patients with severe hypertension may also precipitate cerebral ischemia, angina, cardiac conduction defects and myocardial infarction.[33–35] To avoid complications associated with the sudden lowering of blood pressure, clinical

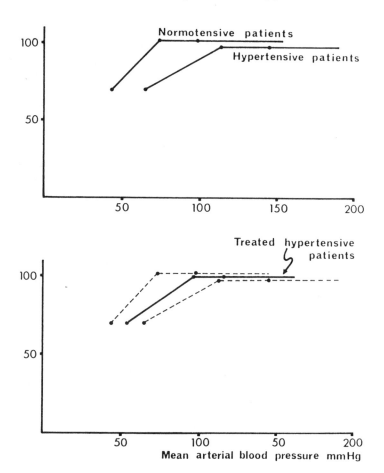

Figure 1: Top panel: *Mean curves of autoregulation of cerebral blood flow (CBF) in normotensive and severely hypertensive human subjects. Each curve is defined by the mean values of resting blood pressure, the lower limit of CBF autoregulation, and the lowest tolerated blood pressure. The curve from the hypertensive patients is shifted to the right on the blood pressure axis.* **Bottom panel:** *Mean curve of CBF autoregulation in patients with a formerly severe hypertension which at the time of the study was effectively controlled by antihypertensive treatment. The curve falls between the two curves above, which are shown by dotted lines. Reproduced with permission from* Circulation 53: 720–727, 1976.

trials or antihypertensive therapy (see below) have been designed to lower blood pressure over several weeks or months.

Excessive long-term lowering of diastolic blood pressure in hypertensive patients with known or unsuspected coronary artery disease may increase the incidence of myocardial infarction and sudden death.[36,37] This paradoxical effect of antihypertensive therapy is known as the J-curve. Among 939 treated hypertensive patients, Cruickshank and colleagues[36] identified 40 deaths from myocardial infarction during a follow-up period of 6.1 years (mean). In patients without prior evidence of coronary artery disease (angina, myocardial infarction, ECG changes, etc.), the incidence of death from myocardial infarction has declined in a linear fashion with lowering of diastolic blood pressure. In contrast, among patients with known ischemic heart disease, lowering of diastolic blood pressure to levels less than 85 mm Hg was associated with an increased incidence of fatal myocardial infarction (Figure 2). Similar observations were made by Alderman and colleagues[39] in their study of 1765 previously untreated hypertensive patients. During 4.2 years (mean) of antihypertensive therapy, the incidence of fatal and nonfatal myocardial infarction was 3–4 times higher in patients who experienced a small (≤6 mm Hg) or a large (≥18 mm Hg) fall in diastolic blood pressure compared with those with a reduction of diastolic blood pressure of 7–17 mm Hg. Patients with high pulse pressure, that is, patients with predominantly systolic hypertension were especially vulnerable to these harmful effects of excessive lowering of diastolic blood pressure.[38] Other data support the view that excessive lowering of blood pressure is paradoxically associated with increased incidence of myocardial infarction and total mortality.[39] The "J-curve" may be one of the reasons why antihypertensive therapy has been generally less effective in preventing coronary events than strokes (see below). It should be noted, however, that in the absence of prospective data, there are still influential voices who question the evidence of the J-curve and continue to advocate aggressive treatment of hypertension.[40]

Among the elderly, excessive lowering of blood pressure with antihypertensive therapy may be also harmful in the secondary prevention of strokes.[41] Hypertensive patients who have suffered a stroke during a 3-month period prior to the study were followed for an average of 38 months. It was found that while moderate reduction of diastolic blood pressure with antihypertensive therapy resulted in reduced recurrence of stroke compared to uncontrolled hypertension, reduction of diastolic blood pressure to less than 80 mm Hg was associated with paradoxical rise in the occurrence of embolic, thrombotic, and lacunar infarcts (J-curve). In contrast, the recurrence rate of hemorrhagic strokes showed a proportional decrease with reduction of diastolic blood pressure. This "J-curve" effect manifests itself during the first year or two of antihypertensive therapy.[42] Thereafter, there is a proportional reduction in blood pressure and complication rate.

There are other pathophysiological alterations in the elderly, but their clinical significance is either minor or unknown.[3] β-adrenergic

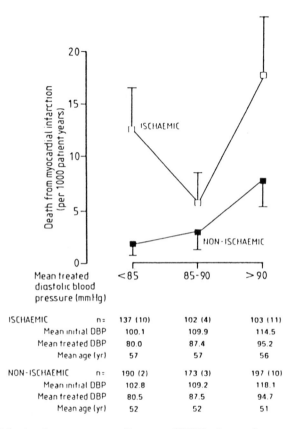

Figure 2: *Relation between mortality rate (SEM) shown from myocardial infarction in ischemic and non-ischemic patients and treated diastolic blood pressure (age-adjusted). Number of deaths given in parentheses. Reproduced with permission from* The Lancet *I:581–584, 1987.*

responsiveness declines with age.[43] In the myocardium, this may contribute to impaired baroreceptor mediated responses of heart rate and cardiac output. Peripherally, impaired β-adrenergic vasodilatation may partially account for elevated vascular resistance. Longitudinal studies indicate that there is a reduction in glomerular filtration rate and creatinine clearance with age, even without renal or vascular disease.[44] The role of hypertension *per se,* without other complications, in this process is controversial. Changes in glomerular filtration rate delay but do not impair the excretion of sodium load in the elderly.[45] The observation that age increases the antihypertensive response to diuretics (but not to nondiuretics) suggests that there may be a subtle, long-term impairment of sodium balance.[46] However, the existence of age-related responsiveness to diuretics has been disputed by some on methodological grounds.[47,48] Finally, the reduction of plasma renin activity with age may be the combined effect of reduced β-adrenergic responsiveness and declining renal function.[3]

Benefits of Treatment

Until recently, intervention trials in hypertension have been confined to patients younger than age 70 years. The small number of elderly patients in these trials has precluded meaningful analysis of results, although the trends were the same as in younger participants.[3] For the subgroup of treated patients aged 60 to 69 years, the Veterans Administration Cooperative Study found a 32% reduction in total cardiovascular morbidity.[49] This was a result of fewer strokes and episodes of congestive heart failure, but the incidence of myocardial infarction was unchanged. However, the number of morbid events was small, and the differences between the treated and untreated groups were not statistically significant.

The results of 6 major intervention trials confined to elderly hypertensives are composed of 4 trials in patients with systolic and diastolic hypertension, and 2 that included patients with isolated systolic hypertension.[7,50–55] The European Working Party on Hypertension in the Elderly was a double-blind, placebo-controlled trial of antihypertensive therapy in patients older than age 60 years (range 60–97).[50] The entry criteria included a sitting diastolic blood pressure in the range of 90–119 mm Hg and a systolic pressure in the range of 160–239 mm Hg. A total of 840 patients was randomly allocated to receive hydrochlorothiazide and triamterene or matching placebo. Methyldopa or matching placebo was added if the blood pressure remained elevated. After an 8-year follow-up, there was a statistically significant reduction in cardiovascular mortality ($-38\%, P = 0.023$), because of a reduction in cardiac deaths ($-47\%, P = 0.48$) and cerebrovascular deaths ($-43\%, P = 0.15$). Nonfatal cerebrovascular events were reduced by 52% ($P = 0.026$), but nonfatal cardiac events were not ($+3\%$). Overall, the treatment resulted in 29 fewer cardiovascular events, mainly strokes, and 14 fewer cardiovascular deaths, mainly coronary events, per 1000 patient-years of treatment. These beneficial effects of treatment on cardiovascular mortality and morbidity were limited to participants younger than age 80 years at entry. Firm conclusions could not be drawn about treatment benefits in the very old because of the relatively small number of participants in this age group and the high rate of noncardiovascular complications in patients older than 80 years.

Coope and Warrender[51] reported a single-blind, randomized trial among elderly hypertensives, aged 60–79 years, in 13 general practices in England and Wales that compared drug treatment (atenolol and bendrofluazide) with observation alone; 884 patients with systolic blood pressure higher than 170 mm Hg or diastolic blood pressure higher than 105 mm Hg were observed for 8 years. In actively treated patients, the rate of combined nonfatal and fatal stroke was reduced by 42% ($P < 0.03$), compared with the observation group. Active treatment did not significantly alter mortality and morbidity as a result of coronary events ($+3\%$).

Two recently published trials provide convincing evidence for the beneficial effects of antihypertensive therapy in patients age 65–80 years. The Swedish Trial in Old Patients with Hypertension examined treatment of diastolic hypertension in the "old elderly" (aged 75.7 years, mean, range: 70–84); 1627 patients were randomly assigned to active treatment with a thiazide diuretic or a β-inhibitor or both, or to placebo treatment.[52] After 25 months (mean) follow-up, in the actively treated group, blood pressure was reduced by 20/8 mm Hg (mean), the incidence of stroke by 47%, and total mortality by 43%. The reduction in incidence of myocardial infarction (-13%) was not statistically significant. This was the first intervention trial in elderly hypertensives that showed a significant reduction in total mortality. Like previous trials, however, the trial lacked sufficient statistical power to prove benefit of treatment in patients older than age 80 years.

The Medical Research Council conducted a randomized placebo-controlled trial comparing the efficacy of antihypertensive therapy with diuretics (hydrochlorothiazide and amiloride) or a β-inhibitor (atenolol) in the prevention of stroke and coronary heart disease in a general practice setting.[53] Compared with placebo, actively treated subjects had a 25% reduction in stroke and a 19% reduction in coronary events. Unexpectedly, these beneficial effects were almost exclusively a result of treatment with diuretics. In the β-inhibitor group, reduction in morbid events was minor and statistically insignificant despite a comparable antihypertensive effect. A subgroup with isolated systolic hypertension (>160 mm Hg) experienced the same benefits as subjects with both systolic and diastolic hypertension. The conclusion drawn from this trial should be interpreted with caution because it was single-blinded, with a high rate of drop-out.

In the Systolic Hypertension in the Elderly Program, 447,921 persons older than age 60 years were screened. Of these, 4736 persons with systolic blood pressure in the range 160–219 mm Hg and diastolic pressure less than 90 mm Hg, were randomly assigned to active treatment or placebo.[54] Active treatment consisted of chlorthalidone, 12.5 or 25 mg per day for step 1, and atenolol 25 or 50 mg per day for step 2. Average follow-up was 4–5 years. The 5-year average systolic and diastolic blood pressure was 155 and 72 mm Hg for placebo and 143 and 68 mm Hg for active treatment. In the treated group, the incidence of fatal and nonfatal stroke was reduced by 36%. In terms of absolute numbers, this represents a reduction of 6 cases per 1000 patient-years, which is about 5 times less than the reduction in incidence of stroke experienced by treated patients with diastolic hypertension. The reduction in fatal and nonfatal coronary events (-26%) did not reach statistical significance. The results of the trial were confounded by a number of findings. Prevention of stroke by active treatment was more effective (48% reduction) in patients receiving antihypertensive therapy at initial contact than in previously untreated patients (27% reduction). It is possible that coexistent diastolic hypertension in previously treated patients did not become apparent during the 2–8 week washout period. This suspicion is confirmed by the finding that at year 5, 44% of placebo-treated patients were receiving active therapy "mostly due to DBP." Treatment of these patients also explains why the diastolic blood pressure of patients in the treatment and control groups was virtually the same (see above). Some of the benefits of treating isolated systolic hypertension may have been due to the prevention of diastolic hypertension.

The Systolic Hypertension in Europe trial was stopped in 1997 after the second interim analysis because the primary end point of stroke prevention had been reached.[7] The trial comprised 4695 patients, 67% women. During an initial run-in placebo-treatment period, their systolic blood pressure, obtained at 3 visits, 1 month apart, ranged between 160–215 mm Hg with diastolic blood pressure lower than 95 mm Hg. The age of participants was 70.2 years (mean). Eligible patients were randomly assigned to treatment with active medication or placebo. The goal of therapy was to reduce systolic blood pressure by at least 20 mm Hg to less than 150. Active treatment was started with nitrendipine 10–20 mg bid and, if necessary, was supplemented or replaced by enalapril 5–20 mg, or hydrochlorothiazide 12.5–25 mg, daily or both. At a median of 2 years follow-up, sitting systolic and diastolic blood pressure had fallen by 13 and 2 mm Hg in the placebo group and by 23 and 7 mm Hg in the active treatment group. Seventy-seven patients on placebo and 47 patients on active treatment had strokes, about 30% fatal in each group. The cumulative rate of strokes were 13.7 and 7.9 per 1000 patient-years, respectively ($P = 0.003$). These results are similar to the ones obtained in the Systolic Hypertension in the Elderly Program (see above). The reduction in the incidence of fatal and nonfatal myocardial infarction by active treatment did not reach statistical significance ($-30\%, P = 0.12$). In the active treatment group, all fatal and nonfatal cardiac end points declined by 26% ($P = 0.03$) due mainly to the reduction in the onset of heart failure, which is not surprising considering that treatment included the use of diuretics and enalapril. It is likely that such treatment would prevent heart failure also in a normotensive cohort of elderly patients.

Meta-analyses of intervention trials in elderly hypertensives show a 36% and 34% reduction in fatal and nonfatal cerebrovascular events respectively, 26% reduction in coronary mortality, but only an insignificant 5% reduction in non-fatal coronary events.[6,55,56] Patients older than 80 years also seem to benefit from antihypertensive therapy.

Evaluation

Diagnosis

The diagnosis and decision to treat hypertension should not be made without at least 3 separate measurements. The routine use of a large cuff is justified because overestimation of blood pressure may occur with an inappropriately small cuff; underestimation of blood pressure with a large cuff is not a problem. Elderly hypertensive patients should have their blood pressure (and heart rate) measured both in the sitting and standing position. The presence of a significant orthostatic drop in pressure before treatment will influence not only the decision to treat but also the choice of antihypertensive medications.

Blood pressures obtained by self-measurements at home are helpful in ruling out hypertension that is predominantly present in the physician's office—so-called "white coat" hypertension.[57] Although "white coat" hypertension is typically found in younger age groups, it is also common in the elderly. It appears to be a conditioned reflex to examination by a physician. Systolic blood pressure is much more likely to be acutely elevated in the clinic setting than diastolic blood pressure.[58] The prevalence of white coat hypertension decreases with increased severity of hypertension (33%, 11%, 3%, and 0% in stage I, II, III, and IV hypertension, respectively).[59] When there is a striking discrepancy between clinic and local or home blood pressures, especially in a patient without target organ damage, 24-hour ambulatory monitoring of blood pressure is indicated. Suggested upper limits for average awake ambulatory blood pressure is 135 mm Hg systolic and 85 diastolic.[60] Additional clinical situations in which ambulatory blood pressure monitoring may be helpful include cases of apparent drug resistance, hypotensive symptoms on antihypertensive medications and episodic hypertension. Occasionally, "fluctuating" blood pressures are a result of discordant readings in the 2 arms, when there is subclavian artery stenosis as a result of atherosclerosis. Measurement of blood pressure in both arms will solve the diagnostic puzzle to the gratification of both patient and examiner.

"Pseudohypertension" is another diagnostic pitfall in evaluation of the elderly.[61,62] It is an overestimation of blood pressure by the indirect cuff method compared with intra-arterial pressure measurement. This occurs when an atherosclerotic brachial artery is not compressed by the inflated cuff. Pseudohypertension should be suspected when hypertension is disproportionate to target organ damage, when patients suffer inordinate postural symptoms despite cautious therapy, and when the brachial and radial arteries feel rigid.

A simple procedure, called the "Osler maneuver" has been used for diagnosis.[62] This is performed by palpating the pulseless radial or brachial artery after inflating the arm cuff above systolic pressure. A normal artery collapses and becomes impalpable under these circumstances. A palpable artery is a positive test. However, in a recent large prospective study of elderly patients, the findings on Osler maneuver were poorly reproducible, making the procedure an inadequate test.[63] If there is strong suspicion of pseudohypertension, the clinician may have to resort to intra-arterial blood pressure measurements to establish the diagnosis. Alternatively, antihypertensive therapy should be reduced.

The prevalence of pseudohypertension in the elderly is controversial. In the original report of Spence et al,[61] 50% of patients suspected of having pseudohypertension because of the absence of target organ damage had false elevation of blood pressure by 30 mm Hg or more by cuff method. In a later report, Spence and coworkers[64] compared intra-arterial (radial) and cuff blood pressure measurements in 55 unselected healthy volunteers, aged 59–80 years (mean 69) and found only 3 subjects (5.4%) with false elevation of systolic blood pressure.[64] The subjects in the study, however, were normotensive.

History

The clinician should assess (1) a history of vascular complications resulting from hypertension itself or atherosclerosis, (2) renal disease that may be the cause of hypertension, and (3) complicating diseases that may influence the choice of antihypertensive medications.

A history of previous cerebrovascular accidents or ischemic heart disease should caution the clinician not to overtreat hypertension. A history of intermittent claudication is a clue that other major arteries may be affected by atherosclerosis. In an elderly hypertensive population, claudication was associated with increased incidence of abdominal aortic aneurysm. Hypertension accompanied by renal insufficiency is usually secondary to either renovascular or renal parenchymal disease. Diabetes mellitus, chronic obstructive lung disease, and gout may be contraindications to specific antihypertensive medications.

Physical Examination

Like the history, physical examination should focus on the cardiovascular system. All readily accessible major arteries including the aorta should be palpated and auscultated. While aortic aneurysm may be primarily a genetic disease, hypertension plays a role in its progression.[65] Among patients with abdominal girth less than 100 cm (40 inches), abdominal aortic aneurysm greater than 3.5 cm is detectable by palpation in almost all cases.[66] In obese patients (abdominal girth greater than 100 cm), abdominal aortic aneurysms are detected by palpation in only about 15% of cases. Cardiomegaly found on physical examination is a strong indication for treatment no matter how mild the hypertension. Finally, the best clue to "silent" cerebrovascular accidents may be the finding of asymmetric deep tendon reflexes.

Laboratory Tests

Recommendations for the initial laboratory evaluation and diagnostic workup of elderly hypertensives are not different from those recommended for hypertensives in general by the National Committee on Detection, Evaluation, and Treatment of High Blood Pressure.[67] A few simple tests should be performed before initiating therapy. Of these, urinalysis and serum creatinine measurements are useful in detecting renal parenchymal and renovascular disease. Hypokalemia (<3.5 mmol/L before therapy) may point to hyperaldosteronism, either primary (adrenal adenoma or hyperplasia) or secondary to hyper-reninemic renovascular disease. Measurements of fasting blood glucose and serum uric acid are helpful guides in the choice of pharmacologic therapy. (In an occasional patient, the correction of severe hyperglycemia is sufficient to control the hypertension.)

LVH by electrocardiographic voltage criteria is an independent cardiovascular risk factor and is considered by some to be an indication for aggressive treatment of hypertension.[10] Measurement of left ventricular (LV) mass by two-dimensional echocardiography is more sensitive and may soon become part of the initial evaluation.[11,68] It should be noted, however, that measurement of LV mass by echocardiography is unsuccessful in 20% of patients.[68] There are also preliminary indications that reduction of LV mass during treatment of hypertension is associated with a more favorable prognosis than persistence or progression of LVH. Converting enzyme inhibitors have been shown to be the most effective drugs for decreasing LV mass in essential hypertension.[69] More extensive workup to rule out renovascular hypertension and pheochromocytoma, which may be correctable surgically is indicated only in cases of severe, refractory hypertension or progressive renal insufficiency (see below under *Renovascular Hypertension*).

Treatment

Nonpharmacological Remedies

In treating cases of mild or moderate hypertension, nonpharmacological interventions have been recommended as the initial approach.[70] Unfortunately, studies of their efficacy have been conducted for the most part in young or middle-aged persons. Of these, only 2 are both practical and beneficial in elderly patients to merit general use, namely, weight reduction in the obese (>150% ideal weight), and cessation or reduction of alcohol consumption for patients who consume more than 2 ounces of ethanol daily (2 drinks of hard liquor or 4 cans of beer). A significant fall of blood pressure may occur with only modest weight reduction. In a study of 301 normotensive and hypertensive, predominantly female patients, with a mean percentage ideal body weight of 164 ± 28% (mean ± SD), a 3–4 kg weight loss during the initial 4–5 weeks of treatment was associated with a 7 mm Hg drop in diastolic blood pressure.[71] In this study, treated hypertensive patients experienced an even larger reduction in diastolic blood pressure (– 10 mm

Hg), but there was no reduction in patients who failed to lose weight. Sodium restriction is not a requirement for reduction of blood pressure by weight loss. In 28 hypertensive men and women aged 60 to 85 years with body weight over 115% of ideal, a 2.1-kg weight loss over 6 months was associated with 6.8 mm Hg diastolic reduction, compared to 1.9 mm Hg reduction in a parallel control group.[72]

Imbibing more than 2 ounces of ethanol per day may be the most common cause of reversible or secondary hypertension in men. Several clinical and epidemiological studies have shown an association between alcohol consumption and hypertension.[70] Amelioration of treated or untreated hypertension after cessation or reduction of alcohol consumption is a common clinical experience but there are few well-controlled clinical studies to document this. Saunders and colleagues[73] followed heavy drinkers (average daily intake of 8.4 ± 3.8, mean ± SD, ounces of ethanol) for 1 year after their hospitalization for detoxification and alcohol-related illnesses. At the time of hospitalization, 51.5% of 132 patients had hypertension. In most patients blood pressure fell to normal after detoxification and only 9% remained hypertensive. Those who remained abstinent stayed normotensive but most of those who reverted to heavy drinking became hypertensive again. Parker and colleagues[74] studied moderate drinkers (6–7 standard drinks per day) who after an initial familiarization period were randomly assigned either to drink a low-alcohol beer alone for 4 weeks or to continue their usual alcohol intake.[74] In those who reduced alcohol intake, there was a fall in supine systolic (−5.4 mm Hg, mean) and diastolic blood pressure (−3.2 mm Hg). Salt restriction did not have an additive effect with reduction of alcohol intake. Small doses of clonidine at bedtime may ease the symptoms of alcohol withdrawal in hypertensive patients.

Pharmacological Agents

Antihypertensive medications are as effective in the elderly as in younger patients.[47,48] There is no ideal medication for the elderly. The choice depends on concomitant diseases and special benefits of each category of agents (Table 1). The emphasis is on once daily treatment to improve compliance, and minidosing to minimize side effects. Because of the greater sensitivity of the elderly to lowering blood pressure, initial doses of medications should be less than in younger individuals (Table 2). While the principal antihypertensive effect of medications is seen within days, a small additional fall in blood pressure may occur during a 3–4 week period that may be sufficient to normalize the blood pressure, thereby sparing the patient from additional medications and overtreatment. In the majority of cases, doubling the recommended initial dose of a given medication has only a modest additional antihypertensive effect. In cases of no or inadequate response, it is generally more efficacious to try a different category of agents or add a second drug. A small dose of thiazide diuretic is recommended in cases of poor

Table 1
Special Benefits and Major Side Effects of Antihypertensive Medications

Category	Benefit	Side Effect
Thiazide diuretics	Prevention of osteoporosis (?) Treatment of hypercalciuric nephrolithiasis	Hypokalemia Hyponatremia Impaired glucose tolerance Hyperuricemia, gout Impotence
β-inhibitors	2° prevention of MI and sudden death Antianginal properties	Reduced exercise tolerance Exacerbation of asthma, COPD Exacerbation of claudication (?) Depression Impotence Masking of hypoglycemia due to insulin
Converting enzyme inhibitors	Cardioprotection, post-MI Treatment of CHF Slowing progression of renal parenchymal disease (?)	Cough Angioedema Hypoglycemia
Ca channel blockers	Antianginal properties Antiatherogenesis	AV block (with β-inhibitor) Edema (dihydropyridines) Constipation (verapamil) Hypotension (dihydropyridines)
α_1-antagonists	Relief of benign prostatic hypertrophy	Hypotension (1st-dose effect) Orthostatic hypotension

(?) Indicates inconclusive evidence
MI, myocardial infarction; CHF, congestive heart failure.

response to nondiuretics because "piling up" of nondiuretic antihypertensives under these circumstances is usually of limited benefit, prone to side effects, and costly. Concern about undesirable side effects of diuretics should not be exaggerated, considering that all the available therapeutic trials in the elderly that showed a reduction in stroke used diuretics. In one trial, treatment with diuretics reduced the incidence of stroke and coronary events, but β-inhibitor treatment in a parallel group of subjects had no beneficial effect despite comparable lowering of blood pressure.[53]

The algorithm (Table 2) for the pharmacological treatment of hypertension in the elderly reflects stated principles, some personal preferences, and cost considerations at our institution; it changes almost yearly as new categories of agents and cheaper, generic versions of older medications become available. Concerning cost, there is a 33-fold difference in cost at our institution between the traditional triple therapy (hydrochlorothiazide, reserpine, hydralazine) and a regimen com-

Table 2
Pharmacological Treatment of Hypertension in the Elderly*

	A	B	C
Step 1	Lisinopril, 5–10 mg daily ↓ 4 weeks	Betaxolol, 10–20 mg daily ↓ 4 weeks	Felodipine, 5–10 mg daily ↓ 4 weeks
Step 2	HCTZ, 12.5–25 mg daily ↓ 4 weeks	HCTZ, 12.5–25 mg daily ↓ 4 weeks	HCTZ, 12.5–25 mg daily ↓ 4 weeks
Step 3	Clonidine, 0.2 mg hs or Doxazosin, 2 mg daily	Hydralazine, 25–50 mg bid or Minoxidil, 5–10 mg daily or Doxazosin, 2 mg daily	Clonidine, 0.2 mg hs or Guanfacine, 1 mg daily

* Assume normal renal function (serum creatinine < 1.5 mg/dL).
A, B, and C represent three approaches to stepped-care. The choice of step 1 medication depends on individual patient considerations (see text).

posed of the more recently marketed antihypertensive agents (hydrochlorothiazide/triamterene, losartan, and amlodipine) for the treatment of severe hypertension. In a patient with hypertension and serum creatinine more than 1.5 mg/dL, a thiazide and loop diuretic is the combination of choice (hydrochlorothiazide 25–50 mg daily and furosemide 10–20 mg b.i.d. or bumetanide 0.5 mg daily), but volume depletion and hypokalemia must be guarded against.

Isolated Systolic Hypertension

Is there a drug of choice for the treatment of isolated systolic hypertension? Theoretically, there are two main approaches: one is to increase large artery compliance with vasodilators and the other is to reduce stroke volume with venodilators or diuretics. To date, the latter approach seems to be more effective than the former. In the Systolic Hypertension in the Elderly Program a diuretic was used with good results.[54] There is also evidence that transdermal or oral nitrates, lower elevated systolic blood pressure without altering diastolic blood pressure.[75,76] In hypertensive patients, the usefulness of nitrates is limited by frequent headache.[75] Among arterial vasodilators, converting enzyme inhibitors have been the most effective in increasing large artery compliance and reducing systolic and diastolic blood pressure proportionately.[77] Aggressive treatment of isolated systolic hypertension poses the danger that diastolic hypotension may lead to hypoperfusion of vital organs in elderly patients with vascular disease (see J-curve effect above).

Special Benefits

There are special ("fringe") benefits of each category of antihypertensive agents that make them the drug of choice in individual patients (Table 1). *Thiazide diuretics* reduce urinary calcium excretion and may, therefore, be considered as therapy to prevent bone fractures secondary to osteoporosis, especially, in elderly women, although randomized prospective clinical trials have not addressed this issue.[78] *β-adrenoceptor antagonists* (β-inhibitors), irrespective of selectivity, are helpful in secondary prevention of myocardial infarction and sudden death.[79,80] In subcategories of hypertensive patients, β-inhibitors may also have a primary cardioprotective effect.[80] Other antihypertensive agents have not been found to be effective in the secondary prevention of cardiovascular morbidity and mortality. β-inhibitors should be part of the antihypertensive regimen of elderly patients with previous ischemic symptoms, signs, or complications, unless there are specific contraindications to their use. *Converting enzyme inhibitors* have been shown experimentally to slow the progression of renal disease, and cardiac dilatation (remodeling) that follows myocardial infarction.[81-83] The extension of these findings to the clinical arena awaits future investigation, but preliminary results are encouraging.[84-86] Administration of long-term converting enzyme inhibitor therapy within days or hours after transmural myocardial infarction attenuates left ventricular dilatation and this may have a long-term beneficial effect on cardiac function.[85,86] After long-term use, converting enzyme inhibitors may also reverse LVH (see above). By all indications, the antihypertensive efficacy and benefits of the recently marketed angiotensin II-receptor antagonists, such as losartan, are comparable to those of converting enzyme inhibitors. *Calcium channel blockers* delay development and limit the extent of atherogenesis in cholesterol-fed animals.[87] The clinical applicability of these beneficial effects of calcium channel blockers is limited. Primary prevention studies are logistically difficult, and secondary prevention trials have been largely negative.[88] Finally, *α₁-receptor antagonists* in large doses relieve the obstructive and irritating symptoms of benign prostatic hypertrophy through their action on the *α₁-receptors* of prostatic smooth muscle.[89]

Side Effects

Among the side effects of antihypertensive medications (Table 1), some are well known and others merit special mention. Among elderly women, thiazide diuretics may cause acute or more insidious development of symptomatic, sometimes life-threatening hyponatremia.[90] Clinicians should be alert to weakness, malaise, and confusion occurring within days after initiation of diuretic therapy. Fortunately, this complication is rare. In an occasional patient with renal insufficiency, the need to control hypertension with diuretics may supersede the risk of attacks of gout. In such a case, diuretics may be administered with allopurinol. β-Inhibitors may aggravate dyspnea in patients with chronic obstructive lung disease without detectable bronchospasm. During long-term follow-up, requirement for antidepressant therapy was greater among patients receiving propranolol than among patients treated with other antihypertensives.[91] This side effect seems to be unique to propranolol, not to β-inhibitors in general, and is encountered mainly in young adults. Insulin therapy is not an absolute contraindication to β-inhibitor therapy provided that the patient is able to recognize symptoms and signs of hypoglycemia. Cough is a side effect (15%) common to all converting enzyme inhibitors and appears to be a result of hypersensitization of the cough reflex.[92] Angioedema, swelling of the mucous membranes of the oropharynx and respiratory tract, is a rare (0.1%) complication of converting enzyme inhibitors, but may lead to respiratory failure and death.[92] There are case reports of symptomatic hypoglycemia after starting converting enzyme inhibitor therapy among diabetic patients treated with insulin or oral hypoglycemic agents that appear to be due to increased insulin sensitivity.[93] In some patients, increased insulin sensitivity during converting enzyme inhibitor therapy may prove to be a special benefit as well as a side effect considering the frequent association of hypertension and insulin resistance. The more costly angiotensin II-receptor antagonists, such as losartan, can be given to patients who have side effects with the use of converting enzyme inhibitors but whose hypertension cannot be controlled without their use. Verapamil or diltiazem in combination with a β-inhibitor is associated with a significant incidence of symptomatic sinus bradycardia and atrioventricular conduction block in patients with underlying coronary artery disease. There has been concern about the possibility of a detrimental effect of the short- and intermediate-acting dihydropyridine-type calcium channel blockers on long-term morbidity and mortality from cardiovascular complications, especially, in patients with previous history of coronary artery disease.[94,95] The underlying mechanism seems to be rapid and excessive drop in blood pressure triggering reflex tachycardia. The jury is still out regarding the safety of the slow- and long-acting dihydropyridines such as amlodipine. In our experience, symptomatic hypotension is a common side effect of both short- and long-acting dihydropyridines in patients 70 years old or older. Another manifestation of the powerful vasodilatory action of dihydropyridines is edema, particularly of the ankles, which may suggest congestive heart failure. With the availability of alternative therapeutic regimens, and in light of the proven benefit of low-dose thiazide diuretics and β-inhibitors in the prevention of cardiovascular complications, it is prudent to avoid the use of dihydropyridines as first or second line agents in the treatment of elderly hypertensives. In contrast, the non-dihydropyridine calcium channel blockers have been shown to be safe in the treatment of hypertensive patients. Finally, α_1-antagonists may cause hypotension either acutely or during long-term use, and should, therefore, be used with caution.

Nonsteroidal Anti-inflammatory Drugs

Nonsteroidal anti-inflammatory drugs (NSAIDs) relieve pain in the elderly, but to the gerontologist, they are a source of headache. Besides their well-known toxic effects on the gastric mucosa and the kidney, most NSAIDs produce mild elevation of normal blood pressure and may partially or completely antagonize the effects of several antihypertensive medications.[96,97] The effect on blood pressure may vary from none to severe elevation. The risk of these interactions increases with age. NSAIDs have been shown to antagonize the antihypertensive effects of thiazide and loop diuretics, β-inhibitors, α-antagonists, and converting enzyme inhibitors. These medications exert their antihypertensive effects in part by promoting natriuresis via prostaglandin-mediated renal mechanisms that NSAIDs antagonize. Interactions have not been reported between NSAIDs and the centrally acting α-agonists (clonidine, methyldopa) or the calcium channel blockers whose principal antihypertensive action is extrarenal. Claims have been made that sulindac and aspirin do not reverse the effects of antihypertensive drugs to the same extent as the other NSAIDs. In the case of sulindac, these claims have been challenged. In large doses, aspirin also attenuates the sodium excretion produced by diuretics. NSAIDs may also interfere with local production of vasodilator prostaglandins elsewhere in the body and with platelet function producing tissue ischemia and microvascular thrombosis. These mechanisms may play a role in the exacerbation of colitis, reported with use of NSAIDs. Theoretically, NSAIDs may also exacerbate angina and peripheral vascular disease, although this has not been documented.

Hypertensive Emergency and Urgency

The diagnosis of hypertensive emergency in the elderly should be made with caution because it mandates intravenous antihypertensive therapy with all the potential dangers inherent in rapid lowering of blood pressure. *Hypertensive emergency* is defined as the absolute need for lowering of blood pressure within 60 minutes to prevent seizure, coma, or death from encephalopathy or cerebral hemorrhage.[98] Diagnosis of hypertensive emergency is made clinically. It is manifested by extreme elevations of diastolic blood pressure, usually exceeding 140 mm Hg, with mental changes that include confusion, somnolence or stupor and neurologic findings such as visual loss or focal deficits, and papilledema. True hypertensive emergency is rare. Much more common is *hypertensive urgency,* when the blood pressure is high (>120 mm Hg diastolic), but the patient is either asymptomatic or has only minor complaints, such as dizziness and a sensation of occipital pressure.[99] Under these circumstances blood pressure should be lowered gradually over several days.

In a true hypertensive emergency, the therapist should retain full control of the rate and extent of lowering of the blood pressure. This can be accomplished only with short-acting intravenous medications such as sodium nitroprusside and nitrates. Optimally, intra-arterial blood pressure should be monitored in an intensive care unit. The goal of therapy is to lower the diastolic blood pressure to about 110 mm Hg during the first few hours. This is usually sufficient to forestall the dreaded complications of hypertensive crisis. If the patient's condition allows, oral medications should be started simultaneously with intravenous therapy so that parenteral medications may be stopped after 1 to 2 hours. Various combinations of oral medications can be used in this setting and in cases of hypertensive urgencies. The simplest is traditional triple therapy for severe hypertension consisting of hydrochlorothiazide 25 mg daily, propranolol 40 mg b.i.d. and hydralazine 25–50 mg b.i.d. Administration of β-inhibitors may help to attenuate the rebound hypertension that follows the discontinuation of sodium nitroprusside.[100] When there is renal insufficiency, furosemide 20–40 mg may have to be added. Recurrence of mental and neurological changes after initial improvement is usually due to rapid lowering of blood pressure and failure of cerebral autoregulation rather than persistent encephalopathy.[101] Reducing antihypertensive therapy may be the treatment of choice.

Preoperative Hypertension

Anesthesia with thiopentone, nitrous oxide, and halothane is accompanied by a severe drop in blood pressure.[102] In normotensive patients, the drop in mean arterial pressure (MAP) may amount to 20–25 mm Hg. The fall of MAP during anesthesia is exaggerated in untreated and treated hypertensive patients, and in patients with moderate to severe hypertension it may drop to 60–70 mm Hg. Such a drastic fall may cause myocardial ischemia, detected by electrocardiographic monitoring, in patients with coronary artery disease. In the elderly, moderate-to-severe hypertension (diastolic blood pressure >110 mm Hg) should be considered a contraindication to elective surgery. Treatment with β-inhibitors attenuates the fluctuation of blood pressure that accompanies intubation and induction of general anesthesia, and this reduces the frequency of cardiac arrhythmias and myocardial ischemia.[103]

One should not attempt to control hypertension a few days or a few hours before surgery because such rapid intervention may produce hypovolemia, especially, when diuretics are used, and result in unstable blood pressure during anesthesia and surgery.[104] In an otherwise healthy patient, it is probably safer to proceed with surgery despite the presence of mild or moderate hypertension (diastolic blood pressure <110 mm Hg) than to lower the blood pressure acutely. By the same reasoning, antihypertensive therapy already in use should not be discontinued before surgery for it may result in rebound hypertension. A short infusion of potassium will raise plasma potassium levels, but may do little to correct chronic potassium depletion in the tissues.[104] More prolonged replacement through several days or weeks before surgery should be administered when there is hypokalemia. Antihypertensive therapy with β-inhibitors and clonidine should be resumed as soon as possible after surgery. If necessary, this should be given intravenously or by nasogastric tube to avoid rebound cardiac excitability or hypertension. Failure to reinstitute β-inhibitors promptly may be one of the causes of myocardial infarction after operation.

Renovascular Hypertension

Because of its importance as a cause of morbidity and mortality in elderly hypertensives, atherosclerotic renovascular hypertension merits special emphasis.[105,106] According to some estimates, renovascular hypertension is responsible for 10%–15% of patients receiving long-term hemodialysis.[21] End-stage renal disease secondary to atherosclerosis is an eminently preventable complication. The key is early diagnosis so that the patient may be treated by angioplasty or surgery while still a reasonable surgical candidate. In the past, emphasis has been on treatment of hypertension itself. Today, emphasis should be on the preservation of renal function. With availability of converting enzyme inhibitors, angiotensin II-receptor antagonists and other powerful antihypertensive medications, control of hypertension is seldom a problem, but this may lull the clinician into complacency, while the underlying disease progresses. It has been noted that the control of hypertension does not have a major impact on the progression of renovascular atherosclerosis.[19-21] By the time symptoms result from renal insufficiency, other atherosclerotic complications may have increased the risk of surgery to unacceptable levels.

Diagnosis

The possibility of renovascular hypertension should be entertained in every elderly patient with hypertension and unexplained renal insufficiency particularly when associated with atherosclerosis (arterial bruits, claudication, transient ischemic attack), or hypertension refractory to pharmacological therapy (Table 3). Screening for renovascular hypertension has been greatly facilitated by captopril renography.[107-109] Of the antihypertensive drugs, only converting enzyme inhibitors have to be stopped 6–7 days before the test. The test takes advantage of the observation that the kidney downstream to a hemody-

Table 3
Indications for Screening for Renovascular Hypertension

1. Hypertension complicated by unexplained renal insufficiency (serum creatinine > 1.5 mg/dL).
2. Moderate to severe hypertension complicated by atherosclerosis (arterial bruits, claudication, TIA).
3. Hypertension refractory to pharmacological therapy (including a diuretic).

namically significant renal artery stenosis (>90%) relies on angiotensin II-mediated glomerular efferent arteriolar constriction to maintain glomerular filtration rate (GFR). Acute administration of captopril drops glomerular filtration pressure and rate by releasing efferent arteriolar constriction.

The sensitivity and specificity of captopril renography is improved by renal imaging on the same day both before and after the administration of 25 mg of captopril orally (Figure 3).[107-109] In this manner, precaptopril and postcaptopril images can be compared during the same physiological conditions. A positive test after administration of captopril is worsening of an abnormality (delay in time to peak activity), or appearance of a new abnormality. If the anatomically identified renal artery stenosis is accompanied by captopril-induced changes on renographic images, then prognosis for reversal or amelioration of hypertension and improvement of renal function after successful intervention, be it angioplasty or surgery is good. What is more important, a hemodynamically significant lesion indicates a high-grade stenosis carrying the threat of imminent complete occlusion, not always reliably identified by radiologic techniques. This constitutes an indication for intervention, especially if there is also arterial disease involving the contralateral kidney, or significant renal insufficiency.

The utility of captopril renography as a screening test is reduced in the presence of bilateral renal disease of any etiology. When one kidney is poorly functioning, captopril renography cannot be relied on to detect hemodynamically significant renal artery stenosis in the contralateral kidney. In recent years, color-coded Doppler ultrasonography has been introduced as an alternative screening test for renovascular disease.[110,111] A number of technical variations have been tried indicating that none of them is entirely satisfactory. Scanning the length of the renal artery is technically difficult and time consuming. Using this approach, there is a high rate of technically inadequate examination, especially in obese subjects. Sampling of arterial waveforms at the renal hilum or in the interlobar arteries from the subject's side is the most promising approach. However, even with this technique, the sensitivity and specificity are diminished in the elderly with reduced arterial compliance, renal insufficiency or severe stenosis. Magnetic resonance angiography and spiral computed tomographic scanning are new

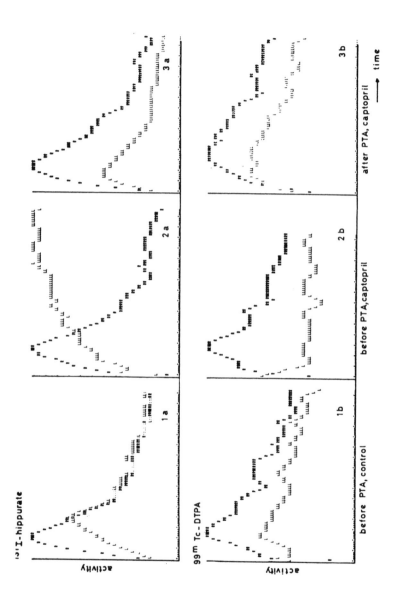

techniques on the horizon that while expensive will facilitate the timely diagnosis of renovascular disease in the elderly.

When captopril renography or Doppler ultrasonography is positive, aortography should be the next step. However, the decision to go ahead with aortography should not be undertaken lightly because of rare, but nevertheless, serious complications. The patient must be agreeable to intervention by angioplasty or surgery, and must be an acceptable risk for elective or, when there are complications of angioplasty, urgent operation. Life expectancy and quality of life are more difficult to define, but are additional considerations in deciding to proceed with aortography and, if necessary, surgery. Apart from bleeding from the puncture site, or thrombosis of the femoral or brachial arteries, aortography may be complicated by cholesterol emboli to the kidneys and lower extremities.[112,113] Radiocontrast material is frequently blamed for deterioration of renal function after aortography, when in fact cholesterol emboli have damaged the kidneys. Cholesterol emboli to the lower extremities may produce livido reticularis, a lace-like purple discoloration of the skin. When extensive, cholesterol emboli may lead to amputation. Fortunately, this dreaded complication of aortography is rare.

Treatment

The primary purpose of treating renovascular disease is preservation of renal function. However, improvement of renal function is not the sole definition of success. Considering the unrelenting course of atherosclerosis, stabilization of renal function during long-term follow-up is an acceptable alternative. Due to a multiplicity of potential influences, blood pressure response is an unreliable indicator of outcome. With rapidly advancing technology and the introduction of intra-arterial stents, angioplasty has become the treatment of choice of renovascular hypertension in the elderly.[114–116] In the best hands, the success rate of treating nonostial renal artery stenoses by balloon angioplasty is over 80%. Recurrence rate of stenoses after 1 year is

◄──────────────────────────────────────

Figure 3: *Renography in a 42-year-old man with hypertension and stenosis of the left renal artery. In 1 (a) lower curve = the left kidney, upper curve = the right kidney. After percutaneous transluminal angioplasty (PTA), his hypertension was cured. The upper half of the figure shows* ^{131}*I-hippurate (a) and the lower half shows* ^{99m}*Tc-diethylenetriamine pentaacetic acid (DTPA) (b) time-activity curves in three different circumstances: (1) before PTA without any medication (control); (2) before PTA but with 25 mg of captopril taken orally 1 hour before the investigation; (3) 6 weeks after PTA with the same captopril pretreatment. Before PTA captopril slowed down the excretion of* ^{131}*-hippurate and reduced the uptake of* ^{99m}*Tc-DTPA only in the left kidney. After PTA this effect disappeared. Reproduced from* Hypertension *9:454–458, 1987. Permission of American Heart Association.*

between 15% to 20%. Renal function is improved or stabilized in about 75% of patients as long as renal function was not severely impaired prior to the procedure. This finding emphasizes the need of timely diagnosis of this condition. The success rate of treating ostial stenoses by balloon angioplasty is low, and stenting is commonly used in the first sitting.

Early results of renal artery stenting are encouraging. In one study conducted in patients with hemodynamically significant renal artery stenosis, restenosis rate was 13% at 6 months.[117] In another study, the rate of restenosis was 11% at 5 years, but functional studies documenting the hemodynamic significance of ostial lesions, which were defined as stenoses of more than 50% of the diameter of the renal artery, were not performed.[118] The outcome of renal artery stenting in older patients (65 and older) with stenoses greater than 85%, which are always hemodynamically significant, is lacking. Anecdotal experience indicates that the restenoses rate in this group of patients at 2 years of follow-up is around 40%. Cholesterol embolization of the kidney during angioplasty and stenting may occur in 5%–10% of patients and may lead to renal impairment.[117]

Close follow-up of patients after angioplasty and stenting of the renal artery is mandatory and is best accomplished by initially semiannual and then annual measurements of serum creatinine.[116] Renography should be repeated 2–3 months after the intervention, when the maximal achievable benefit of the procedure should be apparent, to establish a new baseline. If serial serum creatinine measurements indicate deterioration of renal function, renography should be repeated and, in case of a new abnormality, be followed by aortography. Restenosis of a stented renal artery is amenable to angioplasty.

Surgery is resorted to on an urgent basis when there is dissection or rupture of the renal artery during angioplasty, or after repeated restenosis of the artery despite angioplasty or stenting. The presence of complete occlusion of the main renal artery to a kidney does not preclude the possibility of restoring some of the function of that kidney by surgical revascularization.[119–121] With slow development of stenosis and, ultimately, of closure, collateral circulation to the kidney may be adequate to maintain renal size (>8 cm) and viability. Hypersecretion of renin from a kidney with complete occlusion of the main artery is an indicator of viability. Successful surgery under these circumstances may restore sufficient function to obviate or postpone chronic dialysis. Perioperative mortality following bypass surgery of the renal arteries is about 2% to 3% compared to about 1% with angioplasty.

Conclusions

Hypertension in the elderly should be managed in the context of expected benefits of treatment and of hazards posed by complicating vascular diseases, mainly atherosclerosis. There is evidence that rapid and excessive lowering of blood pressure in elderly hypertensives with cerebrovascular disease may cause stroke, and in the presence of ischemic heart disease may increase the incidence of myocardial infarction and sudden death. Antihypertensive therapy should be introduced gradually, should be based on mini-dosing to minimize side effects, and should be given once a day to improve compliance. The use of diuretics is unavoidable when hypertension is complicated by renal insufficiency and in cases of severe hypertension. Atherosclerotic renovascular hypertension in the elderly is common and a major cause of symptomatic renal insufficiency and failure. The goal of therapy is preservation of renal function. The key to success is early diagnosis, and angioplasty with or without stenting is the primary treatment modality.

References

1. Balsano F, Birkenhäger WH, Marigliano V (eds.): *First International Congress on Hypertension in the Elderly. J Hypertens* 6(suppl 1):S1–S127, 1988.
2. Amery A, Staessen J (eds.): *Hypertension in the Elderly, Handbook of Hypertension,* Vol. 12. Amsterdam, The Netherlands, Elsevier Science Publishers B.V., 1989.
3. Applegate WB: Hypertension in elderly patients. *Ann Intern Med* 110: 901–915, 1989.
4. National High Blood Pressure Education Program Working Group: National high blood pressure education program working group report on hypertension in the elderly. *Hypertension* 23:275–285, 1994.
5. Bulpitt CJ: Definition, prevalence and incidence of hypertension in the elderly. In Amery A, Staessen J (eds): *Hypertension in the Elderly.* Amsterdam, The Netherlands, Elsevier Science Publishers B.V., 1989, pp 153–169.
6. Insua JT, Sacks HS, Lau TS, et al: Drug treatment of hypertension in the elderly: A meta-analysis. *Ann Intern Med* 121:355–362, 1994.
7. Staessen JA, Fagard R, Thijs L, et al: Randomized double-blind comparison of placebo and active treatment for older patients with isolated systolic hypertension. *Lancet* 350:757–762, 1997.
8. Borhani NO, Applegate WB, Cutler JA, et al: Systolic Hypertension in the Elderly Program. Part 1: Rational and design. *Hypertension* 17(suppl II):II-2-II-15, 1991.
9. Vokonas PS, Kannel WB, Cupples LA: Epidemiology and risk of hypertension in the elderly: The Framingham Study. *J Hypertens* 6(suppl 2):53–59, 1988.
10. Kannel WB, Gordon T, Castelli WB, et al: Electrocardiographic left ventricular hypertrophy and the risk of coronary heart disease: The Framingham Study. *Ann Intern Med* 72:813–822, 1970.
11. Levy D, Garrison RJ, Savage DD, et al: Left ventricular mass and incidence of coronary heart disease in the elderly cohort: the Framingham Heart Study. *Ann Intern Med* 110:101–107, 1989.
12. Heikinheimo RJ, Haavisto MV, Kaarela RH, et al: Blood pressure in the very old. *J Hypertens* 8:361–367, 1990.

13. Langer RD, Criqui MH, Barrett-Connor EL, et al: Blood pressure change and survival after age 75. *Hypertension* 22:551–559, 1993.
14. Tervahauta M, Pekkanen J, Enlund H, et al: Change in blood pressure and 5-year risk of coronary heart disease among elderly men: the Finnish cohorts of the Seven Countries Study. *J Hypertens* 12:1183–1189, 1994.
15. Birkenhäger, de Leeuw PW: Systolic blood pressure as a risk factor. In Amery A, Staessen J (eds): *Hypertension in the Elderly*. Amsterdam, The Netherlands, Elsevier Science Publishers B.V., 1989, pp 170–173.
16. O'Rourke M: Arterial stiffness, systolic blood pressure, and logical treatment of arterial hypertension. *Hypertension* 15:339–347, 1990.
17. Lewis RR, Padayachee TS, Ariyanayagram RP, et al: Prevalence of severe internal carotid artery disease in hypertensive elderly patients. *J Hypertens* 6:(suppl 1):S33–S36, 1988.
18. Kaplan NM: *Clinical Hypertension*. Baltimore, MD, Williams & Wilkins, 1990, pp 303–304.
19. Wollenweber J, Sheps S, Davis G: Clinical course of atherosclerotic renovascular disease. *Am J Cardiol* 21:60–71, 1968.
20. Dean R, Kieffer R, Smith B, et al: Renovascular hypertension. *Arch Surg* 116:1408–1415, 1981.
21. Rimmer JM, Gennari FJ: Atherosclerotic renovascular disease and progressive renal failure. *Ann Intern Med* 118:712–719, 1993.
22. Zierler RE, Bergelin RO, Davidson RC, et al: A prospective study of disease progression in patients with atheroslcerotic renal artery stenosis. *Am J Hypertens* 9:1055–1061, 1996.
23. Gribbin B, Pickering TG, Sleight P, et al: Effect of age and high blood pressure on baroreflex sensitivity in man. *Circ Res* 29:424–431, 1971.
24. Karemaker JM, Wieling W, Dunning AJ: Aging and the baroreflex. In Amery A, Staessen J (eds): *Hypertension in the Elderly*. Amsterdam, The Netherlands, Elsevier Science Publishers B.V., 1989, pp 24–38.
25. Shannon RP, Wei JY, Rosa RM, et al: The effect of age and sodium depletion on cardiovascular response to orthostasis. *Hypertension* 8:438–443, 1986.
26. Mathias CJ: Postprandial hypotension. Pathophysiologic mechanisms and clinical implications in different disorders. *Hypertension* 18:694–704, 1991.
27. Lipsitz LA, Nyquist RP, Wei JY, et al: Postprandial reduction in blood pressure in the elderly. *N Engl J Med* 309:81–83, 1983.
28. Vaitkevicius PV, Esserwein DM, Maynard AK, et al: Frequency and importance of post-prandial blood pressure reduction in elderly nursing home patients. *Ann Intern Med* 115:865–870, 1991.
29. Strandgaard S: Autoregulation of cerebral blood flow in hypertensive patients. *Circulation* 53:720–727, 1976.
30. Kaplan NM: *Clinical Hypertension*. Baltimore, MD, Williams & Wilkins, 1990, pp 187–188.
31. Wollner L, McCarthy ST, Soper NDW, et al: Failure of cerebral autoregulation as a cause of brain dysfunction in the elderly. *Br Med J* 1:1117–1118, 1979.
32. Jansen PAF, Gribnau FWJ, Schulte BPM, et al: Contribution of inappropriate treatment for hypertension to pathogenesis of stroke in the elderly. *Br Med J* 293:914–917, 1986.
33. Pitlik S, Manor RS, Lipshitz F, et al: Transient retinal ischemia induced by nifedipine. *Br Med J* 287:1845–1846, 1983.

34. O'Mailia JJ, Sander GE, Giles TD: Nifedipine associated myocardial ischemia or infarction in the treatment of hypertensive urgencies. *Ann Intern Med* 107:185–186, 1987.
35. Zangerle KF, Wolford R: Syncope and conduction disturbances following sublinqual nifedipine for hypertension. *Ann Emerg Med* 14:1005–1006, 1985.
36. Cruickshank JM, Thorp JM, Zacharias FJ: Benefits and potential harm of lowering high blood pressure. *Lancet* 1:581–584, 1987.
37. Alderman, MH, Ooi WL, Madhavan S, et al: Treatment-induced blood pressure reduction and the risk of myocardial infarction. *JAMA* 262: G20–G24, 1989.
38. Madhavan S, Ooi WL, Cohen H, et al: Relation of pulse pressure and blood pressure reduction to the incidence of myocardial infarction. *Hypertension* 23:395–401, 1994.
39. Alderman, MH: Commentary on "How far should blood pressure be lowered? What is the role of the J-curve?" by Lennart Hannson, MD. *Am J Hypertens* 3:730–732, 1990.
40. Hannson L: How far should blood pressure be lowered? What is the role of the J-curve? *Am J Hypertens* 3:726–729, 1990.
41. Irie K, Yamaguchi T, Minematsu K, et al: The J-curve phenomenon in stroke recurrence. *Stroke* 24:1844–1849, 1993.
42. MacMahon S, Rodgers A, Neal B, et al: Blood pressure lowering for the secondary prevention of myocardial infarction and stroke. *Hypertension* 29:537–538, 1997.
43. Nielson CP, Vestal RE: α-adrenoceptors, β-adrenoceptors and aging. In Amery A, Staessen J (eds): *Hypertension in the Elderly*. Amsterdam, The Netherlands, Elsevier Science Publishers B.V., 1989, pp 51–62.
44. Rowe JW, Andres R, Tobin JD, et al: The effect of age on creatinine clearance in men: a cross-sectional and longitudinal study. *J Gerontol* 31: 155–163, 1976.
45. Luft FC, Grim CE, Fineberg N, et al: Effects of volume expansion and contraction in normotensive white, blacks, and subjects of different ages. *Circulation* 59:643–650, 1979.
46. Freis ED: Age and antihypertensive drugs (hydrochlorothiazide, bendroflumethiazide, nadolol and captopril). *Am J Cardiol* 61:117–121, 1988.
47. Thijs L, Amery A, Birkenhäger W, et al: Age-related effects and active treatment in patients beyond the age of 60 years: The need for a proper control group. *J Hypertens* 8:997–1002, 1990.
48. Kaplan NM: Age and the response to antihypertensive drugs. *Am J Hypertens* 2:213–215, 1989.
49. Veterans Administration Cooperative Group: Effects of treatment in hypertension: II. Results in patients with diastolic blood pressure averaging 90 through 114 mmHg. *JAMA* 213:1143–1152, 1970.
50. Amery A, Birkenhäger W, Brixko P, et al: Mortality and morbidity results from the European Working Party on High Blood Pressure in the Elderly trial. *Lancet* 2:1349–1354, 1985.
51. Coope J, Warender TJ: Randomized trial of treatment of hypertension in elderly patients in primary care. *Br Med J* 293:1145–1151, 1986.
52. Dahlöf B, Lindholm LG, Hansson L, et al: Morbidity and mortality in the Swedish Trial in Old Patients with Hypertension (STOP-Hypertension). *Lancet* 338:1281–1285, 1991.
53. MRC Working Party: Medical Research Council trial of treatment of hypertension in older adults: principal results. *Br Med J* 304:405–412, 1992.

54. SHEP Cooperative Research Group: Prevention of stroke by antihypertensive drug treatment in older persons with isolated systolic hypertension. *JAMA* 265:3255–3264, 1991.
55. Beard K, Bulpitt C, Mascie-Taylor M, et al: Management of elderly patients with sustained hypertension. *Br Med J* 304:412–416, 1992.
56. Thijs L, Fagard R, Lijnen P, et al: A meta-analysis of outcome trials in elderly hypertensives. *J Hypertens* 10:1103–1109, 1992.
57. Pickering TG, James GD, Boddie C, et al: How common is white coat hypertension. *JAMA* 259:225–228, 1988.
58. Thijs L, Amery A, Clement D, et al: Ambulatory blood pressure monitoring in elderly patients with isolated systolic hypertension. *J Hypertens* 10: 693–699, 1992.
59. Myers MG: Systolic hypertension and the white coat phenomenon. *Am J Hypertens* 9:938–940, 1996.
60. Pickering T: Recommendations for the use of home (self) and ambulatory blood pressure monitoring. *Am J Hypertens* 9:1–11, 1996.
61. Spence JD, Sibbald WJ, Cape RD: Pseudohypertension in the elderly. *Clin Sci* 55(Suppl) 399s–402s, 1978.
62. Messerli FH, Venturo HO, Amodeo C: Osler's maneuver and pseudohypertension. *N Eng J Med* 312:1548–1551, 1985.
63. Tsapatsaris NP, Napolitana GT, Rothchild J: Osler's maneuver in an outpatient clinic setting. *Arch Intern Med* 151:2209–2211, 1991.
64. Finnegan TP, Spence JD, Wong DG, et al: Blood pressure measurement in the elderly: correlation of arterial stiffness with difference between intra-arterial and cuff pressures. *J Hypertens* 3:231–235, 1985.
65. Kuivaniemi H, Tromp G, Prockop DJ: Genetic causes of aortic aneurysms. Unlearning of what the textbooks say. *J Clin Invest* 88:1441–1444, 1991.
66. Lederle FA, Walker JM, Reinke DB: Selective screening for abdominal aortic aneurysms with physical examination and ultrasound. *Arch Intern Med* 148:1753–1756, 1988.
67. The fifth report of the Joint National Committee on detection, evaluation and treatment of high blood pressure (JNC V). *Arch Intern Med* 153: 154–183, 1993.
68. Dunn FG, Pringle SD: Hypertension and coronary artery disease. Can the chain be broken? *Hypertension* 18(Suppl):I-126–I-132, 1991.
69. Schmieder RE, Martus P, Klingbeil A: Meta-analysis: Blood pressure lowering reduces left ventricular mass index in essential hypertension. *JAMA* 275:1507–1513, 1996.
70. Report of the Joint National Committee on Detection, Evaluation and Treatment of High Blood Pressure. *Arch Intern Med* 153:154–183, 1993.
71. Schotte DE, Stunkard AJ: The effects of weight reduction on blood pressure in 301 obese patients. *Arch Intern Med* 150:1701–1704, 1990.
72. Applegate WB, Miller ST, Elam JT, et al: Non pharmacologic intervention to reduce blood pressure with mild hypertension. *Arch Intern Med* 152: 1162–1166, 1992.
73. Saunders JB, Beever DG, Paton A: Alcohol-induced hypertension. *Lancet* 2:653–656, 1981.
74. Parker M, Puddey IB, Beilin LJ, et al: Two-way factorial study of alcohol and salt restriction in treated hypertensive men. *Hypertension* 16: 398–406, 1990.
75. Simon G, Wittig VJ, Cohn JN: Transdermal nitroglycerin as step 3 antihypertensive agent. *Clin Pharmacol Ther* 40:42–45, 1986.

76. Duchier J, Iannascoli F, Safar M: Antihypertensive effect of sustained-release isosorbide dinitrate for isolated systolic hypertension in the elderly. *Am J Cardiol* 60:99–102, 1987.
77. Perret F, Mooser V, Hayoz D, et al: Evaluation of arterial compliance-pressure curves: Effect of antihypertensive drugs. *Hypertension* 18(Suppl II):II-77–II-83, 1991.
78. Ray WA: Thiazide diuretics and osteoporosis: time for a clinical trial? *Ann Intern Med* 115:64–65, 1991.
79. The Norweigian Multicenter Study Group: Timolol-induced reduction in mortality and reinfarction in patients surviving acute myocardial infarction. *N Engl J Med* 304:801–817, 1981.
80. Wilkstrand J, Warnold I, Olsson G, et al: Primary prevention with metoprolol in patients with hypertension. Mortality results from the MAPHY study. *JAMA* 259:1976–1982, 1988.
81. Remuzzi A, Puntorieri A, Battaglia C, et al: Angiotensin converting enzyme inhibition ameliorates glomerular filtration of macromolecules and water and lessens glomerular injury in the rats. *J Clin Invest* 85:541–549, 1990.
82. Keane WF, Anderson S, Aurell M, et al: Angiotensin converting enzyme inhibitors and progressive renal insufficiency. *Ann Intern Med* 111:503–516, 1989.
83. Pfeffer JM, Pfeffer MA, Braunwald E: Influence of chronic captopril therapy on the infarcted left ventricle of the rat. *Circ Res* 57:84–95, 1985.
84. Ruilope LM, Miranda B, Morales JM, et al: Converting enzyme inhibition in chronic renal failure. *Am J Kidney Dis* 13:120–126, 1989.
85. Pfeffer MA, Lamas GA, Vaughan DE, et al: Effect of captopril on progressive ventricular dilatation after anterior myocardial infarction. *N Engl J Med* 19:80–86, 1988.
86. Oldroyd KG, Pye MP, Ray, SG, et al: Effects of early captopril administration on infarct expansion, left ventricular remodeling and exercise capacity after acute myocardial infarction. *Am J Cardiol* 68:713–718, 1991.
87. Henry PD, Bentley KI: Suppression of atherogenesis in cholesterol fed rabbit treated with nifedipine. *J Clin Invest* 68:1366–1369, 1981.
88. Furberg CD, Psaty BM: Calcium antagonists: Not appropriate as first line antihypertensive agents. *Am J Hypertens* 9:122–125, 1996.
89. Dunzendorfer U: Clinical experience: Symptomatic management of BPH with terazosin. *Urology* 32(Suppl):27–31, 1988.
90. Ashouri OS: Severe diuretic-induced hyponatremia in the elderly. *Arch Intern Med* 146:1355–1357, 1986.
91. Thiessen BQ, Wallace SM, Blackburn JL, et al: Increased prescribing of antidepressants subsequent to β-blocker therapy. *Arch Intern Med* 150:2286–2290, 1990.
92. Israili ZH, Hall WD: Cough and angioneurotic edema associated with angiotensin-converting enzyme inhibitor therapy. A review of literature and pathophysiology. *Ann Intern Med* 117:234–242, 1992.
93. Arauz-Pacheco C, Ramirez LC, Rios JM, Raskin P: Hypoglycemia induced by angiotensin-converting enzyme inhibitors in patients with non-insulin-dependent diabetes receiving sulfonylurea therapy. *Am J Med* 89:811–813, 1990.
94. Psaty BM, Heckbert SR, Koepsell TD, et al: The risk of myocardial infarction associated with antihypertensive drug therapies. *JAMA* 274:620–625, 1995.

95. Laragh JH, Held C, Messerli F, et al: Calcium antagonists and cardiovascular prognosis: a homogeneous group? *Am J Hypertens* 9:95–109, 1996.
96. Oates JA: Antagonism of antihypertensive drug therapy by non-steroidal anti-inflammatory drugs. *Hypertension* 11(suppl II):II-4–II-6, 1988.
97. Houston MC: Non-steroidal anti-inflammatory drugs and antihypertensives. *Am J Med* 90(suppl 5A):42S–47S, 1991.
98. Kaplan NM: *Clinical Hypertension*. Baltimore, MD, Williams & Wilkins, 1990, pp. 268–282.
99. Ferguson RK, Vlasses PH: Hypertensive emergencies and urgencies. *JAMA* 225:1607–1613, 1986.
100. Cottrell JE, Illner P, Kittay MJ, et al: Rebound hypertension after sodium nitroprusside-induced hypotension. *Clin Pharmacol Ther* 27:32–36, 1980.
101. Haas DC, Streeten DHP, Kim RC, Naalbandian AN, Obeid AI: Death from cerebral hypoperfusion during nitroprusside treatment of acute angiotensin-dependent hypertension. *Am J Med* 75:1071–1076, 1983.
102. Prys-Roberts C, Meloche R, Foex P: Studies of anesthesia in relation to hypertension. I: Cardiovascular responses of treated and untreated patients. *Br J Anaesth* 43:122–137, 1971.
103. Prys-Roberts C, Foex P, Biro GP, et al: Studies of anaesthesia in relation to hypertension. V: Adrenergic beta-receptor blockade. *Br J Anaesth* 45:671, 1973.
104. Kaplan NM: *Clinical Hypertension*. Baltimore, MD, Williams & Wilkins, 1990, pp 257–259.
105. Nephrology Forum: Ischemic renal disease: An overlooked clinical entity? *Kidney Int* 34:729–743, 1988.
106. Mann SJ, Pickering TG: Detection of renovascular hypertension. *Ann Int Med* 117:845–853, 1992.
107. Geyskes G, Oei HY, Carl BAJ, et al: Renovascular hypertension identified by captopril-induced changes in the renogram. *Hypertension* 9:451–458, 1987.
108. Setaro JF, Saddler MC, Chen CC, et al: Simplified captopril renography in diagnosis and treatment of renal artery stenosis. *Hypertension* 18:289–298, 1991.
109. Symposium: The role of captopril scintigraphy in the diagnosis and management of renovascular hypertension: a consensus conference. *Am J Hypertens* 4:661S–752S, 1991.
110. Spies K-P, Fobbe F, El-Bedewi M, et al: Color-coded duplex sonography for non-invasive diagnosis and grading of renal artery stenosis. *Am J Hypertens* 8:1222–1231, 1995.
111. Burdick L, Airoldi F, Marana I, et al: Superiority of acceleration and acceleration time over pulsatility and resistance indices as screening tests for renal artery stenosis. *J Hypertens* 14:1229–1235, 1996.
112. Colt HG, Begg RJ, Saporito JJ, et al: Cholesterol emboli after cardiac catheterization—Eight cases and a review of literature. *Medicine* 67:389–400, 1988.
113. Mannesse CK, Blankestijn PJ, Veld AJMI, et al: Renal failure and cholesterol embolization. A report of four surviving cases and a review of literature. *Clin Nephrol* 36:240–245, 1991.
114. Canzanello VJ, Millan VG, Spiegel JE, et al: Percutaneous transluminal renal angioplasty in management of atherosclerotic renovascular hypertension: Results in 100 patients. *Hypertension* 13:163–172, 1989.
115. Jensen G, Zachrisson B-F, Delin K, et al: Treatment of renovascular hy-

pertension: One year results of renal angioplasty. *Kidney Int* 48: 1936–1945, 1995.

116. Baumgartner I, Triller J, Mahler F: Patency of percutaneous transluminal angiography: A prospective sonographic study. *Kidney Int* 51: 798–803, 1997.

117. Van de Ven PJG, Beutler JJ, Kaatee R, et al: Transluminal vascular stent for ostial atherosclerotic renal artery stenosis. *Lancet* 346:672–674, 1995.

118. Blum U, Krumme B, Flugel P, et al: Treatment of ostial renal-artery stenoses with vascular endoprotheses after unsuccessful balloon angioplasty. *N Engl J Med* 336:459–465, 1997.

119. Jamieson GG, Clarkson AR, Woodroffe AJ, et al: Reconstructive renovascular surgery for chronic renal failure. *Br J Surg* 71:338–240, 1984.

120. Dean RH, England R, Dupont WD, et al: Retrieval of renal function by revascularization. *Ann Surg* 202:367–375, 1985.

121. Novick AC, Ziegelbaum M, Vidt DG, et al: Trends in surgical revascularization for renal artery disease: Ten years' experience. *JAMA* 257:498–501, 1987.

Part 3

Congestive Heart Failure

Chapter 18

Heart Muscle Disease

Celia M. Oakley

Cardiomyopathies are heart muscle disorders which are not secondary to coronary disease or hypertension or to congenital valvular or pericardial abnormalities. Classification into hypertrophic, dilated and restrictive forms is based on morphological and functional abnormalities[1] and is still useful despite overlap between types, particularly in the elderly in whom age related changes in the heart significantly modify disease.[2-5]

Cardiomyopathy in Context

Heart failure is the only major cardiovascular disorder that is actually increasing in incidence and in absolute mortality. This is because people are living longer and the prevalence increases dramatically with increasing age.[6,7] Heart failure has a prevalence of 1% in people between the ages of 25 and 54 years, 4.5% between ages 65 and 74 years and 10% over the age of 75 years in the United States.[8] More than 75% of patients with heart failure are over 60 years of age[9] and heart failure is the most frequent cause of hospital admission in this age group but primary cardiomyopathy is numerically only a minor player. Improved survival of patients after myocardial infarction accounts for much of the increase in numbers of heart failure patients, many of whom have more than one chronic cardiac disorder as well as contributory age-related changes. Hypertension is the next most important cause. Systolic hypertension results from increased arterial indistensibility and leads to a wide pulse pressure, myocardial hypertrophy, and greater diastolic stiffness that, in any case, increases with age due to

From *Clinical Cardiology in the Elderly. Second Edition,* edited by Elliot Chesler. © 1999, Futura Publishing Company, Armonk, NY.

greater amounts of collagen in the heart.[10] The duration of both systolic contraction and diastolic relaxation lengthen with intolerance of tachycardia and increased dependence on maintenance of atrial contraction.[11] Degenerative aortic stenosis, mitral ring calcification, and mitral valve prolapse may coexist with hypertension, coronary artery disease and senile amyloid deposition, particularly in patients over the age of 70 years.

The recognition of primary cardiomyopathies amidst these other cardiac pathologies can lead to both under and over-estimation of their frequency and the true prevalence is quite unknown.

Hypertrophic Cardiomyopathy

Hypertrophied Hearts in the Elderly

Hypertrophic cardiomyopathy (HCM) is characterised by hypertrophy of the undilated left ventricle in the absence of pressure overload. Although first recognized in the young and middle aged with a high incidence of sudden death,[12] it has been described with increasing frequency in the elderly[13,14] and with a diversity of cardiac phenotype.[15,16] The disorder carries a dominant inheritance and over half of the younger patients give a family history but in elderly patients this is rare. They usually have no previous history of known cardiac abnormality or murmur and most have a benign prognosis.[17,18] It is still unknown how many have genetic HCM with expression only late in life and how many have senile pseudo-HCM[19] that is age-related changes seen on echo[20] that are misattributed. Hypertensive HCM describes patients with echocardiographic hypertrophy that seems excessive for the amount of blood pressure rise.[21] The elderly heart frequently shows some degree of left ventricular wall thickening and typically the cavity of the left ventricle is small and bent, sometimes with a considerable protrusion of the septum into the outflow tract below the aortic valve. Incorporation of elements of the tricuspid valve or ventricular "strings" or off axis views with M-mode compound the problem. Outflow tract turbulence, a systolic murmur and a variable late systolic gradient provide a murmur[22] and this may be amplified by mitral annular calcification[23] and mitral regurgitation. Both the clinical and echocardiographic features then closely simulate HCM.

Genetic HCM

Family history is very important but takes time and skill to elicit. Patients may lack information after families split up, names change after remarriages and "heart attacks" or road accidents may have been caused by sudden death. Probably less than 10% of cases of HCM are truly sporadic.

At the present time there is no routinely available diagnostic test for HCM. Genetic mutations associated with the disorder were first discovered in 1989 affecting the β-myosin heavy chain gene on chromosome 14 but such mutations only account for about 30% of patients. They usually show the typical cardiac phenotype. Mutations affecting troponin T, α-tropomyosin and the cardiac myosin binding protein C account for an additional 30% (Table 1). All of the mutations so far discovered affect sarcomeric proteins that regulate myocardial contraction.[24,25] Testing for such mutations is not available as a practical means of diagnosis at the present time and in any case, failing to find a mutation does not exclude genetic disease. Increasing research interest has been centered on other genetic and environmental influences that may determine the amount of hypertrophy both in genetic HCM and in other conditions such as aortic stenosis and hypertension which lead to hypertrophy. For example certain polymorphisms of the angiotensin converting enzyme gene have been associated with increased myocardial hypertrophy[26] both in hypertension and in athletes, as well as with diastolic dysfunction[27] and sudden death.[28] Histology shows a distinctive disorganization with fat, misshapen and malaligned myocytes and an excess of extracellular matrix but this disarray is not specific, being found to a much lesser extent in other conditions with myocardial hypertrophy.

Table 1
Known Loci of Mutations Associated with Hypertrophic Cardiomyopathy

Locus		Protein	Frequency
Chromosome	1	Cardiac troponin T	15%
	3	Essential myosin light chain	<3%
	7	(Cardiomyopathy + Wolf-Parkinson-White)	<3%
	11	Cardiac myosin binding protein C	15%
	12	Regulatory myosin light chain	<3%
	14	β cardiac myosin heavy chain	30%
	15	α-tropomyosin	<3%
	19	Cardiac troponin 1	<3%

- Mutations on the three main loci account for 60% of cases
- Myosin heavy chain mutations span a wide range of severity-large gene and many different point mutations.
- Cardiac troponin T mutations show low penetrance but poor prognosis—small gene, easy to test.
    worth screening family after sudden death because only 80% show clinical cardiac abnormality.
- Cardiac myosin binding protein C mutations may not show abnormality until late in life.

Until genetic screening becomes a reality as a clinical test, it will not be possible to distinguish with certainty between age and hypertension related changes and genetic disease. Probably for this reason HCM in the elderly has a mixed reputation. One group found it to be largely benign with a preponderance of females most of whom were asymptomatic.[20] Another group saw it as a cause of intractable heart failure associated with a small left ventricular cavity, marked diastolic dysfunction and only modest hypertrophy but marked outflow tract distortion needing relief by surgery.[29,30] In elderly patients with outflow obstruction and systolic anterior motion (SAM) of the mitral valve the systolic apposition between the mitral leaflets and the septum occurs largely because of excessive posterior systolic movement of the septum together with the angulation and narrowing of the outflow tract. This can be contrasted with younger patients with genetic disease whose hypertrophied septum is largely immobile with vigorous contraction of the posterior wall.

We do not know, therefore, whether genetic HCM in the elderly represents a mild form of the disease with late expression or whether age or high blood pressure may be responsible for expression of a particular phenotype in genetically predisposed individuals. That is for the next edition. As we frequently cannot tell them apart they will be considered together.

Clinical Features

Younger patients with HCM may be asymptomatic or present with syncope, exertional chest pain, breathlessness or palpitation. Elderly patients are no different except that there are many more causes of these symptoms in older subjects. Conduction system dysfunction, vertebrobasilar stenosis, coronary valvular and lung disease need to be considered and may coexist.

Elderly patients frequently have systolic murmurs. These are usually caused by aortic valve stiffening or mitral regurgitation associated with annular calcification or mitral valve prolapse. The diagnosis of HCM is usually based on the echocardiographic features (as it is also in the young) and often comes as a surprise.

Although the changes in the morphology and function of the heart due to ageing and often also hypertension, may closely simulate the clinical and echocardiographic signs genetic HCM is undoubtedly seen in old age. In some the diagnosis is secure because of a family history and 20 or 30 years of medical documentation in the patient. In others the diagnosis seems likely because of marked and asymmetrical hypertrophy in the absence of systolic hypertension even on exercise and in association with a markedly abnormal electrocardiogram (ECG) despite angiographically normal coronary arteries. In most elderly patients in whom the diagnosis is considered but in whom there is no past, personal or family history to suggest the disorder, the diagnosis should be made with caution, especially if the ECG is normal. In genetic HCM there is a 1 in 2 chance of other first degree family members being affected but family clinical screening may be neither possible nor welcome.

Many healthy older patients are regarded as being short of breath by their younger and fitter relations. Chest pain may be caused by accompanying coronary artery disease and the causes of syncope in old age are well known to be legion. In patients with HCM the dyspnea is caused by marked diastolic dysfunction, low cardiac output on exercise and a tendency to hyperventilate. Angina can be related to hypertrophy and microvascular changes with reduced vasodilator reserve even in the absence of disease of the epicardial coronary arteries. Syncope may be caused by arrhythmia, reduced left ventricular stroke volume or inappropriate vasodilatation on exercise. Sudden death may occur in any form of heart disease and is not rare in old age. When related to HCM it is less common in older adults than it is in younger people.[17] Its prevalence is almost certainly inflated by pathologists seeking a cause of sudden death due to natural causes when there is no other apparent explanation. The diagnosis of HCM in a patient who previously believed him or herself to be healthy may lead to avoidance of physical activity, unfitness, hyperventilation and to a perceived disability.

Progressive impairment of diastolic function may be associated with mitral regurgitation and lead to a raised left atrial pressure. If the ventricular cavity remains small, forward stroke volume will be low despite a higher than normal ejection fraction. Systolic murmurs are caused by a narrowed left ventricular outflow tract often associated with mitral regurgitation. The murmur is increased by standing up and momentarily disappears on squatting associated with postural changes in left ventricular volume. Patients with concentric or apical hypertrophy are usually murmur-free.

The ECG

The ECG is rarely normal in genetic HCM beyond early childhood so a normal ECG is strongly against the diagnosis. Abnormalities may result from long-standing hypertension or a previous silent infarct. Left anterior hemi-block is common with increasing age and it is also frequent in HCM. Complete left or right bundle branch block are rare but either can develop with deterioration in the conducting system that may accompany age.

In genetic HCM, the diagnosis can be made from the ECG when the abnormal pattern fails to fit in with any other reasonable diagnosis. The electrical axis may be unusual, there may be abnormal Q-waves in the mid chest leads, deep S-waves or poor R-wave progression in the chest leads or a short PR interval with absent Q-wave with high voltage in the left ventricular leads suggestive of pre-excitation. Features of left ventricular hypertrophy are diagnostic when there is no other discernible cause for them. The voltage is usually high but occasionally is normal or even low. Prominent P-waves are usual and may give a clue to the diagnosis but these of course disappear with loss of sinus rhythm and the onset of atrial fibrillation that is a common cause of deterioration and therefore presentation in older patients. The changes in the ECG are thought to reflect the underlying myocardial disarray that is a cardinal pathological feature of the disease and may cause focally slowed intraventricular conduction leading to ventricular arrhythmias. In familial studies the ECG is a more sensitive indicator of a mutation than echocardiographic abnormality but in old age incomplete penetrance may be associated with very nonspecific abnormalities in the ECG.[31]

Echocardiography

Thickening of the left ventricular wall is mild, severe, global or asymmetric. When it is gross and concentric, the diagnosis is not in doubt except for differentiation from amyloid.[19] The right ventricle may also be thickened in the absence of pulmonary hypertension. Difficulty arises when the thickening is confined to the outflow ventricular septum as protuberance of the septum at this point is common in old people associated with a bend in the long axis of the left ventricular cavity and outflow tract narrowing and less than complete systolic anterior motion of the mitral valve is not specific in old people with increased outflow tract velocity. Continuous wave Doppler shows increased velocity rising to a peak in a scimitar shape both in true HCM and with age-related change.[20] It is not uncommon as in other older patients to see mitral annular calcification with some mitral regurgitation and aortic valve thickening. Previous myocardial infarction may cause focal thinning and akinesia which may bring adjacent hypertrophy into prominence. Diagnosis is therefore more difficult in older patients because of the frequency of other changes in the heart yet the diagnosis of HCM in old people is frequently based on the echocardiographic appearance.

Chest X-ray

There are no specific features on the chest x-ray in most older patients. The heart is not usually enlarged. The left atrium is not dilated unless there is atrial arrhythmia whose onset is frequently a cause of pulmonary congestion.

Exercise Testing

Exercise testing is useful in assessing the origin of symptoms and functional capacity, but may not be successful if there are locomotor problems. Failure of blood pressure to rise or a fall on exercise augures poorly. It may be caused by an inadequate rise in output with inappropriate vasodilation and "an empty heart" and is associated with syncope and sudden death.[32]

Ambulatory Electrocardiography

This is important in patients with intermittent symptoms or syncope. The cause may be tachyarrhythmic or bradycardia but sometimes hypotension despite sinus rhythm at a normal rate. Bursts of self-terminating ventricular tachycardia are typical and may not be perceived by the patient. Atrial arrhythmias usually cause functional deterioration when sustained. High-grade ventricular ectopic activity may be ominous. Short bursts of monomorphic ventricular tachycardia have been associated with sudden death. Ambulatory blood pressure monitoring is needed to document hypotensive episodes.

Natural History

In affected families, HCM is only rarely detected at birth and neonatal HCM frequently regresses. In monitored children hypertrophy is usually only seen to develop towards the end of the first decade. It then often shows marked acceleration around the time of puberty which is the time of greatest risk of sudden death. After that time there is usually stability over decades with little clinical, ECG or echocardiographic change but as the disease was only first recognized clinically 40 years ago and as cross-sectional echocardiography has only been available for half that time, documentation from childhood into old age is never available. In some cases of HCM myocyte loss and fibrous tissue replacement brings about gradual thinning of the left ventricular wall and deterioration in previously good systolic function.[33,34] Stroke volume then falls because of increased residual volume but usually with only mild or moderate dilatation. This leads to low output congestive failure with raised filling pressures and sometimes considerable pulmonary hypertension.

Most of our knowledge of the natural history of HCM has come from interested major centers referred the worst cases. This is because in the earlier years they were the only ones to be recognized and at the present time the indications for referral tend to be recalcitrant symptoms or a "malignant" family history. Their bad experience has greatly exaggerated the malignancy of the disorder. More recent reports from regional centers serving a local population have shown a much better outlook.[35–38] All reports present only a snapshot. Follow-up has been too short to answer questions about time of onset of clinical disease in patients presenting late in life.

Management

Older patients tolerate β-blockers well. They have a track record of more than 30 years in this disease and usually alleviate shortness of breath and angina[39] whether the latter is due to associated coronary artery disease or not. The main benefit is through prolonging diastolic filling and coronary flow time but they also reduce outflow gradients and may improve ventricular compliance. Calcium channel blockers have a more marked myocardial depressant effect and are also vasodilators. Verapamil may precipitate hypotension, pulmonary edema or bradycardia and is not recommended in older patients.[40] Disopyramide has been used to reduce outflow tract gradients but these gradients[41] are poorly correlated either with symptoms or with prognosis and disopyramide is an antiarrhythmic drug with a marked proarrhythmic effect.

Atrial fibrillation brings the risk of thromboembolism as well as functional deterioration and amiodarone is the drug of choice to help to maintain sinus rhythm.[42] Long-term anticoagulant treatment will be needed and repeated DC cardioversion should be carried out for as long as it is followed by reasonably long retention of sinus rhythm. Once this is lost, usually in association with loss of atrial contractile ability and atrial dilatation, atrioventricular nodal ablation and pacing brings regularity and sometimes considerable improvement. Amiodarone may also improve survival in patients prone to ventricular arrhythmia and sudden death.[43]

Antibiotic prophylaxis is needed in patients with outflow tract gradients or mitral regurgitation to prevent infective endocarditis.

Surgical myotomy/myectomy has been carried out in older patients but with quite a high mortality[44-46] and this is true also of mitral valve replacement with a low profile valve.[30,47] The latter is only indicated in rare patients who develop a substantial amount of mitral regurgitation. In recent years surgery has largely receded in favor of medical intervention.[48] Sequential (DDD) pacing to secure early depolarization of the right ventricular septum reduces outflow tract gradients and may improve symptoms but has a marked placebo effect.[49-51] Selective per-catheter infarction of part of the outflow tract septum has been introduced instead of surgical myectomy to reduce its thickness and is achieved by selective occlusion of a septal branch of the left anterior descending coronary artery.[52] Although like spontaneous infarction[53] it has been shown to reduce outflow tract gradients, the size of the infarct is uncontrolled depending on the variable territory of supply of the artery and unlike pacing, the procedure is irreversible. It is particularly inappropriate in older patients who may have atheromatous coronary disease and need to maintain a maximal blood supply.

Transplantation is the last resort for patients in chronic low output congestive failure who are still within the age bracket of the transplant centre.

Dilated Cardiomyopathy

This is a heterogeneous condition with different contributory causes in different patients including coxsackie B virus infection, autoimmunity and heredity.[56–58] Dilated cardiomyopathy is recognized by a dilated and hypokinetic left and/or right ventricle (Table 2). Although by definition the ventricular dysfunction is not the result of hypertension, coronary or valvular disease, the presence of any one or a combination of these in older patients may contribute but seem insufficient to explain the problem. It may be difficult to assign priorities and a combination diagnosis may be reached. When a patient does particularly well on treatment, with considerable improvement and a tendency for the blood pressure to rise rather than fall on medication, a retrospective diagnosis of hypertensive heart failure may be correct. Similarly, mitral regurgitation that diminishes on treatment is probably largely secondary to left ventricular dysfunction. Rare cases may show predominant right ventricular dilatation.

Wall thickness is usually normal or slightly thin but myocardial mass is increased. The trabecular crevices are flattened and often contain small thrombi—this accounting for frequent embolism even in patients with retained sinus rhythm. The myocytes are attenuated and focal fibrosis, the result of excessive apoptosis, is a feature although it is not usually visible macroscopically.

Inheritance

A genetic susceptibility to dilated cardiomyopathy has been recognized in recent years with some abnormality in left ventricular function being found in up to 30% of first-degree relatives when these are systematically investigated by echocardiography.[58] Inheritance is usually dominant but with highly variable penetrance so that many affected family members may be asymptomatic.

X-linked cardiomyopathies with reduced or absent myocardial dystrophin but normal skeletal muscle dystrophin may masquerade as idiopathic as a family history of skeletal myopathy is often absent.[59–61]

Table 2
Possible Contributory Causes to Dilated
Cardiomyopathy in Older People

Hypertension	Heredity
Alcohol	Senile amyloid
Virus infection	Diabetic microvascular disease
Autoimmunity	Tachycardia

Contributory Causes of Heart Failure

Tachycardia Failure

Tachycardia failure is particularly likely to occur in older people whose hearts are more intolerant of a fast rate than in younger people. The onset of atrial fibrillation particularly, may be associated with a rapid ventricular rate that is unperceived by the patient who then presents in failure several days later. The dilated poorly contracting left ventricle may then be misdiagnosed as being caused by a dilated cardiomyopathy. Slowing of the heart will be followed by restoration of left ventricular function (Table 2).[62]

Previous hypertension is a major contributor and with the onset of heart failure and its treatment with diuretics and angiotensive-converting enzyme (ACE) inhibitors, the blood pressure may well become normal and remain low. In patients with unexplained left ventricular failure a specific etiology should always be sought. A family history as well as the examination may highlight hemochromatosis.

Epidemiology

Data on the incidence of dilated cardiomyopathy are unsatisfactory. Its prevalence is largely unknown particularly in the elderly.[63]

Alcohol

Left ventricular dilatation may result from excessive alcohol intake that may contribute to 20% to 30% of patients with dilated cardiomyopathy. These are usually binge drinkers and marked improvement or even return to normal may follow abstinence.[64] Men appear to be more susceptible than women and there may be a familial predisposition. Because the history is often unreliable in such patients, it is important to measure MCV and liver function tests, particularly gamma GT in patients presenting with a dilated cardiomyopathy.

Valve disease may be clinically occult, particularly after the onset of heart failure. Aortic stenosis may be severe yet the murmur may be soft or even absent in an old person with low output left ventricular failure and a thick chest wall. Less often, even severe mitral regurgitation due to degenerative mitral leaflet prolapse may not be clinically prominent or may erroneously be presumed to be secondary if left ventricular function is poor and echocardiographic imaging is poor or misinterpreted. Unlike mitral regurgitation of rheumatic origin in which a central jet is usually clearly seen, the regurgitant jet in mitral prolapse is directed eccentrically against either the septal (in posterior leaflet prolapse) or inferoposterior wall (in anterior leaflet prolapse) of the left atrium and the severity may be seriously underestimated.

Previous cytotoxic treatment particularly with anthracyclines such as doxorubicin or irradiation of the heart may be followed by fibrosis and heart failure.[65] This may have been years before the heart disorder is manifest. A full clinical history is obviously important.

Clinical Features

Most patients with dilated cardiomyopathy notice breathlessness first. This is often attributed to a nonexistent respiratory infection. Chest pain complained of in about 10% of patients may suggest angina or be atypical. Other patients may present with embolism, arrhythmia, a murmur caused by mitral regurgitation or an abnormal "routine" ECG. The condition frequently first presents at an advanced stage.

The possibility of heart failure in someone who has previously seemed to be fit is not always considered and diagnosis at the bedside may not be obvious. Abnormal physical signs are often subtle. Dyspnea and tachycardia of recent onset should alert the physician to the possibility of a cardiac cause. Left ventricular prominence, a third sound gallop or a mitral pansystolic murmur may or may not be elicited. Basal crackles may not be due to heart failure The venous pressure is not usually raised at first (unless the patient has gone into atrial fibrillation) as the right ventricle tends to fail after the left ventricle has failed and sometimes only as a result of pulmonary hypertension. Pedal edema is a very poor indicator of heart failure in the elderly and a cause of overdiagnosis as it is more often caused by stasis associated with relative immobility or varicose veins. Equally its absence is of no importance in excluding a cardiac cause for the patient's symptoms.

Other conditions simulating myocardial failure must be thought of during the clinical examination, particularly constrictive pericarditis and pulmonary thromboembolism.

Atrial fibrillation may precipitate heart failure in a patient with subclinical or even normal left ventricular dysfunction. Because of increased diastolic stiffness, the clinical syndrome of heart failure in elderly people develops without much dilatation and often with an ejection fraction still above 45%. This is in contrast to young people with dilated cardiomyopathy whose ejection fractions may have fallen below 30% with left ventricular diameters of 7 or even 8 cm before symptoms develop.

The ECG

The ECG may show sinus tachycardia, low voltage in standard leads and high voltage in the chest leads with repolarization abnormalities, left anterior hemiblock or complete left bundle branch block is common.

The Chest Radiograph

The chest radiograph may show pulmonary venous congestion but is an insensitive means of detecting left ventricular enlargement. The left atrium is not usually prominent in the absence of atrial arrhythmia.

Echocardiography

Echocardiography provides identification of left ventricular systolic dysfunction and can also be used to exclude structural valvular disease but it cannot exclude a coronary origin for the failure. Left ventricular dysfunction in dilated cardiomyopathy is not always global and homogenous but may appear partly focal. A small excess of pericardial fluid may be seen. The left atrium is dilated. Right ventricular dilatation usually occurs later and is a bad prognostic feature. Mitral and tricuspid regurgitation may be prominent.

Treatment

Patients with recent onset of symptoms, dyspnea, and pulmonary venous congestion usually respond rapidly to diuretics. ACE inhibitors are well tolerated in older patients and combined with diuretics they have been shown to improve the prognosis of patients with heart failure (although most of the trials excluded older patients).[66] Digoxin has been shown to be helpful in advanced cases of heart failure in sinus rhythm[67] and is nearly always needed if atrial fibrillation is present unless the ventricular rate is already sufficiently slow. Anticoagulant treatment should be considered for all patients in atrial fibrillation and the cost-benefit ratio may also be favorable in patients who retain sinus rhythm, although this is has not been submitted to clinical trial in any age group.[68]

β-Blockers have a definite place in the treatment of some (but not all) patients with heart failure but they can be difficult to introduce because the patient's condition may deteriorate before benefit is shown. Improvement is delayed so these drugs need to be introduced in very small doses.[69] Furthermore, each increment in dosage is followed by a further temporary deterioration. Metoprolol is the β-blocker that has been most used. It should be introduced in a dose as little as 6.25 mg daily and gradually increased to 50 mg daily. The patients most likely to benefit are those with a resting tachycardia. They are also the patients most likely to deteriorate abruptly if the β-blocker is introduced in too high a dose. β-Blockers that also have an α-blocking vasodilator action such as carvedilol may be used. Carvedilol, which also has anti-oxidant properties has shown benefit in trials but may cause a marked drop in blood pressure unless introduced with great caution, 6.25 mg daily or less.

Although all of these drugs (except diuretics) have been submitted to clinical trials that showed benefit both reducing hospital admissions and prolonging life, only a small proportion of patients in heart failure, particularly elderly patients in heart failure, are actually prescribed ACE inhibitors and even fewer β-blockers. The reasons given are low blood pressure, cough or deterioration in renal function. Whenever possible diuretics should be stopped 24 or even 48 hours before starting an ACE inhibitor. The initial dose should be of a short-acting drug such as captopril 6.25 mg given at night if treatment is started at home or in the morning if the blood pressure is going to be monitored in hospital. Once the patient is established on captopril three times per day, it should be exchanged for a longer-acting ACE inhibitor such as lisinopril or quinapril. Patients who are already hypotensive before starting ACE inhibitors should not be deprived of them. They stand to benefit most and can be initiated on treatment if this is introduced sufficiently slowly with steady increments.

Losartan, an angiotensin II inhibitor, can be used instead of an ACE inhibitory in patients with intractable cough. Losartan does not cause this side effect and compared favorably with captopril in the ELITE trial (Evaluation of Losartan in the Elderly).[70] Like the ACE inhibitors, losartan has to be introduced cautiously (in incremental doses up to 50 mg daily in the trial) to avoid hypotension and renal dysfunction.

A common problem is overdiuresis particularly in old people whose in-built diastolic dysfunction of aging, further added to by their heart disease, renders them exquisitely sensitive to changes in blood volume and left ventricular filling pressure. The diuretic dosage should be as low as possible and initiated with a loop diuretic as older people do not do well on thiazides. Rather than a steady increase in dosage of frusemide or bumetanide, it is better to combine it with metolazone 2.5 or 5mg once or twice per week. Although a thiazide, the metolazone is usually well tolerated and the intermittency enables dehydration and electrolyte disturbance to be avoided. Patients can be encouraged to participate in their own therapy, timing the metolazone diuresis to their convenience and using weight fluctuations to guide the frequency of dosage. In this way increments in the dose of loop diuretic can be avoided and hospital readmission minimized.

The only inotrope that has not been shown to increase mortality is digoxin. In the DIG trial it reduced the number of hospital admissions for recurrent failure but was not shown to reduce total mortality. This may have been because although it reduced heart failure deaths, it may have increased sudden deaths.[67]

Ventricular arrhythmias usually indicate a poor prognosis and tend to occur pari passu with deteriorating myocardial function. Low-dose amiodarone should be considered for patients with frequent ectopics or tachycardias impairing performance.[71]

Short-term intravenous inotropes, particularly the dobutamine dopamine combination with renal doses of dopamine can bring about temporary improvement. Some patients would prefer improved quality in their lives to prolonged quantity and these drugs may be used to render a patient fit for a forthcoming important event and occasionally to restabilize a patient after deterioration precipitated by a chest infection or even by ill-judged therapy. Recurrent "pulsed" treatment is no longer used.

Other Therapies

The use of growth hormone as a treatment for chronic heart failure has had some encouraging results in short-term use in small numbers of patients.[72] Dual chamber pacing may bring about improvement in patients with chronotropic incompetence and/or prolonged P-R interval.[73]

Transplantation may be available for a few older patients in transplant units using older hearts and having a higher age cutoff. Carefully selected older patients can do well after transplantation.

Mechanical left ventricular assist devices are improving all the time and may soon be sufficiently small, reliable and free from thromboembolic complications to provide an alternative to transplantation rather than simply a bridge to transplantation for patients awaiting hearts. The latter is unjustified as it simply swells the waiting lists for organs which are unlikely to become available.

Natural History

In patients who are first seen at an advanced stage or who respond poorly to initial therapy, the mortality is still high even though modern treatment has greatly improved the outlook. Bad prognostic features are hypotension, hyponatremia, renal impairment and high serum noradrenaline. Older patients tend to do poorly when there is a high element of diastolic failure with greatly elevated left ventricular filling pressure, only slight ventricular dilatation, a very low stroke output and congestive failure.

Specific Heart Muscle Disease

Endocrine Disease

Thyroid function should always be determined in older patients with heart failure that may result both from thyrotoxicosis and in myxedema. Although hyperthyroidism causes a high output failure with warm extremities, bounding pulses and widened pulse pressure in association with an alert and fidgety patient, all of these signs may be absent. Older patients do not usually have Grave's disease with proptosis and obvious eye signs and there may not be a palpable goiter with a bruit over it. Hyperthyroidism is unlikely to be the cause of the failure if the patient is still in sinus rhythm, although a persistent sinus tachycardia, not itself uncommon in heart failure, should initiate a check on thyroid function. Atrial fibrillation is nearly always present and usually with a high ventricular rate that at its onset may have precipitated the failure. About 5% of clinically euthyroid patients with unexplained atrial fibrillation show evidence of hyperthyroidism on routine thyroid function tests.[74]

Prominent venous pulsation, a loud first heart sound and accentuated pulmonary component of the second heart sound with a third heart sound gallop and systolic murmur all tend to be much more prominent in younger patients.

Hyperthyroidism causes some myocardial hypertrophy but the histology of thyrotoxic heart failure is non-specific with some increase in mitochondria even before the development of myocyte hypertrophy. The enhanced sympathetic activity that is apparent cannot be normalized by the use of β-adrenergic blocking drugs, although these are helpful in controlling tachycardia.

In hypothyroidism bradycardia and radiological cardiomegaly with low voltage complexes and flat T-waves on the ECG are typical.[75] Pericardial effusions are common and may be massive with high cholesterol content. When left ventricular function is much disturbed the cause is usually associated coronary disease. Thyroid replacement therapy should be started in low doses and slowly increased until the patient is euthyroid and this includes patients with coronary artery disease and angina.

Diabetes is associated with a cardiomyopathy that causes a further increase in myocardial diastolic stiffness and diabetes is also a major risk factor for the development of coronary atherosclerosis. Heart failure is the leading cause of death in diabetics.[76,77]

The combination of microvascular disease and metabolic derangement leads to an increase in heart weight with excess collagen, thickening of capillary basement membranes, microaneurysms, intimal proliferation and interstitial fibrosis.

Hypertension frequently coexists with noninsulin dependent diabetes in overweight patients with a constellation of risk factors. Diastolic dysfunction can be demonstrated even in younger prediabetics with insulin resistance. Increasing abnormalities in ventricular relaxation increase the tendency of the diabetic heart to develop clinical failure even with small insults due to arrhythmia or coronary disease. Diabetic subjects may show a fall in ejection fraction on exercise even when the resting ejection fraction is normal. Myocardial ischemia and infarction are more apt to be painless in diabetics of any age and these events are also more likely to be silent in older people without diabetes. Heart failure is readily precipitated by coronary bypass surgery in diabetes.

Acromegaly may cause heart failure with a massive increase in myocardial mass and many acromegalics have other contributory causes for heart failure, particularly hypertension and diabetes. It is ironic that while the somatostatin analogue octreotide has been shown to improve cardiac function in acromegalic heart failure,[78] growth hormone is at present under trial for the treatment of idiopathic dilated cardiomyopathy.

Metabolic Disorders

Hemochromatosis

Hemochromatosis is inherited as an autosomal recessive disorder which causes increased absorption of dietary iron. This leads to excessive deposition of iron in multiple organs including the myocardium. Hemochromatosis is a storage disease with deposition of iron within the myocytes. In contrast to amyloid and sarcoid heart diseases the conducting system is largely spared. Because the extracardiac manifestations of hemochromatosis are usually present before myocardial iron toxicity leads to cardiac dysfunction, the clinical diagnosis is usually not difficult with skin pigmentation, diabetes, and testicular atrophy. The ECG becomes abnormal some time before the development of heart failure with low voltage and nonspecific ST and T-wave changes. Cardiac chamber dimensions are increased and the ventricles hypokinetic on echocardiography. Cardiac symptoms may develop before "bronzed diabetes" in a small proportion of younger patients in whom a restrictive pattern of diastolic dysfunction and less dilated ventricles may be striking. In these patients considerable improvement in myocardial function may follow removal of iron but without treatment progressive biventricular failure develops.[79]

Phlebotomy and chelation therapy with desferrioxamine has dramatically improved the outcome for patients diagnosed early. Removal of iron has been demonstrated by serial cardiac biopsy. The mechanism of iron toxicity is not understood.

Autoimmune Diseases

The collagen vascular (autoimmune) diseases are commonly complicated by cardiac involvement which is more often pericardial or endocardial than myocardial but may be combined.

Although cardiac involvement in systemic lupus erythematosus (SLE) mainly causes pericardial effusion and valvular dysfunction, myocardial involvement may also occur. In the Churg-Strauss syndrome, eosinophilic infiltration may cause a myocarditis followed by fibrosis and an associated vasculitis resulting in fibrosis and cardiac failure.

Progressive systemic sclerosis (scleroderma) is associated with a high incidence of cardiac involvement with failure caused largely by myocardial fibrosis with a distinctive contraction band necrosis and fibrosis on histology.

Cancer Chemotherapy and Irradiation

Cytotoxic drugs, particularly anthracycline treatment, widely used in cancer chemotherapy, may cause cardiac toxicity. Doxorubicin causes cardiac failure that is dose- and time-dependent.[65]

Heart failure may develop early after initiation of treatment with recovery and is not then a necessary augury of later chronic heart failure. Children and older people appear to be more sensitive to the toxic effects which may first appear months after discontinuing treatment. Progressive fibrosis may lead to a restrictive syndrome but is always associated with important systolic impairment.

Irradiation for lymphoma or carcinoma of the breast can damage the heart. Pericardial effusion or constriction, coronary artery stenosis, and myocardial fibrosis may result. The risks of cardiac damage are much less with modern radiotherapy.

Restrictive Cardiomyopathy

In restrictive cardiomyopathy diastolic dysfunction predominates in the absence of significant systolic abnormality. The elderly heart shows slow relaxation that is exacerbated by diabetes and hypertension. The atrial contribution to ventricular filling is enhanced and causes an excessive late increment in diastolic pressure. Inflow Doppler velocities show an increased A to E ratio. In restrictive syndromes ventricular filling is early and rapidly completed. There is an excessive rise in ventricular diastolic pressure for any increment in volume. E is enhanced and A suppressed. Amyloid infiltration is the major cause of a severe restrictive syndrome in the elderly. In younger patients restrictive cardiomyopathy may be familial with progressive conduction system dysfunction, atrial dilatation and atrial standstill. Endomyocardial fibrosis in the tropics and Loeffler's endomyocardial disease in the west are restrictive syndromes related to eosinophilia but are rarely seen in the elderly. Hemochromatosis and sarcoid heart disease may present with restrictive features (Table 3).

Table 3
Contributory Causes of Restrictive Syndromes

Primary restrictive cardiomyopathy
Familial restrictive cardiomyopathy with progressive con-
  duction disturbance and atrial standstill
Old age
Amyloid infiltration
Sarcoid granuloma
Hemochromatosis
Endomyocardial fibrosis (tropical)
Loeffler's endomyocardial fibrosis (temperate)

Cardiac Amyloidosis

Amyloidosis is characterized by extracellular deposition of an abnormal fibrillar protein. This differs in the different forms of amyloidosis but in all of them auto-aggregation in association with a non-fibril-
lar glycoprotein, amyloid P and certain glycosaminoglycans leads to
formation of characteristic fibrils (Table 4).[80]
Most patients with amyloid heart disease have an immunocyte
dyscrasia (AL amyloid) although this may be occult (and used to be
called primary amyloidosis). Clinical heart disease is uncommon in AA
amyloid associated with chronic inflammatory conditions (secondary
amyloidosis). Patients should be investigated for myeloma or a monoclonal gamopathy. Senile amyloid is derived from plasma transthyretin
and may be deposited focally in the left and right atrium or may involve
the whole heart, often subclinically but sometimes leading to clinical
heart disease. There are also rare hereditary forms which can first
present with neurological or cardiac problems even in old age, although
usually younger.
Cardiac dysfunction is directly related to the physical presence of

---

Table 4
Acquired Cardiac Amyloidosis

Clinical	Origin of Protein Fibril
• AL amyloidosis associated with overt or occult immunocyte dyscrasia	monoclonal immunoglobulin light chains
• Reactive AA amyloidosis associated with chronic inflammatory diseases	serum amyloid A protein
• Senile amyloidosis focal cardiac atrial amyloid	Transthyretin Atrial natriuretic peptide

---

the amyloid deposits between the myocytes and in the walls of small coronary arteries. This produces increasing diastolic stiffness associated with progressive thickening of the walls of the heart including both ventricles, the atria, atrial septum and valves. Left and right ventricular systolic function are usually preserved but in patients with a predominant deposition in the walls of small arteries systolic failure may predominate. Typically, the heart remains small. At autopsy, the heart is abnormally firm and rubbery sometimes with a pericardial effusion and subserosal petechiae.

The clinical features[81] are of a patient who looks and feels nonspecifically ill but also has dyspnea, fatigue, and sometimes angina. The blood pressure is low and there may be orthostatic hypotension augmented by overenthusiastic diuretic dosage. Sensitivity to digitalis frequently leads to toxicity. The venous pressure is nearly always raised but the heart is quiet. In patients with a very high venous pressure there may be a right ventricular third heart sound gallop, but there is usually no left ventricular gallop. Murmurs are infrequent. The ECG shows low voltage without repolarisation abnormalities and it is this that may first alert the clinician to the diagnosis. Conduction defects and fascicular blocks are common. The chest x-ray may show a heart of normal size (unless there is a pericardial effusion) but with pulmonary venous congestion.

Echocardiography is diagnostic.[81,82] In patients with a known immunocyte dyscrasia in whom the development of cardiac amyloidosis can be predicted,[83] the whole natural history of the disease can be followed by serial echocardiography.[84] This shows that gradually increasing diastolic dysfunction develops pari passu with an increase in ventricular wall thickness. The initial effect of the infiltration is to prolong relaxation but later on this gives way to a restrictive syndrome. The differential diagnosis is from HCM but there are many differences. Patients with HCM do not appear ill, the venous pressure is usually normal, as is the blood pressure. The ECG usually shows increased voltage and repolarization abnormalities which tend to be notably absent in amyloidosis. On echo, thickening of the atrial septum and valves is absent in HCM but characteristic of amyloid. The well-publicized "granular sparkle" seen in amyloidosis, may also be seen in HCM and can be regulated to a considerable extent by manipulating the controls of the echo machine.

The prognosis of cardiac amyloid is very poor with death usually within 2 years of its first evidence on echo and within 1 year of the clinical onset.[81] Although the amyloid material used to be thought to be particularly stable, it is in fact in dynamic equilibrium and if the supply of the precursor protein can be cut off or curtailed, amyloid will regress. Unfortunately this, even when possible, is a slow process. There is no time to wait and transplantation can be very successful in patients who are young enough to be recipients. Although the ideal patients have amyloid that is largely confined to the heart patients with myeloma may also be considered because it is amyloid in the heart that determines their prognosis. Amyloid deposition in the transplanted heart may be seen soon after the transplant but is still compatible with many years of good health before the accumulation causes problems. Aggressive cytotoxic chemotherapy after transplantation can be followed by regression of amyloid infiltration from the other organs.

The medical treatment of amyloidosis is difficult. Digoxin is contraindicated as amyloid patients are abnormally sensitive to it and it may precipitate conduction defects. Diuretics have to be used with circumspection as these patients are exquisitely sensitive to changes in circulating blood volume because of its effects on left ventricular filling pressure, stroke output and blood pressure. Small doses of an ACE inhibitor may be helpful but a dose which causes any degree of peripheral vasodilatation is likely to be detrimental.

Finally, there is no indication for rectal or other non-cardiac biopsies in suspected cardiac amyloidosis. The diagnosis can be made from echocardiography with confidence. Cardiac biopsy is usually unnecessary, although it tends to be particularly easy in amyloidosis.

References

1. Richardson D, McKenna W, Bristow M, et al: WHO/ISFC Task Force definition and classification of cardiomyopathies. *Circulation* 93:23–24, 1996.
2. Waller BF, Morgan R: The very elderly heart. *Cardiovasc Clin* 18:361–410, 1987.
3. Lie JT, Hammond PI: Pathology of the senescent heart: Anatomic observations on 237 autopsy studies of patients 90 to 105 years old. *Mayo Clin Proc* 63:552–564, 1988.
4. Wei JY: Age and the cardiovascular system. *N Engl J Med* 327:1735–1739, 1992.
5. Olivetti G, Melissari M, Capasso JM, et al: Cardiomyopathy of the ageing human heart. Myocyte loss and reactive cellular hypertrophy. *Circ Res* 68:1560–1568, 1991.
6. NHLBI Report of the Task Force on Research in Heart Failure. US Dept of Health and Human Services. PHS-NIH.
7. Massie BM, Packer M: Congestive heart failure: Current controversies and future prospects. *Am J Cardiol* 66:429–430, 1990.
8. Schocken DD, Arrieta ML, Leaverton PE: Prevalence and mortality rate of congestive heart failure in the United States. *J Am Coll Cardiol* 20:301–306, 1992.
9. Klainer LM, Gibson TD, White KL: The epidemiology of cardiac failure. *J Chronic Dis* 18:797–814, 1965.
10. Vasan RS, Benjamin ET, Levy D: Prevalence, clinical features and prognosis of diastolic heart failure. An epidemiological perspective. *J Am Coll Cardiol* 26:1565–1574, 1995.
11. Brutsaert DL, Sys SA, Gillebert TC: Diastolic failure: Pathophysiology and therapeutic implications. *J Am Coll Cardiol* 22:318–325, 1993.
12. Frank S, Braunwald E: Idiopathic hypertrophic subaortic stenosis: Clinical analysis of 126 patients with emphasis on the natural history. *Circulation* 37:759–788, 1968.

13. Pomerance A, Davies M: Pathological features of hypertrophic obstructive cardiomyopathy (HOCM) in the elderly. *Br Heart J* 37:305–312, 1975.
14. Bellone P, Spirito P: Diagnosis of HCM in the elderly. *Cardiol Elderly* 3: 405–408, 1995.
15. Spirito P, Maron BJ: Relation between extent of left ventricular hypertrophy and age in hypertrophic cardiomyopathy. *J Am Coll Cardiol* 13: 820–823, 1989.
16. Lewis JF, Maron BJ: Clinical and morphological expression of hypertrophic cardiomyopathy in patients > or =65 years of age. *Am J Cardiol* 73: 1105–1111, 1994.
17. Fay WP, Taliercio CP, Ilstrup DM, et al: Natural history of hypertrophic cardiomyopathy in the elderly. *J Am Coll Cardiol* 16:821–826, 1990.
18. Peliccia F, Cianfrocca C, Romeo F, et al: Natural history of hypertrophic cardiomyopathy in the elderly. *Cardiology* 78:329–333, 1991.
19. Oakley CM: Aetiology, diagnosis, investigation and management of the cardiomyopathies. *Br Med J* 315:1520–1524, 1997.
20. Agatson AS, Polakoff R, Hippogoankar et al: The significance of increased left ventricular outflow tract velocities in the elderly measured by continuous wave Doppler. *Am Heart J* 117:1320–1326, 1989.
21. Topol EJ, Traill TA, Fortuin NJ: Hypertensive hypertrophic cardiomyopathy. *N Engl J Med* 312:277, 1985.
22. Lever HM, Karam RF, Currie PJ, et al: Hypertrophic cardiomyopathy in the elderly: Distinctions from the young based on cardiac shape. *Circulation* 79:580–589, 1989.
23. Aronow WS, Kronzon L: Prevalence of hypertrophic cardiomyopathy and its association with mitral annular calcification in elderly patients. *Chest* 94:1295–1296, 1988.
24. Schwartz K, Carrier L, Guicheney P, et al: Molecular basis of familial cardiomyopathies. *Circulation* 91:532–540, 1995.
25. Burn J, Camm J, Davies MJ, et al: The phenotype/genotypic relation and the current status of genetic screening in hypertrophic cardiomyopathy, Marfan syndrome and the long QT syndrome. *Heart* 70:110–116, 1997.
26. Schunkert H, Hense HW, Holmer SR, et al: Association between a deletion polymorphism of the angiotensin-converting enzyme gene and left ventricular hypertrophy. *N Engl J Med* 330:1634–1638, 1994.
27. Schunkert H, Paul M: Cardiac angiotensin converting enzyme and diastolic function of the heart. *Agents Action Suppl* 38:119–127, 1992.
28. Marian AJ, Yu QTM, Workman R, et al: Angiotensin-converting enzyme polymorphism in hypertrophic cardiomyopathy and sudden cardiac death. *Lancet* 342:1085–1086, 1993.
29. Davies MJ: The current status of myocardial disarray in hypertrophic cardiomyopathy. *Br Heart J* 51:361–363, 1984.
30. Lewis JF, Maron BJ: Elderly patients with hypertrophic cardiomyopathy: A subset with distinctive left ventricular morphology and progressive clinical course late in life. *J Am Coll Cardiol* 13:36–45, 1989.
31. Ryan MP, Cleland JGF, French JA, et al: The standard electrocardiogram as a screening test for hypertrophic cardiomyopathy. *Am J Cardiol* 76: 689–694, 1995.
32. Frenneaux P, Counihan PJ, Calforio ALP, et al: Abnormal blood pressure response during exercise in hypertrophic cardiomyopathy. *Circulation* 82: 1995–2202, 1991.
33. Spirito P, Bellone P: Natural history of hypertrophic cardiomyopathy. *Br Heart J* 72:510–512, 1994.

34. Spirito P, Maron BJ, Bonow RO, et al: Occurrence and significance of progressive left ventricular wall thinning and relative cavity dilatation in hypertrophic cardiomyopathy. *Am J Cardiol* 60:123–129, 1987.
35. Shapiro LM, Zezulka A: Hypertrophic cardiomyopathy: A common disease with a good prognosis. Five year experience of a district general hospital. *Br Heart J* 50:530–533, 1983.
36. Spirito P, Chiarell AF, Carratino L, et al: Clinical course and prognosis of hypertrophic cardiomyopathy in an outpatient population. *N Engl J Med* 320:749–755, 1989.
37. Maron BJ, Peterson EE, Maron MS, et al: Prevalence of hypertrophic cardiomyopathy in an outpatient population referred for echocardiographic study. *Am J Cardiol* 73:577–580, 1994.
38. Kofflard MJ, Waldstein DJ, Vos J, et al: Prognosis in hypertrophic cardiomyopathy observed in a large clinic population. *Am J Cardiol* 72:939–943, 1993.
39. Alvarez RF, Goodwin JF: Non-invasive assessment of diastolic function in hypertrophic cardiomyopathy on and off beta-adrenergic blocking drugs. *Br Heart J* 48:204–212, 1982.
40. Epstein SE, Rosng DR: Verapamil: Its potential for causing serious complications in patients with hypertrophic cardiomyopathy. *Circulation* 64:437–441, 1981.
41. Pollick C: Muscular subaortic stenosis: Hemodynamic and clinical improvement after disopyramide. *N Engl J Med* 307:997–999, 1982.
42. McKenna WJ, Harris L, Rowland E, et al: Amiodarone for long-term management of patients with hypertrophic cardiomyopathy. *Am J Cardiol* 54:802–810, 1984.
43. McKenna WJ, Oakley CM, Krikler DM, et al: Improved survival with amiodarone in patients with hypertrophic cardiomyopathy and ventricular tachycardia. *Br Heart J* 53:412–416, 1985.
44. Bircks W, Schulte HD: Surgical treatment of hypertrophic obstructive cardiomyopathy with special reference to complications and to atypical hypertrophic obstructive cardiomyopathy. *Eur Heart J* 4:187, 1983.
45. Beahrs MM, Tajik AJ, Seward JB, et al: Hypertrophic obstructive cardiomyopathy. Ten- to 21 year follow-up after partial septal myectomy. *Am J Cardiol* 51:1160, 1983.
46. Robbins RC, Stinson EB: Long-term results of left ventricular myotomy and myectomy for obstructive hypertrophic cardiomyopathy. *J Thorac Cardiovasc Surg* 111:586–594, 1996.
47. Leachman RD, Kragcer Z, Azic T, et al: Mitral valve replacement in hypertrophic cardiomyopathy. Ten year follow-up in 54 patients. *Am J Cardiol* 60:1416, 1987.
48. Chahine RA: Surgical versus medical therapy of hypertrophic cardiomyopathy: Ten year follow-up in 54 patients. *Am J Cardiol* 60:1416, 1987.
49. Fananapazir L, Cannon RO, Tripodi D, et al: Impact of dual-chamber permanent pacing in patients with obstructive hypertrophic cardiomyopathy with symptoms refractory to verapamil and b-adrenergic blocker therapy. *Circulation* 85:2149–2161, 1992.
50. Nishimura RA, Hayes DL, Ilstrup DM, et al: Effect of dual chamber pacing on systolic and diastolic function in patients with hypertrophic cardiomyopathy. *J Am Coll Cardiol* 27:421–430, 1996.
51. Kappenberger L, Linde C, Daubert C, et al: Pacing in hypertrophic obstructive cardiomyopathy. A randomised cross-over study. *Eur Heart J* 18:1249–1256, 1997.

52. Sigwart U: Non-surgical myocardial reduction for hypertrophic obstructive cardiomyopathy. *Lancet* 346:211–213, 1995.
53. Waller BF, Maron BJ, Epstein SE, et al: Transmural myocardial infarction in hypertrophic cardiomyopathy: A cause of conversion from left ventricular asymmetry to symmetry and from normal-sized to dilated left ventricular cavity. *Chest* 79:461, 1981.
54. Goodwin JF, Oakley CM: The cardiomyopathies. *Br Heart J* 34:545–552, 1972.
55. Del GW, Fuster V: Idiopathic Dilated Cardiomyopathy. *N Engl J Med* 331:1564–1575, 1994.
56. Kasper EK, Agema WRP, Hutchins GM, et al: The causes of dilated cardiomyopathy: A clinicopathologic review of 673 consecutive patients. *J Am Coll Cardiol* 72:344–348, 1994.
57. Keeling PJ, Tracy S: Link between enteroviruses and dilated cardiomyopathy in serological and molecular data. *Br Heart J* 72:525–529, 1994.
58. Messtroni L, Krajinovin M, Severini GM, et al: Familial dilated cardiomyopathy. *Br Heart J* 72:S35–41, 1994.
59. Oldfors A, Erikson BO, Kylieman M, et al: Dilated cardiomyopathy and the dystrophin gene: an illustrated review. *Br Heart J* 72:344–348, 1994.
60. Pohtano L, Nigro V, Nigro G, et al: Development of cardiomyopathy in female carriers of Duchenne and Becker muscular dystrophies. *JAMA* 275:1335–1338, 1996.
61. Muntoni F, Di Lenarda A Di, Percu M, et al: Dystrophin gene abnormalities in two patients with idiopathic dilated cardiomyopathy. *Heart* 78:608–612, 1997.
62. Grogan M, Smith HC, Gersh BJ, et al: Left ventricular dysfunction due to atrial fibrillation in patients initially believed to have idiopathic dilated cardiomyopathy. *Am J Cardiol* 69:1570–1573, 1992.
63. Rakar S, Sinagra G, Di Lenarda A, et al: Epidemiology of dilated cardiomyopathy. *Eur Heart J* 18:117–123, 1997.
64. Regan TJ: Alcohol and the cardiovascular system. A review. *JAMA* 264:377–381, 1991.
65. Schwaltz RG, McKenzie WB, Alexander J, et al: Congestive heart failure and left ventricular dysfunction complicating doxorubicin therapy. *Am J Med* 82:1109–1118, 1987.
66. Garg R, Yusuf S: Overview of randomized trials of angiotensin-converting enzyme inhibitors on mortality and morbidity in patients with heart failure. *JAMA* 273:1450–1456, 1995.
67. Yusuf S: Digoxin in heart failure: Results of the recent digoxin investigation group trial in the context of other treatment for heart failure. *Eur Heart J* 18:1685–1688, 1997.
68. Del GW, Fuster V: Idiopathic cardiomyopathy. *N Engl J Med* 331:1564–1575, 1994.
69. Zarembski DG, Nolan PE, Slack MK, et al: Meta-analysis of the use of low dose beta-adrenergic blocking therapy in idiopathic or ischemia dilated cardiomyopathy. *Am J Cardiol* 77:1247–1250, 1996.
70. Pitt B, Segal R, Martnezz FA, et al: On behalf of ELITE Study Investigators. Randomised trial of losartan versus captopril in patients over 65 with heart failure (Evaluation of losartan in the Elderly Study ELITE). *Lancet* 349:747–752, 1997.
71. Stevenson WG: Mechanisms and management of arrhythmias in heart failure. *Curr Opin Cardiol* 10:274–281, 1995.

72. Monson JP, Besser GM: The potential for growth hormone in the management of heart failure 77:1–2, 1997.
73. Brecker SJD, Gibson DG: What is the role of pacing in dilated cardiomyopathy? *Eur Heart J* 17:819–823, 1996.
74. Skelton CL: The heart and hyperthyroidism. *N Engl J Med* 307:1206–1208, 1982.
75. Shenoy MM, Goldman JM: Hypothyroid cardiomyopathy. Echocardiographic documentation of reversibility. *Am J Med Sci* 294:1–9, 1987.
76. Starling MR: Does a clinically definable diabetic cardiomyopathy exist? *J Am Coll Cardiol* 15:1518–1520, 1990.
77. Factor SM, Minnase T, Sonnenblick EH: Clinical and morphological features of human hypertensive-diabetic cardiomyopathy. *Am Heart J* 99: 446–458, 1980.
78. Chanson P, Timsit J, Marquet C, et al: Cardiovascular effects of the somatostatin analog octreotide in acromegaly. *Ann Intern Med* 113:921–925, 1990.
79. Candell-Riera J, Lu L, Seres L, et al: Cardiac hemochromatosis: Beneficial effects of iron removal thereapy. An echocardiographic study. *Am J Cardiol* 52:824–829, 1983.
80. Hawkins DN: The diagnosis, natural history and treatment of amyloidosis. *J R Coll Physicians Lond* 31:552–557, 1997.
81. Oakley CM: Amyloid heart disease and cardiomyopathies difficult to classify. In: J Goodwin, E Olsen, (eds.) *Cardiomyopathies.* Springer-Verlag 1993, pp 193–214.
82. Falk R, Plehn J, Deering T, et al: Sensitivity and specificity of the echocardiographic features of cardiac amyloidosis. *Am J Cardiol* 59:418–422, 1987.
83. Nicolosi GL, Pavan D, Lestuzzi C, et al: Prospective identification of patients with amyloid heart disease by two dimensional echocardiography. *Circulation* 70:432–437, 1984.
84. Klein A, Hatle L, Taliercio C, et al: Prognostic significance of Doppler measures of diastolic function in cardiac amyloidosis. A Doppler echocardiographic study. *Circulation* 83:808–816, 1991.

Chapter 19

Pathophysiology of Chronic Heart Failure

Inder S. Anand

The last two decades have seen remarkable changes in the epidemiology of cardiovascular disease. During this period, whereas the mortality from coronary heart disease, hypertension, and stroke has declined, the incidence and prevalence of chronic heart failure (CHF) have markedly increased.[1-3] The number of new cases of heart failure diagnosed in the United States has increased from 250,000 in 1970 to over 700,000 in 1990. As a result, the prevalence of heart failure has reached 5 million cases, or nearly 1.5% of the United States population. The most striking increase is seen in the aged population, making CHF a disease predominantly of the elderly. More than 80% of patients with CHF in the United States are aged 65 years or older. In a 30-year follow-up study from Framingham,[4] the prevalence of CHF was reported as 1% at 25 to 54 years, 4.5% at 65 to 74 years, and 10% above age 75. Indeed, heart failure has now become the most common cause for admission to hospital in those over 65 years of age.[3] As might be expected, the economic cost of managing heart failure is very high. In 1991, Medicare expenditure on hospitalization for heart failure was $5.45 billion, or more than twice the expenditure for treatment of all types of cancer, and substantially more than the $3.18 billion spent on treatment of myocardial infarction. Estimates of the direct costs of heart failure treatment range from $10 to $40 billion.[5]

There are several factors that contribute to the increased prevalence of CHF; the most important being the increased size of the aging population. Elderly people are at greater risk of developing CHF because of age-related changes in the cardiovascular system and the high

From *Clinical Cardiology in the Elderly. Second Edition,* edited by Elliot Chesler. © 1999, Futura Publishing Company, Armonk, NY.

prevalence of hypertension, coronary artery disease, and valvular heart disease. Also, improved management of myocardial infarction allows patients with left ventricular (LV) dysfunction to survive longer, only to develop CHF at a later date. Similarly, better control of hypertension has resulted in a marked decline in stroke mortality,[2] but these same patients are at risk for CHF. Therefore, the combination of age-related changes in the cardiovascular system and high prevalence of common etiologies of CHF in older people has resulted in an exponential increase in the prevalence of CHF in the elderly.

Age Related Changes in the Cardiovascular System

Aging has profound effects on the cardiovascular system that impairs the ability of the individual to respond normally to physiological (eg, exercise) or pathological (eg, hypertension, myocardial infarction) stress even in the absence of cardiovascular disease.[6,7]

Structural Alterations

The most consistent changes are in the peripheral vasculature, where increased deposition of connective tissue in the walls of large elastic arteries decreases vascular distensibility and compliance. Decreased vascular compliance is manifested as a linear increase in pulse wave velocity with age, which occurs in all populations, irrespective of the presence or absence of atherosclerosis.[7] These changes in vascular compliance increase LV afterload and contribute to the development of isolated systolic hypertension, and LV hypertrophy. Stiffness of the heart is also increased with aging. Several factors contribute to increase in stiffness. With aging there is a progressive attrition of cardiac myocytes due to apoptosis.[6,8] It is estimated that approximately 35% of total cardiac myocytes may be lost with age. Since myocytes are terminally differentiated and cannot be replaced, their place is taken by compensatory hypertrophy of the remaining myocytes and an increase in interstitial connective tissue. This process results in LV hypertrophy, increase in wall thickness, and myocardial stiffness. The LV cavity dimensions usually do not change.[9] Also, thickening and calcification of the aortic and mitral valves may lead to significant valvular stenosis and or regurgitation, contributing further to ventricular afterload.

Physiological Alterations

In rats, progressive changes in several key steps in excitation-contraction coupling lead to a prolongation of contraction and delay in relaxation of senescent cardiac myocytes. Slowed inactivation of the L type sarcolemmal Ca^{++} channels prolongs the transmembrane axon potential, and a reduction in sarcoplasmic reticular Ca^{++}-adenosine triphosphatase (ATPase) contributes to prolongation of cytosolic Ca^{++} transient.[7] Although the capacity of the cardiac muscle to generate force is not altered with age, there is a marked shift in the myosin heavy chain isozymes from the faster α or V_1 isozymes to the slower β or V_3 isozyme in older rats.[7] In addition, the contractile response to β_1-adrenergic receptor stimulation is attenuated with aging, due to molecular and biochemical changes at multiple levels in the adrenergic pathway.[10] In the vasculature, endothelium-dependent vasodilatation is reduced with age, but the endothelium-independent vasodilation is not affected. In the absence of disease, the maximal coronary vasodilating reserve remains unchanged with age.[11]

Functional Alterations

The multiple structural and physiological age-related changes in the cardiovascular system, described above, may have important consequences during stress and with onset of disease. Increase in cardiac stiffness and slow myocardial relaxation result in impaired ventricular filling during diastole. Early ventricular filling is slowed, resulting in delayed upstroke and slow downslope of the E-wave on echo-Doppler mitral filling pattern. The left atrium hypertrophies and enlarges to augment ventricular filling. This is seen in the Doppler signal as a large A-wave. In older people, therefore, the contribution of the atrial "kick" to ventricular filling becomes more important and 30% to 40% of LV filling may be attributable to atrial contraction.[12] These age-related changes in diastolic filling may have other important implications. Impaired diastolic filling raises left atrial pressure. This may explain the increased propensity to develop diastolic heart failure in older patients, with even mild ischemia-induced changes in myocardial relaxation, or with mild increase in blood pressure. Stretch of atrial myocytes also increases the likelihood of atrial arrhythmias and contributes to the high prevalence of atrial fibrillation in the elderly. In contrast to altered diastolic function, the systolic contractile performance of the heart is generally well maintained at rest in the normal elderly individual. However, exercise performance and maximum oxygen consumption is depressed. There are several reasons why elderly patients have poor exercise capacity. The most important factor is a general decrease in β-adrenergic responsiveness that leads to reduced augmentation of heart rate and myocardial contractility, and diminished arterial vasodilatation with exercise. Another important factor is increased impedance to LV ejection due to decreased vascular compliance, and inadequate endothelium-dependent vasodilatation during exercise.[11]

To summarize, age-associated changes in the cardiovascular structure and function combine to reduce the capacity of the older individuals to respond normally to both cardiovascular physiological stress and disease states. These factors greatly increase the risk of developing CHF in the elderly.

Etiology of CHF in the Elderly

The cardiovascular diseases that cause heart failure in the elderly are much the same as in younger patients. The major difference is that the disease processes are superimposed on the age-associated changes described above. Moreover, several diseases often coexist in the same patient. Thus the clinical manifestation of common cardiac diseases may be modified, making diagnosis more difficult.

Hypertension and coronary heart disease still account for more than 70% of all cases of CHF in the elderly.[13] Valvular heart disease is frequently seen, and calcific aortic stenosis is the second most common indication for open heart surgery in patients over 70 years of age.[14] Aortic stenosis is often misdiagnosed because the typical physical signs may be absent. Mitral regurgitation is frequently encountered and may be caused by myxomatous degeneration of the leaflets, ischemic papillary muscle dysfunction, altered ventricular geometry in ischemic, nonischemic dilated cardiomyopathy, and mitral annular calcification. Rheumatic mitral regurgitation is less common, and mitral stenosis rare.

Nonischemic cardiomyopathy is less common among older patients, and when present is either idiopathic or a result of alcohol abuse. With widespread use of echocardiography, hypertrophic cardiomyopathy is increasingly recognized. Senile cardiac amyloidosis, is an occasional cause of restrictive cardiomyopathy; Myocarditis is rare.

High-output failure as a cause of fluid retention in the elderly must always be kept in mind; the diagnosis is often missed because it is uncommon. Chronic anemia, AV fistula (usually a dialysis fistula), hyperthyroidism, and thiamine deficiency are the common causes of high-output failure. Obstructive sleep apnea, because of carbon dioxide retention and hypoxia, often presents with severe fluid retention and may be difficult to manage without continuous positive airways pressure (CPAP).

Finally, a large number of patients with clinical signs and symptoms of CHF have normal systolic function. In these patients, heart failure is often attributed to diastolic dysfunction. The incidence and prevalence of diastolic heart failure is unknown and a prospective study has not been designed to examine this problem. Although some reports state that up to 40% of patients with CHF is a result of diastolic dysfunction, a figure of 20% is probably more realistic.[15,16] Most often, diastolic dysfunction occurs in patients who also have systolic dysfunction.

Contractile Function of the Failing Heart

Hypertension and myocardial infarction are the two important causes of heart failure. In the former, pressure overload leads to concentric left ventricular hypertrophy. Increased LV wall thickness is initially sufficient to maintain systolic wall stress within normal limits.[17] At the cellular level, myofibrils are laid down in parallel and sarcomeres in series, so that both length and cross sectional area of the individual myocytes is increased.[18] At this stage of compensatory hypertrophy, global systolic function may be normal.[19] However, papillary muscle obtained from hearts with pressure overload develop subtle contractile abnormalities even when global function is normal: Maximal isometric force or extent of isotonic shortening remain normal, but the velocity of shortening and relaxation are reduced.[20,21] If severe pressure overload persists, myocardial contractility eventually becomes depressed and the ventricle begins to fail.[19] As the ventricle dilates, wall stress increases further reducing myocardial fiber shortening, leading to more dilatation, initiating a vicious cycle. The transition from hypertrophy to heart failure is accompanied by intrinsic abnormalities of the cardiac muscle[20,22] and myocytes.[23] This process can be delayed, however, by inhibiting the renin-angiotensin-aldosterone system (RAAS) with angiotensin-converting enzyme (ACE) inhibitors.[23] In the senescent heart, drop-out of myocytes due to apoptosis[8] adds an additional stress to pressure overload, and this may hasten the transition to heart failure.

The sequence of events occuring in the heart after myocardial infarction is very different. Unlike pressure overload hypertrophy, global ventricular function is often depressed at the outset, because of myocardial necrosis. Soon after an infarct, the ventricle undergoes a series of complex changes termed remodeling.[24] During the first few days, infarct expansion increases ventricular volume and wall stress that may, in turn, decrease contractile state of the remote normal myocardium because of afterload mismatch.[25] Ventricular hypertrophy that ensues is eccentric and inadequate, so that wall tension remains markedly elevated.[25] At the cellular level, myocyte hypertrophy is characterized by greater increase in myocyte length than cross sectional area.[26] Also, considerable remodeling of the extracellular matrix occurs both at the site of myocardial necrosis and in areas remote from it. RAAS activation plays a prominent role in extracellular matrix remodeling.[27] It is unclear whether the myocardium develops intrinsic contractile abnormality as seen in hearts subjected to pressure overload. Recent data suggest that myocytes isolated from the remote myocardium may remain normal despite global LV dysfunction.[26] Therefore, intrinsic myocyte contractile abnormalities may not be present in the postmyocardial infarction remodeled heart, and nonmyocyte factors such as increased wall stress, interstitial tissue abnormalities, and myocyte loss from necrosis and apoptosis could account for most of the global LV dysfunction. Ventricular remodeling once established, is a self perpetuating process and progresses relentlessly to heart failure. The mechanisms involved in the progression of LV dysfunction remain unclear. However, ACE inhibitors and perhaps even β-adrenergic blockers can arrest or even reverse this process.[28]

Adaptive Mechanisms

When LV dysfunction sets in and cardiac output falls the heart has three important adaptive mechanisms to maintain pump function and restore circulatory homeostasis: (1) activation of neurohormones, that helps to increase cardiac output and maintain blood pressure by causing vasoconstriction, augmenting myocardial contractility, and increasing blood volume through renal retention of salt and water; (2) Frank-Starling mechanism, that utilizes the increased preload to further improve cardiac performance; and (3) myocardial hypertrophy, where increase in contractile mass helps to augment myocardial function.

Neurohormonal Activation

Neurohormonal activation in CHF is initially a beneficial adaptive response. Eventually however, excessive production of neurohormones becomes maladaptive leading to progression of heart failure through a variety of mechanisms including necrotic and apoptotic myocyte death, and myocardial fibrosis with continuous LV remodeling.

Two sets of neurohormones, with opposing effects, are activated in heart failure. The vasoconstrictor hormones are also antinatriuretic and antidiuretic, and generally have growth promoting properties. The vasodilator hormones, on the other hand, are natriuretic and diuretic and have antimitogenic effects. In CHF, the natriuretic and vasodilator

---

Table 1
Neurohormonal Systems Activated in Chronic Heart Failure

Vasoconstrictor Hormones	Vasodilator Hormones
Sympathetic nervous system	Atrial and brain natriuretic peptides
Norepinephrine (NE)	Prostaglandins
Epinephrine	Kallikrein-kinin system
Renin-angiotensin-aldosterone system	
(RAAS)	
Arginine vasopressin (AVP)	

effects are clearly overwhelmed by influences that lead to vasoconstriction, and salt and water retention. We are now beginning to understand some of the other effects of these hormones, especially on cell growth and ventricular remodeling. A better understanding of these actions will help us design novel approaches to the management of heart failure. Table 1 lists the neurohormones that have been well studied in heart failure.

Sympathetic Nervous System

It has been known for many years that there is increased activity of the sympathetic nervous system (SNS) in heart failure demonstrated by an increase in circulating norepinephrine (NE).[29] Levels of epinephrine are usually not elevated in heart failure. The earliest increase in sympathetic activity is detected in the heart, before an increase in renal and muscle sympathetic activity, and precedes the rise in plasma NE.[30] Moreover, myocardial sympathetic activity increases early in the natural history of LV dysfunction, even before an increase in ventricular volume or end-diastolic pressure,[31] and onset of symptoms.[32] Levels of NE are higher in patients with symptomatic heart failure and increase in proportion to the severity of the disease.[32]

Augmented sympathetic activity in heart failure is initially beneficial. It increases cardiac output and redistributes blood flow from the splanchnic area to the heart and skeletal muscles. Renal vasoconstriction leads to salt and water retention which may help improve perfusion of vital organs. However, sustained sympathetic stimulation, as seen in heart failure, activates the RAAS and other neurohormones leading to progressive salt and water retention, vasoconstriction, edema and increased preload and afterload. These developments, in turn, increase ventricular wall stress, resulting in higher myocardial oxygen demand and myocardial ischemia. Excessive sympathetic activity may also predispose to ventricular arrhythmias. Finally, NE has many direct effects on cardiac myocytes including induction of fetal gene programs, down regulation of calcium-regulating genes, myocyte hypertrophy, apoptosis and necrosis. Therefore, although the initial sympathetic nervous system response appears to be adaptive and helps support blood pressure and cardiac output, prolonged and excessive sympathetic activation may have deleterious effects. Indeed, patients with heart failure and high plasma NE have been shown to have a worse prognosis[33] and inhibiting the sympathetic activity is therapeutically beneficial.[34]

The mechanisms responsible for excessive sympathetic activation in heart failure are not entirely clear. The stimulus appears to be an early and sustained attenuation of cardiac and arterial baroreceptor control of sympathetic nerve activity due to a decrease in baroreceptor afferent discharge.[35] When heart failure is established, increased peripheral chemoreceptor sensitivity and augmented muscle mechanoreceptor discharge may further modulate sympathetic activity.[35]

In addition to changes in circulating NE, cardiac stores of NE are also altered in heart failure. Atrial and ventricular stores of NE are reduced due to depletion of the neurotransmitter in the adrenergic nerve ending.[36] Moreover, marked down regulation of the β-adrenergic receptor density and abnormalities in the post-receptor pathway also occur in heart failure.[37] As a consequence of these changes, the failing heart loses an important compensatory mechanism.

RAAS

The importance of RAAS in heart failure has been known for nearly 50 years. Renin is released in response to a number of stimuli, commonly observed in heart failure, eg, reduced renal perfusion pressure, increased renal sympathetic activity, decreased delivery of sodium to the macula densa, and diuretic use. Angiotensin II (A II), the active end product of renin activity is a potent vasoconstrictor. Also, A II augments the presynaptic release of NE, and stimulates release of aldosterone (Aldo), promoting salt and water retention by the kidney. A II also has direct effects on the kidney. A II constricts efferent arterioles and helps maintain the glomerular filtration rate (GFR) and also causes sodium reabsorption by direct action on the renal tubules. Indirectly, through stimulation of thirst and vasopressin release, A II enhances water retention. RAAS is not activated in normal individuals and does not play a significant physiological role. However, in states of volume and salt depletion, as in hypotension, and heart failure, RAAS activity increases and exerts its vasoconstrictor and salt and water retaining effects.

Plasma renin activity (PRA) has generally been used as a measure of RAAS activity because A II is relatively difficult to measure. Levels of PRA vary considerably in heart failure. In patients with asymptomatic LV dysfunction[32] or untreated mild heart failure,[38] PRA is normal, and probably suppressed by atrial natriuretic peptide (ANP) (see later). However, PRA is usually elevated in patients with untreated severe heart failure,[39] and in patients on diuretics.[38] Because PRA is under negative feed-back control through blood volume and arterial blood pressure, its activity depends on the phase of fluid retention. Those who avidly retain salt and water or are hypotensive have higher PRA than those who have reached a new steady state. This explains the great variability of PRA in CHF.

RAAS activation is initially beneficial in heart failure and helps to preserve GFR, and support blood pressure. The same response, however, becomes deleterious if excessive and prolonged, because it may worsen the loading conditions of the heart. In addition, instead of preserving GFR, it reduces it by causing vasoconstriction in the afferent as well as efferent arterioles. In the myocardium, RAAS activity and locally produced A II influence the behavior of the myocytes and fibroblasts, leading to myocyte hypertrophy, necrosis and apoptosis, and increased collagen turnover. Collectively, these adverse effects of RAAS activation may contribute to progressive ventricular remodeling and worsening heart failure.[27] The effectiveness of ACE inhibitors in reducing morbidity and mortality in heart failure may be related to its blocking the deleterious effects of RAAS activity.

Arginine Vasopressin

Arginine vasopressin (AVP), released from the posterior pituitary, is another vasoconstrictor and water retaining hormone with mitogenic properties that may be potentially harmful in CHF. However, relatively little is known about this hormone in heart failure. AVP is increased in some but not all patients with CHF.[32,39,40] Under normal conditions osmoreceptors are the primary determinant of AVP release. In CHF, however, nonosmotic control of AVP release via sympathetic activation becomes more important. Therefore, despite hypo-osmolar hyponatremia, which often occurs in severe CHF and that should suppress AVP, levels remain inappropriately elevated.[39] AVP acts on the vascular smooth muscle V_1 receptors to cause vasoconstriction, and on V_2 receptors in distal tubules and collecting ducts to enhance reabsorption of water. AVP probably contributes to vasoconstriction and fluid retention in heart failure, because infusion of a specific V_1 receptor antagonist, improves hemodynamics. High levels of AVP may also contribute to dilutional hyponatremia in severe heart failure, a feature indicating poor prognosis.

Vasodilator Hormones

A number of endogenous vasodilators are involved in cardiovascular and renal homeostasis in heart failure. These important hormones are released from the heart (natriuretic peptides) and the kidney (prostaglandins and bradykinin). In addition, the vascular endothelium produces a potent vasodilator viz. endothelium-derived nitric oxide. However, the effects of all these endogenous vasodilators are significantly attenuated in CHF.

Atrial and Brain Natriuretic Peptides

ANP and brain natriuretic peptide (BNP) are a family of peptides that are synthesized primarily in atrial myocytes and released in response to atrial stretch. These peptides have natriuretic, vasodilator and antimitogenic properties. They also antagonize most endogenous vasoconstrictors by reducing sympathetic activity, and inhibiting renin and Aldo release. Levels of ANP and BNP are elevated early in heart failure, along with SNS activity, preceding activation of RAAS and before symptoms of LV dysfunction appear.[32,41] Because of these findings, measurement of ANP/BNP is emerging as an important non-invasive marker of LV dysfunction and a screening tool in the general population.[42] Animal studies suggest that the early increase in ANP is responsible for the maintenance of sodium balance and inhibition of RAAS in asymptomatic LV dysfunction.[43] As heart failure progresses, ANP and BNP levels increase, in proportion to the rise in atrial pressure and severity of LV dysfunction.[44,45] However, in severe heart failure, despite greatly increased ANP and BNP, their natriuretic and vasodilator responses are attenuated.[44,46] This may contribute to salt and water retention, and systemic and renal vasoconstriction manifest in severe heart failure. The mechanisms responsible for the attenuated response are unclear, and may be related to a number of factors including decrease in renal blood flow, increased renal sympathetic activity, ANP receptor downregulation, and enhanced enzymatic degradation of the peptides.

Intrarenal Hormones

A number of intrarenal hormonal systems may be activated in CHF. The important ones are the arachidonic acid cascade and the kallikrein-kinin system.

Prostaglandins

The renal arterioles, glomeruli, and some parts of renal tubules and the collecting ducts synthesize the vasodilator prostaglandins PGI_2, PGE_2, and PGF_{2a}.[47] The prominent effect of these prostaglandins is to protect the glomerular microcirculation during states of renal vasoconstriction by causing vasodilation, predominantly in the afferent arterioles, and also through promoting sodium excretion by directly inhibiting sodium transport in the distal tubules. Prostaglandin synthesis is increased during activation of the renin-angiotensin system, and renal sympathetics, and in clinical and experimental heart failure.[48] Prostaglandins probably do not modulate renal hemodynamics or sodium excretion in normal subjects but may play a major role in situations with elevated RAAS and sympathetic activity, as in CHF. Consequently, inhibition of prostaglandins with cyclooxygenase inhibitors may induce marked reduction of cardiac output and renal blood flow, increase in peripheral vascular resistance, and sodium retention.[48] Therefore, nonsteroidal anti-inflammatory drugs (NSAIDs) should be used with caution, particularly in elderly patients with CHF who often also have renal dysfunction.

Kallikrein-kinin System

The distal tubules of the kidney synthesize kallikrein, a protease which cleaves kininogen, to form bradykinin and kalliden. These peptides are degraded by the enzyme kininase II, which is the same as angiotensin converting enzyme. Both bradykinin and kalliden produce vasodilation and natriuresis, and the former also stimulates the production of prostaglandins.[49] Although the exact role of this system in CHF is unknown, there is evidence that at least some of the beneficial effects of ACE inhibitors on ventricular remodeling may be derived from an increase in bradykinin.[50]

Other Hormones

There has been a recent interest in the role of growth hormone (GH) in heart failure. GH is secreted by the anterior pituitary, and mediates its effects via activation of IGF-1. Levels of GH are elevated in the syndrome of severe untreated low and high output heart failure and also in patients with cardiac cachexia.[39,51,52] However, the exact role of GH in heart failure is not known. Treating heart failure with human GH has been shown to be beneficial in some but not all studies.[53] Cortisol is another anterior pituitary hormone which is also elevated in various syndromes of CHF, possibly as part of a general stress response.[39,51]

In addition to the neurohormonal activation described above, it has become evident during the last few years that another class of biologically active molecules, termed cytokines are also over secreted by cells in heart failure. Important among these are endothelins, tumor necrosis factor-α, and interleukin-6. These cytokines appear to exert deleterious effects on the heart and circulation and may be involved in the progression of heart failure.[54]

The neurohormonal responses described above are seen in patients with low output CHF. However, an identical neurohormonal response and retention of salt and water also occurs in a number of conditions where the heart is entirely normal and the cardiac output is even higher than normal. So called "high output congestive heart failure" is seen in diverse conditions including chronic severe anemia, chronic AV fistula, beri-beri, Paget's disease, and chronic obstructive pulmonary disease, states with divergent hemodynamics.[51] The common factor, in all these conditions is a tendency towards low arterial blood pressure. Blood pressure is threatened in low output states because of low cardiac output and in high output states because of decrease in systemic vascular resistance. The neurohormonal response of the body is, however, similar. The same neurohormonal response is also seen whenever blood pressure is reduced; for example, during acute reduction of arterial pressure with nitroprusside,[55] and during physical exercise,[56] where blood pressure is threatened by marked vasodilatation in exercising muscles. These findings, therefore, support the view that the neurohormonal response evoked during CHF is nonspecific and the same that was evolved to support survival of the species under two main circumstances that threaten life, ie, hemorrhage and physical exercise.[57] In these conditions, a short-term threat to blood pressure evokes a baroreceptor-mediated increase in sympathetic activity that causes venoconstriction, tachycardia, stimulation of the myocardium, and regional vasoconstriction. When blood pressure is threatened by reduced cardiac output due to LV dysfunction, the body cannot distinguish whether the threat is from hemorrhage, exercise or heart disease, and therefore uses the same stereotype response for which it is programmed. In heart disease (and other sustained vasodilated high output states), however, blood pressure is threatened over a prolonged period. Therefore, the effector mechanisms continue to operate as long as the threat persists. Unfortunately, prolonged neurohormonal activation is deleterious and may lead to progression of CHF.

Conclusions

CHF has become a major public health problem because of the aging population. As people age, a series of age-associated changes occur in the cardiovascular system. Older people also have a high prevalence of common cardiovascular diseases. When multiple cardiovascular diseases are superimposed on the age-associated changes, LV function is adversely affected, leading to an exponential rise in the prevalence of CHF. Left ventricular dysfunction once established is a progressive process and sets in motion a series of complex changes which are initially adaptive. Central to this is neurohormonal activation that starts early in the natural history of LV dysfunction and helps to maintain circulatory homeostasis. Prolonged neurohormonal activation ultimately becomes deleterious. Progression of heart failure is associated with increased neurohormonal activity. High levels of circulating neurohormones predict a poor prognosis. Drugs like ACE inhibitors and β-blockers that inhibit neurohormones delay the progression of heart failure. Such data support the view that the progression of heart failure is related to the deleterious effects of excessive neurohormonal activation.

References

1. Centers for Disease Control and Prevention: Trends in ischemic heart disease mortality: United States, 1980–1988. *MMWR* 41:548–556, 1992.
2. Centers for Disease Control and Prevention: Cerebrovascular disease mortality and Medicare hospitalization: United States, 1980–1990. *MMWR* 41: 477–480, 1992.

3. Ghali JK, Cooper R, Ford E: Trends in hospitalization rates for heart failure in the United States. *Arch Intern Med* 150:769–773, 1990.
4. Kannel WB, Belanger AJ: Epidemiology of heart failure. *Am Heart J* 121: 951–957, 1991.
5. Konstam M, Dracup K, Baker G, et al: *Heart Failure: Evaluation and Care of Patients with Left Ventricular Systolic Dysfunction. Clinical Practice Guidelines* No. 11. Agency for Health Care Policy and Research, Rockville, MD, 1994.
6. Wei JY: Age and the cardiovascular system. *N Engl J Med* 327:1735–1739, 1992.
7. Lakatta EG. Cardiovascular regulatory mechanisms in advanced age. *Physiol Rev* 73:413–467, 1993.
8. Olivetti G, Giordano G, Corradi D, et al: Gender differences and aging: Effects on the human heart. *J Am Coll Cardiol* 26:1068–1079, 1995.
9. Gerstinblith G, Frederikeriksen J, Yin FC, et al: Echocardiographic assessment of normal adult population. *Circulation* 56:273–278, 1997.
10. Harding SE, Jones SM, O'Gara P, et al: Isolated ventricular myocytes from failing and non-failing heart: The relation of age and clinical status to isoproterenol response. *J Mol Cell Cardiol* 24:549–564, 1992.
11. Lakatta EG, Gerstenblith G, Weisfeldt ML: The aging heart: Structure, function, and disease. In: E Braunwald, eds: *Heart Disease: A Textbook of Cardiovascular Medicine*. 4th ed. W.B. Saunders Co, Philadelphia, 1997, pp 1687–1703.
12. Arora RR, Machac J, Goldman Me, et al: Atrial kinetics and left ventricular diastolic filling in the healthy elderly. *J Am Coll Cardiol* 9:1255–1260, 1987.
13. Ho KKL, Pinsky JL, Kannel WB, et al: The epidemiology of heart failure: The Framingham Study. *J Am Coll Cardiol* 22(Suppl A):6–13A, 1993.
14. Rahimtoola SH, Cheitlin MD, Hutter AM: Valvular and congenital heart disease. *J Am Coll Cardiol* 10(Suppl A):60–62A, 1987.
15. Bonow RO, Udelsen JE: Left ventricular diastolic dysfunction as a cause of congestive heart failure. Mechanisms and management. *Ann Intern Med* 117:502–510, 1992.
16. Vasan RS, Benjamin EJ, Levy D: Prevalence, clinical features and prognosis of diastolic heart failure. An epidemiologic perspective. *J Am Coll Cardiol* 26:1565–1574 1995.
17. Grossman W, Jones D, McLaurin LP. Wall stress and patterns of hypertrophy in the human left ventricle. *J Clin Invest* 56:56–64, 1975.
18. Anversa P, Ricci R, Olivetti G. Quantitative structural analysis of the myocardium during physiologic growth and induced cardiac hypertrophy: A review. *J Am Coll Cardiol* 7:1140–1149, 1986.
19. Aoyagi T, Fujii AM, Flanagan MF, et al: Transition from compensated hypertrophy to intrinsic myocardial dysfunction during development of left ventricular pressure-overload hypertrophy in conscious sheep. Systolic dysfunction precedes diastolic dysfunction. *Circulation* 88:2415, 1993.
20. Spann JF, Buccino RA, Sonnenblick EH, et al: Contractile state of cardiac muscle obtained from cats with experimentally produced ventricular hypertrophy. *Circ Res* 21:34, 1967.
21. Crozatier B, Hittinger L. Mechanical adaptation to chronic pressure overload. *Eur Heart J* 9:7, 1988.
22. Cooper G 4th, Tomanek RJ, Ehrhardt JD, et al ; Chronic pressure overload of the cat right ventricle. *Circ Res* 48:488, 1981.

23. Kagaya Y, Hajjar RJ, Gwathmey JK, et al: Long-term angiotensin-converting enzyme inhibition with fosinopril improves depressed responsiveness to Ca^{2+} in myocytes from aortic-banded rats. *Circulation* 94:2915–2922, 1996.

24. Pfeffer MA, Braunwald E: Ventricular remodeling after myocardial infarction. Experimental observations and clinical implications. *Circulation* 81:1161–1172, 1990.

25. Mitchell GF, Lamas GA, Vaughan DE, et al: Left ventricular remodeling in the year after first anterior myocardial infarction: A quantitative analysis of contractile segment lengths and ventricular shape. *J Am Coll Cardiol* 19:1136–1144, 1992.

26. Anand IS, Liu D, Chugh SS, et al: Isolated myocyte contractile function is normal in postinfarct remodeled rat heart with systolic dysfunction. *Circulation* 96:3974–3984, 1997.

27. Waber KT: Extracellular matrix remodeling in heart failure: A role for de novo angiotensin II generation. *Circulation* 96:4065–4082, 1977.

28. Cohn JN; Overview of the treatment of heart failure. *Am J Cardiol* 80(11A):2L-6L, 1997.

29. Chidsey CA, Harrison DC, Braunwald E; Augmentation of the plasma norepinephrine response to exercise in patients with congestive heart failure. *N Engl J Med* 267:650–655, 1962.

30. Rundqvist B, Elam M, Bergmann-Sverrisdottir Y, et al: Increased cardiac adrenergic drive precedes generalized sympathetic activation in human heart failure. *Circulation* 95:169–175, 1997.

31. Imamura Y, Ando H, Ashihara T, et al: Myocardial adrenergic nervous activity is intensified in patients with heart failure without left ventricular volume or pressure overload. *J Am Coll Cardiol* 28:371–375, 1996.

32. Francis GS, Benedict C, Johnstone DE, et al: Comparison of neuroendocrine activation in patients with left ventricular dysfunction with and without congestive heart failure. A substudy of the Studies of Left Ventricular Dysfunction (SOLVD). *Circulation* 82:1724–1729, 1990.

33. Rector TS, Olivari MT, Levine TB, et al: Predicting survival for an individual with congestive heart failure using the plasma norepinephrine concentration. *Am Heart J* 114:148–152, 1987.

34. Packer M. Effects of beta-adrenergic blockade on survival of patients with chronic heart failure. *Am J Cardiol* 80(11A):46L-54L, 1997.

35. Middlekauff HR. Mechanisms and implications of autonomic nervous system dysfunction in heart failure. *Curr Opin Cardiol* 12:265–275, 1997.

36. Chidsey CA, Sonnenblick EH, Morrow AG, et al: Norepinephrine stores and contractile force of papillary muscle from the failing human heart. *Circulation* 33:43, 1966.

37. Bristow MR: Changes in myocardial and vascular receptors in heart failure. *J Am Coll Cardiol* 22:61A, 1993.

38. Bayliss J, Norell M, Canepa-Anson R, et al: Clinical and neuroendocrine effects of introducing diuretics. *Br Heart J* 57:17–22, 1987.

39. Anand IS, Ferrari R, Kalra GS, et al: Edema of cardiac origin. Studies of body water and sodium, renal function, hemodynamic indexes, and plasma hormones in untreated congestive cardiac failure. *Circulation* 80:299–305, 1989.

40. Goldsmith SR, Francis GS, Cowley AW, et al: Increased plasma arginine vasopressin levels in patients with congestive heart failure. *J Am Coll Cardiol* 1:1385–1390, 1983.

41. Redfield MM, Aarhus LL, Wright RS, et al: Cardiorenal and neurohumoral function in a canine model of early left ventricular dysfunction. *Circulation* 87:2016–2022, 1993.
42. Cowie MR, Struthers AD, Wood DA, et al: Value of natriuretic peptides in assessment of patients with possible new heart failure in primary care. *Lancet* 350:1349–1353, 1997.
43. Stevens TL, Burnett JC Jr, Kinoshita M, et al: A functional role of endogenous atrial natriuretic peptide in a canine model of early left ventricular dysfunction. *J Clin Invest* 95:1101–1108, 1995.
44. Cody JR, Atlas SA, Laragh JH, et al: Atrial natriuretic factor in normal subjects and heart failure patients. *J Clin Invest* 78:1362–1374, 1986.
45. Raine AEG, Erne P, Burgisser E, et al: Atrial natriuretic peptide and atrial pressure in patients with congestive heart failure. *N Engl J Med* 315:553, 1986.
46. Anand IS, Kalra GS, Ferrari R, et al: Hemodynamic, hormonal, and renal effects of atrial natriuretic peptide in untreated congestive heart failure. *Am Heart J* 118:500–505, 1989.
47. Schlondorff D, Ardailloui R: Prostaglandins and other arachidonic acid metabolites in the kidney. *Kidney Int* 29:108–119, 1986.
48. Dzau VJ, Packer M, Lilly LS, et al: Prostaglandins in severe congestive heart failure. *N Engl J Med* 310:347–352, 1984.
49. Stein JH, Congbaly RC, Karsh DL, et al: The effect of bradykinin on proximal tubular sodium reabsorption in the dog. Evidence for functional nephron heterogeneity. *J Clin Invest* 51:1709–1721, 1972.
50. McDonald KM, Garr M, Carlyle PF, et al: Relative effects of a1-adrenoceptor blockade, converting enzyme inhibitor therapy, and angiotensin II subtype 1 receptor blockade on ventricular remodeling in the dog. *Circulation* 90:3034–3046, 19954.
51. Anand IS: Pathogenesis of salt and water retention in the congestive heart failure syndrome. In: PA Poole-Wilson, WS Colucci, BM Massie, et al, eds: *Heart Failure*. Churchill Livingstone, New York, 1997, pp 155–172.
52. Anker SD, Chua TP, Ponikowaki P, et al: Hormonal changes and catabolic/anabolic imbalance in chronic heart failure and their importance in cardiac cachexia. *Circulation* 96:526–534, 1997.
53. Fazio S, Sabatini L, Capaldo B, et al: A preliminary study of growth hormone in the treatment of dilated cardiomyopathy. *N Engl J Med* 334:809–814, 1996.
54. Shan K, Kurrelmeyer K, Seta Y, et al: The role of cytokines in disease progression in heart failure. *Curr Opin Cardiol* 12:218–223, 1997.
55. Ferarri R, Ceconi C, De Guili F, et al: Temporal relations of the endocrine response to hypotension with sodium nitroprusside. *Cardioscience* 3:51–60, 1992.
56. Ferrari R, Ceconi C, Rodella A, et al: Temporal relations of the endocrine response to exercise. *Cardioscience* 2:131–139, 1991.
57. Harris P: Role of arterial pressure in the oedema of heart disease. *Lancet* 1:1036–1038, 1988.

Chapter 20

Management of Congestive Heart Failure

Gordon Pierpont

Although most physicians feel they understand the syndrome of congestive heart failure (CHF), a precise definition can be elusive. A reasonably inclusive description is: *decreased functional capacity due to inability of the heart to circulate blood adequately to meet physiologic demands.* This can occur because of abnormalities of the myocardium, valves, pericardium, or the pulmonary or systemic vasculature. Congenital malformation manifesting for the first time in the elderly is rare, and pericardial disease differs little from that seen in younger adults.[1] This chapter deals with heart failure due to myocardial dysfunction in the absence of severe systemic or pulmonary hypertension.

Mild to moderate aortic stenosis or mitral regurgitation are often present in elderly patients without being the primary cause of CHF. These lesions may be due to intrinsic valvular disease, or, in the case of mitral regurgitation, *secondary* to left ventricular enlargement and dyskinesis. Malalignment of the mitral apparatus leads to inadequate coaptation of the mitral leaflets and allows regurgitation. This secondary mitral regurgitation can be quite dynamic, being sensitive to preload, afterload, and ischemia-induced changes in regional wall motion.[2] Mitral regurgitation attributed to so-called papillary muscle dysfunction is actually a result of coexistent damage to the contiguous left ventricular wall.[3] Such mild to moderate valvular lesions may well contribute to the overall pathophysiology of CHF, but they are not readily amenable to surgical correction. Therapy is therefore oriented toward the same goals discussed below for myocardial failure, accepting the fact that some uncorrectable valve dysfunction may coexist.

From *Clinical Cardiology in the Elderly. Second Edition,* edited by Elliot Chesler. © 1999, Futura Publishing Company, Armonk, NY.

Evaluating Myocardial Dysfunction in the Elderly

The best therapy for most diseases is usually that which most specifically reverses the underlying pathophysiology. It is therefore reasonable to determine the etiology of myocardial dysfunction whenever possible. Unfortunately, this exercise is not as rewarding in geriatric patients with CHF as one would desire. Table 1 lists causes of myocardial dysfunction in the elderly, and it is evident that few are readily reversible. This table does not include all known or suspected causes of cardiomyopathy, only those more likely to be seen in geriatric patients.

Reversible Myocardial Dysfunction

Ischemic heart disease is by far the most frequent cause of myocardial dysfunction, and leads to infarction, scarring and left ventricular dilatation. If reversible ischemia is still present, revascularization can

---

Table 1
**Common Causes of Myocardial Dysfunction
and Heart Failure in the Elderly**

Myocardial Ischemia
   Acute
   Chronic
Idiopathic Cardiomyopathy
   Dilated
   Hypertrophic
   Restrictive
Myocardial Infiltration
   Amyloid
   Hemochromatosis
Toxic
   Alcohol
   Adriamycin
Metabolic
   Thyrotoxicosis
   Myxedema
Myocarditis
   Opportunistic infection in the immunocompromised
   Radiation
Miscellaneous
   Anemia
   Persistent tachycardia
   Arteriovenous shunts

---

be considered, providing the combined risk of older age and left ventricular dysfunction is not prohibitive. Occasionally, stunned or hibernating myocardium may regain function, but in most cases revascularization cannot be expected to improve ejection fraction. Myxedema heart failure can be treated with thyroid hormone replacement, and alcohol induced cardiomyopathy may improve with abstinence.[4] These few examples of potentially reversible heart failure are worth investigating if the clinical presentation warrants. Hypothyroidism, for example, can occur quite insidiously in the elderly, and can be readily diagnosed with standard thyroid function tests. However, in the absence of suggestive evidence of reversible etiology, expensive and/or extensive testing to determine precise myocardial pathology (myocardial biopsy, for example) in elderly patients with CHF is not likely to be fruitful, and therefore is rarely justified. In the absence of angina, or evidence of ischemia on exercise testing, coronary angiography is of questionable value.

Clinical Diagnosis

The manifestations of CHF can vary greatly depending on the nature of the myocardial disease, it's severity, and the relative extent to which other organs are secondarily involved. For this reason clinical criteria for making the diagnosis of CHF can be useful. Criteria established by The Framingham Investigators[5] include information from the medical history (*paroxysmal nocturnal dyspnea,* orthopnea or night cough, or dyspnea on exertion), findings on physical examination (*neck vein distention*, rales, *S3 gallop*, *hepatojugular reflux*, ankle edema, hepatomegaly, or tachycardia) and results of clinical tests (*cardiomegaly, acute pulmonary edema, increased central venous pressure, prolonged circulation time*, pleural effusion, or decreased vital capacity). None of these findings are specific for CHF, and the diagnosis is based on presence of 2 major (major criteria in italics above) or 1 major and 2 minor criteria (minor criteria in roman type). Weight loss of more than 4.5 kg in response to therapy can also be used as a major or minor criteria.

Pathophysiology

The clinical diagnosis of CHF due to myocardial dysfunction can be confirmed by demonstrating abnormal regional or global left ventricular wall motion. As noted previously, extensive diagnostic testing is usually not necessary in the elderly because the etiology is often obvious (ie, old myocardial infarction), or likely to be irremediable. However, it is important to perform those studies needed to fully characterize the cardiac abnormalities in ways that help guide therapy. Toward this end CHF can be considered in 4 categories related to physiology and functional anatomy rather than basic etiology. These are: (1) high versus low cardiac output; (2) right versus left heart failure; (3) dilated vs hypertrophic cardiomyopathy; and (4) systolic versus diastolic dysfunction.

High versus Low Output Failure

High output heart failure is relatively rare, and especially so in the elderly. High output failure does not occur due to intrinsic cardiac muscle dysfunction, but rather to inability of normal or mildly compromised myocardium to keep up with excess demands. As such, high output failure will be discussed only briefly to contrast with the major focus of this chapter, which is the much more common low output failure.

The causes of high output failure are few, and when seen in the elderly, anemia, thyrotoxicosis, or large arteriovenous shunts should be suspected. These conditions usually do not provide a diagnostic challenge, as they are generally both severe and persistent in order to precipitate CHF. Therapy is supportive while the primary problem is being addressed. When severe anemia precipitates CHF, diuretics are often necessary to decrease intravascular volume overload and allow room for red cell replacement. Thyrotoxicosis may be controlled with judicious use of β-adrenergic blockade, until the excess production of thyroxin is eliminated. Peripheral shunting may be correctable, as in the case of atrioventricular (AV) fistulae established for renal dialysis. High output failure may also occur with intrahepatic shunts in patients with cirrhosis of the liver.[6] In this case, therapy is directed at controlling fluid retention with diuretics. The role of digitalis in high output failure is questionable, and since these patients already have a low peripheral vascular resistance, there is little rationale for using vasodilators. Other causes of AV shunting, such as congenital AV malformations, Beriberi, or Paget's disease of bone could be considered in the differential diagnosis of high output CHF, but are unlikely to be seen in the elderly.

Right versus Left Heart Failure

The right and left ventricles are obviously inextricably connected, both anatomically and functionally. As such, whatever adversely effects one ventricle is likely to also alter the function of the other. Indeed, isolated left heart failure suggests a relatively acute or subacute process, as long standing left heart failure usually leads to, and is the most common cause of, right heart failure. Nonetheless, it is clinically useful to assess the relative degree to which each side of the heart is compromised.

The cardinal signs of right heart failure (neck vein distention, large c-v wave, hepatojugular reflux, peripheral edema) are non-specific, but the severity of right heart failure can be readily determined noninvasively using echocardiography. Predominantly right-sided heart failure without left heart failure suggests that the myocardium is not the primary problem. In the elderly, congenital abnormalities causing right heart failure are rare. Right ventricular hypoplasia (Uhl's disease), for example, is a possible cause of dysrhythmias and CHF in adults, but is usually manifest in the young. Most commonly, isolated right heart failure is due to pulmonary hypertension, and the reader is referred to Chapter 7 for additional information on evaluation and treatment. If the right heart failure is secondary to left heart failure (biventricular failure), therapy is essentially the same as for isolated left heart failure.

Hypertrophic Cardiomyopathy

Hypertrophic cardiomyopathy must be distinguished from myocardial hypertrophy secondary to pressure or volume overload. Ventricular hypertrophy is a common component of cardiac disease in the elderly because of the frequency of hypertension and degenerative valvular disease. In contrast, hypertrophic cardiomyopathy is a distinct abnormality characterized by unique histologic abnormalities consisting of disorganized myocardial muscle bundles in whorls, abnormal myofibrils within the cells, and interstitial fibrosis.[7,8] The precise etiology of hypertrophic cardiomyopathy is unknown, but it is familial, with heterogeneous genetic cause and variable expression.[9] Although originally felt to be a disease of the young and middle aged, a population based study in Olmsted County (Figure 1) documented a high incidence of hypertrophic cardiomyopathy in patients over 74 years old.[10]

Physiological dysfunction in hypertrophic cardiomyopathy includes both systolic and diastolic abnormalities. Abnormal stiffness and impaired relaxation compromise left ventricular filling. As a result, end-diastolic pressure is elevated, contributing to pulmonary congestion and symptoms of dyspnea. Systolic dysfunction is not due to inadequate contraction, but rather due to dynamic outflow obstruction. A pressure gradient develops within the ventricle because the disproportionately thickened septum touches the displaced anterior mitral valve leaflet in mid-systole and narrows the left ventricular (LV) outflow tract. The resultant high-velocity ejection of blood produces a murmur that mimics aortic stenosis. This murmur can usually be distinguished from that of aortic stenosis on physical examination by the characteristic rapid carotid upstroke. However, in the elderly, hardened carotid arteries alter the frequency response of transmitted pulses. This makes differentiation of clinical conditions effecting pulse contour more difficult. Significant aortic stenosis, for example, can occur without the usual slowed upstroke (pulsus tardus) detectable in younger patients.[11] The ausculatory findings of a louder murmur with Valsalva maneuver, or when arising from a squatting position, can assist in diagnosing obstructive hypertrophic cardiomyopathy. However, if either aortic ste-

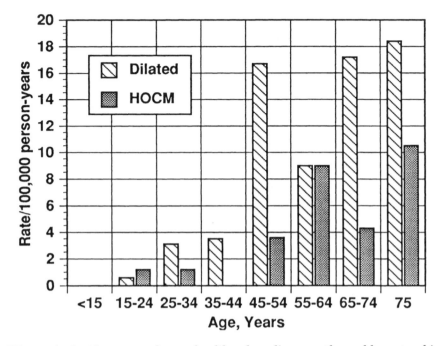

Figure 1: *Incidence rates by age for dilated cardiomyopathy and hypertrophic obstructive cardiomyopathy (HOCM) in Olmsted County. Reproduced with permission from Backes R, Gersh B: Cardiomyopathies in the elderly. In Lowenthal,* ed. Geriatric Cardiology. *F.A. Davis Company, Philadelphia, 1992, pp 105–125.*

nosis or obstructive hypertrophic cardiomyopathy is suspected, an echocardiogram readily distinguishes the two and helps assess severity of either abnormality.

Therapy of hypertrophic cardiomyopathy targets both systolic and diastolic abnormalities, with much the same considerations in the elderly as younger patients. β-adrenergic blockers reduce symptoms, predominantly by controlling heart rate, and thus providing adequate time to overcome restricted filling caused by decreased ventricular compliance.[7,8,12] Negative inotropic activity may also contribute to the beneficial effects achieved with β-blockers. Negative chronotropic and inotropic activity likely explain the beneficial effects of calcium antagonists such as verapamil.[13-16] Since the direct myocardial effects of calcium antagonists impair relaxation,[17,18] the mechanisms for improvement of clinical indices of diastolic function, such as rate of ventricular filling, must be indirect. Interestingly, diastolic filling is improved by nifedipine[19,20] and nicardipine[21] as well as verapamil[22] and diltiazem.[23,24] β-Blockers and calcium antagonists are often combined, but close observation for potential side effects, particularly severe bradycardia, is needed. Disopyramide has also been used, more for its negative inotropic effect than antiarrhythmic potential.[25] Diuretics should be used with caution, and only if symptoms of dyspnea predominate.

Surgical treatment with septal myomectomy, with or without mitral valve replacement,[26] is usually reserved for younger patients, but older patients are not necessarily excluded from consideration. Williams et al[27] and Krajcer et al[28] included patients as old as 76 in their series, and patients up to 83 years old have had surgery for obstructive cardiomyopathy at the Mayo Clinic.[29] A potential benefit has been described using AV sequential pacing to alter the dynamics of ventricular contraction in hypertrophic cardiomyopathy and thereby reduce the gradient,[30,31] but experience with this technique is not large enough to warrant routine use.

Systolic versus Diastolic Dysfunction

CHF is usually associated with systolic dysfunction, but abnormalities of relaxation in diastole can also be important, and in some cases predominate. It is therefore useful to consider diastolic dysfunction of the heart as a distinct component of CHF.

As discussed in Chapter 2, the natural aging process alters diastolic function, and ventricular compliance progressively decreases. This loss of compliance can be aggravated by scarring from ischemic heart disease, hypertrophy from longstanding hypertension or valvular heart disease, or infiltrative diseases such as amyloidosis or hemochromatosis. Peripheral vascular compliance also decreases with advanced age, so that the whole cardiovascular system operates on a steeper pressure volume curve (Figure 2). Consequently, elderly patients are much more sensitive to changes in intravascular volume. A small amount of fluid retention, for example, can cause a disproportionate increase in intravascular pressure, particularly cardiac filling pressures. Dietary indiscretion or medical non-compliance can lead directly to progressive dyspnea (increased left heart filling pressure) and/or peripheral edema (increased right heart filling pressure). Alternatively, overly aggressive diuresis has exaggerated effects of decreasing cardiac output and/or systemic blood pressure because the stiff heart is dependent on a higher than normal filling pressure to maintain a normal stroke volume. Orthostatic symptoms such as lightheadedness, dizziness, or syncope can appear with a relatively small decrease in blood volume when poor vascular compliance is accompanied by delayed or diminished peripheral reflex adjustments. Managing fluid and electrolyte homeostasis clearly presents a major challenge in the care of elderly patients with CHF.

Quantification of diastolic dysfunction is not as straight forward as that of systolic dysfunction. Physicians are well acquainted with ejection fraction, obtained by echocardiography, radionuclide gated blood pool angiography, or dye contrast left ventriculography, as readily available measures of systolic function. However, there is no equivalent

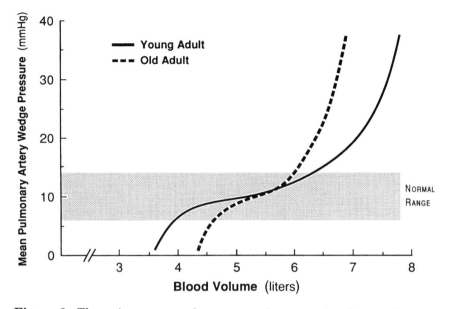

Figure 2: *Theoretic pressure volume curves demonstrating decreased cardio-vascular compliance (ie, steeper curve) in the elderly.*

universally accepted measurement analogous to ejection fraction that quantitatively describes diastolic dysfunction. Clues to the presence of significant diastolic dysfunction begin with a history of known cardiac disease likely to cause scarring, hypertrophy, or cardiac infiltration. Evidence of ventricular hypertrophy on physical examination (sustained apical impulse), electrocardiogram, or echocardiogram, provide additional evidence of diastolic dysfunction.

The most widely accepted method for assessing diastolic function utilizes Doppler echocardiographic measurement of ventricular inflow across the mitral valve. Early diastolic flow is reduced, and the "atrial kick" is increased. This can be expressed as the ratio of the maximum early filling velocity (E point) to the atrial filling velocity (A point). This E/A ratio is normally greater than 1 (ie, E > A), but is reversed (A > E) with diastolic stiffening. Radionuclide gated blood pool angiography provides a volume-time curve of left ventricular filling during the cardiac cycle. A decreased peak filling rate or delayed time to peak filling indicates diastolic dysfunction. Intracardiac hemodynamic pressure recordings can also provide evidence of diastolic dysfunction. The slope of the pressure rise during left ventricular filling, ("h wave") is increased, and the "a" wave due to atrial contraction exaggerated.

Studies of diastolic dysfunction are rarely requested specifically to assess diastolic function alone. However, echocardiograms, radionuclide angiograms, and heart catheterizations are often part of the overall evaluation of patients with CHF sometime during the course of their disease. Specific attention to diastole in such studies can provide the treating physician with additional insight into the pathophysiology of their patient's disease.

Understanding the pathophysiology of diastolic dysfunction leads directly to appreciation of the difficulties of treating this condition. Pharmacological agents that specifically improve ventricular compliance without other cardiovascular effects are not available. Calcium antagonists have been recommended,[32] and verapamil has been shown to improve diastolic filling in patients with CHF and normal systolic function.[33] The mechanism for improved diastolic filling is likely indirect, as direct cardiac effects of calcium antagonists impair ventricular relaxation (see previous discussion of hypertrophic cardiomyopathy). Moreover, diastolic dysfunction in elderly patients is often accompanied by abnormal systolic function, and the negative inotropic effects of calcium antagonists are cause for concern. The major focus of therapy must therefore be directed at controlling the brittle volume status of such patients. Moderation in diet and consistent salt and fluid intake are essential adjuncts to judicious use of diuretics. Proper management usually requires frequent clinic visits to assess clinical and electrolyte status, and adjustments of drug dosage may often be needed. Training the patient and/or home health care provider to use daily weighing to monitor volume status can be invaluable. Many patients do well if they are given the responsibility of adjusting their diuretic dose to maintain a constant weight. Physician visits are still necessary to assure that the target weight is appropriate for the patient's clinical status.

It should be evident that the 4 pathophysiological classifications described above are not distinct entities. Patients with hypertrophic cardiomyopathy can suffer myocardial infarction. Both systolic and diastolic dysfunction commonly contribute to the syndrome of CHF, and the right and left ventricles are frequently both abnormal. However, after assessing each abnormality separately, the knowledge can be integrated to better understand the overall problems of a specific patient with CHF. This information must be supplemented with thorough analysis of the extent to which other organ systems are compromised. Pulmonary and renal abnormalities are particularly important, and it is not always easy to determine how much dysfunction is due to intrinsic disease in the lungs or kidneys compared to secondary effects from the cardiovascular disease. Despite its importance, a complete treatise on evaluating the pulmonary and renal response to CHF is beyond the scope of this chapter. Subsequent sections will be devoted to short- and long-term therapy of CHF caused predominately by left ventricular systolic dysfunction.

Treatment of Acute Decompensation of CHF

Acute decompensation of heart failure in elderly patients frequently presents more of a therapeutic than diagnostic challenge. An antecedent history of heart disease is often present, and the nature and extent of the problem may be well defined in records available to the treating physician. Symptoms of dyspnea are usually due to elevated left heart filling pressure causing pulmonary congestion or pulmonary edema. Occasionally, right-sided symptoms predominate, with fluid retention, peripheral edema, and sometimes ascites. Symptoms of low cardiac output such as weakness and fatigue are frequent. Rarely, the combination of passive congestion plus inadequate perfusion produce presenting symptoms of end organ damage such as renal failure or "shock liver." If the diagnosis of CHF is not evident following the initial history and physical examination, results of basic laboratory studies, chest x- ray, and electrocardiogram usually provide enough information to direct initial therapy, even if additional studies such as an echocardiogram are still needed for a complete workup.

Several of the major therapeutic decisions to be made when elderly patients present with acute decompensation of CHF involve assessing the need for invasive measures. Early inquiry should be made to the patient and/or accompanying relatives or friends about Advanced Directives or Living Wills that may limit the use of mechanical support. When respiratory distress is severe, intubation and artificial respiration must be considered. If the patient is unable to communicate, and no other information is readily available to guide the physician, the decision regarding intubation becomes very difficult. As noted above, it is likely that any therapy offered will be supportive, but not curative of the underlying etiology of the CHF. Despite this fact, in many cases the vicious cycle of progressively decompensating heart failure can be reversed by positive pressure ventilation, and the patient stabilized with aggressive medical therapy. Consequently, in the absence of advanced directives stating otherwise, artificial respiration is sometimes applied in situations where physicians are not able to anticipate the outcome with reasonable assurance. Since there are no specific guidelines that are universally applicable to severely ill patients unable to participate in critical care decisions, physicians must rely on their best knowledge and judgment in each individual case.

Invasive hemodynamic monitoring provides valuable information to guide therapy, and decisions regarding use of pulmonary artery and/ or intra-arterial catheters should be made early in the course of evaluation and treatment of acute CHF. Because invasive hemodynamic monitoring is not therapeutic, the ominous possibility that the patient may become dependent on continued use is not of concern. This makes the decision about invasive monitoring much easier than that regarding intubation. The benefits of data available from pulmonary artery catheterization in acutely decompensated CHF are well appreciated when choosing drugs and titrating their doses to optimal levels. Intra-arterial pressure monitoring is particularly valuable because brachial cuff measurements may be inaccurate. Peripheral vasoconstriction can decrease limb blood flow, thereby diminishing the Korotkoff sounds and result in an underestimate of true intra-arterial pressure.[34] Alternatively, the stiff, noncompliant atherosclerotic brachial vessels encountered in the elderly may resist compression by a pneumatic cuff to the extent that a significant overestimate of intra-arterial pressure results.[35] In addition to improved accuracy of pressure measurements, intra-arterial lines provide continuous blood pressure readings that are useful when titrating vasoactive drugs, and ready access to arterial blood for blood gas analysis.

In a large group of critically ill patients with multiple presenting diagnoses, the benefits of right heart catheterization have been questioned.[36] The complications of pulmonary artery catheters and arterial cannulae are discussed in Chapter 10, and adequate time should be taken to carefully weigh the relative risks and benefits of invasive hemodynamic monitoring The decision regarding right heart catheterization in the elderly patient with acute cardiac decompensation can be facilitated more by considering what impact the information provided will have on guiding important therapeutic decisions, rather than whether or not it will improve long term survival. When invasive monitoring is used, care must be taken to ensure that reasonable therapeutic intervention proceeds unhindered by the procedure of placing the catheters. It is all too easy for catheter insertion to become an end in itself that diverts time and attention from other therapeutic aspects of acute care. Clinical and x-ray findings of pulmonary edema, for example, present sufficient evidence of severely elevated pulmonary artery wedge pressure to begin appropriate therapy without waiting for hemodynamic documentation. "Fine tuning" of therapy can proceed more electively as additional information becomes available. Finally, despite the advantages of invasive hemodynamic monitoring, physicians should not withhold aggressive use of intravenous vasoactive drugs when a reasonable chance of favorable clinical response can be expected, even when invasive studies are not indicated or not desired by the patient.

Severe dysrhythmias often occur in decompensated CHF,[37] and it is estimated that 33% to 47% of patients with CHF die suddenly,[38] presumably due to arrhythmia. Factors contributing to arrhythmogenesis in CHF must therefore be sought and corrected as soon as possible. Standard care calls for continuous electrocardiographic monitoring, during which time electrolyte imbalance, hypoxia, acidosis, possible drug toxicity, etc. are reversed. Oxygen is best provided by a mask, because mouth breathing often decreases the efficiency of nasal prongs in tachypneic patients. Such procedures are standard intensive care unit measures, and need not be detailed further.

The remainder of this section will focus on medical measures used for acute heart failure, including diuretics, inotropic agents, and vasodilators.

Diuretics

Fluid retention is not a universal finding in acute CHF. Occasional patients can be relatively dehydrated and present with problems related solely to inadequate cardiac output. However, fluid overload with pulmonary edema and/or peripheral edema is commonly evident, and consequently diuretics remain the cornerstone of therapy. Unless the patient is minimally symptomatic, diuretics should be given intravenously to assure adequate drug delivery without concern for delayed or incomplete intestinal absorption. A prompt diuresis usually results and left heart filling pressure begins to decrease. The Frank-Starling mechanism would predict that a decrease in cardiac filling pressure should result in a decrease in left ventricular function. This response has indeed been documented to occur early in the course of diuretic therapy.[39] Usually, this initial decrease in cardiac output is not large enough to cause severe adverse effects. However, since cardiac output often is low, concomitant therapy that improves cardiac output is generally indicated.

Inotropic Drugs

Although digoxin has a fairly rapid onset of action when given intravenously, it is a relatively weak inotropic agent. As such, in the absence of atrial fibrillation, digoxin is not a therapeutic agent of choice for acutely decompensated CHF. More potent drugs for this role include sympathomimetic amines and phosphodiesterase inhibitors.

Table 2 lists currently available inotropic drugs of potential use in decompensated CHF. Although several sympathomimetic drugs are listed, the preferred agent is generally a choice between dopamine and dobutamine. Because of its severe peripheral vasoconstrictor effects, norepinephrine is generally used only during resuscitation. Epinephrine, isoproterenol, and metaraminol also have significant undesirable

---

Table 2
Inotropic Drugs for Congestive Heart Failure

Digitalis Glycosides
   Digoxin
   Digitoxin
Sympathomimetic Amines
   Dobutamine
   Dopamine
   Epinephrine
   Norepinephrine
   Isoproterenol
   Metaraminol
   Phenylephrine
Phosphodiesterase inhibitors
   Amrinone
   Milrinone

effects that limit their use. Epinephrine has a poorly predictable dose response curve in different vascular beds, and tachyphylaxis limits sustained use. The tachycardia and peripheral vasodilator effects of isoproterenol can be detrimental, and it is very arrhythmogenic. Metaraminol acts by releasing endogenous catecholamines, which reduces its effectiveness for sustained use, and phenylephrine has predominantly peripheral vascular effects with only slight cardiac stimulation.

Information directly applicable to choosing between dopamine and dobutamine was obtained by Leier et al[40] using a crossover study design. Dose-response data were obtained for the effects of each drug on systemic hemodynamics in 13 patients (age 30 to 70 years) with low-output heart failure (Figure 3). Drug response was not reported by age, but the relative effects would likely be similar in a group of elderly patients as in this mixed group.

The dose-dependent increase in systemic blood pressure with dopamine, not seen with dobutamine, makes dopamine the drug of choice if blood pressure is dangerously low. However, when blood pressure is

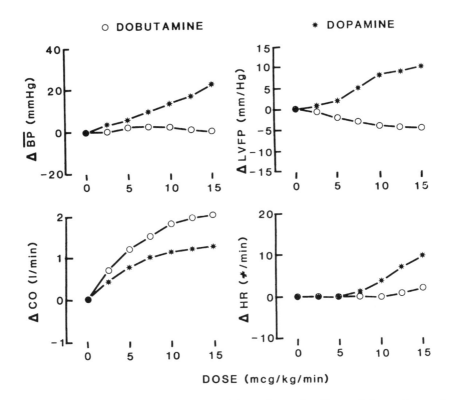

Figure 3: *Comparison of the expected hemodynamic effects of dopamine and dobutamine at increasing doses in patients with congestive heart failure (CHF).*[40]

adequate to maintain cerebral and renal blood flow (even if lower than usual normal values) the added work load created by dopamine-induced peripheral vasoconstriction would make dobutamine the preferable drug. It is also evident that the increase in blood pressure with dopamine occurs at the expense of a rise in left ventricular filling pressure, and an increase in heart rate. Also, ventricular irritability (premature ventricular complexes per minute [PVCs/min]) was more prominent with dopamine.

The effect of these 2 drugs on regional blood flow is more difficult to predict because comparative dose-response curves are not available. In the study by Leier et al,[40] renal function was examined once for each drug, after a stable maintenance infusion was achieved. Both drugs tended to improve urine flow, creatinine clearance and renal blood flow, and a clear difference between the 2 was not evident. Sato et al[41] studied several doses of dopamine and dobutamine in patients after open heart surgery and found renal blood flow increased with dobutamine in proportion to cardiac output, whereas low-dose dopamine increased renal blood flow more than cardiac output. It is known that the kidneys have specific dopaminergic receptors that can preferentially vasodilate renal vessels, with the optimal response occurring at low doses, usually below 3 to 5 mg/kg per minute.[42]

In summary, dobutamine is generally the sympathomimetic inotrope of choice for acute decompensation of CHF. Invasive hemodynamic monitoring assists in titrating to optimal dosage, but is not absolutely required. Dobutamine has also been used as intermittent maintenance therapy in patients with severe chronic CHF.[43,44] Although some beneficial effects may last for several weeks,[45] long-term benefits of such "prophylactic" use of dopamine infusion have not been demonstrated adequately to consider it for routine use, particularly in the elderly. Dopamine should be used if blood pressure is dangerously low, and small doses of dopamine may provide benefit through selective renal vasodilatation.

Phosphodiesterase Inhibitors

Phosphodiesterase is the enzyme that breaks down cyclic adenosine monophosphate (cAMP). Inhibiting this enzyme therefore increases the concentration of intracellular cAMP. cAMP is the "second messenger" that also mediates the inotropic response to stimulation of β-adrenergic receptors. Amrinone and milrinone are phosphodiesterase inhibitors currently approved for use in the United States. These drugs are structurally related dipyridines and have similar hemodynamic effects. Both exert inotropic effects on the heart, but milrinone is 15 to 20 times more potent.[46] They are also peripheral vasodilators and improve diastolic relaxation (lusitropic effect) with minimal chronotropic response.[47,48] As a result, pulmonary wedge pressure decreases and cardiac output increases with minimal change in myocardial oxygen consumption in patients with CHF.[49–51] Side effects with short-term use of these drugs are minimal, although they can be arrhythmogenic in a small percent of patients. Hypotension may occur, and occasional patients experience headaches.

Since milrinone and amrinone have beneficial hemodynamic effects comparable in many ways to dobutamine, choosing an agent can be problematic. This choice is further complicated by the fact that vasodilators are also beneficial in acute heart failure. It is difficult therefore, to assess the relative contribution made by vasodilator versus inotropic versus lusitropic actions of either milrinone or amrinone toward the overall response. It has been argued that the major benefit of amrinone is through its vasodilator effect rather than its inotropic effect.[52] To the extent that this is true, the drug should be compared more to vasodilators such as nitroprusside than to other inotropic agents.

Direct comparisons among these drugs have been made by several investigators. Gage et al[53] compared dobutamine to amrinone in 11 patients aged 35 to 73 years with CHF. Unfortunately, the order of drugs was not randomized, but dobutamine was titrated first to a plateau cardiac output or maximum dose of 15 mg/kg per minute. After hemodynamic measurements, the drug was stopped and amrinone given in a bolus of 1.5 mg/kg, with a second bolus of 0.75 mg/kg if the response was inadequate. Both drugs increased LVdp/dt and cardiac output equivalently, with a similar reduction in ventricular end-diastolic pressure, whereas amrinone but not dobutamine reduced systemic arterial pressure. Milrinone may also cause a greater decrease in systemic vascular resistance than dobutamine at doses that raise cardiac output equivalently.[54–56] When milrinone is compared to nitroprusside,[57,58] similar decreases in systemic vascular resistance and cardiac output can be achieved, but milrinone increases indices of myocardial contraction such as LVdp/dt, while nitroprusside does not. Collectively, these studies support the thesis that vasodilator effects are indeed a very prominent component determining the overall response of CHF patients to phosphodiesterase inhibitors.

Although adverse effects of phosphodiesterase inhibitors are few when used short term, long term infusions may become more toxic. The possibility has been raised that there may be a direct myocardial toxicity.[59] It is particularly pertinent to note that although oral forms of both amrinone and milrinone have been studied, both have been withdrawn from clinical trials due to unacceptable side affects such as thrombocytopenia and ventricular arrhythmias.[60] Milrinone given orally resulted in more deaths than placebo in a recent randomized double-blind trial.[61] It therefore appears reasonable to reserve phosphodiesterase inhibitors for short-term use in patients not responding adequately to dobutamine. Since the inotropic response to dobutamine appears to be diminished in patients with higher levels of circulating norepinephrine,[62] it is possible that the response to dobutamine may be decreased in the elderly. Aging increases plasma norepinephrine[63,64] and decreases adrenergic responsiveness,[65,66] and heart failure exacerbates both of these changes. Whether or not this phenomenon provides a relative advantage for using amrinone or milrinone in geriatric practice is uncertain.

Vasodilators

Low-output congestive heart failure is characterized in part by elevated systemic vascular resistance. It now appears quite logical that when left ventricular function is compromised, intervention that decreases peripheral vascular resistance produces beneficial effects by decreasing the work required to circulate blood effectively. However, because systemic blood pressure is also frequently below normal in patients with CHF, the administration of an agent that further lowers blood pressure was not always considered reasonable therapy. In the early 1970s the demonstration that infusion of nitroprusside could produce dramatic and rapid hemodynamic improvement in patients with acute myocardial infarction was instrumental in promoting afterload reduction as a useful therapeutic strategy in CHF.[67]

The expected hemodynamic response of patients with CHF to nitroprusside depicted in Figure 4 is now well known. Cardiac output is

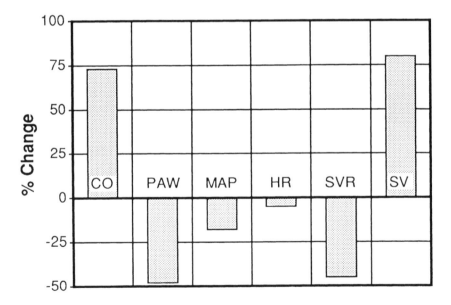

Figure 4: *Hemodynamic response of patients with congestive heart failure (CHF) to titrated doses of nitroprusside. Data from Guiha et al.[104] CO, cardiac output; PAW, pulmonary artery wedge pressure; MAP, mean arterial pressure; HR, heart rate; SVR, systemic vascular resistance; SV, stroke volume.*

increased and pulmonary artery wedge pressure decreased, with only a modest decrease in arterial pressure and minimal change in heart rate. As a result, calculated systemic vascular resistance is significantly reduced, and stroke volume greatly improved.

Nitroprusside is the vasodilator of choice for acutely decompensated CHF because it has a rapid onset of action, is predictable, can be titrated to achieve reasonable therapeutic goals, has few side effects, and is inexpensive. Hypotension can occur if the dose is excessive, and long term infusion can result in build up of thiocyanate.[68] In rare cases, intrapulmonary vasodilatation can lead to ventilation/perfusion mismatch and a decrease in arterial oxygen saturation.[69,70] Since the drug has a very short half-life of only approximately 2 minutes, decreasing the dose or stopping the drug usually reverses these few undesirable effects should they occur. In patients where active myocardial ischemia is contributing to acute decompensation in left ventricular function, intravenous nitroglycerin is a reasonable alternative. However, tolerance to nitroglycerin can occur within 24 hours,[71] with consequent loss of beneficial affects. Intravenous nitroprusside (or nitroglycerin) can be replaced by oral vasodilators electively after the patient has been stabilized.

Combination Therapy

There is strong rationale for combining sympathomimetic inotropic support with vasodilators in acute CHF. The 2 types of drugs act through separate mechanisms, and there is potential for offsetting adverse hemodynamic effects while augmenting favorable responses. Combining dopamine with nitroprusside is particularly attractive. Dopamine provides positive inotropic effect that nitroprusside lacks, while proper titration of nitroprusside counteracts the peripheral vasoconstrictor effects of dopamine. Nitroprusside can be expected to decrease left ventricular filling pressure, a desirable effect that dopamine lacks. Indeed, there is clinical evidence suggesting that these goals can be achieved.[72,73] A reasonable application of this combination is in patients with low cardiac output in whom vasodilators cannot be given because of inadequate blood pressure. Initial therapy with dopamine would improve cardiac output and increase systemic pressure. Nitroprusside can then be added as tolerated to further increase cardiac output and decrease left ventricular filling pressure, as long as adequate systemic pressure is maintained.

Because dobutamine does not induce a pressor response, the need for adding nitroprusside is not as obvious. Indeed, the overall effect of dobutamine has been compared to that of combining dopamine with nitroprusside.[74] However, dobutamine does have a direct inotropic effect that nitroprusside lacks. It is therefore reasonable to add dobutamine infusion to patients receiving nitroprusside if the improvement in cardiac output is inadequate. Nitroglycerin[75] as well as nitroprusside[76] have been successfully combined with dobutamine to augment cardiac output.

The phosphodiesterase inhibitors amrinone and milrinone, as noted above, have fairly potent vasodilator effects on their own. As such, combining either of these agents with a vasodilator has less rationale than the combination of a sympathomimetic amine and a vasodilator.

It is also possible to consider combining a phosphodiesterase inhibitor with a sympathomimetic amine. The peripheral vasodilator effects of the phosphodiesterase inhibitor would tend to produce effects similar to combining nitroprusside with a sympathomimetic amine as described above. However, the direct cardiac effects of combining the two types of agents would be more difficult to predict. Both types of drugs increase myocardial cAMP albeit by different mechanisms (beta adrenergic stimulation vs phosphodiesterase inhibition). This raises the possibility that any adverse myocardial effects (metabolic, arrhythmogenic, toxic) might be multiplied by combining these agents. Despite these considerations, amrinone has been successfully combined both with dobutamine[53,77-79] and dopamine.[80] When other combinations fail, a phosphodiesterase inhibitor combined with a sympathomimetic amine can be given a trial.

In summary, the drugs used to treat acute decompensation of CHF in the elderly do not differ from those used in younger patients. Their application to elderly patients requires defining reasonable goals and expectations, and careful consideration of adjunctive measures. The risk portion of the risk benefit ratio is generally higher for any intervention as age increases.

Chronic Congestive Heart Failure

In Chapter 9 it was pointed out that prognosis is worse in the elderly who suffer acute myocardial infarction than in younger patients. It is of equal interest to determine the effect of age on prognosis of patients with heart failure. The incidence of heart failure increases with age,[81,82] and the Department of Veterans Affairs Cooperative Vasodilator-Heart Failure Trial Investigators used their data from V-HeFT I and V-HeFT II to ascertain if this is due to more severe underlying disease, or to the coexistence of heart disease with the cardiovascular effects of aging.[83] They found that the slope of the survival curves did not increase with age, and although the oldest patients did have the poorest survival, this was due to interaction with presence of coronary artery disease and randomization to placebo. These findings are consistent with those of Cody et al,[84] who found that elderly patients with heart failure had a greater incidence of ischemic heart disease than younger patients with CHF. There was an age related decrease in glomerular filtration rate, increase in blood urea nitrogen and creatinine, increase in systemic vascular resistance, decrease in heart rate and heart rate response to tilt, and increases in circulating norepinephrine. These findings are consistent with superimposition of an aging effect on the CHF process. Such studies suggest that caution must be used when attempting to interpret results of heart failure trials that exclude the elderly by extrapolating from younger patients to older patients. In the following discussions of therapy, specific attempts will be made to note any analysis done according to age in the studies cited.

Digitalis

Digitalis has been used to treat CHF for over 200 years, and has been the subject of innumerable investigations throughout the world. Despite this wealth of experience, the proper role for digitalis in therapy of CHF remains controversial. There is general agreement that digitalis is important therapy for CHF patients in chronic atrial fibrillation requiring control of their ventricular rate. For patients in sinus rhythm, the role of digitalis is less clear. This controversy surrounding digitalis is in part due to the availability of alternate therapy with diuretics and/or vasodilators. As will be discussed below, convincing evidence is now available that vasodilators can prolong life for patients with CHF.

Because no large prospective randomized trials have shown that routine use of digitalis prolongs life of patients with CHF, the question remains as to whether adding digitalis to vasodilator therapy is warranted. This question was recently addressed in the DIG trial, an international study sponsored jointly by the U.S. National Heart, Lung and Blood Institute and the Department of Veterans Affairs Cooperative Studies Program.[85] In this double-blind, randomized, controlled trial of 8000 patients with CHF, digoxin failed to reduce overall mortality. However, it did reduce the rate of hospitalization both overall and for worsening heart failure. As such, it is reasonable to consider digitalis as potentially beneficial in patients with severe chronic CHF where hospitalization may be anticipated in the near future. This outlook is supported by evidence that switching patients with CHF from digoxin to placebo results in a higher incidence of decompensation than those maintained on active drug.[86] Recognition that elderly patients are likely to be more sensitive to digitalis toxicity should lead to careful monitoring of patients receiving this drug. It is important to document serum levels of digitalis in older patients as soon as the dose is stabilized, to insure that expected values have been achieved without "overshooting." Drug levels can easily change should gastrointestinal problems arise that alter absorption, the patient become dehydrated, renal function become impaired, or drugs that interact with digitalis be instituted. Such events should readily trigger repeat analysis of serum levels to insure safety is maintained.

Diuretics

Diuretics remain a cornerstone of therapy for chronic CHF. Large randomized trials demonstrating prolonged survival are not necessary because physicians treating heart failure patients are quite aware of the importance of diuretics in controlling fluid retention and the symptoms that fluid retention causes. The need to closely monitor elderly patients receiving diuretics was discussed earlier in this chapter, and need not be reiterated here.

β-Adrenergic Blockers and Calcium Antagonists

Ischemic heart disease is present in the vast majority of elderly patients with CHF, and it is important to recognize that we are often treating intermittent ischemia at the same time we are treating left ventricular dysfunction. Specific considerations on the role of β-blockers and calcium antagonists when heart failure is present are discussed in Chapter 12.

Vasodilators

The beneficial hemodynamic effects of intravenous vasodilators demonstrated in the early 1970s led directly to attempts to reproduce such effects with oral agents. Nitrates, hydralazine, and prazosin were among the first drugs tried in this regard. Prazosin demonstrated an initial hemodynamic benefit,[87] but tolerance to the drug was considered a potential problem.[88] Nitrates produced predominantly venodilator effects,[89] while hydralazine was more potent as an arterial dilator.[90] Combining these latter 2 drugs produced the expected additive beneficial effects, and the results were comparable to those attainable with nitroprusside.[91]

Long-term benefits of oral vasodilators in CHF were more difficult to demonstrate, and several studies suggested efficacy was maintained, while others found no detectable long-term improvement.[92] The question of long-term efficacy of oral vasodilators in CHF was first addressed in a large randomized clinical trial by the V- HeFT I.[93,94] This study randomly assigned 642 men with CHF up to age 75 to either placebo, prazosin, or hydralazine/nitrate combination. Prior therapy with digitalis and diuretics was continued during the trial. Mortality rate was reduced in the group receiving hydralazine/nitrate combination compared to placebo, but no benefit was seen with prazosin.

V-HeFT II was designed in follow-up of V-HeFT I, to determine if an angiotensin converting enzyme (ACE) inhibitor would demonstrate long term benefit as vasodilator therapy for CHF. Because V-HeFT I showed hydralazine/nitrate to be efficacious, ACE inhibitor was compared to this known beneficial combination rather than placebo. Again the upper age limit was 75 years, and traditional therapy with digitalis and diuretics was continued. Results in 804 men demonstrated an 18% improvement in 2-year survival with ACE inhibition compared to hydralazine/nitrate. Additional data comes from the Hy-C trial,[95] where a titrated dose of hydralazine was compared to captopril in patients with severe CHF referred for cardiac transplantation. Hydralazine was combined with isosorbide dinitrate if tolerated, and isosorbide was added together with captopril if coronary artery disease was present, or the pulmonary artery wedge pressure remained greater than 20 mm Hg on captopril. One-year survival was 81% in the captopril group, but 51% in the hydralazine group ($P = 0.05$), results consistent with V-HeFT I.

Other studies have compared ACE inhibition to placebo in CHF. The CONSENSUS- I trial (Cooperative North Scandinavian Enalapril Survival Study)[96] showed a 31% decrease in one year mortality using enalapril compared to placebo. This study was limited to severe CHF (NYHA class IV), but had no age limit. As a result, the average age of participants in this study was 70 to 71 years, compared to 58 years in V-HeFT I and 61 in V-HeFT II. In the Studies of Left Ventricular Dysfunction (SOLVD) trial,[97] enalapril improved survival and decreased hospitalizations. The patients enrolled in SOLVD had ejection fractions 35% or less, and an upper age limit of 80 years (average 61 years). There was a 16% reduction in mortality in those with symptomatic CHF, and 8% in those with asymptomatic LV dysfunction.

Data that symptoms of CHF need not be present in order to warrant therapy with ACE inhibitors comes from the Survival and Ventricular Enlargement (SAVED) trial.[98] Patients under 80 years of age were randomly assigned to captopril or placebo within 3 to 16 days after a myocardial infarction if their ejection fraction was less than 40%, independent of symptoms of CHF. The all-cause mortality was 5% lower in the captopril group (20% compared to 25% for placebo). Both fatal and nonfatal major cardiovascular events were consistently reduced by captopril. Similarly positive results were reported by the SOLVD investigators using enalapril in asymptomatic patients with ejection fractions 0.35 or less.[99]

The renin-angiotensin system is susceptible to intervention by blocking angiotensin-II receptors as well as by ACE inhibition. The orally active, nonpeptide, angiotensin II type 1 receptor antagonist losartan has been studied in elderly patients with CHF for safety and efficacy compared to the ACE inhibitor captopril. Results of the ELITE trial (Evaluation of Losartan in the Elderly Study) of 722 previous patients aged 65 or older without prior exposure to ACE inhibitors, demonstrated a benefit of losartan on all cause mortality.[100] There was no difference between losartan and captopril effects on renal function, but no losartan patients required discontinuation due to cough, whereas cough required discontinuation of captopril in 14 patients. It is likely that the cough side effect of ACE inhibitors is due to increased bradykinin, and this is avoided by losartan.[101] The antiotensin-II receptor antagonists irbesartan and valsartan are also available in the United States, but are only indicated for treating hypertension.

In the aggregate these studies clearly demonstrate that chronic oral vasodilator therapy improves symptoms and prolongs life in patients with left ventricular dysfunction. Currently, ACE inhibitors are the vasodilators of choice if tolerated by the patient. Unfortunately, several of these studies had upper age limits. Nonetheless, enough elderly patients were included to suggest that the elderly are as likely to benefit from vasodilator therapy as younger patients. Hopefully, future large clinical trials will refrain from putting arbitrary upper age limits on participants. For additional opinion on therapy of CHF the reader is referred to the Guidelines for the Evaluation and Management of Heart Failure published by the American College of Cardiology/American Heart Association Task Force on Practice Guidelines.[102]

References

1. Wenger N: Pericardial disease in the elderly. In DT Lowenthal (ed): *Geriatric Cardiology*. Philadelphia, PA, F.A. Davis Co, 1992, pp 97–103.
2. Pierpont G, Talley R: Pathophysiology of valvar heart disease: The dynamic nature of mitral valve regurgitation. *Arch Intern Med* 142: 998–1001, 1982.
3. Tsakiris A, Rastelli G, Amorim D, et al: Effect of experimental papillary muscle damage on mitral valve closure in intact anesthetized dogs. *Mayo Clinic Proc* 45:275–285, 1970.
4. Pavan D, Nicolosi G, Lestuzzi C, et al: Normalization of variables of left ventricular function in patients with alcoholic cardiomyopathy after cessation of excessive alcohol intake: An echocardiographic study. *Eur Heart J* 8:535–540, 1987.
5. McKee P, Castelli W, McNamara P, et al: The natural history of congestive heart failure: The Framingham Study. *N Engl J Med* 285:1441–1446, 1971.
6. Murray J, Dawson A, Sherlock S: Circulatory changes in chronic liver disease. *Am Med* 24:358–367, 1958.
7. Maron B, Bonow R, Cannon R, et al: Hypertrophic cardiomyopathy: Interrelations of clinical manifestations, pathophysiology, and therapy (first of two parts). *N Engl J Med* 316:780–789, 1987.
8. Maron B, Bonow R, Cannon R, et al: Hypertrophic cardiomyopathy: Interrelations of clinical manifestations, pathophysiology, and therapy (second of two parts). *N Engl J Med* 316:844–852, 1987.
9. Maron B: The genetics of hypertrophic cardiomyopathy. *Ann Intern Med* 105:610–613, 1986.
10. Codd M, Sugrue D, Gersh B, et al: Epidemiology of idiopathic dilated and hypertrophic cardiomyopathy: A population-based study in Olmsted County, Minnesota, 1975–1984. *Circulation* 80:564–572, 1989.
11. Flohr K, Weir E, Chesler E: The diagnosis of aortic stenosis in older age groups using external carotid pulse recording and phonocardiography. *Br Heart J* 45:577–582, 1981.
12. Bonow R, Maron B, Leon M, et al: Medical and surgical therapy of hypertrophic cardiomyopathy. *Cardiovasc Clin* 19:221–239, 1988.
13. Kaltenbach M, Hopf R, Kober G, et al: Treatment of hypertrophic obstructive cardiomyopathy with verapamil. *Br Heart J* 42:35–42, 1979.
14. Rosing D, Kent K, Borer J, et al: Verapamil therapy: A new approach to the pharmacologic treatment of hypertrophic cardiomyopathy: I. Hemodynamic effects. *Circulation* 60:1201–1207, 1979.

15. Rosing D, Kent K, Maron B, et al: Verapamil therapy: A new approach to the pharmacologic treatment of hypertrophic cardiomyopathy: II. Effects on exercise capacity and symptomatic status. *Circulation* 60: 1208–1213, 1979.
16. Rosing D, Condit J, Maron B, et al: Verapamil therapy: A new approach to the pharmacologic treatment of hypertrophic cardiomyopathy: III. Effects of long-term administration. *Am J Cardiol* 48:545–553, 1981.
17. Gelpi R, Mosca S, Rinaldi G, et al: Effect of calcium antagonism on contractile behavior of canine hearts. *Am J Physiol* 244:H378-H386, 1983.
18. Walsh R, O'Rourke R: Direct and indirect effects of calcium entry blocking agents on isovolumic left ventricular relaxation in conscious dogs. *J Clin Invest* 75:1426–1434, 1985.
19. Lorell B, Paulus W, Grossman W, et al: Modification of abnormal left ventricular diastolic properties by nifedipine in patients with hypertrophic cardiomyopathy. *Circulation* 65:499–507, 1982.
20. Yamakado T, Okano H, Higashiyama S, et al: Effects of nifedipine on left ventricular diastolic function in patients with asymptomatic or minimally symptomatic hypertrophic cardiomyopathy. *Circulation* 81:593–601, 1990.
21. Rodrigues E, Lahiri A, Raftery E: Improvement in left ventricular diastolic function in patients with stable angina after chronic treatment with verapamil and nicardipine. *Eur Heart J* 8:624–629, 1987.
22. Bonow R, Ostrow H, Rosing D, et al: Effects of verapamil on left ventricular systolic and diastolic function in patients with hypertrophic cardiomyopathy: Pressure-volume analysis with a nonimaging scintillation probe. *Circulation* 68:1062–1073, 1983.
23. Suwa M, Hirota Y, Kawamura K: Improvement in left ventricular diastolic function during intravenous and oral diltiazem therapy in patients with hypertrophic cardiomyopathy: An echocardiographic study. *Am J Cardiol* 54:1047–1053, 1984.
24. Iwase M, Sotobata I, Takagi S, et al: Effects of diltiazem on left ventricular diastolic behavior in patients with hypertrophic cardiomyopathy: Evaluation with exercise pulsed doppler echocardiography. *J Am Coll Cardiol* 9:1099–1105, 1987.
25. Sherrid M, Delia E, Dwyer E: Oral disopyramide therapy for obstructive hypertrophic cardiomyopathy. *Am J Cardiol* 62:1085–1088, 1988.
26. McIntosh C, Maron B: Current operative treatment of obstructive hypertrophic cardiomyopathy. *Circulation* 78:487–495, 1988.
27. Williams W, Wigle E, Rakowski H, et al: Results of surgery for hypertrophic obstructive cardiomyopathy. *Circulation* 76:V-104-V-108, 1987.
28. Krajcer Z, Leachman R, Cooley D, et al: Mitral valve replacement and septal myomectomy in hypertrophic cardiomyopathy: Ten-year follow-up in 80 patients. *Circulation* 78:I-35-I-43, 1988.
29. Mohr R, Schaff H, Danielson G, et al: The outcome of surgical treatment of hypertrophic obstructive cardiomyopathy: Experience over 15 years. *J Thorac Cardiovasc Surg* 97:666–674, 1989.
30. Fananapazir L, Cannon R, Tripodi D, et al: Impact of dual-chamber permanent pacing in patients with obstructive hypertrophic cardiomyopathy with symptoms refractory to verapamil and b-adrenergic blocker therapy. *Circulation* 85:2149–2161, 1992.
31. Jeanrenaud X, Goy J, Kappenberger L: Effects of dual-chamber pacing in hypertrophic obstructive cardiomyopathy. *Lancet* 339:1318–1323, 1992.

32. Wei J: Use of calcium entry blockers in elderly patients: Special consideration. *Circulation* 80:IV-171-IV-177, 1989.
33. Setaro J, Zaret B, Schulman D, et al: Usefulness of verapamil for congestive heart failure associated with abnormal left ventricular diastolic filling and normal left ventricular systolic performance. *Am J Cardiol* 66: 981–986, 1990.
34. Cohn J: Blood pressure measurement in shock: Mechanism of inaccuracy in ausculatory and palpatory methods. *JAMA* 199:972–976, 1967.
35. Taguchi J, Suwangool P: Pipe-stem brachial arteries: A cause of pseudohypertension. *JAMA* 228:733, 1974.
36. Conners AF, Speroff T, Dawson NV, et al: The effectiveness of right heart catheterization in the initial care of critically ill patients. *JAMA* 276: 889–897, 1996.
37. Francis G: Should asymptomatic ventricular arrhythmias in patients with congestive heart failure be treated with antiarrhythmic drugs? *J Am Coll Cardiol* 12:274–283, 1988.
38. Packer M: Sudden unexpected death in patients with congestive heart failure: A second frontier. *Circulation* 72:681–685, 1985.
39. Francis G, Siegel R, Goldsmith S, et al: Acute vasoconstrictor response to intravenous furosemide in patients with chronic congestive heart failure: Activation of the neurohumoral axis. *Ann Intern Med* 103:1–6, 1985.
40. Leier C, Heban P, Huss P, et al: Comparative systemic and regional hemodynamic effects of dopamine and dobutamine in patients with cardiomyopathic heart failure. *Circulation* 58:466–475, 1978.
41. Sato Y, Matsuzawa H, Eguchi S: Comparative study of effects of adrenaline, dobutamine and dopamine on systemic hemodynamics and renal blood flow in patients following open heart surgery. *Jpn Circ J* 46: 1059–1072, 1982.
42. Hollenberg N, Adams D, Mendell P, et al: Renal vascular responses to dopamine: Haemodynamic and angiographic observations in normal man. *Clin Sci Mol Med* 45:733–742, 1973.
43. Applefeld M, Newman K, Grove W, et al: Intermittent, continuous outpatient dobutamine infusion in the management of congestive heart failure. *Am J Cardiol* 51:455–458, 1983.
44. Krell M, Kline E, Bates E, et al: Intermittent, ambulatory dobutamine infusions in patients with severe congestive heart failure. *Am Heart J* 112:787–791, 1986.
45. Liang C, Sherman L, Doherty J, et al: Sustained improvement of cardiac function in patients with congestive heart failure after short-term infusion of dobutamine. *Circulation* 69:113–119, 1984.
46. Alousi A, Stankus G, Stuart J, et al: Characterization of the cardiotonic effects of milrinone, a new and potent cardiac bipyridine, on isolated tissues from several animal species. *J Cardiovasc Pharmacol* 5:804–811, 1983.
47. Monrad E, McKay R, Baim D, et al: Improvement in indexes of diastolic performance in patients with congestive heart failure treated with milrinone. *Circulation* 70:1030–1037, 1984.
48. Alousi A, Johnson D: Pharmacology of the bipyridines: amrinone and milrinone. *Circulation* 73:III-10-III-24, 1986.
49. Benotti J, Grossman W, Braunwald E, et al: Hemodynamic assessment of amrinone: A new inotropic agent. *N Engl J Med* 299:1373–1377, 1978.
50. Benotti J, Grossman W, Braunwald E, et al: Effects of amrinone on myo-

cardial energy metabolism and hemodynamics in patients with severe congestive heart failure due to coronary artery disease. *Circulation* 62: 28–34, 1980.

51. Anderson J, Baim D, Fein S, et al: Efficacy and safety of sustained (48 hour) intravenous infusions of milrinone in patients with severe congestive heart failure: A multicenter study. *J Am Coll Cardiol* 9:711–722, 1987.

52. Wilmshurst P, Thompson D, Juul S, et al: Comparison of the effects of amrinone and sodium nitroprusside on haemodynamics, contractility, and myocardial metabolism in patients with cardiac failure due to coronary artery disease and dilated cardiomyopathy. *Br Heart J* 52:38–48, 1984.

53. Gage J, Rtuman H, Lucido D, et al: Additive effects of dobutamine and amrinone on myocardial contractility and ventricular performance in patients with severe heart failure. *Circulation* 74:367–373, 1986.

54. Colucci W, Wright R, Jaski B, et al: Milrinone and dobutamine in severe heart failure: Differing hemodynamic effects and individual patient responsiveness. *Circulation* 73:III-175-III-183, 1986.

55. Grose R, Strain J, Greenberg M, et al: Systemic and coronary effects of intravenous milrinone and dobutamine in congestive heart failure. *J Am Coll Cardiol* 7:1107–1113, 1986.

56. Biddle T, Benotti J, Creager M, et al: Comparison of intravenous milrinone and dobutamine for congestive heart failure secondary to either ischemic or dilated cardiomyopathy. *Am J Cardiol* 59:1345–1350, 1987.

57. Jaski B, Fifer M, Wright R, et al: Positive inotropic and vasodilator actions of milrinone in patients with severe congestive heart failure: Dose-response relationships and comparison to nitroprusside. *J Clin Invest* 75: 643–649, 1985.

58. Monrad E, Baim D, Smith H, et al: Milrinone, dobutamine, and nitroprusside: Comparative effects on hemodynamics and myocardial energetics in patients with severe congestive heart failure. *Circulation* 73:III-168-III-174, 1986.

59. Franciosa J: Intravenous amrinone: An advance or a wrong step? *Ann Intern Med* 102:399–400, 1985.

60. Massie B, Boukassa M, DiBianco R, et al: Long-term oral administration of amrinone for congestive heart failure: Lack of efficacy in a multicenter controlled trial. *Circulation* 71:963–971, 1985.

61. Packer M, Carver J, Rodeheffer R, et al: Effect of oral milrinone on mortality in severe chronic heart failure. *N Engl J Med* 325:1468–1475, 1991.

62. Colucci W, Denniss A, Leatherman G, et al: Intracoronary infusion of dobutamine to patients with and without severe congestive heart failure: Dose-response relationships, correlation with circulating catecholamines, and effect of phosphodiesterase inhibition. *J Clin Invest* 81:1103–1110, 1988.

63. Ziegler M, Lake C, Kopin I: Plasma noradrenaline increases with age. *Nature* 261:333–335, 1976.

64. Saar N, Gordon R: Variability of plasma catecholamine levels: Age, duration of posture and time of day. *Br J Clin Pharmacol* 8:353–358, 1979.

65. Lakatta E: Age-related alterations in the cardiovascular response to adrenergic mediated stress. *Fed Proc* 39:3173–3177, 1980.

66. Krall J, Connelly M, Weisbart R, et al: Age-related elevation of plasma catecholamine concentration and reduced responsiveness of lymphocyte adenylate cyclase*. *J Clin Endocrinol Metab* 52:863–867, 1981.

67. Franciosa J, Guiha N, Limas C, et al: Improved left ventricular function during nitroprusside infusion in acute myocardial infarction. *Lancet* 1: 650–654, 1972.

68. Page I, Corcoran A, Dustan H, et al: Cardiovascular actions of sodium nitroprusside in animals and hypertensive patients. *Circulation* 11: 188–198, 1955.

69. Mookherjee S, Keighley J, Warner R, et al: Hemodynamic, ventilatory and blood gas changes during infusion of sodium nitroferricyanide (nitroprusside)*: Studies in patients with congestive heart failure. *Chest* 72: 273–278, 1977.

70. Pierpont G, Hale K, Franciosa J, et al: Effects of vasodilators on pulmonary hemodynamics and gas exchange in left ventrical failure. *Am Heart J* 99:208–216, 1980.

71. Elkayam U, Kulick D, McIntosh N, et al: Incidence of early tolerance to hemodynamic effects of continuous infusion of nitroglycerin in patients with coronary artery disease and heart failure. *Circulation* 76:577–584, 1987.

72. Miller R, Awan N, Joye J, et al: Combined dopamine and nitroprusside therapy in congestive heart failure: Greater augmentation of cardiac performance by addition of inotropic stimulation to afterload reduction. *Circulation* 55:881–884, 1977.

73. Stemple D, Kleiman J, Harrison D: Combined nitroprusside-dopamine therapy in severe chronic congestive heart failure: Dose-related hemodynamic advantages over single drug infusions. *Am J Cardiol* 42:267–275, 1978.

74. Keung E, Siskind S, Sonneblick E, et al: Dobutamine therapy in acute myocardial infarction. *JAMA* 245:144–146, 1981.

75. Meretoja O: Haemodynamic effects of combined nitroglycerin-and dobutamine- infusions after coronary by-pass surgery: With one nitroglycerin-related complication. *Acta Anaest Scand* 24:211–215, 1980.

76. Pomer S, Sarai K, Krause E, et al: Hemodynamic equivalence of automated nitroglycerin-and nitroprusside-infusions combined with dobutamine for augmentation of cardiac output in patients following aorta coronary bypass- operation. *Int J Clin Pharm Ther Toxicol* 22:602–607, 1984.

77. Guimond J-G, Matuschak G, Meyers F, et al: Augmentation of cardiac function in end-stage heart failure by combined use of dobutamine and amrinone. *Chest* 90:302–304, 1986.

78. Uretsky B, Lawless C, Verbalis J, et al: Combined therapy with dobutamine and amrinone in severe heart failure: Improved hemodynamics and increased activation of the renin-angiotensin system with combined intravenous therapy. *Chest* 92:657–662, 1987.

79. Sundram P, Reddy H, McElroy P, et al: Myocardial energetics and efficiency in patients with idiopathic cardiomyopathy: Response to dobutamine and amrinone. *Am Heart J* 119:891–898, 1990.

80. Olsen K, Kluger J, Fieldman A: Combination high dose amrinone and dopamine in the management of moribund cardiogenic shock after open heart surgery. *Chest* 94:503–506, 1988.

81. Ghali JK, Cooper R, Ford E: Trends in hospitalization rates for heart failure in the United States, 1973–1986. *Arch Intern Med* 150:769–773, 1990.

82. Sutton GC: Epidemiologic aspects of heart failure. *Am Heart J* 120: 1538–1546, 1990.

83. Hughes CV, Wong M, Johnson G, et al: Influence of age on mechanisms and prognosis of heart failure. *Circulation* 87:VI-111-VI-117, 1993.
84. Cody RJ, Torre S, Clark M, et al: Age-related hemodynamic, renal, and hormonal differences among patients with congestive heart failure. *Arch Intern Med* 149:1023–1028, 1989.
85. The Digitalis Investigation Group: The effect of digoxin on mortality in patients with heart failure. *N Engl J Med* 336:525–533, 1997.
86. Packer M, Gheorghiade M, Young J, et al: Withdrawal of digoxin from patients with chronic heart failure treated with angiotensin-converting-enzyme inhibitors. *N Engl J Med* 329:1–7, 1993.
87. Miller R, Awan N, Maxwell K, et al: Sustained reduction of cardiac impedance and preload in congestive heart failure with the antihypertensive vasodilator prazosin. *N Engl J Med* 297:303–333, 1977.
88. Packer M, Meller J, Gorlin R, et al: Hemodynamic and clinical tachyphylaxis to prazosin-mediated afterload reduction in severe chronic congestive heart failure. *Circulation* 59:531–539, 1979.
89. Miller R, Vismara L, Williams D, et al: Pharmacological mechanisms for left ventricular unloading in clinical congestive heart failure: Differential effects of nitroprusside, phentolamine, and nitroglycerin on cardiac function and peripheral circulation. *Circ Res* 39:127–133, 1976.
90. Franciosa J, Pierpont G, Cohn J: Hemodynamic improvement after oral hydralazine in left ventricular failure: A comparison with nitroprusside infusion in 16 patients. *Ann Intern Med* 86:388–393, 1977.
91. Pierpont G, Cohn J, Franciosa J: Combined oral hydralazine-nitrate therapy in left ventricular failure: Hemodynamic equivalency to sodium nitroprusside. *Chest* 73:8–13, 1978.
92. Taylor S: Promises and disappointments of vasodilator treatment of chronic heart failure. In H Just, W-D Bussmann (eds.) *Vasodilators in Chronic Heart Failure.* Springer-Verlag, Berlin, 1983, pp 93–111.
93. Cohn J, Archibald D, Ziesche S, et al: Effect of vasodilator therapy on mortality in chronic congestive heart failure: Results of a Veterans Administration Cooperative Study. *N Engl J Med* 314:1547–1552, 1986.
94. Cohn J, Johnson G, Ziesche S, et al: A comparison of enalapril with hydralazine- isosorbide dinitrate in the treatment of chronic congestive heart failure. *N Engl J Med* 325:303–310, 1991.
95. Fonarow G, Chelimsky-Fallick C, Stevenson L, et al: Effect of direct vasodilation with hydralazine versus angiotensin-converting enzyme inhibition with captopril on mortality in advanced heart failure: The Hy-C trial. *J Am Coll Cardiol* 19:842–850, 1992.
96. CONSENSUS Trial Study Group: Effects of enalapril on mortality in severe congestive heart failure: Results of the cooperative north Scandinavian enalapril survival study (CONSENSUS). *N Engl J Med* 316:1429–1435, 1987.
97. SOLVD Investigators: Effect of enalapril on survival in patients with reduced left ventricular ejection fractions and congestive heart failure. *N Engl J Med* 325:293–302, 1991.
98. Pfeffer M, Braunwald E, Moye L, et al: Effect of captopril on mortality and morbidity in patients with left ventricular dysfunction after myocardial infarction: Results of the survival and ventricular enlargement trial. *N Engl J Med* 327:669–677, 1992.
99. SOLVD Investigators: Effect of enalapril on mortality and the development of heart failure in asymptomatic patients with reduced left ventricular ejection fractions. *N Engl J Med* 327:685–691, 1992.

100. Pitt B, Segal R, Martinez FA, et al: Randomized trial of losartan versus captopril in patients over 65 with heart failure (Evaluation of Losartan in the Elderly Study, ELITE). *Lancet* 349:747–752, 1997.
101. Israili ZH, Hall WD: Cough and angioneurotic edema associated with angiotensin-converting enzyme inhibitor therapy. *Ann Intern Med* 117: 234–242, 1992.
102. ACC/AHA Task Force: Guidelines for the evaluation and management of heart failure. *Am J Cardiol* 26:1376–1398, 1995.
103. Backes R, Gersh B: Cardiomyopathies in the elderly. In Lowenthal , (ed.) *Geriatric Cardiology*. F.A. Davis Company, Philadelphia, 1992, pp 105–125.
104. Guiha N, Cohn J, Mikulic E, et al: Treatment of refractory heart failure with infusion of nitroprusside. *N Engl J Med* 291:587–592, 1974.

Chapter 21

Physical Exercise and Training in Congestive Heart Failure

Andrew L. Clark, Andrew J.S. Coats

The pharmacological management of chronic heart failure (CHF) has improved dramatically over recent years with the introduction of drugs that not only improve symptoms, but improve survival. From the patients' perspective, CHF remains a disease characterized by exercise limitation, and despite the therapeutic advances, CHF is accompanied by high levels of morbidity as well as mortality,[1] and objective measures suggest considerable reductions in levels of everyday activity reflecting reductions in quality of life.[2,3] Some novel approaches to treatment, for example β- blockade, even raise the possibility that treatments aimed at increasing survival may worsen symptoms,[4] and conversely, treatments that improve symptoms may worsen prognosis.[5]

Training in the Elderly

The formal studies of training in CHF, as in many clinical studies, have focused on small numbers of carefully selected patients. It is difficult to be certain whether results obtained in these circumstances can be extrapolated to a wider population. Heart failure is, of course, predominantly a disease of the elderly, and yet the average age of patients included in research work has been less than 60. Training has been shown to improve left ventricular systolic function in a population of "normal" older men.[6] Rehabilitation has been shown to be helpful after

From *Clinical Cardiology in the Elderly. Second Edition,* edited by Elliot Chesler. © 1999, Futura Publishing Company, Armonk, NY.

cardiac events in older people[7,8] and is associated with a greater apparent improvement in submaximal endurance exercise than in peak exercise capacity.[9] Training may be helpful more widely in an aging population, particularly as a means of improving muscle strength and bulk.[10]

Why Train in Heart Failure?

Traditional cardiological management of CHF has emphasized the importance of rest as part of an overall treatment strategy.[11] There has been little published evidence of the therapeutic effect of rest other than in acute pulmonary edema. The little evidence that exists for rest as a specific therapy comes from studies of long term (up to 589 days) strict bed rest conducted in the 1960s.[12–14] In these studies, there was a high dropout rate and high mortality, and the end point was a decrease in heart size in some patients. It is easy to be critical of studies conducted in the days before modern treatment with loop diuretics and angiotensin-converting enzyme inhibitors, but there have been no comparable studies in the modern era.

Many of the changes seen in the periphery in patients with CHF are similar to those seen in detrained normal subjects. There is activation in the renin-angiotensin[15] and sympathetic[16] systems, loss of skeletal muscle, and depletion of oxidative enzymes.[17,18] Some of these features, such as loss of muscle bulk, are reversible with training in normal subjects, but are associated with a poor prognosis in CHF.[19]

Modest gains in exercise capacity are worth pursuing in their own right and by analogy with the benefits of exercise training in ischemic heart disease,[20] and after myocardial infarction,[21,22] it seems worthwhile to investigate the role of training in heart failure. Early uncontrolled work showed promising results.[23,24]

Safety Concerns

A note of caution should be introduced in considering exercise training. A potential worry in heart failure is the possible deleterious effects of increased stress on the myocardium itself, and the potential for causing cardiac dilation. In an influential paper, Jugdutt et al[25] reported the effects of a low level training program beginning 15 weeks after moderate sized anterior infarcts. Using echocardiographic techniques to define left ventricular contraction pattern abnormalities, they reported that patients with initial asynergy developed increased asynergy with training and worsened functional class despite an increase in exercise capacity. Further work in an animal model has also suggested that training can cause aggravation of left ventricular dilation after infarction and decreased survival.[26]

These findings are clearly worrying if exercise training is to be widely applicable in CHF. Judgutt's study was uncontrolled and in a relatively small number of patients. It also used a very strenuous program early after myocardial infarction. To address this point further, Gianuzzi et al[27] conducted a larger scale study in 95 patients randomly assigned to either training or control after anterior myocardial infarction (the EMI trial). Patients with lower left ventricular ejection fractions at entry demonstrated ventricular enlargement after 6 months, but there were no differences between the control and training groups.[27] In a small study conducted over a year, Enhance et al[28] found no deterioration in cardiac performance. Further data from the much larger ELVD trial, as yet unpublished, suggest that there may indeed be a slight improvement in left ventricular size and function related to training.

The studies to be considered in this chapter have selected patients carefully, and often supervised them closely during their training regimes (Tables 1 and 2). So far, there have been no adverse events directly related to exercise training. Certainly, formal exercise testing[29]

Table 1
Characteristics of Patients Entered into Selected Clinical Trials of Exercise Training in Chronic Heart Failure

Authors	Age of Patients (y)	n Study Design	LV Ejection Fraction	Initial peak Vo_2 (ml/kg/min)	NYHA
Sullivan[30]	54 (10)	24 all trained	24 (10) (9%–33%)	16.8 (3.8)	I–2 II–8 III–6
Coats[33]	61.8 ± 1.5	17 crossover	19.6 ± 2.3	13.2 ± 0.9	II–10 III–7
Meyer[34]	52 ± 2	18 crossover	21 ± 1	12.2 ± 0.7	II–8 III–10
Kiilavuorr[43]	52 (8)	27; randomized 12 trained	24 (5)[a]	19.3 ± 1.6[a]	II–15 III–12
Keteyian[44]	56 (11)	40; randomized 21 trained	21 (7)	14.7 ± 1.1	II–27 III–13
Kavanagh[49]	62 (6)	17 trained	21.4 ± 1.5	15.6 ± 3.5	II–2 III–19
Hambrecht[73]	51 (10)	22; randomized 12 trained	26 (9)[a]	17.5 (5.1)[a]	II–12 III–10
Belardinelli[94]	57 (6)	27; 18 trained; 9 matched controls	30 (5) (19%–38%)	16.1 (2)[a]	II–17 III–10
Demopoulos[95]	61 ± 2	16; all trained	21 ± 2	11.5 ± 0.4	II–6 III–7 IV–3

n is the number of patients entered into each study. NYHA in New York Heart Association classification of symptoms in heart failure. Figures in brackets are standard deviations; figures as ± are standard errors.
[a] Training group only

Table 2
Training Regimes and Improvement in Peak Exercise Capacity Seen in Selected Exercise Training Studies in Chronic Heart Failure

Authors	Type of Training	Intensity of Training	Frequency	Duration	S/U	↑ Peak Vo_2
Sullivan[30]	Cycle, walking	75%	60/min, 3–5/week	16–24 w	S	23%
Coats[33]	Cycle	60%–80%	20 min, 5/ week	8 w	U	18%
Meyer[34]	Cycle, walking (interval[a])	50%	45 min, 11/ week	3 w	S	20%
Kiilavuori[43]	Walking, cycling	55%	30 min, 3/ week	6 mo	S-3 mo U-3 mo	12%
Keteyian[44]	Treadmill, cycle, rowing	60%–80%	45/min, 3/ week	24 w	S	16%
Kavanagh[49]	Walking	55%	10–21 km per week	52 w	initially S[b]	17%
Hambrecht[73]	Cycle	near max	40/min daily	6 mo	S-3w U-6 m[c]	33%
Belardinelli[94]	Cycle	40%	30/min, 3/ week	8 w	S	17%
Demopoulos[95]	Cycle	<50%	60/min, 4/ week	12 w	S	22%

S/U refers to supervised or unsupervised training. ↑ peak Vo_2 is the percentage increase in peak oxygen consumption (ml/kg/min) seen after training.
[a] Interval training is characterized by repeated short bursts of exercise with recovery periods between.
[b] Initially supervised, but then mainly home-based with regular review visits.
[c] Additional twice weekly supervised group sessions.

has been found to be safe in a range of different patients, but the safety of unsupervised training in unselected patients has not as yet been directly addressed.

Training Benefits

Exercise Capacity

Depending on the method of assessment chosen, exercise training produces an improvement of about 20% in exercise capacity. The first investigators to examine training effects systematically were Sullivan et al.[30,31] They reported an increase in peak oxygen consumption of 23%, with no change in central hemodynamics at matched workloads,

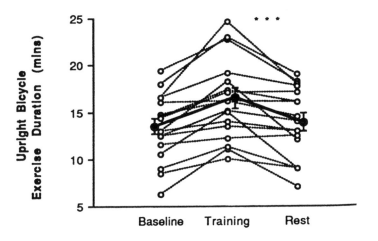

Figure 1: *Individual and mean responses to 8 weeks cycle training as assessed by upright incremental exercise testing before and after training, and following 8 weeks de-training (rest). Reproduced with permission from Coats AJS, Adamopoulos S, Radaelli A, et al: Controlled trial of physical training in chronic heart failure: Exercise performance, hemodynamics, ventilation, and autonomic function. Circulation 85:2119–31, 1992.*

but a trend towards an increase in peak cardiac output. The anaerobic threshold was delayed, and there was an increase in constant load exercise duration, as well as improvements in peak exercise leg blood flow.

A more rigorous approach using a randomized cross-over design and an 8-week home based exercise program[32,33] demonstrated an increase in peak oxygen consumption of 18% with a small increase in submaximal cardiac output (Figure 1). A second crossover study demonstrated similar benefits,[34] and emphasizes the potential importance of continuing to train once started; in the detraining phase, patients' exercise capacity returned to baseline. Further work has emphasized the increases in peak oxygen consumption possible with training.[35–37] Anaerobic and ventilatory thresholds are also consistently found to be increased following training.[31,34] In terms of the improvement in exercise capacity, training is better than, and additive to, the effects of angiotensin-converting enzyme inhibition.[38]

Ventilatory Response

The breathlessness of CHF is associated with an excessive ventilatory response in relation to carbon dioxide production which correlates inversely with exercise capacity.[39,40] Unlike the situation in normal subjects, where training does not affect ventilatory responses,[41] training in heart failure results in a reduction in the slope of the ventilatory

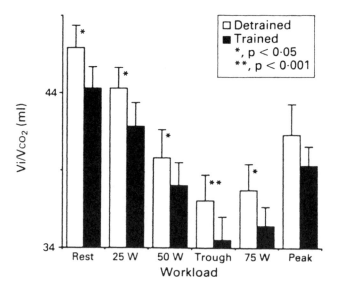

Figure 2: *Training results in a reduction in the ventilatory response to exercise. Vi/VCO₂ is ventilation per unit carbon dioxide production; after training, it can be seen that ventilation at matched workloads is reduced for a given level of carbon dioxide production. Reproduced with permission from Davey P, Meyer T, Coats A, et al: Ventilation in chronic heart failure: Effects of physical training. Br Heart J 68:473–4777, 1992.*

response,[42] with a reduction in ventilation at matched submaximal workloads (Figure 2).[31,43] There is an increase in peak exercise ventilation,[44] reflecting the increase in total exercise capacity and duration.

Sympathovagal Balance

Sympathetic activation and parasympathetic withdrawal is one of the characteristic features of chronic heart failure, and is associated with an adverse prognosis.[45] Coats et al[33] were able to examine the effects of training on sympathovagal balance, finding an improvement in heart rate variability and norepinephrine spillover suggesting a shift from sympathetic towards vagal activity. Training also improves circadian heart rate variability,[45,46] although Kiilavuori[47] reported an increase in heart rate variability during the day, but not at night, during both rest and exercise.

Quality of Life

From the patients' perspective, quality of life is vital, and may be of greater importance than increases in abstract measurements of maximal exercise capacity in the artificial setting of a laboratory exercise test. Improvements in patients' self-assessment symptom scores of breathlessness, fatigue and daily activity have been reported,[33] and reductions in perceived lag fatigue and dyspnea during exercise testing.[34] Using the CHF questionnaire,[48] Kavanagh[49] showed that improvements were maintained over a years' training program, with improvements most marked in those with the worst initial quality of life. There are also improvements in depression and anxiety scores.[37] Koch et al[36] reported that 80% of patients in their study requested that training should be prolonged.

An oblique way of considering quality of life issues in an objective manner is in responses to submaximal exercise (which more accurately reflect the day-to-day activities of patients than maximal testing), and in performance at self selected walking speeds. Patients choose electively to walk more slowly than normal subjects, although at a similar proportion of peak exercise capacity.[50] After training, there are increases in exercise duration at fixed workloads[31] and increases in the distance covered in a 6-minute walk test.[49,51] Interestingly, Beneke and Meyer[52] have reported that some of the improvements are due to an improvement in walking *efficiency*, in other words, a net decrease in the energy cost of walking.

Hemodynamic Response to Training

The central hemodynamic response to exercise training is somewhat controversial. Most investigators have reported no change in submaximal responses to training. Sullivan et al[30] found no change in cardiac filling pressures, pulmonary and systemic arterial pressures or cardiac output after training, a finding also shown by Jette et al,[28] Ehansi et al,[35] and Killavuori et al,[43] who in addition found no change in left ventricular ejection fraction. In contrast, Coats et al[33] showed small increases at submaximal workloads. Most investigators have found reductions in submaximal heart rates,[30,33,34,44] a commonly seen training effect in normals, but peak heart rate,[33,44] and in some studies, peak cardiac output,[53] is increased, reflecting the greater duration of exercise and increased peak exercise load, following training. The differing effects of posture on exercise hemodynamics may be one explanation for these differences, with a greater cardiac output response to training when assessed by supine exercise testing.

Belardinelli et al[54,55] have drawn attention to the possible beneficial effects of training on left ventricular diastolic rather than systolic function, finding increases in early diastolic filling and increases in peak filling rates at matched heart rates during exercise.

It seems unlikely that improvements in systolic function are likely to be of prime importance. Patients with chronic heart failure usually have normal submaximal cardiac output responses[56,57] and it is difficult to see how normal responses could be improved. Wilson et al[58] reported that training benefits were restricted to those patients with normal responses and that those patients with subnormal responses before a training program were unlikely to benefit. This conflicts with Meyer's work,[34] which suggests that the greatest benefits from training are gained by those patients with the worst pre-training function. These contrasting findings have yet to be resolved. Much more careful selection and classification of CHF patients based on the pathophysiology of their limiting symptoms may be necessary.

Mechanisms of Benefit

If training results in an increase in exercise capacity, but no change in central hemodynamics, how are the benefits mediated? The implication is that changes in the periphery are predominant in the training effect, presumably due to changes in skeletal muscle.

Peripheral Changes

Peripheral blood flow, measured as leg blood flow, is also unchanged by training, at least at matched workloads.[30] There may be a reduction in leg vascular resistance, and a tendency for leg arteriovenous oxygen difference to increase after training at matched submaximal workloads, although this did not achieve formal statistical significance.[30] Maximal arteriovenous oxygen difference is increased,[53] but this may simply reflect an increase in exercise duration. There is a reduction in submaximal arterial and venous lactate at matched exercise.[30,34] Studies in a rat model of chronic heart failure have shown reduced responses to endothelium-dependent vasodilatation with acetylcholine with no improvement with training,[59] but training may beneficially affect endothelial function, by causing an increase in flow-dependent dilation.[60]

Skeletal Muscle in CHF

Skeletal muscle in CHF is abnormal. Early in the progression of the disease, there is loss of muscle bulk,[61] and exercise capacity is related to both muscle strength and bulk.[62] Muscle strength is reduced,[63] as is endurance.[64] Skeletal muscle becomes histologically abnormal with a shift towards type II muscle fibers (Table 3).[65,66] Mitochondrial structure is abnormal,[67] with a reduction in volume of the cristae, and there are reductions in enzyme content, particularly of the enzymes of the Kreb's cycle and in the oxidative chain.[68,69]

Some of these changes are similar to those seen in normal subjects undergoing detraining, with generalized muscle wasting, although

Table 3
Skeletal Muscle Fiber Types

Fiber Type	Color, Function	Glycolytic Capacity	Oxidative Capacity
I	Red; slow oxidative	Medium	High
IIa	Red; fast oxidative	High	High
IIb	White; fast glycolytic	High	Low

In chronic heart failure, there is a shift in fiber distribution away from type I, oxidative fibers towards type II fast twitch glycolytic fibers with reduced oxidative enzyme levels.

with no change in muscle fiber type distribution.[70,71] Training can, however, result in a shift toward type I muscle fiber in normals.[72]

Training and Skeletal Muscle

Hambrecht et al[73] reported findings from muscle biopsies taken from vastus lateralis after a 6-month intensive training regime. There was an increase in the volume density[a] of mitochondria, and more specifically, an increase in the volume density of cytochrome c oxidase positive mitochondria. Although there were no changes in central hemodynamics, there was an increase in leg oxygen consumption.

Hambrecht et al[74] also showed a shift from type 11 to type I fibers, and increase in the surface density[a] of cytochrome c oxidase positive mitochondria, and in the surface density of mitochondrial cristae. The changes in cytochrome c oxidase positive mitochondria correlated closely with the change in peak oxygen consumption.[73,74] A further study has used vastus lateralis biopsy specimens coupled with same-site magnetic resonance images to calculate muscle cross-sectional area.[75] After training, there was a small increase in the muscle cross-sectional area and of isometric quadriceps strength. There was a rise in the ratio of capillaries to muscle fibers, and the endurance trained legs demonstrated a rise in citrate synthase and hydroxyacyidehydrogenase. It must be kept in mind, however, that most training studies to date have been predominantly of aerobic training regimes far less likely to increase muscle bulk compared to isometric training. This latter form of exercise training has been little studied in heart failure.

The changes in muscle structure and ultrastructure are reflected in changes in muscle metabolism. Magnetic resonance spectroscopy can be used to examine intracellular phosphate metabolism, which has been shown to be abnormal in CHF with more rapid depletion of phos-

[a] Volume density is the fraction of total tissue volume accounted for by mitochondrial volume. Surface density is measured as the number of intersections of the membrane in question with a test line as a proportion of the length of the test line.

phocreatine and early acidosis compared with normals.[76,77] Minotti et al[78,79] showed improvements in forearm metabolism after training both in normals and in patients with CHF in the absence of any systemic training effect.

Adamopoulos et al[80] have examined the effects of training on calf muscle metabolism in patients with CHF, showing partial reversal of MR abnormalities. There was a decrease in phosphocreatine depletion and a shortening in the recovery time of phosphocreatine following exercise, although no change in intracellular pH.[80] The results of forearm training are similar, with an improved pH response to exercise.[81] In an animal model, the skeletal muscle metabolic benefits are shown to be independent of changes in muscle bulk.[82] Taken together, these results suggest that training may have a profound effect on skeletal muscle metabolism without any changes in hemodynamics, and without the mechanism simply reflecting muscle hypertrophy in response to exercise.

Respiratory Muscle

Respiratory muscle is involved in the changes affecting skeletal muscle more generally. Respiratory muscle becomes histologically abnormal,[83] with reduced endurance[84] and strength[85] and early respiratory muscle deoxygenation during exercise.[86] The work of breathing is increased in heart failure, which may equate with the sensation of breathlessness.[87] Some of the histological changes seen in diaphragmatic muscle suggest a pre-existing training effect, perhaps due to chronic hyperventilation.[88] Despite this finding, selective training of respiratory muscle alone can result in ventilatory improvements and an improvement in exercise capacity.[89]

The Ergoreflex

Ergoreflex is the term used to describe the neural reflex originating in exercising skeletal muscle that drives, at least in part, the ventilatory and hemodynamic responses to exercise. Its stimulation also results in sympathetic activation.[90] Abnormal activation of the ergoreflex, perhaps due to abnormal skeletal muscle responses to exercise, may be responsible for much of the abnormal exercise response seen in chronic heart failure (Figure 3).[91,92]

The ergoreflex can be shown to be abnormally active in CHF.[93] Training partially reverses the ergoreflex responses, with an attenuation of the ergoreflex-driven ventilatory, blood pressure and peripheral blood flow responses of CHF. This mechanism, the reduced ergoreflex activation, may explain how changes in muscle metabolism and structure produce the wider beneficial effects of the training response.

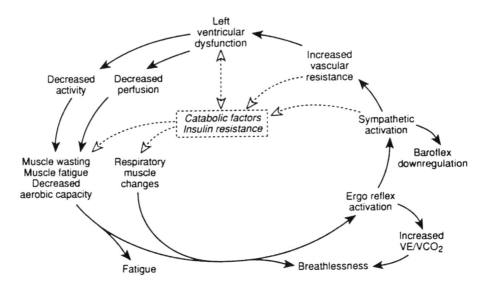

Figure 3: *The muscle hypothesis of symptom generation in chronic heart failure. The abnormal skeletal muscle response to exercise results in excessive ergoreflex activation with resultant sympathetic activation and thus increased vascular resistance. The symptom of fatigue arises from abnormal muscle, and breathlessness from the increased ventilatory response to exercise (seen as the slope of the ventilation-carbon dioxide production (VE/VCO$_2$) slope. Reproduced with permission from Clark AL, Poole-Wilson PA, Coats AJS: Exercise limitation in chronic heart failure: The central role of the periphery. J Am Coll Cardiol 28:1092–1102, 1996.*

Patient Selection and Level of Training

The formal studies of training in CHF discussed have used carefully selected patients in closely supervised training protocols. The types of exercise used range from home cycling[33] to supervised intensive training using cycle treadmill and rowing.[44] Similarly, patients with a range of left ventricular dysfunction and ages has been included in studies (Table 1).

The intensity of training has usually been at levels of approximately 60%–80% of maximal capacity, which raises questions as to safety and the need for supervision. There is some evidence that this intensity of exercise may not be necessary. Belardinelli et al[94] studied 27 patients with mild CHF, 18 of whom underwent supervised low-intensity training at 40% of peak oxygen consumption, with an increase in peak oxygen consumption of 17%. Demopoulos et al[95] studied patients with more severe heart failure who trained at low workloads (<50% of maximal) using supine cycle exercise in a deliberate attempt to minimize ventricular wall stress. Peak oxygen consumption increased by 30% following 12 weeks of training. The principal training methods have concentrated on endurance training. There is some provisional evidence that interval training may be more appropriate; that is, short periods of high-intensity exercise interspersed with periods of rest. These exercise protocols allow higher levels of exercise to be attained, while not producing increased cardiac stress.[96] Strength versus resistance training is another possible avenue to be explored. In patients with coronary artery disease, a training regime of endurance and weightlifting improved both peak exercise capacity and submaximal endurance more effectively than endurance training alone.[97] *Isometric* exercise is associated with adverse hemodynamic effects in heart failure,[98,99] but *resistance* exercise appears to be safe with no adverse change in cardiac function.[100] A small study has shown that resistance training alone improves endurance although not peak performance.[101] Recent reports suggest that improvement may follow localized muscle training.[102] Further work is needed to define the type of exercise and relative contributions to be made by endurance and resistance training.

Time Course of Benefits

While training of as short a duration as 4 weeks[35] results in improvements in exercise capacity, the duration of training required for maximal benefit. Most of the possible improvement has occurred by 12 weeks.[44] The longest term formal study of training over 12 months suggests that the training effects reach a plateau at about 16 to 26 weeks, and persist while training continues (Figure 4).[49] Conversely, the crossover studies of training suggests that the benefits reverse quickly if training is stopped,[33,34] and the training benefit has been shown to be related to the level of compliance.[33] Once undertaken, it appears that training should be continued for life.

Prognosis as a Result of Training

There are, as yet, no data on the effects of exercise training in CHF and prognosis. Multinational studies are now being mounted to examine this question. Training has already been shown to improve features of the heart failure syndrome associated with an adverse prognosis. Thus, decreased exercise capacity,[103,104] the excessive ventilatory response to exercise,[105,106] sympathetic activation,[104,107] and reduction in muscle bulk,[19] which are all associated with an adverse prognosis, are all at least partially reversed by training. A definitive judgement as to the survival benefits of training will have to await trial results.

The work to date suggests that in selected patients, training can improve exercise capacity by about 20% with improved quality of life and decrease in the ventilatory response to exercise. These changes

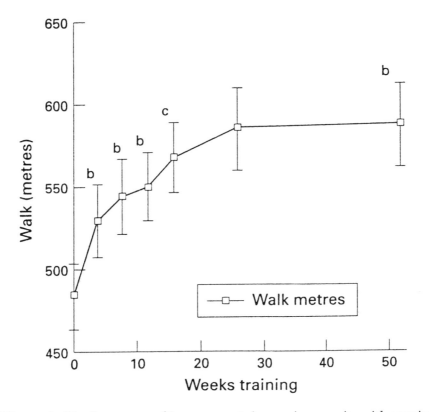

Figure 4: *The time course of improvements in exercise capacity with exercise training assessed as the distance covered in a 6 minute walk test. Reproduced with permission from Kavanagh T, Myers MG, Baigrie RS, et al: Quality of life and cardiorespiratory function in chronic heart failure: Effects of 12 months' aerobic training.* Heart 76:42–49, 1996.

may be associated with an improvement in outcome; certainly, the benefits seen are in addition to any benefits gained from conventional drug therapy.

In contrast to the advice previously given for the management of chronic heart failure, we would now recommend that patients are encouraged to exercise. With the present state of knowledge, a regime of 20 minutes aerobic exercise at least 3 times per week is appropriate. As further information becomes available, the prescription may need to be refined.

References

1. Stewart AL, Greenfield S, Hays RD, et al: Functional status and well-being of patients with chronic conditions. *JAMA* 262:907–913, 1989.

2. Davies SW, Jordan SL, Lipkin DP: Use of limb movement sensors as indicators of the level of everyday physical activity in chronic congestive heart failure. Am J Cardiol 69:1581–1586, 1992.
3. Oka RK, Stotts NA, Dae MW, et al: Daily physical activity levels in congestive heart failure. Am J Cardiol 71:924–925, 1993.
4. Australia/New Zealand Heart Failure Research Collaborative Group: Randomised, placebo-controlled trial of carvedilol in patients with congestive heart failure due to ischaemic heart disease. Lancet 349:375–380, 1997.
5. Cowley AJ, Skene AM, on behalf of the Enoximone Investigators. Treatment of severe heart failure: Quantity or quality of life? A trial of enoximone. Br Heart J 72:226–230, 1994.
6. Ehansi M, Ogawa T, Miller TR, et al: Exercise training improves left ventricular systolic function in older men. Circulation 83:96–103, 1991.
7. Lavie CJ, Milani RV: Effects of cardiac rehabilitation and exercise training programs in patients 75 years of age. Am J Cardiol 78:675–677, 1996.
8. Levine CJ, Milani RV: Benefits of cardiac rehabilitation and exercise training in elderly women. Am J Cardiol 79:664–666, 1997.
9. Ades PA, Waldmann ML, Poehiman ET, et al: Exercise conditioning in older coronary patients: Submaximal lactate response and endurance capacity. Circulation 88:572–575, 1993.
10. Fielding RA: Effects of exercise training in the elderly: Impact of progressive resistance training on skeletal muscle and whole-body protein metabolism. Proc Nutr Soc 54:665–675, 1996.
11. Braunwald E, (ed) Heart Disease. 3rd ed. Philadelphia, WB Saunders Co., 1988, p 488.
12. Burch GE, Walsh JJ, Black WC: Value of prolonged bed rest in management of cardiomegaly. JAMA 183:81–87, 1963.
13. Burch GE, McDonald CD: Prolonged bed rest in the treatment of ischemic cardiomyopathy. Chest 60:424–430, 1971.
14. McDonald CD, Burch GE, Walsh JJ: Prolonged bed rest in the treatment of idiopathic cardiomyopathy. Am J Med 52:41–50, 1972.
15. Hespel P, Lijnen P, Faggard R, et al: Effects of physical endurance training on the plasma renin-angiotensin-aldosterone system in normal man. J Endocrinol 116:443–449, 1988.
16. Cooksey JD, Reilly P, Brown S, et al: Exercise training and plasma catecholamines in patients with ischemic heart disease. Am J Cardiol 42:372–376, 1978.
17. Holloszy JO: Adaptations of muscular tissue to training. Prog Cardiovasc Dis 18:445–458, 1976.
18. Refenberick DH, Gamble JG, Max SR: Response of mitochondrial enzymes to decreased muscular activity. Am J Physiol 225:1295–1259, 1973.
19. Anker S, Ponikowski P, Varney S, et al: Wasting as an independent risk factor for mortality in chronic heart failure. Lancet 349:1050–1053, 1997.
20. Clausen JP. Circulatory adjustments to dynamic exercise and effect of physical training in normal subjects and in patients with coronary artery disease. Prog Cardiovasc Dis 18:459–495, 1976.
21. Oldridge NB, Guyatt GH, Fisher ME, et al: Cardiac rehabilitation after myocardial infarction: Combined experience of randomized clinical trials. JAMA 260:945–950, 1988.
22. O'Connor GT, Buring JE, Yusuf S, et al: An overview of randomized trials of rehabilitation with exercise after myocardial infarction. Circulation 80:234–244, 1989.

23. Lee AP, Ice R, Blessey R, et al: Long term effects of physical training on coronary patients with impaired LV function. *Circulation* 60:1519–1526, 1978.
24. Conn EH, Williams RS, Wallace AG: Exercise responses before and after physical conditioning in patients with severely depressed left ventricular function. *Am J Cardiol* 49:296–300, 1982.
25. Jugdutt BI, Michorowski BL, Kappagoda CT: Exercise training after anterior Q wave myocardial infarction: Importance of left ventricular function and topography. *J Am Coll Cardiol* 12:362–372, 1988.
26. Gaudron P, Hu K, Schamberger R, et al: Effect of endurance training early or late after coronary artery occlusion on left ventricular remodelling, hemodynamics, and survival in rats with chronic transmural myocardial infarction. *Circulation* 89:402–412, 1994.
27. Gianuzzi P, Tavazzi L, Temporelli PL, et al, for the EAMI study group. Long-term physical training and left ventricular remodelling after anterior myocardial infarction (EAMI) trial. *J Am Coll Cardiol* 22:1821–1829, 1993.
28. Ehansi AA, Miller TR, Miller TA, et al: Comparison of adaptations to a 12-month exercise program and late outcome in patients with healed myocardial infarction and ejection fraction <45% and >50%. *Am J Cardiol* 79:1258–1260, 1997.
29. Tristani FE, Hughes CV, Archibald DG, et al: Safety of graded symptom-limited exercise testing in patients with congestive heart failure. *Circulation* 76(suppl VI):54–58, 1987.
30. Sullivan MJ, Higginbotham MB, Cobb FR: Exercise training in patients with severe left ventricular dysfunction: Hemodynamic and metabolic effects. *Circulation* 78:506–516, 1988.
31. Sullivan MJ, Higginbotham MB, Cobb FR: Exercise training in patients with chronic heart failure delays ventilatory anaerobic threshold and improves submaximal exercise performance. *Circulation* 79:324–329, 1989.
32. Coats AJS, Adamopoulos S, Meyer T, et al: Physical training in chronic heart failure. *Lancet* 335:63–66, 1990.
33. Coats AJS, Adamopoulos S, Radaelli A, et al: Controlled trial of physical training in chronic heart failure: Exercise performance, hemodynamics, ventilation, and autonomic function. *Circulation* 85:2119–2131, 1992.
34. Meyer K, Schwaibold M, Westbrook S, et al: Effect of short-term exercise training and activity restriction on functional capacity in patients with severe chronic congestive heart failure. *Am J Cardiol* 78:1017–1022, 1996.
35. Jette M, Heller R, Landry F, et al: Randomised 4-week exercise program in patients with impaired left ventricular function. *Circulation* 84: 1561–1567, 1991.
36. Koch M, Douard H, Broustet J-P: The benefit of graded physical exercise in chronic heart failure. *Chest* 101(suppl):231S–235S, 1992.
37. Kostis JB, Rosen RC, Cosgrove NM, et al: Nonpharmacologic therapy improves functional and emotional status in congestive heart failure. *Chest* 106:996–1001, 1994.
38. Meyer TE, Casadei B, Coats AJS, et al: Angiotensin-converting enzyme inhibition and physical training in heart failure. *J Intem Med* 230: 407–413, 1991.
39. Buller NP, Poole-Wilson PA: Mechanism of the increased ventilatory response to exercise in patients with chronic heart failure. *Br Heart J* 63: 281–283, 1990.

40. Davies SW, Emery TM, Watling MIL, et al: A critical threshold of exercise capacity in the ventilatory response to exercise in heart failure. *Br Heart J* 65:179–183, 1991.
41. Clark AL, Skypala I, Coats AJS: Ventilatory efficiency is unchanged after physical training in health persons despite an increase in exercise tolerance. *J Cardiovasc Risk* 1:347–351, 1994.
42. Davey P, Meyer T, Coats A, et al: Ventilation in chronic heart failure: Effects of physical training. *Br Heart J* 68:473–477, 1992.
43. Kiilavuori K, Sovijarvi A, Naveri H, et al: Effect of physical training on exercise capacity and gas exchange in patients with chronic heart failure. *Chest* 110:985–991, 1996.
44. Keteyian SJ, Levine AB, Brawner CA, et al: Exercise training in patients with heart failure. *Ann Intern Med* 124:1051–1057, 1996.
45. Cohn JN, Johnson GR, Shabetai R, et al, for the V-HeFT VA Cooperative Studies Group: Ejection fraction, peak exercise consumption, cardiothoracic ratio ventricular arrhythmias, and plasma norepinephrine as determinants of prognosis in heart failure. *Circulation* 87(suppl Vl):VI-5-VI-16, 1993.
46. Adamopoulos S, Ponikowski P, Cerquetani E, et al: Circadian patterns of heart rate variability in chronic heart failure patients: Effects of training. *Eur Heart J* 16:1380–1386, 1995.
47. Killavuori K, Tolvonen L, Naveri H, et al: Reversal of autonomic derangements by physical training in chronic heart failure assessed by heart rate variability. *Eur Heart J* 16:490–495, 1995.
48. Guyatt GH, Nogradi S, Halcrow S, et al: Development and testing of a new measure of health status for clinical trials in heart failure. *J Gen Intern Med* 4:101–107, 1989.
49. Kavanagh T, Myers MG, Baigrie RS, et al: Quality of life and cardiorespiratory function in chronic heart failure: Effects of 12 months' aerobic training. *Heart* 76:42–49, 1996.
50. Clark AL, Rafferty D, Arbuthnott K: Exercise dynamics at submaximal workloads in patients with chronic heart failure. *J Cardiac Failure* 3:15–19, 1997.
51. Meyer K, Schwalbold M, Westbrook S, et al: Effects of exercise training and activity restriction on 6-minute walking test performance in patients with chronic heart failure. *Am Heart J* 133:447–453, 1997.
52. Beneke R, Meyer K: Walking performance and economy in chronic heart failure patients pre and post exercise training. *Eur J Appl Physiol* 75:246–251, 1997.
53. Dubach P, Myers J, Dziekan G, et al: Effect of high intensity exercise training on central hemodynamic responses to exercise in men with reduced left ventricular function. *J Am Coll Cardiol* 29:1591–1598, 1997.
54. Belardinelli R, Georgiou D, Cianci G, et al: Exercise training improves left ventricular diastolic filling in patients with dilated cardiomyopathy. Clinical and prognostic implications. *Circulation* 91:2775–2784, 1995.
55. Belardinelli R, Georgiou D, Cianci G, et al: Effects of exercise training on left ventricular filling at rest and during exercise in patients with ischemic cardiomyopathy and severe left ventricular dysfunction. *Am Heart J* 132:61–70, 1996.
56. Wilson JR, Mancini DM, Dunkman WB: Exertional fatigue due to skeletal muscle dysfunction in patients with heart failure. *Circulation* 87:470–475, 1993.

57. Wilson JR, Rayos G, Yeoh TK, et al: Dissociation between peak exercise oxygen consumption and hemodynamic dysfunction in potential heart transplantation candidates. *J Am Coll Cardiol* 26:429–435, 1995.
58. Wilson JR, Groves J, Rayos G: Circulatory status and response to cardiac rehabilitation in patients with heart failure. *Circulation* 94:1567–1572, 1996.
59. Lindsay DC, Jiang C, Brunotte F, et al: Impairment of endothelium dependent responses in a rat model of chronic heart failure: Effects of an exercise training protocol. *Cardiovasc Res* 26:694–697, 1992.
60. Hornig B, Maier V, Drexler H: Physical training improves endothelial function in patients with chronic heart failure. *Circulation* 93:210–214, 1996.
61. Mancini DM, Walter G, Reichnek N, et al: Contribution of skeletal muscle atrophy to exercise intolerance and altered muscle metabolism in heart failure. *Circulation* 85:1364–1373, 1992.
62. Volterrani M, Clark AL, Ludman PF, et al: Determinants of exercise capacity in chronic heart failure. *Eur Heart J* 15:801–809, 1994.
63. Buller NP, Jones D, Poole-Wilson PA: Direct measurements of skeletal muscle fatigue in patients with chronic heart failure. *Br Heart J* 65:20–24, 1991.
64. Minotti JR, Pillay P, Chang L, et al: Neurophysiological assessment of skeletal muscle fatigue in patients with congestive heart failure. *Circulation* 86:903–908, 1992.
65. Lipkin D, Jones D, Round J, et al: Abnormalities of skeletal muscle in patients with chronic heart failure. *Int J Cardiol* 18:187–195, 1988.
66. Mancini DM, Coyle E, Coggan A, et al: Contribution of intrinsic skeletal muscle changes to 31P NMR skeletal muscle abnormalities in patients with chronic heart failure. *Circulation* 80:1338–1346, 1989.
67. Drexler H, Riede U, Munzel T, et al: Alterations of skeletal muscle in chronic heart failure. *Circulation* 85:1751–1759, 1992
68. Wilson JR, Martin JL, Ferraro N: Impaired skeletal muscle nutritive flow during exercise in patients with congestive heart failure: Role of cardiac pump dysfunction as determined by the effect of dobutamine. *Am J Cardiol* 53:1308–1315, 1984.
69. Sullivan MJ, Green HJ, Cobb FR: Skeletal muscle biochemistry and histology in ambulatory patients with long-term heart failure. *Circulation* 81:518–527, 1990.
70. Green HJ, Thomson JA, Daub BD, et al: Biochemical and histochemical alterations in skeletal muscle in man during a period of reduced activity. *Can J Physiol Pharmacol* 58:1311–1316, 1980.
71. Patel A, Razzack Z, Dastir D: Disuse atrophy of human skeletal muscles. *Arch Neurol* 20:413–421, 1969.
72. Holloszy JO, Coyle EF: Adaptations of skeletal muscle to endurance exercise and their metabolic consequences. *J Appl Physiol* 56:831–838, 1984.
73. Hambrecht R, Niebauer J, Fiehn E, et al: Physical training in patients with stable chronic heart failure: Effects on cardiorespiratory fitness and ultrastructural abnormalities of leg muscles. *J Am Coll Cardiol* 25: 1239–1249, 1995.
74. Hambrecht R, Fiehn E, Yu J, et al: Effects of endurance training on mitochondrial ultrastructure and fiber type distribution in skeletal muscle of patients with stable chronic heart failure. *J Am Coll Cardiol* 29: 1067–1073, 1997.

75. Magnusson G, Gordon A, Kaijser L, et al: High intensity knee extensor training in patients with chronic heart failure. *Eur Heart J* 17:1048–1055, 1996.
76. Massie BM, Conway M, Yonge R, et al: Skeletal muscle metabolism in patients with congestive heart failure: Relation to clinical severity and blood flow. *Circulation* 76:1009–1019, 1987.
77. Massie BM, Conway M, Yonge R, et al: ^{31}P nuclear magnetic resonance evidence of abnormal skeletal muscle metabolism in patients with congestive heart failure. *Am J Cardiol* 60:309–315, 1987.
78. Minotti JR, Johnson EC, Hudson TL, et al: Training-induced skeletal muscle adaptations are independent of systemic adaptations. *J Appl Physiol* 68:289–294, 1990.
79. Minotti JR, Johnson EC, Hudson TL, et al: Skeletal muscle responses to exercise training in chronic heart failure. *J Clin Invest* 86:751–758, 1990.
80. Adamopoulos S, Coats AJS, Brunotte F, et al: Physical training improves skeletal muscle metabolic abnormalities in patients with chronic heart failure. *J Am Coll Cardiol* 23:1101–1106, 1993.
81. Stratton JR, Dunn JF, Adamopoulos S, et al: Training partially reverses skeletal muscle metabolic abnormalities during exercise in heart failure. *J Appl Physiol* 76:1575–1582, 1994.
82. Brunotte F, Thompson CH, Adamopoulos S, et al: Rat skeletal muscle metabolism in experimental heart failure: Effects of physical training. *Acta Physiol Scand* 154:439–447, 1995.
83. Lindsay DC, Lovegrove CA, Dunn MJ, et al: Histological abnormalities of muscle from limb, thorax and diaphragm in chronic heart failure. *Eur Heart J* 17:1239–1250, 1996.
84. Walsh JT, Andrews R, Johnson P, et al: Inspiratory muscle endurance in patients with chronic heart failure. *Heart* 76:332–336, 1996.
85. Hammond MD, Bauer KA, Sharp JT, et al: Respiratory muscle strength in congestive heart failure. *Chest* 98:1091–1094, 1990.
86. Mancini DM, Ferraro N, Nazzaro D, et al: Respiratory muscle deoxygenation during exercise in patients with heart failure demonstrated with near-infrared spectroscopy. *J Am Coll Cardiol* 18:492–498, 1991.
87. Mancini DM, Henson D, LaManca J, et al: Respiratory muscle function and dyspnea in patients with chronic congestive heart failure. *Circulation* 86:909–919, 1992.
88. Tikunov B, Levine S, Mancini D: Chronic congestive heart failure elicits adaptations of endurance exercise in diaphragmatic muscle. *Circulation* 95:910–916, 1997.
89. Mancini DM, Henson D, LaManca J, et al: Benefit of selective respiratory muscle training on exercise capacity in patients with chronic congestive heart failure. *Circulation* 91:320–329, 1995.
90. Piepoli M, Clark AL, Coats AJS: Muscle metaboreceptors in the hemodynamic, autonomic and ventilatory responses to exercise in man. *Am J Physiol* 269(Heart Circ Physiol 38):H1428-H1436, 1995.
91. Coats AJS, Clark AL, Piepoli M, et al: Symptoms and quality of life in heart failure: The muscle hypothesis. *Br Heart J* 72(suppl):36–39, 1994.
92. Clark AL, Poole-Wilson PA, Coats AJS: Exercise limitation in chronic heart failure: The central role of the periphery. *J Am Coll Cardiol* 28:1092–1102, 1996.
93. Piepoli M, Clark AL, Volterrani M, et al: Contribution of muscle afferents to the hemodynamic, autonomic, and ventilatory responses to exercise in

patients with chronic heart failure: Effects of physical training. *Circulation* 93:940–952, 1996.

94. Belardinelli R, Georgiou D, Scocco V, et al: Low intensity exercise training in patients with chronic heart failure. *J Am Coll Cardiol* 26:975–982, 1995

95. Demopoulos L, Bijou R, Fergus I, et al: Exercise training in patients with severe congestive heart failure: Enhancing peak aerobic capacity whilst minimizing the increase in ventricular wall stress. *J Am Coll Cardiol* 29: 597–603, 1997.

96. Meyer K, Samek L, Schwaibold M, et al: Interval training in patients with severe chronic heart failure: Analysis and recommendations for exercise procedures. *Med Sci Sports Exerc* 29:306–312, 1997.

97. McCartney N, McKelvie RS, Haslam DRS, et al: Usefulness of weightlifting training in improving strength and maximal power output in coronary artery disease. *Am J Cardiol* 67:939–945, 1991.

98. Elkayam U, Roth A, Weber L, et al: Isometric exercise in patients with chronic advanced heart failure: Hemodynamic and neurohormonal evaluation. *Circulation* 72:975–981, 1985.

99. Reddy HK, Weber KT, Janicki JS, et al: Hemodynamic, ventilatory and metabolic effects of light isometric exercise in patients with chronic heart failure. *J Am Coll Cardiol* 12:353–358, 1988.

100. McKelvie RS, McCartney N, Tomlinson C, et al: Comparison of hemodynamic responses to cycling and resistance exercise in congestive heart failure secondary to ischemic cardiomyopathy. *Am J Cardiol* 76:977–979, 1995.

101. Hare DL, Ryan TM, Selig SE, et al: Effects of resistance weight training in patients with chronic heart failure. *Circulation* 94(suppl I):1–192, 1996.

102. Ohtsubo M, Yonezawa K, Nishijima H, et al: Metabolic abnormality of calf skeletal muscle is improved by localised muscle training without changes in blood flow in chronic heart failure. *Heart* 78:437–443, 1997.

103. Parameshwar J, Keegan J, Sparrow J, et al: Predictors of prognosis in severe chronic heart failure. *Am Heart J* 123:421–426, 1992.

104. Cohn JN, Johnson GR, Shabetai R, et al: Ejection fraction, peak exercise consumption, cardiothoracic ratio, ventricular arrhythmias, and plasma norepinephrine as determinants of prognosis in heart failure. *Circulation* 87(suppl VI):5–16, 1993.

105. MacGowan GA, Janosko K, Cecchetti A, et al: Exercise-related ventilatory abnormalities and survival in congestive heart failure. *Am J Cardiol* 79: 1264–1266, 1997.

106. Chua TP, Ponikowski P, Harrington D, et al: Clinical correlates and prognostic significance of the ventilatory response to exercise in chronic heart failure. *J Am Coll Cardiol* 29:1585–1590, 1997.

107. Cohn JN, Levine BT, Olivari MT, et al: Plasma norepinephrine as a guide to prognosis in patients with chronic congestive heart failure. *N Engl J Med* 311:819–823, 1984.

Chapter 22

Cardiac Transplantation

Alfredo Rego, Sara J. Shumway,
Norman E. Shumway

As heart transplantation has evolved into a routine clinical option, so the guidelines for recipient age have become more lenient. Originally, cardiac transplants were offered to patients 18 to 55 years of age. Improved immunosuppression and experience in dealing with these patients intraoperatively and postoperatively have extended the age range from the newborn to patients over age 60, but there are few heart transplant recipients older than 70 years. For the purposes of this review, we shall consider patients over age 55 to be elderly with respect to heart transplantation. This group constitutes 10%–20% of all patients awaiting cardiac transplantation. Approximately 50% have ischemic cardiomyopathies, many having had multiple angioplasties or coronary artery bypass grafting. Nonischemic dilated cardiomyopathy, primary restrictive cardiomyopathy and primary valvular disease are less frequent.

The elderly have always been thought of as a high-risk group due to more frequent coexisting premorbid conditions that would limit survival and negatively impact the potential for life-years served. Nevertheless, survival rates among the elderly have been found, in several clinical series, to be comparable to younger patients undergoing heart transplantation, therefore age is no longer considered a contraindication to the procedure.[1–9] However, the acute shortage of donor hearts has focused attention on the selection criteria for transplantation, particularly on the upper age limit. Providing the benefits of heart transplantation to an increasing number of older individuals has raised some ethical issues. Should a scarce source of donor hearts be made available to individuals whose life expectancy, even with good graft function, is

From *Clinical Cardiology in the Elderly. Second Edition,* edited by Elliot Chesler. © 1999, Futura Publishing Company, Armonk, NY.

only 5 to 10 years, when a younger recipient may benefit for several decades? Such issues become relevant when one considers that the elderly is the largest growing demographic group in this country. It is estimated that by early next century, the elderly will comprise more than 15% of the United States population. Consequently, it will be patients between the ages of 65 to 74 years who will be asking for a larger share of limited donor resources, as well as health care dollars.[10]

In dealing with the complex issues surrounding heart transplantation in the elderly, this chapter will address some of the most controversial questions on the subject: Should the elderly undergo more stringent pretransplant evaluation? What comorbidities should exclude heart transplantation? Are they more at risk for certain complications after cardiac transplantation? Are older donors a viable option for the older cardiac recipient? What is their overall survival? Is the immune response in the elderly different than in younger patients?

Patient Selection

The most common diagnosis in elderly patients referred for heart transplantation is heart failure due to ischemic coronary artery disease. Nonischemic dilated cardiomyopathy, primary restrictive cardiomyopathy and primary valvular disease are less frequent. In general, elderly patients with irreversible heart disease will be considered candidates for heart transplantation if they are found to have one of the following: severe activity-limiting ischemia not amenable to revascularization; recurrent ventricular arrhythmias refractory to all therapeutic modalities; persistent or labile cardiac failure despite tailored medical therapy and compliance; peak oxygen consumption below 14 mL/kg per minute with limitation of daily activities.

Evaluation for transplantation includes a careful search for any noncardiac condition that limits life expectancy or increases the risk of complications from the procedure and particularly from immunosuppression. Thus, when selecting older patients for heart transplantation, greater attention needs to be paid to concomitant diseases than in younger individuals. The workup should ensure that the candidate is free of neoplasms commonly found in older individuals such as carcinoma of the bronchus, prostate, breast, colorectum and uterine cervix. Other comorbid conditions such as cholecystitis may lead to dangerous complications in elderly individuals, especially diabetics. It is wise, therefore, to perform gallbladder ultrasound examination in elderly transplant candidates; whether preoperative cholecystectomy should be performed in patients with asymptomatic cholelithiasis depends on the judgment and experience of the transplant surgeon.[11] The same applies to the need for routine barium enema and surgery for patients with asymptomatic diverticular disease of the colon. Colonic perforation in immunosuppressed recipients is associated with a mortality of 60% and is usually caused by diverticulitis. It has been suggested however that pretransplant colonic resections should be reserved for patients with symptomatic diverticular disease.[11,12] Earlier publications have indicated that older recipients were at increased risk for infection and had decreased long-term survival.[8-9] This is no longer true with modified immunosuppression regimens free of induction therapy and more effective therapy for cytomegalovirus infection.[2]

The same exclusion principles apply to the elderly as for any would be cardiac transplant recipient. Diseases of the lungs, liver, or kidneys are contraindications. The presence of any two comorbid factors such as severe peripheral vascular disease or significant cerebrovascular disease contraindicates transplantation. Active infection, active peptic ulcer disease and uncontrolled insulin-dependent diabetes should also be considered relative contraindications. Age alone is rarely the deciding factor. Every patient is evaluated on an individual basis. Medical compliance is mandatory and the elderly should be potentially capable of cardiac rehabilitation.

Donor Selection

The selection of suitable donor hearts remains one of the key points in the efficacy and success of transplant programs. The number of donors in the United States has remained unchanged in the past 5 years. In contrast, recipient waiting lists for solid organs have grown exponentially, as documented by statistics from the United Network for Organ Sharing (UNOS). Because of the ever-increasing demand for cardiac transplant donors, and the seemingly fixed donor pool, donor acceptance has been extended to older individuals. The urgent need for more heart transplant donors and the lack of well defined contraindications based on increasing age, has resulted in the extension of the traditional guidelines to include donors aged 35 years and above. Acceptable age limits of donors has gradually risen over the past decade from age 35 to 55 years.[13-16] Extending the donor age, however, carries the risk of accepting hearts with coronary artery disease that, if transplanted, could be associated with increased perioperative morbidity and mortality and poor long-term graft survival. Accordingly, echocardiography and coronary angiography is mandatory when considering male donors over the age of 40 to 45 and female donors over the age of 45 to 50.

In response to the urgent need for transplantable organs, Alexander and Vaughn[17] carried out a critical analysis of the influence of donor age on outcomes of all kidney, heart, and liver transplants performed in the United States between 1987 and 1989, using the UNOS database. With respect to heart transplants (n = 3,026), survival at the end of 1 year was significantly inferior in recipients of hearts from donors aged 16 to 45 years compared with hearts from donors aged 46 to 55 years. However, the difference was small (8.4%) and was associated with a relative risk of 0.8.[17] The authors do not provide a clear explanation for this finding. Adverse mortality statistics for older donor hearts probably reflects that these hearts are often used in more marginal, high-risk recipients, thus predisposing to a worse outcome.

In larger studies with sufficiently long follow-up, older donor age has been shown to impact survival negatively and increase the risk of coronary atherosclerosis in the graft. Increased rates of fatal cerebrovascular accidents and acute graft failure have been documented in patients receiving hearts from older donors (more than 45 years of age) despite comparable 5-year actuarial survival and graft function.[18] In addition, there appears to be a higher prevalence of coronary artery disease (CAD) in hearts from older donors, an observation that has been confirmed in several studies, including those using intravascular ultrasound to determine the severity of coronary artery intimal thickening.[19]

The management of coronary atherosclerosis in older donor hearts was addressed in a study by Drinkwater et al.[20] Simultaneous coronary artery bypass grafting (CABG) was performed in ten of 52 patients receiving heart transplants from donors over the age of 45 years. Among the recipients of hearts from older donors, actuarial survival at 1 year was lower in patients undergoing bypass than in patients not undergoing bypass (60% vs 84%). Comparing the entire group of recipients of older hearts with those of younger hearts there was a higher incidence of transplant-associated CAD at 5 years in the older donor hearts. However, if the ten patients who had undergone CABG at the time of heart transplantation were excluded, no significant differences in the 5-year incidence of transplant-associated CAD was discernible.[20] Despite its retrospective design, this study is of particular importance for several reasons. First, the incidence of angiographic CAD at 5 years posttransplantation was only 20% in older donor hearts that did not have severe disease at the time of transplantation. This is much lower than the rates reported from other centers, and likely reflects the focus of this center on early corticosteroid withdrawal and an aggressive approach to prevention and management of lipoprotein abnormalities.[3]

Recently, Drinkwater's group reported that pravastatin, a 3-hydroxy-3-methylglutaryl coenzyme A (HMG-CoA) reductase inhibitor, started early after transplantation, decreased mortality and reduced coronary artery intimal thickening at 1 year. This finding is consistent with the protective effect of HMG-CoA reductase inhibitors seen in several large clinical trials studying the primary and secondary prevention of atherosclerosis in native vessels. Second, this study reports that the use of CABG for the management of coronary stenosis in donor hearts is associated with only a slight diminution of survival compared with the expected results in nonbypassed grafts. Given the limited donor supply and the attrition rate of patients waiting for heart transplantation, it would seem that the use of older donor hearts, combined with treating recipients with lipid-lowering drugs, may be an option for improving survival of grafts from so-called "marginal donors." It has been proposed that organs from marginal donors be allocated specifically to older recipients. While the study by Drinkwater et al,[20] demonstrated that this approach results in medically acceptable outcomes, the widespread application of this intuitively correct compromise to donor shortage requires much deeper philosophical and ethical consideration.[3]

The current practice is to consider hearts for donation up to the age of 55, with more careful screening given to hearts from all donors over the age of 40, including the request for coronary angiography when appropriate. Hearts from donors 55 to 65 years of age are considered on a case by case basis depending on the age of recipient and urgency of the recipient's medical situation.[3,21-24]

Survival Rates and Outcomes

The survival rate after heart transplantation appears to be negatively affected by recipient age at both the very young and the very old ends of the spectrum. The mortality risk is particularly marked in patients over the age of 65. In this group the increased mortality is evident within 3 months of transplantation and remains significantly elevated throughout the first 36 months.[25] The presence of concomitant vascular disease or predisposition to diabetes mellitus and greater susceptibility to infection, probably contribute to the increased mortality.

One of the largest studies, from the Utah Heart Transplantation Program, which included 101 patients older than 60 years of age at the time of transplantation, revealed that actuarial survival was decreased in older patients as soon as 3 months post-transplantation and are more pronounced at 1 year. At 6 years posttransplantation, survival was 54% in patients older than 60 years of age, compared with 72% in patients age 60 years or less.[2] When Stanford reviewed their own series of patients undergoing heart transplantation, ages 50 to 59, compared with ages 60 to 69, their experience was consistent with that from Utah.[3,26] One-year survival for the 50 to 59 year group was 80%, and 1-year survival for the older group (6069 years) was 73%. The real dropoff was at 3 years, when survival for the age 50 to 59 group fell to 60% and for the age 60 to 69 group to just over 40%. This has not been our experience at the University of Minnesota. Recently, we analyzed the outcome of 31 patients over age 60; the mean follow-up time was 50 months. The 1- year and 5-year survival rates of 90% and 85% were not significantly different to that for patients ages 18 to 59.[27] These findings are in accordance with those reported by Robin and his group[28] on 48 patients older than 60 years. Their actuarial survival in this group approached 70% versus 88.5% in the group aged 20 to 59.

Conversely, when the results from the Stanford series are compared decade by decade, there appears to be an age-dependent effect on survival. Patients aged 60 to 69 years had decreased survival compared with patients in all other groups. Patients aged 50 years or older had a 5-year survival rate of 49% compared to a 5-year survival rate of 62% for patients less than 50 years of age.[3] In support of these findings, the Transplant Cardiologist's Research Database Group found a slight, but progressive, increase in the mortality rate for patients over age 50, but age was only one of several factors that influenced death in the multivariable analysis. Other significant factors included lower pretransplant cardiac output, ventilator support at the time of transplantation, longer donor ischemic time, older donor age, blood type of the donor and recipient and abnormal renal function.[25]

Importantly, the data from these studies must be considered in light of the immunosuppressive protocols used before we can determine if the experience is widely applicable to other centers. At Stanford and Utah, antilymphocyte antibodies were used prophylactically in all patients. Because we now recognize that the use of these agents can influence outcome, we must consider whether the same results would be observed in the absence of these agents. There are few reports and no randomized prospective studies to address these questions because of the widespread prophylactic use of antilymphocyte antibody therapies during the 1980s. It is interesting to note that in the small study by Aravot et al,[29] in which antilymphocyte antibodies prophylaxis was not administered, the 2-year survival for patients over the age of 60 years was 100%. This observation becomes even more relevant when one considers that the major causes of death after heart transplantation in older patients are infection and malignancy, both of which may be direct complications of immunosuppression. Late sudden death, usually due to fatal arrhythmias, is seen more frequently in the younger patients.

Immune Function in the Elderly

Rejection

A consistent and favorable observation in many reports is the finding that the incidence of acute rejection is lower in heart transplant recipients over 60 years of age than in younger recipients. Alterations in macrophage activity, partly account for the decreased immune reactivity in the elderly. Peripheral blood monocytes from older patients express decreased levels of HLA-DR antigens when compared to younger individuals. Lymphocytes from older individuals have decreased proliferative responses to T-cell mitogens. In addition, the production of interleukin-2 and interleukin-2 receptor decreases with age. This decrease in immune reactivity results in decreased rates of rejection in the elderly.[30] These findings are consistent with previous studies by Renlund et al,[31] who reported a nearly 100%, 12-month actuarial survival rate in patients 54 years of age or older. These studies suggest that decreased rejection in the older recipient is likely a manifestation of an age-associated decline in immune function and might represent an advantage in transplantation for the elderly. In reviewing most of the recent age series of cardiac transplantation in patients over 55 years of age, it appears that the incidence of rejection in this group is in the average of 0.8 to 1.9 episodes per patient per surgical year.[1-2]

In the Utah study, older patients whose prophylactic immunosuppressive regimens included antilymphocyte antibody had significantly fewer rejection episodes than did younger patients. Similar results were observed in a study by Heroux[32] in which older patients did not receive antilymphocyte antibody prophylaxis. An important implication of this lower rejection rate in older patients is that corticosteroids may be withdrawn from their maintenance immunosuppressive regimens, thereby preventing adverse effects, such as hypertension, diabetes mellitus, musculoskeletal complications, and infection.[3]

Infection

It now appears that the major survival benefit from immunosuppressive drugs is a decreased rate of fatal infection. Following the introduction of cyclosporin A during the early 1980s, studies have consistently reported that patients over the age of 60 years are at an increased risk of developing fatal infections; the Stanford experience indicates an age-related increase in all infections.[3] In the Utah study there was not a statistically significant difference in the number of infections between older and younger patients, but fatal infections accounted for 18% of deaths in older patients compared with only 7% of deaths in younger patients. The majority of these infections were opportunistic (eg, *Aspergillus, Nocardia, Candida*), as might be expected in patients with impaired T-cell function, thus implicating the effects of immunosuppressive agents.[2]

The importance of cytomegalovirus (CMV) infection in older patients has been emphasized in several reports. In the study by Heroux et al,[32] patients over the age of 65 years demonstrated a higher frequency of CMV infections than did younger patients (50% vs. 19%). Several studies have suggested that one of the major risk factors for CMV infection following heart transplantation is the use of antilymphocyte antibodies. Therefore, it is interesting to note that in the Heroux study, conducted prior to the widespread use of CMV prophylaxis, an increased risk of CMV infection was observed despite the fact that antilymphocyte antibodies were not used in older patients. This emphasizes the need for optimal CMV prophylaxis in the elderly, particularly seronegative recipients of hearts from seropositive donors whose risk of developing CMV disease is markedly increased. It is important to note that in a randomized, double-blinded study, a 28-day course of intravenous ganciclovir did not prevent CMV disease in this high-risk group of patients, indicating that additional strategies such as the administration of CMV hyperimmune globulin may be needed.[3]

CMV infection is of particular relevance because it has been implicated in the pathophysiology of accelerated atherosclerosis. This becomes even more important in the elderly, because of issues related to the use of the older donor heart, which has been associated with an increased risk of atherosclerosis. Clearly, strategies for minimizing immunosuppression and optimizing CMV prophylaxis are critical in older recipients of heart transplants. Adequate prophylaxis against CMV, fungal and pneumocystic infections should be given. In addition, ganciclovir or CMV immunoglobulin, or both, should be given during periods of increased immunosuppression.[3]

Immunosuppressive Therapy

Another consequence of decreased immune activity in the elderly is an increased incidence of viral, mycobacterial and fungal infections. Death from infection appears to be related to the intensity of immunosuppressive therapy. Lower doses of immunosuppressive agents should, therefore, be used in older patients. Older patients have reduced P-450 microsomal enzymes, leading to diminished cyclosporin A metabolism and higher blood concentrations of the drug. Consequently, a higher incidence of cyclosporine-induced nephrotoxicity is encountered in these patients. Cyclosporin A, however, remains the mainstay of immunosuppressive therapy in combination with azathioprine and Prednisone. As mentioned previously, doses should be adjusted according to age and renal function. Newer drugs such as Tacrolimus (FK-506) and mycophenolate mofetil (MMF) appear to have less toxic effects. However, their use in older patients is not yet well characterized.

Elderly cardiac transplant recipients are at an increased risk of developing osteopenic bone disease. When severe enough, this complication may cause early disability and may preclude adequate rehabilitation. Prolonged periods of physical inactivity, poor nutritional status and immunosuppressive therapy are the most common etiologic factors.[33–34] Severe osteopenia may be present as early as the time of hospital discharge after transplantation and further bone loss occurs at a considerable rate during the first postoperative year.[35] Thus, older patients should have a much faster tapering of prednisone to avoid the damaging effects of steroids, especially to soft tissue and bone. Some authors even advocate single drug therapy in older transplant patients leading to adequate survival rate but less risk of infectious and metabolic complications.

Bridge to Cardiac Transplantation in the Elderly

Recent estimates indicate that 20% to 30% of all patients listed for cardiac transplantation die each year waiting for a suitable donor heart. Consequently, many centers have developed successful programs to bridge patients to transplantation using mechanical circulatory support devices. The benefits of Left Ventricular Assist Systems (LVAS) in improving hemodynamics, renal, hepatic and cerebral function, and overall physical condition before transplantation has been well documented.[36,37] Outcome, in terms of success of bridge to transplant, post-transplant survival, and pretransplant mortality have all improved with the use of LVAS; recent reports document 80%–90% surviving to transplantation, and post-transplant survival of almost 100%. In evaluating the experience with a variety of devices, the overall rate of success has been 61% of patients successfully bridged to transplantation and 85%–95% successfully discharged.[38–41] As the population of elderly cardiac transplant candidates continues to grow, the need to extend the use of mechanical circulatory support to these patients has become a reality. The available data is very encouraging. In a recent report by Van Meter et al,[40] the worldwide registries for three different ventricular assist devices (HeartMate, Abiomed BV5000 and Thoratec) were reviewed and the results in the elderly population were analyzed. Patients over 60 years of age fared as well as the overall population. Successful bridge to transplantation was achieved in 70%, with 63% post-transplant survival. Despite the general impression of many practitioners, it is safe to conclude that age alone is not a significant risk factor. Retrospective univariant and multivariant analysis of pre-implantation risk factors has failed to identify specific characteristics of the elderly population that place them at greater risk of complications during support with a ventricular assist device. In addition, the overall rate of infectious, thromboembolic and other complications associated with long-term mechanical cardiac support is not different in patients over 60 when compared with a younger population.[40] It must be recognized, however, that results are influenced by patient selection prior to mechanical cardiac support to exclude comorbidities that would put them at increased risk for complications. Thus, to ensure successful outcome, patients should be selected on the basis of their functional status (physiological age) rather than their chronological age. Smedira, et al.[41] recently reported on the age-related outcome after LVAS support at the Cleveland Clinic. The authors conclude that the survival rate to transplantation in patients over 60 years of age, after left ventricular assistance, is comparable to the younger group.[41] Thus, age does not appear to be a significant risk factor for outcome after LVAS support.

Increasing use of LVAS has aggravated the donor shortage by including recipients who otherwise would not have survived. This observation, combined with the high success in rehabilitating terminal cardiac patients, has been used to support the concept of mechanical assistance as an alternative to cardiac transplant in the elderly. Comprehensive medical management of heart failure may include years of extensive medication, clinical evaluations and repeated hospitalizations. Mechanical assistance could become a long-term therapeutic option, proving to be more cost effective and provide better quality of life to elderly patients who otherwise may die awaiting transplantation.

Furthermore, patients with relative contraindications for transplantation may be offered a reasonable therapeutic option. To this end, the initial results from the Cleveland Clinic and Columbia University are encouraging. Both institutions have recently reported their experience with extended cardiac support with portable LVAS at home. It appears that this is a safe and more economical approach, with minimal rate of mechanical, physiological and infectious complications.[43-45] Further studies are needed to identify the long-term risks and benefits of such a therapeutic approach.

Rehabilitation

The improvement in quality of life in patients with heart failure who undergo cardiac transplantation has been well documented.[46-49] Rehabilitation, however, plays a pivotal role in maintaining good quality of life. Cardiac rehabilitation consists of comprehensive long-term services involving medical evaluation, prescribed exercise, cardiac risk factor modification, and education, counseling and behavioral interventions. This is designed to limit the adverse physiological and psychological effects of cardiac illness, reduce the risk of sudden death, control symptoms and enhance the patient's psychological and vocational status. Here, we present a summary of the guidelines provided by the U.S. Department of Health and Human Services for rehabilitation of the cardiac patient,[47] as well as comprehensive recent reviews by Joshi and Kevorkian.[48]

The positive effect of exercise after cardiac transplantation in the postoperative period is well documented in the literature. Most studies demonstrate improved exercise capacity in these medically complex patients, who are often markedly deconditioned prior to cardiac transplantation. Rehabilitative exercise training following cardiac transplantation improves exercise tolerance and elderly patients benefit in the same way as younger patients. Also, pretransplantation rehabilitative strength training may enhance preoperative status and operative recovery. The primary physiological goals of cardiac rehabilitation are to maximize oxygen uptake, increase anaerobic threshold, maximize minute ventilation, increase exercise blood pressure, thus reducing resting systemic pressures, increasing maximal heart rate, and decreasing resting heart rate. A secondary benefit of rehabilitation is improved blood lipid profiles and reduced body fat stores, resulting in controlled weight loss in obese patients. In addition, cardiac rehabilitation improves psychological well-being, social adjustment and functioning, and provides ample opportunity for continuing education.

The rehabilitation period after cardiac surgery is generally grouped into phases that have implicit activities and precautions. Phase I inpatient rehabilitation describes activity in the perioperative period beginning with range-of-motion exercises. Phase II rehabilitation begins at discharge with supervised therapy lasting for approximately 6 months. Phase III rehabilitation follows this and is described as the late recovery period, during which the patient continues to gain endurance and exercise tolerance. Phase IV, the maintenance phase, lasts indefinitely.

A lower intensity, more gradually progressive, and more protracted course of exercise training, is usually recommended for the elderly patient. The exercise program for the elderly should begin in the period following endotracheal extubation, but in the event of complications only gentle passive exercises should be continued. During the first few days after surgery, the goal is to stand and ambulate short distances with assistance. After the patient is able to tolerate walking, an evaluation of exercise parameters is determined using data from ergonomic stress testing. After discharge, activities should include increasing amounts of ambulation, preferably supervised by a rehabilitation team. Specific instructions should deal with: (1) symptoms and early signs of rejection, such as orthopnea and lower limb edema; (2) mode of exercise, which must be aerobic; (3) duration of exercise, which should occur for a minimum of 60 minutes to allow time for the denervated heart to respond to metabolic demands, (4) frequency of exercise, which should be between 4 and 6 times per week; (5) intensity of exercise, which involves training the patient to correctly use exercise scales; (6) progression, with an adequate warm-up and cool-down period; and (7) risk factor modification and guidelines for returning to usual activities of daily living.

A number of mechanisms interact to varying degrees to bring about the training effect in transplant patients. Strengthening of peripheral muscles plays a pivotal role in returning to optimal function. The use of steroids may, however, result in severe skeletal muscle atrophy and weakness, and steroid-induced obesity. In addition, the higher incidence of osteoporosis in the elderly population may compound this steroid myopathy, resulting in lower exercise tolerance and protracted rehabilitation. High doses of prednisone may significantly impede healing and contribute to sternal dehiscence. Therefore, pushing, pulling or heavy lifting during the first 3 to 6 months after surgery should be prohibited.

Generally, rehabilitation after heart transplantation is similar to that of other cardiac rehabilitation except for several differences in hemodynamics resulting from the denervated transplanted heart. Thus, heart rate, stroke volume, cardiac output and diastolic volumes are established primarily through intrinsic cardiovascular mechanisms. The heart rate response to exercise is delayed in part because of the lack of cardiac innervation. The peak heart rate in response to maximal effort is reduced, and this response remains essentially unchanged even years after transplantation.

Resting heart rate is higher after transplantation than in other cardiac subjects because of the higher intrinsic rate of the denervated sinoatrial node but this decreases as the patient ages. There is a normal demand for peripheral blood flow at rest and the cardiac output is maintained with a resting tachycardia and smaller stroke volume. During light exercise the Frank Starling mechanisms (increase in left ventricular end-diastolic volume and pressure) can increase cardiac output sufficiently to meet peripheral requirements. However, during vigorous exercise activity, further increase in cardiac output depends on chronotropic and inotropic central responses, induced by catecholamines. Despite near-normal resting hemodynamics, most transplant patients have a marked degree of exercise intolerance due to several factors that initially are related to post surgical status and prolonged functional disability. A long history of congestive heart failure with associated chronic elevation of catecholamine concentrations, may result in receptor desensitization and down regulation due to chronic hyperstimulation. This state will result in altered responses to exercise.

Transplant patients, regardless of age, should resume activity as completely as possible and increase activity as quickly as tolerated, with early addition of low weight, high repetition resistance exercises. Stair climbing should be incorporated and is important at home because managing stairs is a major barrier to many elderly patients even in the late recovery period. Special attention to psychosocial issues is also crucial to ensure successful rehabilitation of the elderly transplant patient.

Summary and Conclusions

Taken as a whole, it would appear that the elderly are not as likely to reject a transplanted heart. They appear to be at increased risk to develop infection and malignancy after transplantation, and osteoporosis and steroid-induced diabetes are expected complications. It is reasonable to expect the elderly to be challenging patients to treat after heart transplantation. Immunosuppression should be scaled down, surveillance for infection should be vigilant, and every precaution should be taken to avoid problems related to osteoporosis and steroid-induced diabetes. Most patients after cardiac rehabilitation can resume normal lives. Age alone is not an adequate criterion for exclusion from heart transplantation.

References

1. Frazier OH, Macris MP, Duncan JM, et al: Cardiac transplantation in patients over 60 years of age. *Ann Thorac Surg* 64:1866–1867, 1997.
2. Bull DA, Karawande SV, Hawkins JA, et al: Long-term results of cardiac transplantation in patients older than sixty years. *J Thorac Cardiovasc Surg* 111:423–428, 1996.
3. Valentine HA, Reitz BA: Heart transplantation in the elderly. *Transplant Immunol Lett* 13(1):1–13, 1997.

4. Defraigne JO, Demoulin JC, Van Damme H, et al: Cardiac transplantation in patients older than 55 years. *Acta Chir Belg* 91:38–42, 1991.
5. Defraigne JO, Demoulin JC, Beaujean MA, et al: Cardiac transplantation beyond 55 years of age. *Transplant Int* 3:59–61, 1990.
6. Aravot DJ, Banner NR, Khaghani A, et al: Cardiac transplantation in the seventh decade of life. *Am J Cardiol* 63:90–93, 1989.
7. Olivari MT, Antolick A, Kaye MP, et al: Heart transplantation in elderly patients. *J Heart Transplant* 7:258–264, 1988.
8. Miller LW, Vitale-Noedel N, Pennington G, et al: Heart transplantation in patients over age fifty-five years. *J Heart Transplant* 7:254–257, 1988.
9. Copeland JG: Cardiac transplantation after 60 years of age. *Ann Thorac Surg* 45:115–116, 1988.
10. Rudich SM, Busutill RW: Orthotopic liver transplantation in the elderly. *Transplant Immunol Lett* 13(1):1–13, 1997.
11. Ismail N, Hakim RM, Helderman H: Renal replacement therapies in the elderly. *Am J Kidney Dis* 23:1–15, 1994.
12. Church JM, Fazio VW, Braun WE, et al: Perforation of the colon in renal homograft recipients. *Ann Surg* 203:69–76, 1986.
13. Schuler S, Warnecke H, Lobe M, et al: Extended donor age in cardiac transplantation. *Circulation* 80(suppl III):III-133-III-139, 1989.
14. Mulvagh SL, Thornton B, Frazier OH, et al: The older cardiac transplant donor: Relation to graft function and recipient survival longer than 6 years. *Circulation* 80(suppl III):III-126-III-132, 1989.
15. Fields BL, Hoffmann RM, Berkoff HA: Assessment of the impact of recipient age and organ ischemic time on heart transplant mortality. *Trans Proc* 20:1035–1037, 1988.
16. Schuler S, Parnt R, Warnecke H, et al: Extended donor criteria for heart transplantation. J Heart Transplant 7:326–330, 1988.
17. Alexander JW, Vaughn WK: The use of "marginal" donors for organ transplantation. The influence of donor age on outcome. *Transplantation* 51:135–141, 1991.
18. Livi V, Bartolotti V, Luciani GB, et al: Donor shortage in heart transplantation. Is extension of donor age limits justified? *J Thorac Cardiovasc Surg* 107:1346–1354, 1994.
19. Rickembacher PR, Pinto FJ, Lewis NP, et al: Correlation of donor characteristics with transplant coronary artery disease as assessed by intracoronary ultrasound and angiography. *Am J Cardiol* 76:340–345, 1995.
20. Drinkwater DC, Laks H, Blitz A, et al: Outcomes of patients undergoing transplantation with older donor hearts. *J Heart Lung Transplant* 15:684–691, 1996.
21. Laske A, Niederhauser V, Larrel T, et al: Are elderly organ donors acceptable for heart transplantation? *Transplant Proc* 24(6):2679–2680, 1992.
22. El Oakley RM, Yonan NA, Simpson BM, et al: Extended criteria for cardiac allograft donors: A consensus study. *J Heart Lung Transplant* 15:255–259, 1996.
23. Hauptman PJ, Kartashov AI, Couper GS, et al: Changing patterns in donor and recipient risk: A 10-year evolution in one heart transplant center. *J Heart Lung Transplant* 14:654–658, 1995.
24. Young JB, Naftel DC, Bourge RC, et al: Matching the heart donor and heart transplant recipient. Clues for successful expansion of the donor pool: A multivariable, multi-institutional report. *J Heart Lung Transplant* 13:353–365, 1994.

25. Cinguegran MP, Hosenpud JD: Results of cardiac transplantation and factors influencing survival based on the Registry of the International Society for Heart and Lung Transplantation and The Cardiac Transplant Research Database. In: DKC Cooper, LW Miller, GA Patterson, (eds.) *The Transplantation and Replacement of Thoracic Organs*. Boston, MA. Kluwer Academy Publishers 1996, pp 409–416.

26. Sarris GE, Moore KA, Schroeder JS, et al: Cardiac transplantation: The Stanford experience in the cyclosporine era. *J Thorac Cardiovasc Surg* 108: 240–252, 1994.

27. Everett JE, Djalilian AR, Kubo SH, et al: Heart transplantation for patients over age 60. *Clin Transplant* 10(6)Part 1:478–481, 1996.

28. Robin J, Ninet J, Tronc F, et al: Long-term results of heart transplantation deteriorate more rapidly in patients over 60 years of age. *Eur J Cardiothorac Surg* 10(4):259–263, 1996.

29. Aravot DJ, Banner NR, Khayhani A, et al: Cardiac transplantation in the seventh decade of life. *Am J Cardiol* 63:90–93, 1989.

30. Penn I: Renal transplantation in the elderly. *Transplant Immunol Lett* 13(1):1–13, 1997.

31. Renlund DG, Gilbert EM, O'Connell JB, et al: Age-associated decline in cardiac allograft rejection. *Am J Med* 83:391–398, 1987.

32. Heroux Al, Constanzo-Nordin MR, O'Sullivan JE, et al: Heart transplantation as a treatment option for end-stage heart disease in patients older than 65 years of age. *J Heart Lung Transplant* 12:573–578, 1993.

33. Thiebaud D, Kreig MA, Gillard-Berguer D, et al: Cyclosporine induces high bone turnover and may contribute to bone loss after heart transplantation. *Eur J Clin Invest* 26:659, 1996.

34. Rich GM, Mudge GH, Laffel GL, et al: Cyclosporine A and prednisone-associated osteoporosis in heart transplant recipients. *J Heart Lung Transplant* 11:950–958, 1992.

35. Van Cleemput J, Daenen W, Nijs J, et al: Timing and quantification of bone loss in cardiac transplant recipients. *Transplant Int* 8:196–200, 1995.

36. Frazier OH, Rose EA. McCarthy P, et al: Improved mortality and rehabilitation of transplant candidates treated with a long-term implantable left ventricular assist system. *Ann Surg* 222:327–338, 1995.

37. McCarthy PM, Sabik JF: Implantable circulatory support devices as a bridge to heart transplantation. *Semin Thorac Cardiovasc Surg* 6:174–180, 1994.

38. Massad MG, McCarthy PM, Smedira NG, et al: Does successful bridging with the implantable left ventricular assist device affect cardiac transplantation outcome? *J Thorac Cardiovasc Surg* 112:1275–1283, 1996.

39. Pennington DG, McBride LR, Peigh PS, et al: Eight years' experience with bridging to cardiac transplantation. *J Thorac Cardiovasc Surg* 107: 472–481, 1994.

40. Van Meter CH Jr, Smart FW, Stapleton DD, et al: Mechanical assistance of the failing heart in the elderly. *Cardiol Elderly* 4:28–31, 1996.

41. Smedira NG, Dasse KA, Patel AN, et al: Age related outcome after implantable left ventricular assist system support. *ASAIO J* 42:M570-M573, 1996.

42. Oz MC, Argenziano M, Catanese KA, et al: Bridge experience with long-term implantable left ventricular assist devices: Are they an alternative to transplantation? *Circulation* 95:1844–1852, 1997.

43. Myers TJ, Catanese KA, Vargo RL, et al: Extended cardiac support with a portable left ventricular assist system in the home. *ASAIO J* 42:M576-M579, 1996.

44. McCarthy PM, James KB, Savage RM, et al: Implantable left ventricular assist device: Approaching an alternative for end-stage heart failure. *Circulation* 90(suppl II):II-73-II-86, 1994.
45. Catanese KA, Goldstein DJ, Williams DL, et al: Outpatient left ventricular assist device support: A destination rather than a bridge. *Ann Thorac Surg* 62:646–653, 1996.
46. Grady KL, Jalowiec A, White-Williams C. Improvement in quality of life in patients with heart failure who undergo transplantation. *J Heart Lung Transplant* 15:749–757, 1996.
47. Wenger NK, Froelicher ES, Smith LK, et al: Cardiac rehabilitation as secondary prevention. *Agency for Health Care Policy and Research and National Heart, Lung, and Blood Institute. Clinical Practice Guidelines-Quick Reference Guide for Clinicians* 17:1–23, 1995.
48. Joshi A, Kevorkian CG. Rehabilitation after cardiac transplantation: Case series and literature review. *Am J Phys Med Rehabil* 76:249–254, 1997.
49. Coffman KL, Valenza M, Czer LSC, et al: An update on transplantation in the geriatric heart patient. *Psychosomatics* 38:487–496, 1997.

Part 4

Cardiac Surgery

Chapter 23

Cardiac Surgery

Luis F. Santamarina, Herbert B. Ward

Open heart surgery can be gratifying, intriguing, frustrating, or disappointing and, when the patient is elderly, all of the above emotions tend to apply simultaneously. A 93-year-old man with critical aortic stenosis convinced us to replace his valve by telling us that he recently became too short of breath to continue dancing. Believing that this robust nonagenarian really had something to live for, we consented to perform his operation. When asked about his ability to waltz 6 months after his successful valve replacement, he informed us that now his feet hurt too much to dance.

Cardiac surgery in patients over 70 years of age has changed dramatically during the past two decades. Prior to 1975, septuagenarians, octogenarians, and nonagenarians were routinely considered to be too high a risk or lacking sufficient life expectancy for open heart surgery. Because of their decreased longevity and inability to take anticoagulant medications, patients older than 70 years who did undergo valve replacement were automatically assigned a bioprosthesis. When the internal mammary artery (IMA) became the bypass graft of choice because of its long-term patency, its use was routinely restricted to patients less than 70 years of age.

In 1971, only 2% of a large series of patients undergoing heart surgery at the Texas Heart Institute were over 70 years of age.[1] By 1982, the frequency had increased to 9%. Currently, we are far more liberal in our treatment of elderly people who need cardiac surgery and this trend is still increasing. In 1991, at the Minneapolis Veterans Affairs Medical Center (MVAMC), 31% of patients undergoing open heart surgery were older than 70 years of age. In 1997, 43% of patients undergoing open heart surgery at the MVAMC were older than 70 years

From *Clinical Cardiology in the Elderly. Second Edition,* edited by Elliot Chesler. © 1999, Futura Publishing Company, Armonk, NY.

of age and 80% of those who underwent coronary artery bypass grafting (CABG) received an IMA graft.

Findings from many centers have documented that the life expectancy of elderly patients after open heart operations approximates, or even exceeds the life expectancy of age- and sex-matched controls.[2,3] Given that the *average* life expectancy of an octogenarian is approximately 7 years, it is hard to justify withholding an IMA graft or a valve that lasts longer than 10 years, or even a surgical procedure itself based on age alone.[4] Despite these data, the risk of dying or suffering a disabling complication during cardiac surgery is much higher in the aged. Cerebral vascular accidents are far more frequent and technical or judgmental errors are poorly tolerated.[5]

The complication of cerebral vascular accident in elderly patients deserves special consideration. A stroke during heart surgery may be caused by many factors including:

1. Hypotension during induction of anesthesia or during the cardiopulmonary bypass (pump) run;
2. Hypoperfusion during the pump run because of fixed cerebral arterial stenosis or low flow rates from the pump;
3. Intracerebral bleeding secondary to systemic heparinization;
4. Atheromatous emboli from the ascending aorta.[5]

The incidence of stroke is often reported to be in the 1% to 2% range overall regardless of the patient's age. Other studies dispute these reports. The incidence of stroke rate in patients over age 70 years who had cardiac operations at the Cleveland Clinic between 1970 and 1982 was 4.5%.[6] From 1974 to 1983, the incidence of stroke in patients undergoing coronary bypass procedures at the Johns Hopkins Hospital increased nearly linearly with age.[7] Patients aged 51 to 60 years had a 1% risk of stroke, while patients over age 75 years had a 7% risk. In a more recent report of 2211 patients undergoing cardiac operations the incidence of stroke was 2%.[8] Patients with stroke were older and had higher rates of preoperative transient ischemic attack, congestive heart failure, and peripheral vascular disease. Overall, older patients show a greater incidence of deficits in neuropsychological functioning following both valve and coronary bypass procedures.[9] In 3030 patients undergoing open heart surgery at the MVAMC from 1988–1997, the incidence of stroke was 2%.

The increased risk of stroke in the elderly undergoing cardiac surgery is usually caused by severe atherosclerosis in the ascending aorta.[5] Echocardiography, either by the transesophageal or the direct handheld approach, is far superior to x-ray or direct palpation of the aorta in identifying the soft protuberant mobile type of aortic plaque most likely to embolize.[5] There is increasing evidence that localizing these plaques will allow the operating surgeon to alter cannulation techniques or the position of bypass grafts to hopefully avoid the occurrence of cerebral emboli. Radical debridement of the aorta under profound hypothermia and circulatory arrest has even been advocated in an effort to reduce the incidence of stroke in high-risk patients with mobile atheromas.[10,11] Techniques to avoid manipulation of the ascending aorta in patients with severe atherosclerosis have also been proposed to decrease the rate of embolic strokes.[12] The contribution of extracranial large artery stenosis to the incidence of stroke during cardiac operations and the timing of surgical management of the lesions remains controversial.[13]

Myocardial Revascularization

Myocardial revascularization remains the most freuently performed thoracic surgical procedure in the United States. Given the almost exponential growth expected in the United States geriatric population, from 26.8 million (11.6% of the population) older than 65 years of age in 1982 to 65 million (21%) older than 65 years of age by 2030, the issue of coronary bypass grafting in the elderly is not trivial.[14,15] A recent report from the Society of Thoracic Surgeons National Database revealed that currently more than half of bypass procedures are performed in patients older than 65 years of age.[16] There are multiple reports on the experiences of various centers with coronary bypass grafting in the elderly.[17-27] By examining these, some of the risk factors peculiar to the elderly patient that increase both the operative morbidity and mortality can be examined.

The decision to surgically revascularize a patient depends on the risk of operation compared to other forms of therapy.[26-29] This is no different for the elderly patient. A review of 24,461 octogenarians undergoing angioplasty, revealed a mortality of 7% as opposed to 1.8% in patients 65 to 69 years of age.[26] In addition, other factors must be put into the equation to realistically appraise the patient and the family of the anticipated outcome. These range from tangible factors such as the support system available to the patient during recovery to intangible estimates of the patient's physiological age and ability to stand up to the rigors of the operation and postoperative convalescence. This evaluation may be difficult because elderly patients tend to be considered for surgery at a more advanced stage of their disease and their daily routines cannot be accurately established. The most important questions to ask, therefore, are:

1. What is the proper time to offer surgical revascularization to the elderly patient who is disabled by angina?
2. What are the mortality and morbidity risks of operation in the elderly as compared to younger patients?
3. What is the long-term function and survival of elderly patients after myocardial revascularization?

Timing of Surgery and Operative Risk

Surgical revascularization is frequently not offered to the elderly patient until late in the course of the disease, often after medical therapy has failed.[17–19,21] Although risk factors for death are generally similar in young and elderly patients, the prevalence of these risks factors is significantly higher in the elderly. A group of 6635 CABG patients younger than 75 years were compared to a group of 469 CABG patients older than 75 years at the same institution over an identical time.[17] There was a significantly higher percentage of urgent or emergent operations ($P < 0.01$) and a more severe New York Heart Association (NYHA) Functional Class ($P < 0.001$) in the older group. Another series reported that 44% of coronary revascularizations in 121 septuagenarians were either urgent or emergent.[21] An analysis of Medicare data on 24,461 patients age 80 years and older between 1987 to 1990 demonstrated a significantly higher incidence of preoperative acute myocardial infarction, congestive heart failure, and cerebral vascular disease at the time of coronary revascularization when compared with patients 67 to 70 years of age.[26]

Despite these reports, myocardial revascularization can be performed in the elderly with acceptable, albeit higher, mortality. Univariate analysis identifies history of renal disease, higher preoperative left ventricular end diastolic pressure, acute myocardial infarction, reoperation, and urgency of operation as important factors in increasing hospital mortality.[18,19,21–23] Table 1 demonstrates the combined mortality statistics of seven series of elderly patients undergoing coronary revascularization. Although increasing age appears to increase hospital mortality, a more critical influence is timing of operation as shown in Table

Table 1
Hospital Survival After Coronary Revascularization by Age

Author	Year	Age (years)	Number	Hospital Deaths	Hospital Survival (%)
Salomon[17]	1989	≥ 75	469	32	93.2
Ko[18]	1990	≥ 80	100	12	88.0
Edwards[21]	1991	≥ 70	121	9	92.6
Cane[22]	1995	≥ 80	84	5	94.0
Talwalkar[23]	1996	≥ 80	100	8	92.0
Canver[24]	1996	≥ 70	218	7	96.8
Ward‡	1997	≥ 70	733	38	95.0
Total			1825	111	93.9

‡ unpublished data Minneapolis VA Medical Center (1988–1997), includes 11.3% reoperative coronary artery bypass grafting.

Table 2
Hospital Mortality Following Coronary Revascularization by Urgency of Operation

			Operative Classification					
			Elective		Urgent		Emergent	
Author	Age (year)	Total Number	Number	Deaths (%)	Number	Deaths (%)	Number	Deaths (%)
Salomon[17]	≥ 75	469	365	6.0	104	9.6	—	—
Ko[18]	≥ 80	100	36	2.8	52	13.5	12	33.3
Edwards[21]	≥ 70	121	68	2.9	35	8.6	18	22.0
Talwalkar[23]	≥ 80	100	39	0.0	—	—	61	13.1

2. Patients considered to be *elective* had a 0% to 6% overall mortality. The mortality risk increased in the range of 8% to 13.5% in urgent revascularizations and up to 33% in emergency operations.

Perioperative Morbidity

The incidence of perioperative complications after bypass surgery tends to increase with increasing age (Table 3). The overall incidence of nonfatal complications in the elderly ranges from 30% to 73% in different series.[18,21,22,27] Salomon et al[17] reported a significantly higher rate of major complications in the group older than 75 years. For 569 patients, these complications resulted in statistically longer stays in the intensive care unit, longer stays in the hospital and greater overall cost.[17,18]

Of the major complications, cerebral vascular accident is the most devastating and appears to be more frequent in the elderly with an incidence of approximately 4%.[17,19,28] Atrial arrhythmias have been

Table 3
Major Morbidity After Coronary Revascularization in the Elderly

Author	Year	Age (year)	Number	Major Morbidity (number patients)	Major Morbidity (%)
Ko[18]	1990	≥ 80	100	32	32.0
Edwards[21]	1991	≥ 70	121	47	39.0
Cane[22]	1995	≥ 80	121	59	49.0
Talwalkar[23]	1996	≥ 80	100	32	32.0
Boucher[25]	1997	≥ 70	329	177	53.8

reported in 20% to 60%, renal insufficiency 5% to 13%, prolonged ventilatory support 4% to 13%, congestive heart failure 11% to 29%, and
perioperative myocardial infarction 1.3% to 16%.[27] Hemorrhage requiring reoperation is reported to occur in 5% to 12% of elderly patients
and may be due to the fragile nature of their tissues or to a less active
coagulation system.[19,21] Osteoporosis may lead to increased bleeding
from the sternum or to sternal fracture during harvesting of the mammary artery. The elderly also experience a loss of tissue elasticity, which
may lead to avulsion of the epicardium or even perforation of the ventricle during retraction of the heart. Atrial tissue is especially friable and
the utmost of care is required to avoid a severe laceration during cannulation.

As described above, the use of the IMA as a bypass conduit in the
elderly appears to be increasing. Salomon et al[17] reported using an IMA
graft in 41.6% (195/465) of his patients over 75 years of age. Canver et
al[24,30] utilized IMA in 36% of patients over 70 years, and reported an
improvement in survival in these patients as compared to patients receiving only vein grafts. Gardner et al[29] reports its use in more than
90% of elderly patients. There appears to be no increase in perioperative
morbidity or mortality associated with the use of the mammary artery
during elective revascularization and the consensus of the reported series is that age alone is not a contraindication to its use.[29]

Long-Term Function and Survival

Improvement in functional status and independent living may be
more important to elderly patients than long-term survival (Table 4).
Despite the higher morbidity and mortality seen in elderly patients
undergoing CABG, relief of symptoms and return to improved functional status is quite good. Multiple studies report significant improvement in relief of angina and quality of life.[18,19,23,25] In a group of 121
octogenarians undergoing CABG at the Deborah Heart Center, 92%
were discharged home, with only 6% requiring transfer to a specialized
nursing facility.[22]

Table 4
Results of Coronary Revascularization in the Elderly

Author	Age	Follow-up period (months)	Patients evaluated (number)	NYHA Functional Class		P Value
				Preoperative	Postoperative	
Freeman[19]	≥ 80	22.6	54	3.6	1.6	P < 0.0001
Ko[18]	≥ 80	22.0	63	3.8	1.1	P < 0.00001
Boucher[25]	≥ 70	31.2	266	3.2	1.6	P < 0.001

NYHA, New York Heart Association.

These results indicate that older people are relieved of angina as frequently as younger patients. Preoperative variables unfavorably influencing a successful functional outcome in a multivariable analysis of 266 patients include hypertension and cerebrovascular disease.[25]

Long-term survival in elderly patients after myocardial revascularization also appears to be improved. Actuarial survival of patients discharged from the hospital is reported to be better than that of age-matched controls. In a series of 469 patients over 75 years of age, the 5-year survival rate (80%) was statistically less than the survival rate of 6635 patients younger than age 75 years, but exceeded the predicted five-year survival for age-matched controls.[17] In a study of 100 consecutive patients aged 80 or older following CABG, Talwalkar et al[23] reported an actuarial survival of 87%, 80%, 77% and 73% at 1, 2, 3 and 4 years, respectively, with only 2 cardiac related deaths. A report of 1689 consecutive patients undergoing CABG included 218 patients older than 70 years of age.[24] Analysis of the 10-year survival revealed no difference between these patients and their age-matched control population (42.7% vs. 45.9%). Opposite results were found in the younger patients, where patients undergoing CABG had a significantly lower 10-year survival than their age-matched counterparts (74.2% vs. 93.4% in patients 50 years and younger and 67.5% vs. 75% in patients 51 to 70 years).[24] An examination of Medicare data on 24,461 patients older than 80 years confirms that despite a higher initial surgical risk, octogenarians who underwent CABG had a long-term survival rate similar to that of the general US octogenarian population (71.2% vs. 73.3% at 3 years).[26]

Caution should be exercised in interpreting these statements as the findings may contain an inherent selection bias toward otherwise healthy persons. Patients with liver, pulmonary, and peripheral or cerebral vascular diseases, who make up a large portion of the elderly population and account for increased noncardiac deaths, may have been excluded from consideration for myocardial revascularization.

In summary, chronological age *per se* is not a contraindication to myocardial revascularization. Careful patient selection and frank discussion about the perceived outcome of the procedure will benefit both the patient and family. Because the operative mortality for elective cases is much lower than mortality in urgent or emergent cases, one might argue that earlier consideration of surgical revascularization will lead to better overall results. For the elderly patient who survives the perioperative period, the long-term functional results and improved survival statistics appear to justify the added risk of the procedure.

Valve Operations

Valve operations are a major undertaking regardless of age, despite technical improvements in myocardial preservation in valvular repair and replacement. Valve operations are recommended when the risks of surgery (operative mortality/morbidity and long-term valve-related complications) are outweighed by the benefits of surgery (improved long-term survival and, more importantly for the aged, improved quality of life). There are many excellent current reviews in the literature detailing the results of valve operations in the elderly.[2,31–41] Using these data, we are now able to divide elderly patients into subgroups, and this can be used to predict short- and long-term outcome with valve replacement or repair. These results can be compared to known results with medical treatment and an honest recommendation made to the patient and family.

The most important questions to be asked are:

1. What are the chances of the patient surviving the procedure (based on age, ejection fraction, coronary artery disease, type and position of the valve lesion, type of prosthesis to be used, and presence of calcium in the valve or ascending aorta), without having a serious perioperative complication (such as a stroke or renal failure) that would degrade rather than improve the quality of life?

2. What are the long-term sequelae (valve failure, reoperation, endocarditis, thromboembolism and hemorrhage) of a mechanical versus a biological prosthesis in the aortic versus the mitral position?

3. What will be the influence of valve repair procedures in the aortic versus the mitral position?

Chances of Survival

The short- and long-term survival data for elderly patients after valve surgery are presented in Table 5. The hospital mortality from

Table 5
Hospital and Five-Year Survival After Valve Surgery in the Elderly

Author	Procedure	Year	Age (years)	Number	Hospital Deaths	Hospital Survival (%)	5-Year Survival (%)
Jamieson[32]	AVR or MVR*	1989	≥ 65	1127	107	90.5	72.0
Bergus[37]	AVR	1992	≥ 70	126	4	97.0	75.0
Gehlot[38]	AVR	1996	≥ 80	322	44	86.3	70.3
Lee[39]	MVR or MVRP	1997	≥ 70	190	7	96.3	—
Ward‡	AVR or MVR*	1997	≥ 65	359	35	90.0	67.0
Total				2124	197	92.0	71.0

MVRP, mitral valve repair; MVR, mitral valve replacement, AVR, aortic valve replacement; *: includes multiple valve replacement; †: includes hospital deaths; and ‡: unpublished data, includes mitral valve repair.

these combined series of 2124 elderly patients was 8%. This compares with a 6.1% hospital mortality for 2000 patients of all ages undergoing aortic (AVR) or mitral (MVR) valve replacement at the University of Alabama and Green Lane Hospital as reported by Kirklin and Barratt-Boyes, respectively.[42] In a review article of mortality for cardiac valve surgery in patients of all ages, Sethi et al[43] found a hospital mortality rate between 5% and 12%.

The 5-year survival for patients over age 65 years in the combined series was 66.4%. This can be compared to an 80% to 85%–5-year survival for patients of all ages undergoing AVR or MVR and a 25% to 35%–5-year survival in patients with nonoperated symptomatic aortic or mitral valve disease.[42] The noncardiac-related death rate in elderly patients is much higher than in younger patients. The 5-year freedom from cardiac-related death in elderly patients (80%) approximates the 5-year survival found in patients of all ages undergoing valve surgery and equals or even exceeds the survival reported in age- and sex-matched controls.[2]

The hospital mortality rate associated with valve surgery is not only higher in the aged patient, but also increases incrementally with age (Table 6). In a study of 322 patients over 80 years undergoing AVR, Gehlot et al[38] reported independent predictors of operative mortality to be: female gender ($P = 0.0001$), renal impairment ($P = 0.001$), bypass grafting ($P = 0.005$), ejection fraction less than 0.35 ($P = 0.01$) and chronic obstructive pulmonary disease ($P = 0.028$). In a 10-year experience with MVR in the elderly, Nair et al[40] reported presence of aortic

Table 6
Hospital and Five-Year Survival by Age

Author	Procedure	Age (years)	Hospital survival (%)	5-Year survival (%)
Scott[36]	MVRP	65–69	92.6	—
		≥ 70	76.2	—
Antunes[34]	AVR or MVR*	65–74	93.5	62.0
		≥ 75	90.9	49.0
Jamieson[32]	AVR or MVR*	65–69	92.7	79.0
		70–79	89.3	69.0
		≥ 80	84.6	30.0
Ward‡	AVR or MVR or MVRP*	65–69	95.0	64.0
		70–79	89.0	71.0
		≥ 80	81.0	45.0
Nair[40]	MVR	< 70	88.0	65.0 (4 yrs.)
		≥ 80	73.0	46.0 (4 yrs.)

MVRP: mitral valve repair; MVR: mitral valve replacement; AVR: aortic valve replacement; *: includes multiple valve replacement; and ‡: unpublished data.

calcification and prolonged pump time as independent predictors of operative mortality.

The influence of coexistent coronary artery disease and the need for combined coronary bypass with valve surgery requires special consideration. Gehlot et al[38] reported increased operative mortality in octogenarians undergoing combined CABG and AVR (18%) when compared with patients undergoing isolated AVR (10%) (P = 0.005). Galloway et al[2] also reported an increased operative mortality in elderly patients undergoing AVR with concomitant myocardial revascularization compared with isolated AVR (14.3% vs. 8.2%). Other reports have shown operative mortality for AVR with and without coronary revascularization to be equivalent,[31] or have no influence on late survival.[44] These results need to be analyzed with caution because patients undergoing combined CABG/AVR may have less severe or borderline aortic valve disease with the main indication for the operation being coronary revascularization.

Coexistent coronary disease appears to have a more significant impact in mitral valve surgery particularly in patients with ischemic mitral regurgitation. Davis et al[41] reported significantly lower mortality in patients over 70 undergoing AVR (5.3%) as compared with MVR (20.4%). Ischemic mitral pathology was an independent predictor of increased operative mortality.

Hospital and 5-year survival may be affected by the intracardiac position of the valve to be replaced. The mitral valve is more difficult to expose than the aortic valve and the risk of MVR has been higher than the risk of AVR in some series.[32,33] In aged patients, however, the ascending aorta contains more atheromatous plaque than in younger patients and this can be the source of increased morbidity/mortality.[10] In the combined series presented in Table 7, there appears to be no significant difference in the hospital mortality rate for elderly patients undergoing MVR versus AVR, but the 5-year survival appears to be decreased in patients after MVR. The hospital survival for double valve replacement approximates that of single valve surgery, however, at 5 years, survival appears to be worse. Important factors that influence long-term freedom from cardiac death are NYHA class and left ventricular ejection fraction.[40-44]

Tissue versus Mechanical Valve

The age of the patient at the time of valvular replacement has remained an important determinant in the selection of the most appropriate prosthetic valve. The excellent performance and reliability of mechanical prosthesis has been proven in several studies.[45-48] Mechanical valves, however, require lifetime anticoagulation with potential higher risk of bleeding complications. The main concern regarding bioprosthesis is the possibility of structural valve degeneration, which has been shown to be less of an issue with increasing age. In a study on

Table 7
Hospital and Five-Year Survival in the Elderly by Position of Valve

	AVR		MVR/MVRP		DVR	
Author	Hospital Survival (%)	5-Year Survival (%)	Hospital Survival (%)	5-Year Survival (%)	Hospital Survival (%)	5-Year Survival (%)
Borkon[33]	81.6	64.0	—	—	—	—
Galloway[2]	87.6	60.0	—	—	—	—
Gehlot[38]	86.3	70.0	—	—	—	—
Nair[40]	—	—	73.0	46.0	—	—
Davis[41]	94.7	68.0	80.0	75.0	—	—
Antunes[34]	93.9	66.0	95.2	49.0	78.9	44.0
Jamieson[32]	93.7	74.0	86.5	69.0	86.3	73.0
Ward‡	91.0	69.0	89.0	65.0	86.0	40.0

AVR, aortic valve replacement; MVRP/MVR: mitral valve repair/replacement; DVR, double valve replacement; and ‡: unpublished data.

the influence of age on later results of valve replacement with porcine bioprosthesis, Pelletier et al[49] reported incremental improvement in freedom from valve degeneration at 10 years with increasing age (57% for patients younger than 45 years of age, 70% for patients between 45 and 54 years of age, 79% for patients 55 to 64 years of age and 93% for those older than 65 years of age). Similar results were reported by Jamieson et al[32] with a 10-year freedom from valve degeneration of less than 30% among patients younger than 30 years of age to more than 95% after 69 years of age.

Table 8 shows the results of combined series of elderly patients

Table 8
Hospital and Five-Year Survival in the Elderly by Type of Prosthesis

		Mechanical Valve		Tissue Valve	
Author	Procedure	Hospital Survival (%)	5-Year Survival (%)	Hospital Survival (%)	5-Year Survival (%)
Borkon[33]	AVR	82.0	61.0	81.0	67.0
Galloway[2]	AVR	88.0	67.0	88.0	58.0
Antunes[34]	AVR or MVR	93.0	60.0	—	—
Jamieson[32]	AVR or MVR	—	—	90.0	72.0

AVR, aortic valve replacement; MVR, mitral valve replacement.

Table 9
Freedom from Bleeding or Thrombotic Complication at Five Years
by Type of Prosthesis

	Mechanical Valve		Tissue Valve	
Author	Bleeding (%)	Thrombosis (%)	Bleeding (%)	Thrombosis (%)
Borkon[33]	65.0	82.0	96.0	78.0
Galloway[2]	91.0	100.0	95.0	89.0
Antunes[34]	97.0*	85.0	—	—
Jamieson[32]	—	—	97.0	88.0

* fatal bleeding complications only.

who underwent valve replacement with mechanical versus bioprosthetic valves. Although not randomized, the report of Borkon et al[33] is the only one to directly compare tissue and mechanical valves in the elderly. In their analysis, there was no statistical difference in short- or long-term survival for either type of valve, but there was a significantly higher incidence of anticoagulant-related hemorrhage in the group receiving mechanical valves (Table 9). Because there was no valve-related failure in either group at nine years, Borkon et al[33] recommends a tissue valve for patients over 70 years of age.

Galloway et al[2] reported equivalent short-term survival in patients receiving a tissue versus mechanical valve. Although long-term survival tended to be better in patients receiving a mechanical prosthesis, the difference was not significant and overall valve- related complications were similar in both groups. Antunes et al[34] and Thulin et al[35] used exclusively mechanical valves in their elderly patients and have had excellent short- and long-term results without increased anticoagulant-related complications. Jamieson et al[32] used porcine valves exclusively in over 1000 patients and states that "structural valve deterioration is essentially nonexistent at 10 and 12 years in patients 70 years of age or older." He also reported excellent short- and long-term survival without significant valve-related complications.

Experience with the Ionescu-Shiley bovine pericardial valve was very discouraging with early valve degeneration and high rates of reoperation when compared to porcine valves.[50] Better results, however, have been obtained with the newer Carpentier Edwards pericardial valve. Pelletier et al[51] has reported freedom from valvular deterioration and reoperation at 10 years of 96% and 93% in the aortic position and 84% and 77% at 8 years in the mitral position. This valve also appears to have an advantage in hemodynamic performance particularly for small aortic roots.

The most recent approach to improve the hemodynamics of tissue valves has been the development of the stentless porcine valve. Stented porcine valves have higher resting gradients than mechanical valves which may result in slower regression of left ventricular hypertrophy and shorter long-term survival. Stentless aortic valves have a low transvalvular gradient, large effective orifice area, good hemodynamic efficacy, but require more technical expertise to implant.[52] David et al[53] reported actuarial survival rates of 84% at 8 years in 2002 patients with stentless aortic valves compared with 68% in patients with stented valves ($P < 0.01$). The freedom from cardiac death was 97% versus 89% ($P < 0.03$) and the freedom from all valve-related complications was 88% versus 71% ($P < 0.02$). These valves have been recommended for older patients with small aortic roots.[54] In a recent personal communication, Dr. David informed us that freedom from structural valve deterioration is equivalent in stented and nonstented tissue valves.

The choice of valve in the elderly patient must be individualized. Patients with a small aortic root who are able to take medications appropriately or those with risk factors for thromboembolism, such as chronic atrial fibrillation, where permanent anticoagulation is necessary, could be selected for mechanical prosthesis. There is general agreement, however, that a bioprosthesis is probably the best choice for patients 70 years of age or older.[55] Clearly, valve replacement in the elderly is a safe and satisfying procedure that improves both the quality and length of life.

Valve Repair and Balloon Valvuloplasty

Stenotic lesions of the aortic valve are repaired using either ultrasonic debridement or careful sharp dissection to decalcify the valve. This allows the valve tissues to become more compliant and permits greater excursion of the leaflets. The initial results of this procedure were promising, but the long-term follow-up has been disappointing. While outflow gradients are significantly reduced initially, restenosis occurs. There is also a high rate of aortic regurgitation following decalcification and this often leads to reoperation and valve replacement.[56,57] Open valvotomy, which is highly successful in infants and children, is rarely indicated in the elderly. Balloon valvuloplasty for aortic stenosis in the elderly had widespread appeal and was enthusiastically supported when it was first attempted, however, long-term results were found to be disappointing. The 1-year mortality in a recent multicenter report of 674 elderly patients was 45%.[58] Severe restenosis has been found to occur within 3 to 18 months in the majority of the patients.[59,60] Subsequently, balloon aortic valvuloplasty should be viewed as a palliative procedure in the following categories:[61]

1. Patients who refuse surgery;
2. Patients with major functional defects that would contraindicate surgery;

3. The need for major noncardiac emergency surgery in a patient with tight aortic stenosis; and

4. Patients with poor left ventricular function, low transvalvular gradient and significantly reduced valvular orifice.

Repair of aortic regurgitation is being attempted with more frequency, but almost exclusively in younger patients. Methods include subcommissural annuloplasty, cusp resuspension and cusp extension. Duran et al[62] reported that repair was attempted in 107 (42.6%) of 251 patients with aortic disease (mean age of 23 years), 77 (72%) of whom had pure regurgitation. There were 2 operative deaths and 12 reoperations (16%) for failed repair. More recently Cosgrove[63] reported his experience with 88 patients undergoing an AVR with no operative deaths and 89% freedom from reoperation at three years. The long-term outcome of these patients is unknown and the current recommendation is to apply these methods in younger patients in whom other options for valve replacement may be less satisfactory.[63]

Mitral valve repair and balloon valvuloplasty in the elderly have a much better and longer record than aortic repair or valvuloplasty. Repair techniques pioneered by Carpentier et al[64] have proven to be safe, effective and reproducible. Jebara et al[65] reported the experience with 79 patients greater than 70 years undergoing mitral valve repair with an operative mortality of 3.8%. Actuarial analysis of the results revealed overall survival at 5 years of 81% with freedom from thromboembolism, hemorrhage and reoperation of 96%, 97%, and 98% respectively. The author concludes that mitral valve repair should now be considered the procedure of choice in patients of any age referred for mitral insufficiency.

Balloon valvuloplasty for mitral stenosis is reported to be successful in selected patients. The appearance of the stenotic mitral valve is graded echocardiographically by:

1. Mobility of the leaflets;
2. Amount of valvular and subvalvular thickening;
3. Degree of calcification; and
4. Presence of regurgitation.

Vahanian et al[66] reported the results of balloon commissurotomy in 200 patients with severe mitral stenosis. The result was considered to be good in 162 (86%) of the 189 successfully completed procedures, while in 27 patients (14%) the outcome was poor (final mitral valve area <1.5 cm^2 or mitral regurgitation of >2+ or both). Fifteen of the 200 patients were over 70 years in age and increased age was a predictor of poor outcome ($P < 0.001$, by multivariate analysis).

Cardiac Transplantation

Marked improvement in survival rates after heart transplantation have caused transplant surgeons to liberalize upper age limits for this procedure.[67] Patients 50 to 60 years of age currently represent about one-third of the transplant population.[67] Favorable results have been reported in patients 60 years of age or greater.[68,69] The most frequent indication for transplantation in this elderly population is ischemic cardiomyopathy.[69] Operative mortality is not significantly increased in patients over age 60 years when compared with an overall patient mortality of 10%.[70]

The long-term survival decreases with increasing age. A recent report on 23,132 heart transplants from the Registry of the International Society of Heart and Lung Transplantation[71] revealed a statistically significant decrease in long-term survival in patients 65 years or older ($P = 0.006$). Bull et al[69] recently reported on the experience with 101 heart transplant patients older than 60 years. Their data reveal that both the short- and long-term survival for these patients was significantly lower when compared with a younger group of heart transplant recipients. The 6-year actuarial survival for patients older than 60 years of age was 54% compared with 72% for patients younger than 60 years of age ($P < 0.05$). Rejection episodes are decreased in the elderly population,[69,72] but infectious complications and malignant disease have been reported to be more prevalent with increasing age.[69] Quality of life after cardiac transplantation in the elderly is significantly improved and supports the recommendation to perform cardiac transplantation in adequately selected patients.[69,72]

Conclusion

Although cardiac surgery in the elderly can be both frustrating and disappointing, in our experience, it is more frequently gratifying and intriguing. Oliver Wendell Holmes stated on his 91st birthday that "The riders in a race do not stop short when they reach the goal. There is a little finishing canter before coming to a standstill."[28] It is in this light that the elderly patient with cardiac disease should be evaluated.[28]

Clearly, elderly patients undergoing cardiac surgery have a higher morbidity and mortality with a shorter long-term survival than their younger counterparts. Nevertheless, in *carefully selected patients*, the operative morbidity and mortality is not prohibitive and the subsequent quality of their lives is markedly improved. The criteria used for operating on a patient who is 40 or 50 years old should not be applied to the octogenarian. An elderly patient with renal insufficiency, peripheral vascular disease, and Alzheimer's disease who is confined to a nursing home and does not ambulate is clearly not a candidate for coronary revascularization or valve replacement. On the other hand, a robust octogenarian with critical aortic stenosis or tight proximal coronary artery stenosis with good ventricular function should not be denied the likely improvement in the quality of life that can be gained with open heart surgery. Careful consultation with the patient and his family should lead the practitioner to a scientifically and ethically correct recommendation. As Maurice Chevalier is reported to have said, "Old age is not so bad when you consider the alternative."[28]

References

1. Hall RJ, Elayda MA, Gray A, et al: Coronary artery bypass: Long-term follow-up of 22,284 consecutive patients. *Circulation* 68(suppl II):II-20-II-26, 1983.
2. Galloway AC, Colvin SD, Grossi EA, et al: Ten-year experience with aortic valve replacement in 482 patients 70 years of age or older: Operative risk and long-term results. *Ann Thorac Surg* 49:84–93, 1990.
3. Center for Disease Control and Prevention: *Vital Statistics of the United States Life Tables*. Washington, DC: US Department of Health and Human Services, 1989. Vol. II, Section 6.
4. National Center for Health Statistics: *United States Life Tables: US Decennial Life Tables for 1979–1981*. Government Printing Office, Washington, DC: US Department of Health and Human Services; 1985. DHHS Publication No. (PHS) 85–1150–1, Vol. 1. No. 1.
5. Katz ES, Tunick PA, Rusinek H, et al: Protruding aortic atheromas predict stroke in elderly patients undergoing cardiopulmonary bypass: Experience with intraoperative transesophageal echocardiography. *J Am Coll Cardiol* 20:70–77, 1992.
6. Cosgrove DM, Loop FD, Lytle BW, et al: Primary myocardial revascularization: Trends in surgical mortality. *J Thorac Cardiovasc Surg* 88:673–684, 1984.
7. Gardner TJ, Horneffer PH, Manolio TA, et al: Stroke following coronary artery bypass grafting: A ten-year study. *Ann Thorac Surg* 40:574–581, 1985.
8. Libman RB, Wirkowski E, Neystat M, et al: Stroke associated with cardiac surgery: Determinants, timing and stroke subtypes. *Arch Neurol* 54:83–87, 1997.
9. Smith PL, Taylor KM: *Cardiac Surgery and the Brain: Neuropsychological Changes*. Boston, MA, Little Brown and Company, 1993, p 39.
10. Culliford AT, Colvin SB, Rohrer K, et al: The atherosclerotic ascending aorta and transverse arch: A new technique to prevent cerebral injury during bypass: Experience with 13 patients. *Ann Thorac Surg* 41:27–35, 1986.
11. Wareing TH, Davila-Roman VG, Barzilai B, et al: Management of the severely atherosclerotic ascending aorta during cardiac operations: A strategy for detection and treatment. *J Thorac Cardiovasc Surg* 103:453–462, 1992.
12. Mills NL, Everson CT: Atherosclerosis of the ascending aorta and coronary artery bypass: Pathology, clinical correlates and operative management. *J Thorac Cardiovasc Surg* 102:546–553, 1991.
13. Gerraty RP, Gates PC, Doyle JC: Carotid stenosis and perioperative stroke risk in symptomatic and asymptomatic patients undergoing vascular or coronary surgery. *Stroke* 24:1115–1118, 1993.
14. Bureau of Census: *Projections of the Population of the United States by Age, Sex and Race: 1983–2080. Current Population Reports, Series P-25, No. 952*. Government Printing Office, Washington, DC: 1984.

15. Elder AT, Cameron EWJ: Cardiac surgery in the elderly can produce substantial benefits at the price of a moderately increased risk. *Br Med J* 299: 140–141, 1989.
16. Edwards FH, Clark RE, Schwartz M: Coronary artery bypass grafting: The Society of Thoracic Surgeons National Database Experience. *Ann Thorac Surg* 57:12–19, 1994.
17. Salomon NW, Page US, Bigelow JC, et al: Coronary artery bypass grafting in elderly patients: Comparative results in a consecutive series of 469 patients older than 75 years. *J Thorac Cardiovasc Surg* 101:209–218, 1991.
18. Ko W, Krieger KH, Lazenby WD, et al: Isolated coronary artery bypass grafting in one hundred consecutive octogenarian patients: A multivariate analysis. *J Thorac Cardiovasc Surg* 102:532–538, 1991.
19. Freeman WK, Schaff HV, O'Brien PC, et al: Cardiac surgery in the octogenarian: Perioperative outcome and clinical follow-up. *J Am Coll Cardiol* 18: 29–35, 1991.
20. Horvath KA, DiSea VJ, Peigh PS, et al: Favorable results of coronary artery bypass grafting in patients older than 75 years. *J Thorac Cardiovasc Surg* 99:92–96, 1990.
21. Edwards FH, Taylor AJ, Thompson L, et al: Current status of coronary artery operation in septuagenarians. *Ann Thorac Surg* 52:265–269, 1991.
22. Cane ME, Chen CH, Bailey B, et al: CABG in octogenarians: Early and late events and actuarial survival in comparison with a matched population. *Ann Thorac Surg* 60:1033–1037, 1995.
23. Talwalkar NG, Damus PS, Durban LH, et al: Outcome of isolated coronary artery bypass surgery in octogenarians. *J Cardiac Surg* 11:172–179, 1996.
24. Canver CC, Nichols RD, Cooler SD, et al: Influence of increasing age on long- term survival after coronary artery bypass grafting. *Ann Thorac Surg* 62:1123–1127, 1996.
25. Boucher JM, Dupras A, Jutras N, et al: Long-term survival and functional status in the elderly after cardiac surgery. *Can J Cardiol* 13(7):646–652, 1997.
26. Peterson ED, Cowper PA, Jollis JG, et al: Outcomes of coronary artery bypass graft surgery in 24,461 patients aged 80 years or older. *Circulation* 92(suppl II):II-85-II-91, 1995.
27. Alexander KP, Peterson ED: Coronary artery bypass grafting in the elderly. *Am Heart J* 134:856–864, 1997.
28. Mannion JD, Armenti FR, Edie RN: Cardiac surgery in the elderly patient: Therapy considerations. In: DT Lowenthal (ed.) *Geriatric Cardiology*. Philadelphia, PA, FA Davis Co, 1992, p 189.
29. Gardner TJ, Greene PS, Rykiel MF, et al: Routine use of the left internal mammary artery graft in the elderly. *Ann Thorac Surg* 49:188–194, 1990.
30. Canver CC, Kronke GM, Nichols RD, et al: Coronary artery bypass surgery in older patients. *Cardiol Elderly* 2:442–447, 1994.
31. Bessone LN, Pupello DF, Hiro SP, et al: Surgical management of aortic valve disease in the elderly: A longitudinal analysis. *Ann Thorac Surg* 46: 264–269, 1988.
32. Jamieson WRE, Burr LH, Munro AI, et al: Cardiac valve replacement in the elderly: Clinical performance of biological prostheses. *Ann Thorac Surg* 48:173–185, 1989.
33. Borkon AM, Soule LM, Baughman KL, et al: Aortic valve selection in the elderly patient. *Ann Thorac Surg* 46:270–277, 1988.
34. Antunes MJ: Valve replacement in the elderly: Is the mechanical valve a good alternative? *J Thorac Cardiovasc Surg* 98:485–491, 1989.

35. Thulin LI: Age-related complications and optimal choice of artificial heart valves in elderly patients. *J Cardiovasc Surg* 32:497, 1991.
36. Scott ML, Stowe CL, Nunnally LC, et al: Mitral valve reconstruction in the elderly population. *Ann Thorac Surg* 48:213–217, 1989.
37. Bergus BO, Feng WC, Bert AA, et al: Aortic valve replacement: Influence of age on operative morbidity and mortality. *Eur J Cardiothorac Surg* 6: 118–121, 1992.
38. Gehlot A, Mullany CJ, Ilstrup D, et al: Aortic valve replacement in patients aged eighty years and older: Early and long-term results. *J Thorac Cardiovasc Surg* 111:1026–1036, 1996.
39. Lee EM, Porter JN, Shapiro LM, et al: Mitral valve surgery in the elderly. *J Heart Valve Dis* 6:22–31, 1997.
40. Nair CK, Biddle WP, Kaneshige A, et al: Ten-year experience with mitral valve replacement in the elderly. *Am Heart J* 124:154–159, 1992.
41. Davis EA, Gardner TJ, Gillinor AM, et al: Valvular disease in the elderly: Influence on surgical results. *Ann Thorac Surg* 55:333–338, 1993.
42. Kirklin JW, Barratt-Boyes BG: *Cardiac Surgery. Morphology, Diagnostic Criteria, Natural History, Techniques, Results and Indications.* New York, NY, John Wiley & Sons, 1986, p 1550.
43. Sethi GK, Miller DC, Souchek J, et al: Clinical, hemodynamic, and angiographic predictors of operative mortality in patients undergoing single valve replacement. *J Thorac Cardiovasc Surg* 93:884–897, 1987.
44. He GW, Grunkemeier GL, Starr A: Aortic valve replacement in elderly patients: Influence of concomitant coronary grafting on late survival. *Ann Thorac Surg* 61:1746–1751, 1996.
45. Arom KV, Nicoloff DM, Kersten TE, et al: Ten years experience with the St. Jude Medical Valve prosthesis. *Ann Thorac Surg* 47:831–837, 1989.
46. Baudet EM, Puel V, McBride JT, et al: Long-term results of valve replacement with the St. Jude Medical prosthesis. *J Thorac Cardiovasc Surg* 109: 858–870, 1995.
47. Nitter-Hauge S, Abdelnoor M: Ten-year experience with the Medtronic Hall valvular prosthesis: A study of 1104 patients. *Circulation* 80(suppl I):I-43-I-48, 1989.
48. Cobanoglu A, Fessler CL, Guvendik L, et al: Aortic valve replacement with the Starr-Edwards prosthesis: A comparison of the first and second decades of follow-up. *Ann Thorac Surg* 45:248–252, 1988.
49. Pelletier LC, Carrier M, Le Clerc Y, et al: Influence of age on later results of valve replacement with porcine bioprosthesis. *J Cardiovasc Surg* 33: 526–533, 1992.
50. Reul GJ Jr, Cooley DA, Duncan JM, et al: Valve failure with the Ionescu-Shiley bovine pericardial bioprosthesis: Analysis of 2680 patients. *J Vasc Surg* 2:191–204, 1985.
51. Pelletier LC, Carrier M: Bioprosthetic heart valves: 25 years of development and clinical experience. In: J Acar, E Bodnar (eds.) *Textbook of Acquired Heart Valve Disease.* London, UK, ICR Publishers, 1995, pp 937–938.
52. David TE, Pollick C, Bos J: Aortic valve replacement with stentless porcine aortic bioprosthesis. *J Thorac Cardiovasc Surg* 99:113–118, 1990.
53. David T, Bos J, Feindel C, et al: VII *International Symposium Cardiac Bioprostheses* (abstract). Barcelona, Spain, June 1997.
54. Sintek C, Fletcher AD, Khonsari S: Stentless porcine aortic root: Valve of choice for the elderly patient with small aortic root? *J Thorac Cardiovasc Surg* 109:871–876, 1995.

55. Pelletier LC, Carrier M, Le Clerc Y, et al: Porcine versus pericardial bio-prostheses: A comparison of late results in 1593 patients. *Ann Thorac Surg* 47:352–361, 1989.
56. Craver JM: Aortic valve debridement by ultrasonic surgical aspirator: A word of caution. *Ann Thorac Surg* 49:746–753, 1990.
57. Craver JM, Weintraub WS, Jones EL, et al: Predictors of mortality, complications, and length of stay in aortic valve replacement for aortic stenosis. *Circulation* 78(suppl I):I-85-I-90, 1988.
58. Otto CM, Mickel MC, Kennedy JW, et al: Three-year outcome after balloon aortic valvuloplasty: Insight into prognosis of valvular aortic stenosis. *Circulation* 89:642–650, 1994.
59. Kuntz RE, Leonard BM, Erny RE, et al: Follow-up of balloon aortic valvuloplasty: Results in 192 cases (abstract). *J Am Coll Cardiol* 13(suppl A): 16A, 1989.
60. Robicsek F, Harbold NB Jr, Daugherty HK, et al: Balloon valvuloplasty in calcified aortic stenosis: A cause for caution and alarm. *Ann Thorac Surg* 45:515–525, 1988.
61. Vahanian A, Nullet O, Elias J: Percutaneous balloon valvuloplasty. In J Acar, E Bodnar (eds.) *Textbook of Acquired Heart Valve Disease*. London, UK, ICR Publishers, 1995, pp 763–764.
62. Duran C, Kumar N, Gometza B, et al: Indications and limitations of aortic valve reconstruction. *Ann Thorac Surg* 52:447–454, 1991.
63. Fraser CD, Cosgrove DM: Aortic valve reparative procedures. In RB Karp, H Laks, AS Wechsler (eds.) *Advances in Cardiac Surgery*. Chicago, IL, 1996, pp 82–83.
64. Carpentier A, Chauvaud S, Fabiani JN, et al: Reconstructive surgery of mitral valve incompetence: Ten-year appraisal. *J Thorac Cardiovasc Surg* 79:338–348, 1980.
65. Jebara V, Dervanian P, Acar C, et al: Mitral valve repair using Carpentier techniques in patients more than 70 years old: Early and late results. *Circulation* 86(suppl II):II-53-II-59, 1992.
66. Vahanian A, Michel PL, Cormier B, et al: Results of percutaneous mitral commissurotomy in 200 patients. *Am J Cardiol* 63:847–852, 1989.
67. Kaye MP: The Registry of the International Society for Heart and Lung Transplantation: Ninth Official Report - 1992. *J Heart Lung Transplant* II:599–606, 1992.
68. Blanche C, Matloff JM, Denton TA, et al: Heart transplantation in patients 70 years of age and older: Initial experience. Ann Thorac Surg 1996; 62: 1731–1736.
69. Bull DA, Shreekanth V, Karwande, et al: Long-term results of cardiac transplantation in patients older than sixty years. *J Thorac Cardiovasc Surg* 111:423–428, 1996.
70. Amrein C, Vulser C, Farge D, et al: Is heart transplantation a valid therapy in elderly patients? *Transplant Proc* 22:1454–1456, 1990.
71. Hosenpud JD, Novick RJ, Breen TJ, et al: The Registry of the International Society of Heart and Lung Transplantation: Twelfth Official Report. *J Heart Lung Transplant* 14:805–815, 1995.
72. Rickenbacher PR, Lewis NP, Valantine HA, et al: Heart transplantation in patients over 54 years of age: Mortality, morbidity and quality of life. *Eur Heart J* 18:870–878, 1997.

Chapter 24

Mitral Valve Repair in the Elderly

Eugene A. Grossi, Martin J. Sussman, A.C. Galloway, Stephen B. Colvin

The population of the United States is growing older. In a recent review Atkins et al[1] stated that by the year 2000, 6% of the population will be above age 80 years and although their life expectancy exceeds an additional 8 years, more than 25% suffer from cardiovascular disease. Most of these patients have coronary artery and aortic valve disease; mitral valve disease accounts for a minority of those requiring cardiac surgery. Age remains a significant risk factor in open heart surgery but improvements in techniques of cardiopulmonary bypass and cardiac anesthesia have significantly reduced the risk, and operating upon octagenarians is now part of everyday practice.

To illustrate how rapidly progress has been made in this regard, an editorial in the *British Medical Journal* of 1968[2] stated that "surgical treatment for valve disease is not at present feasible in elderly patients." By 1978, as safety of heart surgery and valve prosthesis technology improved, it became apparent that elderly patients could indeed benefit from valve surgery. Initially, the benefits were reported for aortic valve replacement, but benefits for those with mitral valve disease also became apparent. Although elderly patients had, and still do have, a greater operative risk than their younger counterparts the benefits to the survivors are comparable in terms of improved ventricular function and symptomatic improvement. Their *late* survival, however, is not improved because both cardiac and non-cardiac deaths are more frequent in elderly patients compared with a younger cohort.[3] In this

From *Clinical Cardiology in the Elderly. Second Edition,* edited by Elliot Chesler. © 1999, Futura Publishing Company, Armonk, NY.

chapter we will review the results of mitral valve repair in the elderly patient in the modern era of cardiac surgery.

It is generally accepted that mitral valvuloplasty (MV) is superior to mitral valve replacement (MVR) for most patients in terms of operative risk, valve related morbidity and late mortality. Possible exceptions to this include acute ischemic mitral regurgitation, rheumatic disease with stiff or calcified valve leaflets and patients with severe hemodynamic instability when repair is judged to be complex and time consuming. Most reports in this regard do not differentiate outcome according to age, but there are some which confirm the safety and efficacy of MV in elderly patients.[4] Reports of MVR in the elderly still show high operative mortality, but there is some bias in terms of patient selection as most surgeons now choose repair over replacement in all age groups, so that those receiving MVR tend to be a higher preoperative risk.

The reasons for MV being superior to MVR include better postoperative left ventricular function, and avoidance of foreign material in the heart. There is some evidence[5-7] that MVR even with chordal preservation is still inferior to MV in terms of preserving left ventricular performance; this may be due to the presence of a rigid structure in the mitral annulus that precludes changes in annulus shape and size during the cardiac cycle. Stenting the ventricle open with a bioprosthesis may also contribute by preventing ventricular remodeling.

The potential disadvantages of MV relate to its predictability and durability. However, the efficacy of MV has been reported in many series, including elderly patients despite their more fragile tissues and higher incidence of coexisting disease. Different pathologies are variably repairable and durable, and as a rule myxomatous mitral valve disease is more easily repaired than rheumatic or ischemic disease. The high incidence of other disease is reflected in the frequency of multiple procedures in these patients. At NYU we evaluated the results of MV in 243 patients older than age 70 (34 were older than 80 years at the time of surgery). Comparing the results of MV in these patients with patients younger than 70 years showed significantly greater frequency of angina, previous myocardial infarction, and hypertension in those over age 70 years. Preoperative cerebrovascular accidents were also more frequent in this group, but this does not reach statistical significance. Among older patients the incidence of associated procedures was 74.1%, with 53.9% requiring coronary artery surgery. The presence of co-existent disease, and hence greater operative risk, in fact serves to increase the difference in outcomes between MV and MVR, with MV being superior in terms of early and late mortality and morbidity, despite MV being more complex and time-consuming.[8]

While actuarial analysis is the standard tool for comparing the long-term outcome of valve operations, it probably is not the analysis of choice in an elderly population. Actuarial analysis overestimates the risk of late valve degeneration because it assumes that dead patients are still at risk. Grunkemeier in 1994[9] demonstrated that actuarial analysis is misleading in the elderly, because it does not properly take into account the large competing risks of death when we look at freedom from valve related complications. He advocated the use of cumulative incidence or *"actual analysis"* that would not lead to exaggerated estimations of various complication rates because it acknowledges that patients who die have no risk of valve degeneration. We demonstrated a similar phenomenon[10] while examining the freedom from reoperation for valve failure in our elderly population. Actuarial analysis improperly overestimated by 3-fold the failure rate of tissue valves in the elderly, and a similar analysis for patients over 70 years undergoing MV showed a less marked but still apparent difference. All events in this chapter analyzing NYU data are based on *actual* analyses where appropriate. Obviously, as this new technique for statistical analysis becomes more popular, it should help us correctly interpret the long-term sequelae to the various valve operations among elderly patients.

In a report by Cohn et al.[11] in which only myxomatous mitral valve disease was examined, 36% of the patients were over age 70 years and failure rates were low. Operative mortality although 5.1% in those over 70 versus 0.7% in the younger patients, was not statistically significantly different. Late survival was similarly worse in the elderly (84% versus 87% at 5 years) but again not statistically significant. Late valve failures were related to operator experience with the procedure, not age of the patient. They concluded that long term results in patients with myxomatous mitral valves undergoing MV are excellent in terms of survival and freedom from valve related problems, even in the elderly patient.

Myxomatous degeneration, however, is not the only cause of mitral valve disease in the elderly. Although the frequency increases with age in males, in our experience myxomatous degeneration accounts for just under half the causes of mitral valve disease in those above age 70 years (49.8%).[8] Ischemia accounts for 31.3%, rheumatic heart disease for 7.8%, infection for 5.8%, and 2.9% have other miscellaneous causes.[8] All causes other than myxomatous degeneration make MV technically more difficult and the results are less favorable in terms of freedom from valve related events. These factors plus coexisting diseases combine to make MV in the elderly less successful than in younger patients but still an excellent, reproducible option.

At NYU,[8] hospital mortality is 5.7% for isolated MV, but 16.0% for those requiring concomitant coronary artery surgery, 12.2% when a second valve is operated on, and 11.5% overall. The respective figures for those patients under 70 years old are likewise listed (Table 1). Among patients older than 70 years the 5-year freedom from late cardiac death is 100% for isolated MV and 79.2% when combined with another procedure. For those younger than 70 years at the time of operation, the 5-year freedom from late cardiac death is 97.6% for isolated MV and 85.8% when combined with another procedure. This difference in mortality, although small, does not appear to be related to valve failure, as freedom from reoperation is very similar in both age groups:

Table 1
Comparison of Operative Mortality for Mitral Valve Repair

Patient Age	Less than 70 Years Old	Greater or Equal to 70 Years Old
Procedure		
Isolated mitral repair	1.4%	5.7%
Concomitant CABG	7.4%	16.0%
Concomitant Valve	3.0%	12.2%
Overall	3.5%	11.9%

92.0% in those older than 70 years versus 92.7% in those younger than 70 years. Freedom from late events was also similar in both groups: thromboembolism, 88.5% versus 94.5%; anticoagulant-related problems, 97.5% versus 98.2%; endocarditis, 96.1% versus 97.8%. Overall freedom from late cardiac death, reoperation, and all valve-related complications at 5 years was 65.2% for those over 70 years old, (77.5% for patients with isolated mitral disease) and 73.7% for those under 70 years. This probably reflects the impact of the higher incidence of coexistent disease among the older population. Thus, although MV appears safe in the elderly, the risk is still greater than for those younger than 70 years for both early and late outcome. Reparability and durability of the procedure do not appear to be affected by advancing age. Symptomatic improvement is also impressive: preoperatively 91.7% were in NYHA class III or IV, whereas postoperatively 89.0% were in NYHA class I or II. This corresponds to an improvement in mean NYHA functional class in those older than 70 years from 3.34 to 1.70.

Lee et al[12] in a review of mitral valve surgery in the elderly stated that although the risks are increased in the elderly, particularly for postoperative myocardial failure, late referral for operation contributed far more than age itself to poor outcome. Interestingly, in their review myocardial failure was included in the analysis of outcomes and proved to be the most important risk factor among the elderly. In most series, myocardial failure is excluded from this type of valve-related event analysis, in accordance with the guidelines for reporting results of heart valve surgery.[13] Although co-existing, noncardiac disease affects the elderly more than the younger patients, complications, particularly heart failure, are the main cause for the higher mortality among elderly patients undergoing mitral valve surgery. The non-surgical related deaths in those over 70 years old, although more frequent, were far less significant numerically than heart failure, which had a 30% higher frequency in the elderly at 7 years. In their analysis, age itself was not a risk for operative mortality, but late referral was, and more elderly patients were referred later in the disease process than younger patients. It is important to note that in the elderly who were referred early, when relatively asymptomatic with well-preserved ventricular function, had low operative risk not significantly different from younger patients. Lee et al[12] concluded that just as early surgery is now recommended for younger patients with severe mitral regurgitation, particularly if judged repairable, advanced age should not be a reason to deny early referral. There was no difference in valve repair failure rates between patients younger than 70 years and those older than 70 years. Early referral in MV rather than MVR results in an excellent outcome in both old and young.

Two situations warrant special mention when considering MV *viz* heavy mitral valve annular calcification associated with mitral regurgitaiton (MR), and ischemic MR. Heavy calcification of the mitral annulus was considered a contraindication to MV[14], but this has been disputed, and it is now generally accepted that mitral annular calcification does not preclude successful MV.[15] In our NYU report there was no significant difference in success of repair and survival between those patients who required debridement of calcium as part of MV and those who did not. Freedom from reoperation at 5 and 10 years for the 2 groups was 92.1% and 88.0% versus 89.3% and 82.6%, respectively. Importantly, many of the young patients had rheumatic heart disease, where the pattern of calcification is different from annular calcification in older patients. Carpentier[16] reported on how to manage these cases with mitral annular calcification. Even extensive deposition of annular calcium can be successfully removed leaving pliable leaflets (unlike rheumatic disease) which can be securely sutured and an annuloplasty performed. Carpentier concluded that "extensive calcification of the mitral valve annulus does not preclude the use of reconstructive techniques because, in the majority of the cases, the process of calcification does not involve the other components of the mitral valve apparatus." Others recommend removal of just enough calcium to enable the repair to be completed, thus reducing the risk of injuring the adjacent circumflex artery, but the conclusions are similar.

The second special situation, ischemic mitral insufficiency, covers a large spectrum of conditions and patients requiring mitral valve and coronary artery surgery should be divided into 2 groups: those with ischemic mitral insufficiency and those with mitral insufficiency and unrelated coronary artery disease. The latter group has an inherently lower risk and studies reporting results of MV or MVR and CABG must be interpreted in this light. Differentiating between them may be more difficult than initially apparent as Bolling and coworkers[6] point out even the histological appearance may be similar. The mere presence of coronary artery disease, more common in the elderly, still increases risk of mitral valve surgery, but less so with MV than MVR. Despite the high reported risk of surgery in this subgroup of patients (operative mortality approximately 20% is usual) nonsurgical treatment has a worse outcome. In addition, the symptomatic improvement in the survivors is dramatic, so surgery, although high risk, is still indicated, and MV compared to MVR has a better early and late outcome.

Conclusion

Older patients are referred for mitral valve surgery with increasing frequency, and reports of acceptable outcome in these patients are now the rule. Improvements in preoperative management, anesthesia and surgical techniques, and cardiopulmonary bypass combine to reduce the risks to an acceptable level, such that age itself is no longer a contraindication. Despite many reports claiming favorable outcomes in these patients, age persists as a risk factor in most studies, for both early and late morbidity and mortality. Nevertheless, late survival rates are reported as matching those of age, sex, and race-matched populations, even when hospital deaths are included.[17] It is important when reviewing data on this topic to keep populations as homogeneous as possible. Great differences in outcomes probably relate to patient differences, not surgical, as illustrated in the differences between the results reported by Carpentier's group,[4] and our own.[8] The most striking difference relates to the frequency of associated procedures in the 2 groups, and this translates into higher risk in the NYU group.

In summary, advances in cardiac surgery and allied disciplines involved in the care of these patients have progressed to the extent where MV is now a frequently performed procedure in the elderly patient. It should be considered early before onset of left ventricular dysfunction as the procedure of choice for patients with severe mitral regurgitation. Improvement in quality of life is good; most patients being in functional class I or II following operation.

References

1. Akins CW, Vlahakes GJ, et al: Cardiac operations in patients 80 years old and older. *Ann Thorac Surg* 64:606–615, 1997.
2. Editorial. Systolic murmurs in the elderly. Br Med J 4:530–531, 1968.
3. Nair CK, Kaneshige A, et al: Ten-year experience with mitral valve replacement in the elderly. *Am Heart J* 124:154–159, 1992.
4. Jebara VA: Mitral valve repair using Carpentier techniques in patients more than 70 years old: Early and Late Results. *Circulation* 86:II-53-II-59, 1992.
5. Lee EM, Well FC: Importance of subvalvular preservation and early operation in mitral valve surgery. *Circulation* 94:2117–2123, 1996.
6. Bolling, SF, Bach DS: Mitral valve reconstruction in elderly, ischemic patients. *Chest* 109:35–40, 1996.
7. Antunes MJ: Valve replacement in the elderly: Is the mechanical valve a good alternative? *J Thorac Cardiovasc Surg* 98:485–491, 1989.
8. Grossi EA, LeBoutillier M, Steinberg B, et al: Mitral valve repair in the elderly. *Cardiol Elderly* 3:269–272, 1995.
9. Grunkemeier GL, Miller C: Actuarial versus actual risk of porcine structural valve deterioration. *J Thorac Cardiovasc Surg* 108:709–718, 1994.
10. Grossi EA, Zakow PK, Miller JS, et al: Choice of mitral prosthesis in the elderly: An analysis of "actual" outcome. *Circulation* 96(8):I-683, 1997.

11. Cohn LH, Aranki SF et al: Long-term results of mitral valve reconstruction for regurgitation of the myxomatous mitral valve. *J Thorac Cardiovasc Surg* 107:143–151, 1994.
12. Lee EM, Porter JN, Shapiro L, et al: Mitral valve surgery in the elderly. *J Heart Valve Dis* 6:22–31, 1997.
13. Edmunds LH Jr, Cohn LH, et al: Guidelines for reporting morbidity and mortality after cardiac valvular operations. *J Thorac Cardiovasc Surg* 96:351–353, 1988.
14. Oury JH, Folkert TL, et al: Mitral valve replacement versus reconstruction. Analysis of indications and results of mitral valve procedures in a consecutive series of 80 patients. *J Thorac Cardiovasc Surg* 73:825–835, 1977.
15. Grossi EA, Galloway AC, Steinberg BM, et al: Severe calcification does not affect long-term outcome of mitral valve repair. *Ann Thorac Surg* 58(3):685–687, discussion 688, 1994.
16. Carpentier AF, Fuzellier J: Extensive calcification of the mitral valve annulus: Pathology and surgical management. *J Thorac Cardiovasc Surg* 111:718–730, 1996.
17. Adkins MS, Harnum N, et al: Efficacy of combined coronary revascularization and valve procedures in octogenarians. *Chest* 108:927–931, 1995.

Chapter 25

Quality of Life after Cardiac Surgery in Patients Older Than Seventy Years of Age

Jonathan Unsworth-White, Tom Treasure

Publications attesting to the ability of cardiac surgeons to operate on elderly patients are now commonplace.[1,2] In our own practice, the proportion of patients coming to cardiac surgery aged 70 years and older now exceeds 30% and octogenarian patients are not uncommon (Figure 1). Elderly patients form a distinct group within the practice of adult cardiac surgery, presenting particular challenges and dilemmas that are simply not issues among younger patients. Comorbidity is common, making intervention more hazardous and costly. There is a relatively greater proportion presenting for valve replacement operations (Figure 2) and more of the patients are female. The patients are keenly aware that quality of remaining life is paramount. Their clinicians are concerned about resource allocation and value for money.

These patients are highly selected by the time they come to the operating room, both from self selection and from that of their referring physicians. This selection process can act in opposite directions. On the one hand, patients must be tough to make it to their eighth and ninth decades and physicians generally do not refer "no-hopers" for elective cardiac surgery. On the other hand, an increasing proportion of the elderly work load is made up of emergency referrals; patients with unstable angina on nitrate and heparin infusions who are blocking medical beds (Figure 3). These patients are a particular concern, being much more likely to have left main stem coronary disease with impaired left

From *Clinical Cardiology in the Elderly. Second Edition,* edited by Elliot Chesler. © 1999, Futura Publishing Company, Armonk, NY.

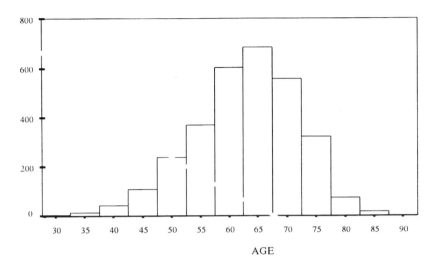

Figure 1: *Age distribution of patients undergoing only coronary artery surgery at St. George's Hospital 1990–1995 (n = 3036).*

ventricular function in association with serious comorbidity in the form of respiratory and renal compromise and even malignancy.

The diverse and conflicting pressures within health care systems worldwide make it beholden upon us to ensure that when taking these elderly patients to the operating room, we are improving the quality

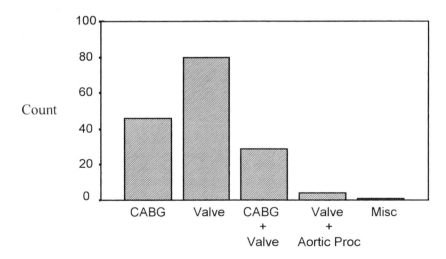

Figure 2: *Operative procedure in patients over the age of 80 at St. George's Hospital 1990–1995. Aortic proc, ascending aortic replacement.*

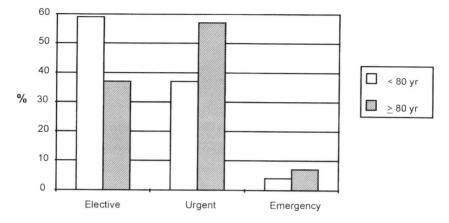

Figure 3: *Priority of coronary surgery in patients older and younger than 80 years of age. Chi squared* P = 0.009. *(Data from St. George's Hospital database 1990–1995).*

in addition to the duration of their lives. This chapter examines the issues concerning both the patients and their medical teams and highlights the sparse quality of life data applicable to this challenging group of patients.

Issues

What is Quality of Life?

Indiscriminate use of the phrase "quality of life" is common, especially in the cardiothoracic literature. In cardiac surgery descriptions of angina and dyspnea scores and incorrect applications of these scores to quality of life issues has been widespread. While angina grade has been shown to correlate well with quality of life in a younger population of patients,[3] in themselves such scores describe only 2 symptoms of cardiac disease. One should remain cautious before assuming that they tell us much about older patients' responses to them or indeed about any other aspect of their lives at that time. Reports of improvements in angina and dyspnea scores are all very well but must not purport to tell the reader anything about changes in the patients' perception of their quality of life.

In its broadest sense, the term quality of life is a catch-all phrase that means all things to all people. An individual rendered paraplegic after aortic surgery might be said to have no life quality left to him and yet the patient may feel otherwise. It is important to dispel such differences between observer and individual interpretation if treatments are not to be denied to deserving patients. Equally it is important to appreciate that an intervention that fails to add quality to life should be questioned. Patients will judge the outcome of the medical intervention in their lives according to the impact it has on their general sense of well being. After all a sense that all is not well is what usually brings them to medical attention in the first place. This is not always the case, as will be discussed further below. Cardiovascular diseases are not uncommonly asymptomatic and may be identified during routine screening programs or during workup for other unrelated conditions. Such asymptomatic patients are especially justified in asking to what degree their quality of life is to be enhanced when the proposed remedy for their cardiovascular condition is likely to leave them with new symptoms. From the medico-political point of view, an intervention that cannot be justified from the quality of life standpoint is unlikely to be sanctioned in today's health care systems.

Measures of Quality

Assessment of the impact of medical interventions on life quality is achieving ever more prominence. Life quality is of course a subjective state, but researchers have attempted to quantify it by breaking it down into "dimensions" that can be measured. Typical dimensions and subdimensions are given in Table 1. The questionnaires or techniques used to examine them are referred to as instruments. In general terms in-

---

Table 1
Essential Dimensions of Quality of Life and Examples of Subdimensions

Social function
    Participation in social events
    Contact with friends or relatives
    Quality of family and social relationships
    Marital satisfaction
    Performance of usual social role (eg, work, parent)
Physical function
    Aspects of everyday living (eg, self-care, shopping, housework, home repairs)
    Physical aspects of leisure-time pursuits or work
    Physical symptoms (eg, pain, fatigue)
Psychological function
    Mood (eg, depression, anxiety)
    Cognition (eg, memory, concentration)
    Overall feeling of well being

Reproduced with permission from Wilson A, Wiklund I, Lahti T, et al: A summary index for the assessment of quality of life in angina pectoris. *J Clin Epidemiol* 44:981–988, 1991.

Table 2
Instruments for the Assessment of Quality of Life

General	Disease-specific	Attribute-specific
Nottingham Health Profile[34] The University of York questionnaire[8]	Angina-specific Quality-of-Life Questionnaire[35]	Beck Depression Inventory[36] Karnofsky Performance Status Scale[13]

struments are categorized into 3 types depending on whether they are general, disease specific or attribute specific (Table 2). Each has its merits depending on the outcome of interest. Many studies use a combination of all 3. Mangione et al[4] used a combination of global and specific measures in a cross-section of adults undergoing major elective noncardiac surgery. This study revealed that elderly patients had similar perceptions of their global health to younger patients even though registering lower scores in their specific health dimensions of physical, role and social functions, mental health, energy, and pain. This group concluded that either global health was the result of different factors in the elderly or their expectations of health were lower. The study is useful in 2 ways. Firstly it emphasises the importance of specific measures of life quality, but secondly, it raises the interesting question of what is more valid in determining a patient's quality of life. Because the less physically and socially able elderly still registered similar global scores to their younger counterparts, who can say that their perceived life quality is less important than their reduced, but measured, quality?

Quality of Life/Cost versus Benefit

Quality adjusted life-years or QALYs are an attempt to rationalize the apportionment of health care resources. It is an intriguing concept that by combining duration with quality of life, seeks to account for cost effectiveness, the available choice between therapeutic options and the fact that many treatments do not cure but instead provide alleviation of symptoms. Each year after an intervention is multiplied by a fraction of 1, depending on the quality of each year where 1 equals a year of healthy life. In this way the impact of an intervention can be compared with that of another intervention in the same group of patients or the same intervention can be compared across different groups of patients. Where resources are limited, allocation might be limited to those interventions with the least cost per QALY.

Such a policy is controversial, even "ageist,"[5] because elderly patients cannot hope to gain as many years postoperatively as younger patients. Handicapped patients are also dealt a blow by this system because quality in each year is already compromised. Perhaps the use of QALYs to discriminate against particular groups of patients (elderly or handicapped) should be avoided, their use reserved instead for the comparison of treatment options for individual patients.[6] Clearly important is the quality of data on which such calculations are based. Consequently there is an increasing interest in quality of life and ways to measure it.

Apart from quality of life issues, other theories also govern the allocation of health care resources. They are briefly described below to highlight the current dilemma faced by all of us and thence to emphasise the need for the collection of better information on quality of life to make rational choices more of a possibility.

Fair Innings/Sanctity of Life

If elderly patients are considered to be less deserving of medical expenditure on the basis that they have lived out their "fair innings," one is obviously favoring treatment of younger patients who have more potential years to gain. This ignores the supposition that all life is valuable. Such a supposition puts greater emphasis on patients in imminent danger irrespective of age. To some extent this is the current situation in the United Kingdom. Elderly patients are less likely to be referred for elective cardiac surgery until their disease becomes critical and they are blocking a medical bed. At this stage the risk of their surgery is much greater and a self perpetuating cycle is set up.

Market Forces

The cycle is broken when patients are self-funding. In other words allocation of surgical time is more likely led by market forces provided the surgeon is willing to take the patient on. This system now favors the wealthy and is irrespective of age, putting poorer patients at a distinct disadvantage.

Quality of Life Studies

As stated above, decisions based on quality of life data are only as good as the data available. There is precious little relating specifically to the older population. Four representative studies are outlined below.

St. George's Study

This is a study of elderly patients who underwent cardiac surgery between the years 1987–1989 at St. George's Hospital in London.[7] All surviving patients who were 70 years or older at the time of their surgery were sent questionnaires at a mean follow-up of 3 years asking them to compare their preoperative and postoperative life qualities. The University of York questionnaire[8] based on the Rosser-Kind health-related quality of life scale was used. This is a general questionnaire which considers the broad domains of distress and disability. Being retrospective in nature the study relied on the patients' recollections of their preoperative state and as such was a bit like asking them whether they would choose to undergo the same procedures again.

Of the patients undergoing coronary bypass surgery (Figure 4), only 1 patient was more distressed after surgery and 80% of patients were in the lowest 2 grades of "distress" at follow-up. Disability was also much decreased after surgery with 86% of patients registering 1 of the top 3 grades of mobility.

Although these figures seemed very encouraging, further analysis revealed that 24% of patients had not registered an improvement in distress (7% were in the lowest distress group to start with) and 32% had not registered improvement in mobility (8% were in the most mobile grade to begin with).

Results were a little disappointing for those patients who underwent valve surgery (with or without bypass surgery). In this group only 45% and 50% of patients registered improvements in mobility and distress respectively (Figure 5). However the instrument chosen to measure their quality of life had upper and lower limits and many patients registered close to the top of the relevant scales preoperatively. Therefore, the majority of patients were not in fact able to register improvements. This emphasises the point that elderly patients with valve lesions frequently perceive only mild symptoms even when their prognosis is impaired by damaged left ventricular function. In contrast to surgery for coronary disease, valve surgery is often indicated more for prognosis than symptoms, even in elderly patients. Having received an operation to improve their longevity, they may now complain of a sore chest from the sternotomy!

Nevertheless, although perceived benefit was less in the valve replacement patients than in the coronary artery bypass patients, the proportion of patients in the upper 2 categories of mobility and distress at follow-up was encouraging and mirrored findings of other groups[9] who used the New York Heart Association Class (NYHA) as the yard stick[10,11] (see below).

Duke University Study

Glower et al[12] published another retrospective study focusing on the functional outcome of octogenarians after coronary surgery. Performance status was assessed using the Karnofsky scoring system.[13] This grades an individual's ability to work, their level of activity and their

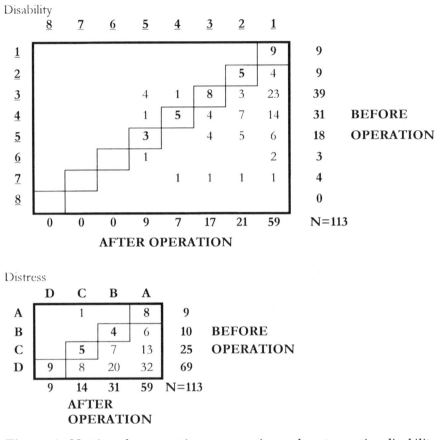

Figure 4: *Matrices demonstrating preoperative and postoperative disability and distress scores in a consecutive series of 113 patients who were over the age of 70 at the time of coronary artery bypass surgery. The numbers along the left and upper borders represent the possible preoperative and postoperative scores, respectively, while the numbers along the right and lower borders represent the numbers of patients falling into each score group preoperatively and postoperatively. Thus, for example, 39 patients had a disability score of 3 preoperatively and 8 of them remained in this group postoperatively; 23 had improved to a score of 1 and 4 had deteriorated to a score of 5. Reproduced with permission from Unsworth-White MJ, Kallis P, Treasure T, et al: Quality of life after cardiac surgery in patients over 70 years of age. Cardiol Elderly 2:133–138, 1994.*

requirements for support from others. Preoperative scores were compared with those achieved at discharge.

Over an 8-year period from 1983, 86 octogenarians underwent coronary surgery at Duke University Medical Center. Karnofsky Scores were significantly improved postoperatively, the median change being 40% with 89% of survivors improving by at least 20%. However, 29%

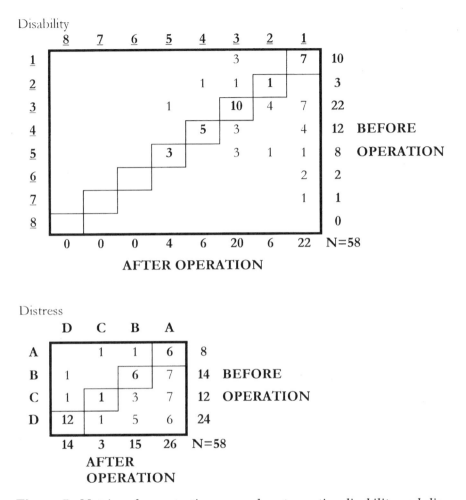

Figure 5: *Matrices demonstrating pre and postoperative disability and distress scores in a consecutive series of 58 patients who were over the age of 70 at the time of aortic valve surgery (with or without concomitant coronary artery surgery). Reproduced with permission from Unsworth-White MJ, Kallis P, Treasure T, et al: Quality of life after cardiac surgery in patients over 70 years of age. Cardiol Elderly 2:133–138, 1994.*

of patients incurred a "significant" postoperative complication and 1 in 5 patients either died before discharge or required a nursing home placement. Overall the authors suggest that 70% of their octogenarians had a favorable outcome, having postoperative Karnofsky scores of at least 60% and 20% greater than the preoperative score. Interestingly they correlated unfavourable outcomes with preoperative comorbid conditions. They stressed however that avoiding such patients may make one's surgical mortality figures look better at the expense of consigning them to a higher risk strategy of nonsurgical management.

Swedish Study

A comprehensive prospective study by Sjöland et al[14] is one of only a few prospective quality of life studies to compare outcomes in patients older and younger than 65 years of age. Although 65 is not considered old in today's society, the study is nevertheless important in providing information on quality of life issues in patients who are past retirement age.

Of more than 2000 consecutive patients undergoing coronary bypass surgery in the University Hospital at Sahlgrenska and the Scandinavian Heart Centre in Göteborg, almost 1400 patients completed a preoperative questionnaire encompassing the Nottingham Health Profile (NHP), the Psychological General Well-being Index and the Physical Activity Score. One thousand seven hundred forty-five patients completed the questionnaires 2 years after the operation.

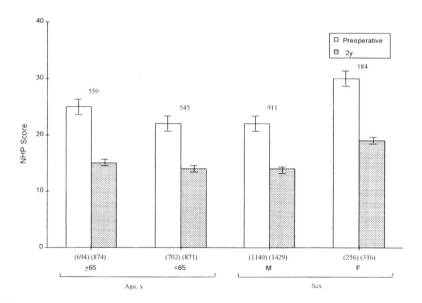

Figure 6: *Nottingham Health Profile (NHP) score (±SEM) in relation to age and sex. The NHP change score correlation with age was not significant (P = 0.12), but that with sex was (P < 0.001). Numbers in parentheses below bars represent total numbers of patients; numbers above bars, patients with paired preoperative and postoperative assessment. Reproduced with permission from Sjöland H, Wiklund I, Caidahl K, et al: Improvement in quality of life and exercise capacity after coronary bypass surgery. Arch Intern Med 156:265–271, 1996.*

There were considerable improvements in quality of life scores at 2 years, returning toward those of an age matched population. This was especially evident in the energy and pain scores of the NHP. As in the St. George's study (above), patients with the worst scores preoperatively gained the most. Importantly, quality of life results were similar between the over and under 65 year old age groups (Figure 6) and there were also comparable improvements in workload measures.

Baltimore Study

A study from Kumar et al[15] describes 68 octogenarians undergoing a variety of cardiac procedures during two time periods (1986 and 1991). Independence of living, ease of life and Karnofsky dependency categories were improved postoperatively but differences were not as great in patients followed up for longer (Figure 7). Nevertheless 75% and 84% of the patients respectively from the 2 time periods said that they would have made the same decision to opt for surgery again in retrospect. However, only 53% of the longer follow-up group and 72% of the more recent group were available for follow-up assessment because of the high rates of late mortality in this age group. The "missing" patients (and their physicians) might have made different choices if they had known what their outcome would be!

NYHA

NYHA class is a crude but frequently used indicator of life quality after cardiac surgery. It is worth including here if only to partially make up for the lack of good information in the elderly cardiac surgical population.

A typical study is that from Gehlot et al[11] who collected NYHA data from 322 octogenarian patients undergoing aortic valve replacement surgery (with or without coronary bypass surgery) during a 21-year time period. At 1-year of follow-up, just 3% of patients were in NYHA classes III and IV but this had increased to 18% by last follow-up at an average of 47 months postoperatively. As an indicator of "global health," the patients were asked at 1 year whether they felt that they had benefited from the operation. Five percent felt that they were unchanged, 2% felt worse, and 92% thought they were better off. Unfortunately, the exercise was not repeated at 47 months.

Cane et al[1] studied 121 octogenarian patients undergoing primarily coronary bypass surgery. Sixty-nine percent were experiencing class III or IV symptoms prior to surgery, compared with just 16% at a mean of just over 2 years postoperatively. These and other similar series attest to the good functional results that are now routinely experienced in patients of this age group but they add little understanding to the finer details of quality of life.

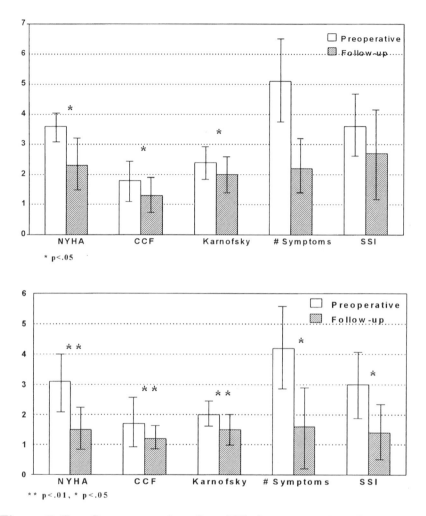

Figure 7: Top, *Parameters of quality of life for octogenarians from 1986 at follow-up compared with the preoperative status. Bottom, the same for octogenarians operated on in 1991. NYHA, New York Heart Association angina functional class; CCF, congestive cardiac failure functional class; # symptoms, number of cardiovascular symptoms experienced; Karnofsky, Karnofsky dependency category; SSI, social support index for activities of daily living. Reproduced with permissin from Kumar P, Zehr KJ, Chang A, et al: Quality of life in octogenarians after open heart surgery.* Chest 108:919–926, 1995.

Neurological End Points

Stroke

Neurological and cognitive functions are unquestionably vital qualities of life. For patients suffering perioperative strokes, the postoperative quality of life is seriously impaired. In a large prospective study of cerebral damage after coronary bypass surgery[16] only 32% of patients suffering major in-hospital neurological events were discharged to their homes. The remainder either died or required intensive nursing facilities.

Consequently a great deal of research effort has gone into examining the neurological impact and outcomes of cardiac surgery. Many elderly patients are prepared to accept even a high risk of operative death in their quest for an improvement in the quality of what life they have left. "After all, I won't know anything about it if I die on the operating table will I doctor?" is a phrase that many of us will have heard from our older patients. However they, and their clinicians, may be much more concerned about the possibility of a debilitating stroke during the peri-operative phase than from death on the operating table.

The incidence of perioperative stroke after cardiac surgery is related to age[16,18] and is approximately 6.5% for octogenarian patients (Table 3). This was confirmed in a review of the St. George's Hospital database,[19] which also revealed the strong association with operation type (Figure 8) and pre-existing hypertension. Thus, patients undergoing valve surgery were more than twice as likely to suffer a perioperative stroke than patients undergoing coronary surgery alone ($P < 0.05$). Patients suffering perioperative strokes spend longer on the intensive care unit (Figure 9) and in the hospital over all, and are much more likely to die.[16,18-21] A previous history of stroke or transient ischemic attack, longer bypass and cross-clamp times[17,21] and the presence of

---

Table 3
Incidence of Perioperative Stroke in Octogenarian Patients
Undergoing Cardiac Surgery

Data Source	Number of Patients Older Than 80 Years	Perioperative Stroke (%)
37	103 CABG or AVR ± CABG	6
24	474 CABG	6.3
11	322 AVR	8
15	64 CABG or AVR ± CABG	4.7
1	121 CABG	5.0
Total	**1084**	**6.5**

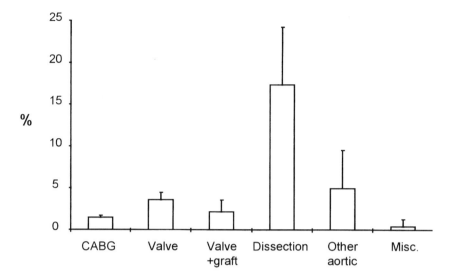

Figure 8: *Incidence of stroke (with upper 70% confidence limit) after cardiac surgery, subdivided by operation type. (Data from St. George's Hospital database 1990–1995).*

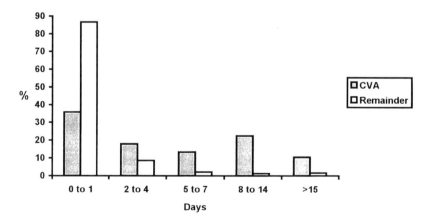

Figure 9: *Duration of ITU stay among patients undergoing cardiac surgery with or without a perioperative stroke. (Data from St. George+s Hospital 1990–1995).*

ascending aortic atheroma[16,21,22] have also been shown to increase the risk. Transesophageal identification of ascending aortic atheroma followed by replacement of the affected portion when indicated has been shown to reduce the likelihood of perioperative stroke.[23] The position regarding concomitant carotid endarterectomy remains controversial. Although carotid arteries are undoubtedly the source of some embolic strokes, the aorta seems much the more likely source during manipulation for cardiac surgery. Some support for this comes from the study of the use of mammary artery grafts in octogenarians.[24] In this study not only was a survival advantage evident after just 2 years in the internal mammary artery group, but the incidence of stroke was also less albeit not statistically significant (5.8% vs. 7.5%, $P > 0.2$), possibly because of the reduced need for ascending aortic manipulation in this group. Data from another group[25] revealed that carotid stenoses greater than 75% were not associated independently with strokes and the side of the stenosis did not correlate with that of the cerebral event. Furthermore, while some surgeons report excellent results from synchronous carotid endarterectomy and coronary surgery,[23] this is not universal.[21,26] Nevertheless, females with left main stem disease, peripheral vascular disease, a history of smoking, stroke or transient ischemic events are very likely to have significant carotid artery disease,[27] which may warrant synchronous surgery.

Cognitive Impairment

While the incidence of stroke is approximately 6.5% as described above, the incidence of perioperative cognitive impairment is much higher, depending on definitions and how closely one looks for it.[28] Like stroke, cognitive impairment is related to the patient's age.[29] This comprehensive prospective study by Newman et al[29] found that deteriorations in 7 of 9 cognitive measures (such as visuomotor speed and function, mood and memory) were related to the patient's age and that short-term memory was especially affected in this age group. The etiology of this impairment however remains elusive. Newman's group found that although temperature on bypass profoundly affected metabolic demand and cerebral blood flow autoregulation (metabolism-flow coupling), these changes were independent of age. Nevertheless the evidence did support the relationship between impairment of oxygen extraction and cognitive impairment.

Emboli are accepted as a cause of stroke, but other work from the Middlesex Hospital suggests an important link with neuropsychological dysfunction.[30] In this work, high-intensity transcranial Doppler signals, believed to represent embolic load, were much reduced in the group of patients who had a 40-μm filter on the arterial side of the cardiopulmonary bypass circuit. These patients performed significantly better than nonfiltered patients in a range of neuropsychological tests at both 8 days and 8 weeks after surgery. In addition there were more patients with soft neurological signs such as drowsiness and depressed reflexes in the nonfiltered group. Furthermore the likelihood of neuropsychological deficit at 8 weeks was related to the number of signals during surgery. Interestingly the incidence of depression was also more common among unfiltered patients at 8 weeks (Pugsley, personal communication). What this study also showed was the 27% incidence of measurable deficits in the non-filtered group, persisting at 8 weeks even in this group of patients who were all less than 70 years of age at the time of their surgery.

Another study from the Middlesex group[31] highlights the frequent perception of cognitive impairment in cardiac surgical patients which might considerably reduce a patients perception of their quality of life. Twenty-eight percent of patients reported impaired memory function 1 year after coronary surgery. Other frequent complaints were with problem solving in 18%, clarity of thinking in 16%, and concentration in 16%. Interestingly there was little relation between these subjective reports of cognitive deficit and measured changes. Instead they found that where deficits were reported, especially regarding deterioration of memory, they correlated instead with the occurrence of depression and low mood.

Conclusion

Although the title of this chapter refers to patients over the age of 70 years, the real dilemmas concern the treatment of a slightly older age group. Patients up to the age of 75 are now considered routine and make up a significant proportion of surgical practice. As we face the prospect of still older patients on the waiting list, information is urgently needed to inform us about realistic outcomes in terms of quality of life. This is often what concerns the patients most of all and it is vital to aid decisions about resource allocation.

As information slowly becomes available, these resource questions look to become more, rather than less, difficult. Elderly patients would appear to perceive just as much gain in their quality of life as their younger counterparts, albeit at greater risk. This implies that resources will have to be spread ever more thinly in the future. Clinicians must carefully select those elderly patients who have the most to gain at the most acceptable risk. It is clear that more research is required in order to provide the necessary data for these decisions to be made. As neatly summarized by Sprigings and Forfar[32] we need to be " . . .guided by science rather than prejudice."

References

1. Cane ME, Chen C, Bailey BM, et al: CABG in octogenarians: Early and late events and actuarial survival in comparison with a matched population. *Ann Thorac Surg* 60:1033–1037, 1995.

2. Williams DB, Carrillo RG, Traad EA, et al: Determinants of operative mortality in octogenarians undergoing coronary bypass. *Ann Thorac Surg* 60: 1038–1043, 1995.
3. Pocock SJ, Henderson RA, Seed P, et al: Quality of life, employment status, and anginal symptoms after coronary angioplasty or bypass surgery. 3-year follow-up in the Randomized Intervention Treatment of Angina (RITA) Trial. *Circulation* 94:135–142, 1996.
4. Mangione CM, Marcantonio ER, Goldman L, et al: Influence of age on measurement of health status in patients undergoing elective surgery. *J Am Geriatr Soc* 41:377–383, 1993.
5. Harris J: Unprincipled QALYs. *J Med Ethics* 17:185–188, 1991.
6. Hope T, Sprigings D, Crisp R. "Not clinically indicated": Patients' interests or resource allocation? *Br Med J* 306:379–381, 1993.
7. Unsworth-White MJ, Kallis P, Treasure T, et al: Quality of life after cardiac surgery in patients over 70 years of age. *Cardiol Elderly* 2:133–138, 1994.
8. Gudex C, Kind P: The QALY Tool Kit. Discussion Paper 38, 1–36. 1988. University of York, Centre for Health Economics.
9. Teoh KH, Fulop JC, Weisel RD, et al: Aortic valve replacement with a small prosthesis. *Circulation* 76:III-123-III-131, 1987.
10. Pupello DF, Bessone LN, Hiro SP, et al: Bioprosthetic valve longevity in the elderly: An 18-year longitudinal study. *Ann Thorac Surg* 60:S270-S275, 1995.
11. Gehlot A, Mullany CJ, Ilstrup D, et al: Aortic valve replacement in patients aged eighty years and older: Early and long-term results. *J Thorac Cardiovasc Surg* 111:1026–1036, 1996.
12. Glower DD, Christopher TD, Milano CA, et al: Performance status and outcome after coronary artery bypass grafting in persons aged 80 to 93 years. *Am J Cardiol* 70:567–571, 1992.
13. Karnofsky DA, Burchenal JH: The clinical evaluation of chemotherapeutic agents in cancer. In: CM Macleod (ed.) Symposium held at New York Academy of Medicine, New York 1948. New York, Columbia University Press, 1949, pp 191–205.
14. Sjöland H, Wiklund I, Caidahl K, et al: Improvement in quality of life and exercise capacity after coronary bypass surgery. *Arch Intern Med* 156: 265–271, 1996.
15. Kumar P, Zehr KJ, Chang A, et al: Quality of life in octogenarians after open heart surgery. *Chest* 108:919–926, 1995.
16. Roach GW, Kanchuger M, Mangano CM, et al: Adverse cerebral outcomes after coronary bypass surgery. *N Engl J Med* 335:1857–1863, 1996.
17. Frye RL, Kronmal R, Schaff HV, et al: Stroke in coronary bypass surgery: An analysis of the CASS experience. *Int J Cardiol* 36:213–221, 1992.
18. Tuman KJ, McCarthy RJ, Najafi H, et al: Differential effects of advanced age on neurologic and cardiac risks of coronary artery operations. *J Thorac Cardiovasc Surg* 104:1510–1517, 1992.
19. Unsworth-White MJ, Valencia O, Murday AJ, et al: Cerebral events after cardiac surgery. *Heart* 75(Suppl1):P83, 1996.
20. Fessatidis I, Prapas S, Hevas A, et al: Prevention of perioperative neurological dysfunction. A six year perspective of cardiac surgery. *J Cardiovasc Surg* 32:570–574, 1991.
21. Cernaianu AC, Vassilidze TV, Flum DR, et al: Predictors of stroke after cardiac surgery. *J Cardiac Surg* 10:334–339, 1995.
22. Marschall K, Kanchuger M, Kessler K, et al: Superiority of transesophageal

echocardiography in detecting aortic arch atheromatous disease: Identification of patients at increased risk of stroke during cardiac surgery. *J Cardiothorac Vasc Anesthes* 8:5–13, 1994.

23. Wareing TH, Davila-Roman VG, Daily BB, et al: Strategy for the reduction of stroke incidence in cardiac surgical patients. *Ann Thorac Surg* 55: 1400–1407, 1993.

24. Morris RJ, Strong MD, Grunewald KE, et al: Internal thoracic artery for coronary artery grafting in octogenarians. *Ann Thorac Surg* 62:16–22, 1996.

25. Ricotta JJ, Faggioli GL, Castilone A, et al: Risk factors for stroke after cardiac surgery: Buffalo Cardiac- Cerebral Study Group. *J Vasc Surg* 21: 359–363, 1995.

26. Vermeulen FE, Hamerlijnck RP, Defauw JJ, et al: Synchronous operation for ischemic cardiac and cerebrovascular disease: Early results and long-term follow-up. *Ann Thorac Surg* 53:381–389, 1992.

27. Berens ES, Kouchoukos NT, Murphy SF, et al: Preoperative carotid artery screening in elderly patients undergoing cardiac surgery. *J Vasc Surg* 15: 313–321, 1992.

28. Treasure T, Smith PLC, Newman S. Impairment of cerebral function following cardiac and other major surgery. *Eur J Cardiothorac Surg* 3: 216–221, 1989.

29. Newman MF, Croughwell ND, Blumenthal JA, et al: Effect of aging on cerebral autoregulation during cardiopulmonary bypass. Association with postoperative cognitive dysfunction. *Circulation* 90:II-243-II-249, 1994.

30. Pugsley WB, Klinger L, Paschalis C, et al: The impact of microemboli during cardiopulmonary bypass on neuropsychological functioning. *Stroke* 25: 1393–1399, 1994.

31. Newman S, Klinger L, Venn G, et al: Subjective reports of cognition in relation to assessed cognitive performance following coronary artery bypass surgery. *J Psychosom Res* 33:227–233, 1988.

32. Sprigings D, Forfar JC: How should we manage symptomatic aortic stenosis in the patient who is 80 or older? *Br Heart J* 74:481–484, 1995.

33. Fletcher A. Quality-of-life measurements in the evaluation of treatment: Proposed guidelines. *Br J Clin Pharmacol* 39:217–222, 1995.

34. Hunt SM, McEwan J, McKenna SP: *Measuring Health Status*. London, Groom Helm, 1986.

35. Wilson A, Wiklund I, Lahti T, et al: A summary index for the assessment of quality of life in angina pectoris. *J Clin Epidemiol* 44:981–988, 1991.

36. Beck AT, Ward CH, Mendolson J, et al: An inventory for measuring depression. *Arch Gen Psychiatr* 4:561–571, 1961.

37. Naunheim KS, Dean PA, Fiore AC, et al: Cardiac surgery in the octogenarian. *Eur J Cardiothorac Surg* 4:130–135, 1990.

Part 5

Noncardiac Surgery

Chapter 26

Abdominal Aortic Aneurysm

Frank A. Lederle

An aneurysm is a failure of the arterial wall resulting in a balloon-like dilatation of a segment of the artery. Once formed, aneurysms tend to progress and may ultimately rupture, usually with disastrous consequences. Aortic aneurysms constitute the 14th leading cause of death in the United States,[1] and the 10th leading cause of death in older men, their principal victims.[2] Approximately 80% of aortic aneurysms occur between the renal arteries and the aortic bifurcation. These abdominal aortic aneurysms (AAA) are responsible for more than 10,000 deaths per year in the United States.[3] Death results from either rupture of the aneurysm or as a consequence of elective treatment of an unruptured aneurysm, and should be preventable in many cases. Aortic aneurysms are also a leading cause of sudden death[4] and often remain undiagnosed even after death, with the result that physicians may not get the necessary feedback to increase their vigilance for this disease.

Pathophysiology

The integrity of the aortic wall is maintained by concentric lamellae of the structural proteins elastin and collagen located in the arterial media. Elastin, which bears the principal elastic load of the pulse pressure, is not synthesized in the adult aorta and degrades slowly over decades. Collagen forms a strong inelastic reinforcement layer and is synthesized throughout life. Gradual destruction of this lamellar architecture results in aneurysmal dilatation, associated with reduced elastin concentration and increased collagen turnover. These changes also occur in nonaneurysmal segments of the arteries of affected persons, suggesting that the process represents a systemic defect.

From *Clinical Cardiology in the Elderly. Second Edition,* edited by Elliot Chesler. © 1999, Futura Publishing Company, Armonk, NY.

Aneurysms tend to form upstream of an arterial bifurcation, where the pulse pressure wave reflected back by the bifurcation encounters an oncoming wave and the additive effects create an area of increased wall stress.[5] The particular susceptibility of the abdominal aorta to aneurysmal disease is believed to reflect not only its location upstream of a bifurcation, but also a paucity of structural lamellae to support the load carried, and of the vasa vasorum that supply nutrients to the arterial wall.

Once an aneurysm is formed, dilatation tends to be progressive both because medial degeneration is progressive and also because of several physical factors, including: (1) increased wall stress generated by turbulence in the dilated segment; (2) increased force of the pulse wave reflected by a bifurcation as the upstream segment widens; and (3) Laplace's law that relates wall tension to the product of arterial pressure and radius. Because aneurysms are not always circular in cross section, it is worth noting that the radius term in Laplace's law refers to the radius of curvature at a given point on the wall,[6] and not to half the distance to the opposite wall as is sometimes assumed.[7]

Why this process of medial degeneration and progressive dilatation is initiated in susceptible persons remains unclear. The traditional view of aneurysmal disease as simply a manifestation of atherosclerosis appears to be inadequate for a variety of reasons, many of them epidemiological, as discussed below. It now appears that multiple factors combine to cause aneurysm formation, including atherosclerosis, genetic factors (although a specific defect has not been identified), and, perhaps most importantly, smoking.[8]

Epidemiology

Unlike atherosclerosis, which has been declining in incidence for the past 30 years, the incidence of AAA appears to be increasing even beyond what can be attributed to improved diagnostic techniques.[9] The prevalence of AAA depends both on the population considered and on how AAA is defined. There is no widely accepted method of defining the cutoff point between AAA and normal. Most authors have used unadjusted aortic diameter (eg, ≥ 3.0 cm), which is known to be associated with the risk of rupture.[10] While such a "one-size-fits-all" method could exaggerate the prevalence of AAA in larger people, we have found that age, gender, race, and body size have little influence on normal aortic diameter, suggesting that their use in defining AAA may not offer sufficient advantage to be warranted.[11]

Small AAA are much more common than large AAA. Data from a large screening study conducted in older veterans[8] show that with each 1-cm decrease in AAA diameter, the number of prevalent AAA of that diameter or larger more than doubles (Table 1).

Men are affected 4 times as often as women, whites twice as often as blacks, and the incidence increases steeply with age. Smoking is the

Table 1
Prevalence of Abdominal Aortic
Aneurysm (AAA) by Diameter
in a Veteran Population*

AAA Diameter (cm)	Prevalence (%)**
≥8.0	.03
≥7.0	.06
≥6.0	.19
≥5.0	.50
≥4.0	1.4
≥3.0	4.6

* Adapted from Lederle et al.[8]

** Percent of population with AAA of diameter shown or larger.

strongest risk factor for AAA, with smokers having more than 5 times the risk of nonsmokers.[8] The excess prevalence associated with smoking accounted for 78% of all the AAA ≥ 4.0 cm in a veteran population.[8] The effects of age and smoking on the prevalence of AAA are shown in Figure 1.

A family history of AAA is uncommon, but when present, doubles the likelihood that AAA will be present. Other risk factors include height, coronary artery disease, any atherosclerosis, high cholesterol,

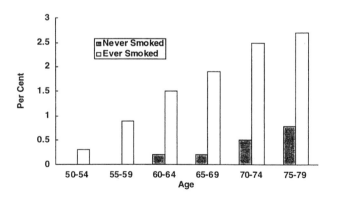

Figure 1: *Prevalence of abdominal aortic aneurysm ≥4.0 cm in men by age and smoking history. Adapted from Lederle FA, Johnson GR, Wilson SE, et al, for the Aneurysm Detection and Management (ADAM) Veterans Affairs Cooperative Study Group: Prevalence and associations of abdominal aortic aneurysm detected through screening. Ann Intern Med 126:441–449, 1997.*

and hypertension. AAA appears to be less common in diabetics, a curious finding that further distinguishes AAA from atherosclerosis.[8]

Natural History

The natural history of AAA is usually one of progressive slow growth with the risk of rupture increasing with the size of the aneurysm. The mean growth rate of AAA has been reported to be 0.2-0.5 cm per year,[10,12] but there is considerable individual variation. Less than one-third of AAA eventually rupture, and most patients with AAA die of other causes, especially coronary artery disease.[13]

Reliable estimates of AAA rupture rates by AAA diameter, though essential to rational management, have been difficult to obtain. Three population-based studies have reported rupture rates of less than 0.5% per year in AAA ≤ 5.0 cm.[10,14,15] These studies have been criticized for dependent censoring, ie, the selective removal, through elective surgery, of the patients most likely to rupture. However, if elective surgery was performed only because of AAA diameter and on asymptomatic patients, then the results should be valid up to the diameter at which elective surgery was offered.

The annual risk of rupture for AAA 5.0–5.9 cm was 3.4% in a study from Kingston, Ontario,[16] but the natural history of larger AAA is poorly documented. As a result, when vascular surgeons were asked for their estimates of the 1-year rupture rates for AAA 6.5 cm and 7.5 cm in diameter, the responses spanned a remarkably large range and reflected profound lack of consensus.[17] More accurate information on rupture rate by AAA diameter is currently being collected in 2 VA Cooperative Studies.

Diagnosis

A diagnosis can be made (1) in response to symptoms; (2) incidentally; or (3) by screening asymptomatic individuals. AAA usually remain asymptomatic until rupture, and the diagnosis of rupture will be discussed in a later section. Traditionally, diagnosis of asymptomatic AAA has usually been incidental, as the result of a physical examination or imaging test done for reasons other than to detect AAA. More recently, some physicians have begun screening for AAA with physical examination or ultrasound, and this too will be discussed in a later section.

Abdominal palpation is the original method of AAA detection. Few aneurysms will be found by "routine" 4-quadrant palpation of the abdomen,[1] but deliberate and careful evaluation of the aorta will detect most clinically important AAA. The patient should be supine with knees raised and the abdomen relaxed. The examiner places both hands palms down on the abdomen a few centimeters cephalad of the umbilicus (remembering that the aorta bifurcates at about the level of the umbilicus), and feels deeply for the pulsatile aorta between the 2 index fingers. A generous amount of abdominal skin should be included between the 2 index fingers, and it is often helpful initially to probe for 1 side of the aorta at a time.

It is the width, and not the intensity, of the aortic pulsation that determines the diagnosis; a normal aorta is often readily palpable in thin patients or those with loose abdominal muscles. The aorta is normally less than one inch in diameter (2.5 cm), and aortas larger than this (after allowing for skin thickness) warrant further investigation, usually with ultrasound. Findings of abdominal or femoral bruits or absent femoral pulses do not contribute to the diagnosis of asymptomatic AAA.[1] As Osler[18] observed, "no pulsation, however forcible, no thrill, however intense, no bruit, however loud—singly or together—justify the diagnosis of an aneurysm of the abdominal aorta, *only the presence of a palpable expansile tumour.*"

The sensitivity of abdominal palpation for detecting AAA depends on the size of the aneurysm and the size of the patient. Three fourths of AAA $\geq$ 5.0 cm in diameter are detectable by abdominal palpation whereas less than one third of AAA 3.0–3.9 cm are palpable. The sensitivity of palpation is also much lower in patients with an abdominal girth of more than 100 cm (a 40-inch waist) compared with thinner patients.[1] Less than half of elderly men suspected of having an enlarged aorta on abdominal palpation will be found to actually have AAA. This number (the positive predictive value) is much lower in women and young men,[1,19] but is not of great concern because ultrasound provides a safe and inexpensive confirmatory test.

Several imaging procedures have important roles in the initial detection or confirmation of AAA. Ultrasound is particularly useful because of its accuracy, low cost, patient acceptance, lack of radiation exposure, and general availability. A variety of studies have shown the sensitivity and specificity of ultrasound for AAA to be nearly 100%.[1,20] Computerized tomography (CT) is also highly accurate for detecting AAA, but is more expensive than ultrasound and involves some radiation exposure. The more detailed information provided by CT is useful for preoperative evaluation and diagnosis of AAA rupture.

A high degree of precision has been demonstrated for CT measurement of AAA diameter when carefully done using calipers and a magnifying glass and a defined protocol, but this precision is not often obtained in practice because of rounding errors and disagreement over how to measure AAA.[21] Ultrasound is associated with somewhat lower precision, and differences between imaging modalities further increase variability. Variations in AAA measurement of 0.5 cm or more are not uncommon, and this should be taken into account in management decisions.[21]

Plain radiography is a common means of incidental diagnosis of AAA and often provides diagnostic clues to rupture, eg, calcification, soft tissue mass, or loss of psoas or renal outlines.[22] However, plain radiography should not be used to confirm or exclude the diagnosis because many AAA will be missed due to insufficient calcification. Several other procedures, including angiography, magnetic resonance imaging, and spiral or helical CT angiography, have little role in initial diagnosis but can be useful for preoperative evaluation.

Management

The only currently established treatment for AAA is open surgical repair, a procedure first performed in 1951.[23] Aneurysm repair offers the only chance of survival for patients whose AAA has ruptured, as discussed in a later section. Elective repair is considered when the diagnosis is made before symptoms of rupture develop, with the goal of preventing the very high mortality associated with rupture (about 80%[24]). However, autopsy studies indicate that most AAA never rupture, suggesting that a selective approach to elective surgery should be taken. AAA diameter is the strongest known predictor of rupture,[10] so AAA diameter and the patient's operative risk are normally used to guide the decision of when to operate.

Because the number of AAA available for surgery increases markedly as the diameter selected for surgery decreases (Table 1), the AAA diameter at which patients are referred has a large impact on the number of operations performed. Operating on aneurysms that are "too small" is likely to result in excess mortality due to operative deaths, whereas waiting until the aneurysm is "too large" could to lead to excess deaths from rupture. When surgery is deferred, follow-up imaging, usually with ultrasound, every 6–12 months is essential to detect AAA enlargement that would warrant repair.

There is general agreement (but only indirect evidence) that a large aneurysm ($\geq$ 6.0 cm) in a patient with low surgical risk should be repaired. Whether elective repair should be performed on small AAA (4.0–6.0 cm) is an area of current debate. Data from randomized trials are not yet available to help determine the optimum diameter for elective surgery. The considerably less satisfactory alternative is to compare data from published case series of patients undergoing elective repair with those managed with follow-up imaging.

The operative mortality of elective AAA repair is well known. The two largest series, reporting statewide data from New York,[25] and Michigan,[26] yielded an identical overall operative mortality rate of 7.5%. When these and other population-based series are limited to high volume surgeons and hospitals, the rates fall to 4.5% to 6.5%.[2] Late mortality from repaired AAA (due to complications and recurrence) is more difficult to determine, but has been reported to be about 2%.[2] Adding this 2% to the operative mortality rate yields a total AAA-related mortality for patients treated with elective resection of about 10%, or 6%–9% in high volume centers.

For comparison, several studies have described patients who were followed with periodic imaging for AAA measurement and operated on if and when their AAA reached a predetermined diameter (usually 6 cm), grew rapidly, or became symptomatic. Summarizing these studies, after a mean 2–4 years of follow-up, 40%–45% of patients required surgery, 3%–9% died from AAA-related causes (rupture or surgery deaths), 20%–35% died of other causes, and 20%–35% were alive without operation. Assuming that the latter group continued to undergo elective surgery and/or suffer AAA-related death at the same rate after the study period, a final AAA-related death rate of 4%–13% can be projected for these series, with 53%–66% having surgery.[2] This AAA-related mortality is similar to the 6%–10% estimated above for immediate surgery, indicating that an optimal management strategy cannot be determined from published data for AAA of 4.0–6.0 cm.

The result has been a wide range of recommendations. A subcommittee appointed by the Society for Vascular Surgery and the International Society for Cardiovascular Surgery has recommended elective surgery for AAA ≥4.0 cm.[27] A RAND/Academic Medical Center Consortium expert panel produced recommendations in numerous patient subgroups, but basically recommended operating on AAA ≥5.0 cm.[28] The directors of the Chichester screening program have demonstrated that AAA can be observed with apparently comparable safety until they reach 6.0 cm.[29]

These unresolved questions in the management of small AAA led to the development of two randomized clinical trials that are currently underway, the UK Small Aneurysm Trial (UK SAT)[30] and the VA Cooperative Study Program's Aneurysm Detection and Management (ADAM) Study.[31] In both studies, patients with AAA 4.0–5.4 cm who are not at high surgical risk are randomized to either immediate surgery or to observation with imaging every 6 months until the aneurysm has enlarged to 5.5 cm or greater or becomes symptomatic, at which time surgery is offered. The UK SAT and the ADAM Study, respectively, began in 1991 and 1992, have completed enrollment with 1090 and 1136 patients, and are scheduled to complete follow-up in 1998 and 2000.

Although surgery is the only accepted treatment for AAA at present, several experimental therapies have generated considerable interest and deserve mention here. First is the method of endovascular grafting. Endovascular stent grafts were designed to serve as a new lumen for the dilated arterial segment, thereby shielding the aneurysmal wall from the blood pressure load. When successful, endovascular grafting is clearly associated with less morbidity than surgery, but postoperative mortality and cost have not yet been shown to be reduced. In addition, many patients are ineligible for currently available grafts because they lack a sufficient length of normal aorta below the renal arteries for cephalad anchoring, or because their iliac arteries are too tortuous or stenotic to permit passage of the graft. The most important concern regarding endovascular treatments is that long-term safety and ability to prevent rupture have not been demonstrated,[32] whereas decades of experience have shown surgical repair to be effective at preventing rupture. By the end of 1997, no endovascular graft was approved for use in the United States.

Also under investigation is medical therapy in the form of β-blocking drugs, intended to slow AAA growth. β-Blockers reduced aortic root dilation in a 10-year randomized trial of 70 patients with Marfan syndrome, [33] suggesting a possible role in the management of AAA. Several small cohort studies showed β-blockers to be associated with substantially slower growth rates of AAA, but the differences did not reach statistical significance.[12,34] A larger cohort study reported a P value less than 0.05 for a reduction in growth rate with β-blocker use when the analysis was limited to large aneurysms, but the results in the entire study were nonsignificant and the effect in the large aneurysm subgroup does not remain significant when corrected for multiple comparisons.[35] Also worrisome was a 2-fold higher rupture rate in the β-blocker group. β-Blockers appear promising for the management of small asymptomatic AAA, but cannot yet be generally recommended. A randomized trial of the influence of β-blockers on AAA expansion rate is currently in progress in Canada.[36]

Diagnosis and Management of Ruptured AAA

There are few conditions encountered in the practice of medicine that require accurate diagnosis more urgently than does AAA rupture. In many patients, ruptured AAA presents as sudden vascular collapse, in which case the need for emergency surgery may be obvious but the likelihood of a successful outcome is low. In other patients, an AAA may become symptomatic prior to rupture or an aneurysmal leak may be contained in the retroperitoneum for hours to weeks. These cases present more difficult diagnostic problems but also better chance of success if prompt action is taken. Unfortunately, the diagnosis is often missed, largely due to a lack of awareness of the various presentations. When shock develops during the resulting treatment delay, the chance of survival is markedly reduced.

Recognition of the diagnostic difficulties associated with ruptured AAA is not new. Osler noted that the diagnosis of retroperitoneal rupture was particularly difficult and frequently overlooked.[18] Ruptured AAA commonly present with abdominal, back, flank, or groin pain, abdominal distention, tenderness in any abdominal quadrant, constipation, urinary retention, transient hypotension and syncope, ecchymoses of the lower trunk or genitalia, leukocytosis, and anemia (which may be mild or absent). Less frequent presentations include inguinal hernia, femoral neuropathy, melena caused by aortoenteric fistula, and high output heart failure with hematuria caused by rupture into the vena cava.

Many of these characteristic findings of contained rupture are often misinterpreted as evidence against the diagnosis. Common misdiagnoses of ruptured AAA include urinary tract obstruction or infection, diverticulitis, and benign or malignant spinal disease.[37] Pain may precede rupture, presumably due to acute expansion of the aneurysm or partial disruption of the vessel wall, and a CT scan showing AAA without leakage in a symptomatic patient does not exclude imminent rupture.

The "classic triad" of abdominal pain, pulsatile mass and hypotension is problematic for the diagnosis of rupture. Palpation of a pulsatile mass can be an important clue, but although aneurysms that rupture are usually large, they may not be easily palpable because of obesity, abdominal distention, guarding, or loss of integrity of the aneurysm. Hypotension often occurs as a late finding and marks the end of the best opportunity for a successful outcome, and abdominal pain has a long differential diagnosis which may lead the clinician away from urgent evaluation of the abdominal aorta.

The following strategy can be recommended for the diagnosis and management of ruptured AAA[37]: (1) All physicians who provide care to older patients should become proficient at measuring the width of the aorta between the 2 index fingers. (2) Physicians should lower their threshold for obtaining abdominal ultrasound in elderly patients with symptoms of abdominal or back pain. Screening asymptomatic elderly men for AAA with ultrasound has been seriously debated (see below), so it is difficult to justify failure to obtain ultrasound in a patient with symptoms that could be caused by rupture or imminent rupture of AAA. (3) A patient with abdominal pain and shock should be taken directly to the operating room with ultrasound obtained while resuscitation procedures are underway. (4) When ruptured AAA is suspected in a hemodynamically stable patient, an immediate CT scan is generally considered to be safe and appropriate, though cardiovascular collapse in the radiology suite does occasionally occur. (5) When a CT scan shows leakage from an AAA, the patient should be taken to the operating room immediately. (6) A CT scan demonstrating AAA without leakage in a symptomatic patient should not be dismissed as "negative" because the symptoms may mean that rupture is imminent. These cases represent a difficult clinical decision in which urgent surgery must be carefully considered in view of the symptoms, AAA diameter and other CT scan findings, and the general health of the patient.

The Question of Screening

Screening for AAA was first proposed by Schilling and colleagues 30 years ago.[38] The idea is appealing because AAA appears to meet the criteria for an acceptable target of a screening program: (1) it is an important cause of death; (2) there is a long asymptomatic period during which elective repair can be carried out with acceptable operative mortality, whereas after symptoms of rupture develop, only one-fifth of patients survive[24]; and (3) the proposed screening tests (ultrasound or abdominal palpation with confirmatory ultrasound) are safe, inexpensive and acceptable to patients.

The Vascular Surgery Society of the United Kingdom has recommended a national ultrasound screening program for AAA,[39] and a review of periodic physical examination found abdominal palpation for AAA to be one of the few maneuvers that could be recommended for older men.[40] The Canadian Task Force on the Periodic Health Examination noted that abdominal palpation of men over age 60 was "prudent" and that ultrasound "could be considered" in obese or high risk patients,[41] but both the Canadian and the U.S. Preventive Services Task Forces gave AAA screening a "C" rating (poor evidence to include or exclude from the periodic health examination), apparently because they considered the effectiveness and cost-effectiveness of screening to be uncertain.

In the only randomized trial of screening versus no screening reported to date, from Chichester UK, AAA screening and elective repair in men resulted in a significant 55% reduction in AAA ruptures, and a 41% reduction in AAA-related deaths that did not reach statistical significance despite a sample size of over 15,000.[42] There were no operative deaths in 33 elective repairs in this study and repair was offered only for AAA ≥6 cm or rapid growth; 2 factors crucial to the success of the program but unlikely to be replicated in general practice. A more definitive assessment of screening may be difficult because of the very large numbers of patients required and the difficulty of ascertaining AAA-related deaths, particularly in the unscreened group,[43] but other large randomized trials are currently underway in Denmark and western Australia.

At least 5 cost-effectiveness analyses of ultrasound screening for AAA have been published for men over age 60.[44] One concluded that screening did more harm than good; the others found screening to be beneficial at costs ranging from about $2,000 to $41,550 per year of life saved. Cost effectiveness ratios up to $40,000 per year of life saved are consistent with currently funded programs and those under $20,000 are considered to be "very attractive", so screening for AAA looks very promising in this regard.[44]

Most of these analyses assumed that all AAA over 4.0 cm would be repaired, which is a more expensive policy than operating only on aneurysms at the larger end of the size range currently under study by the two randomized treatment trials described above. The only analysis to look at the cost effectiveness of operating at different AAA diameters found that increasing the diameter at which AAA were electively repaired from 5.0 cm to 6.0 cm reduced the cost per year of life saved of the screening program by more than 90%.[45]

Screening with abdominal palpation and confirmatory ultrasound has been calculated to be more cost effective than screening with ultrasound.[46] The principal drawback of this screening method is the lower sensitivity of palpation, as discussed above. Larger AAA are preferentially detected by palpation, however, accounting in part for the improved efficiency.

That aortic aneurysm remains a leading cause of death attests to the inadequacy of the present situation in which many small AAA are detected incidentally and repaired while many large AAA remain undetected until rupture. Only about 15% of the cost of AAA screening accrues from diagnosis with most of the rest coming from treatment,[46] so the Chichester policy of screening the population and operating only on large AAA[42] appears to be a better use of resources. If ultrasound screening is undertaken, it should be focused on men over age 60, particularly smokers and former smokers. When screening ultrasound is not readily available, abdominal palpation with confirmatory ultrasound is an efficient alternative.

References

1. Lederle FA, Walker JM, Reinke DB: Selective screening for abdominal aortic aneurysms with physical examination and ultrasound. *Arch Intern Med* 148:1753–1756, 1988.
2. Lederle FA: Management of small abdominal aortic aneurysms. *Ann Intern Med* 113:731–732, 1990.
3. Gillum RF: Epidemiology of aortic aneurysm in the United States. *J Clin Epidemiol* 48:1289–1298, 1995.
4. Thomas AC, Knapman PA, Krikler DM, et al: Community study of the causes of "natural" sudden death. *BMJ* 297:1453–1456, 1988.
5. Johansen K: Aneurysms. *Scientific American* 247:(1):110–25, 1982.
6. Burton AC: The importance of the shape and size of the heart. *Am Heart J* 54:801–810, 1957.
7. Elger DF, Blackketter DM, Budwig RS, et al: The influence of shape on the stresses in model abdominal aortic aneurysms. *J Biomech Eng* 118:326–332, 1996.
8. Lederle FA, Johnson GR, Wilson SE, et al, for the Aneurysm Detection and Management (ADAM) Veterans Affairs Cooperative Study Group: Prevalence and associations of abdominal aortic aneurysm detected through screening. *Ann Intern Med* 126:441–449, 1997.
9. Melton LJ, Bickerstaff LK, Hollier LH, et al: Changing incidence of abdominal aortic aneurysms: A population-based study. *Am J Epidemiol* 120:379–386, 1984.
10. Nevitt MP, Ballard DJ, Hallett JW: Prognosis of abdominal aortic aneurysms: A population-based study. *N Engl J Med* 321:1009–1014, 1989.
11. Lederle FA, Johnson GR, Wilson SE, et al, and the ADAM VA Cooperative Study Investigators: Relationship of age, gender, race, and body size to infrarenal aortic diameter. *J Vasc Surg* 26:595–601, 1997.
12. Cronenwett JL, Sargent SK, Wall WH, et al: Variables that affect the expansion rate and outcome of small abdominal aortic aneurysms. *J Vasc Surg* 11:260–269, 1990.
13. Darling RC, Messina CR, Brewster DC, et al: Autopsy study of unoperated abdominal aortic aneurysms: The case for early resection. *Circulation* 56(suppl 2):161–164, 1977.

14. Glimaker H, Holmberg L, Elvin A, et al: Natural history of patients with abdominal aortic aneurysm. *Eur J Vasc Surg* 5:125–30, 1991.
15. Guirguis EM, Barber GG: The natural history of abdominal aortic aneurysms. *Am J Surg* 162:481–483, 1991.
16. Brown PM, Pattenden R, Vernooy C, et al: Selective management of abdominal aortic aneurysms in a prospective measurement program. *J Vasc Surg* 23:213–222, 1996.
17. Lederle FA: Risk of rupture of large abdominal aortic aneurysms: Disagreement among vascular surgeons. *Arch Intern Med* 156:1007–1009, 1996.
18. Osler W: Aneurysm of the abdominal aorta. *Lancet* 1905; 1089–96.
19. Beede SD, Ballard DJ, James EM, et al: Positive predictive value of clinical suspicion of abdominal aortic aneurysm: Implications for efficient use of abdominal ultrasonography. *Arch Intern Med* 150:549–551, 1990.
20. Nusbaum JW, Freimanis AK, Thomford NR: Echography in the diagnosis of abdominal aortic aneurysm. *Arch Surg* 102:385–388, 1971.
21. Lederle FA, Wilson SE, Johnson GR, et al, for the Abdominal Aortic Aneurysm Detection and Management Veterans Administration Cooperative Study Group. Variability in measurement of abdominal aortic aneurysms. *J Vasc Surg* 21:945–952, 1995.
22. Loughran CF: A review of the plain abdominal radiograph in acute rupture of abdominal aortic aneurysms. *Clin Radiol* 37:383–387, 1986.
23. Dubost C, Allary M, Oeconomos N: Resection of an aneurysm of the abdominal aorta: Reestablishment of the continuity by a preserved human arterial graft, with result after five months. *Arch Surg* 64:405–408, 1951.
24. Ingoldby CJH, Wujanto R, Mitchell JE: Impact of vascular surgery on community mortality from ruptured aortic aneurysms. *Br J Surg* 73:551–553, 1986.
25. Hannan EL, Kilburn H, O'Donnell JF, et al: A longitudinal analysis of the relationship between in-hospital mortality in New York State and the volume of abdominal aortic aneurysm surgeries performed. *Health Serv Res* 27:517–542, 1992.
26. Katz DJ, Stanley JC, Zelenock GB: Operative mortality rates for intact and ruptured abdominal aortic aneurysms in Michigan: An eleven-year statewide experience. *J Vasc Surg* 19:804–817, 1994.
27. Hollier LH, Taylor LM, Ochsner J: Recommended indications for operative treatment of abdominal aortic aneurysms. *J Vasc Surg* 15:1046–1056, 1992.
28. Ballard DJ, et al: Abdominal Aortic Aneurysm Surgery: A Literature Review and Ratings of Appropriateness and Necessity. Santa Monica, California: RAND publication. JRA-04;1992.
29. Scott RAP, Wilson NM, Ashton HA, et al: Is surgery necessary for abdominal aortic aneurysm less than 6 cm in diameter? *Lancet* 342:1395–1396, 1993.
30. Powell JT, Greenhalgh RM, Ruckley CV, et al: The UK small aneurysm trial. *Ann NY Acad Sci* 800:249–251, 1996.
31. Lederle FA, Wilson SE, Johnson GR, et al, for the ADAM VA Cooperative Study Group. Design of the abdominal aortic Aneurysm Detection and Management (ADAM) Study. *J Vasc Surg* 20:296–303, 1994.
32. Parodi JC, Barone A, Piraino R, et al: Endovascular treatment of abdominal aortic aneurysms: Lessons learned. *J Endovasc Surg* 4:102–10, 1997.
33. Shores J, Berger KR, Murphy EA, et al: Progression of aortic dilatation and the benefit of long-term β-adrenergic blockade in marfan's syndrome. *N Engl J Med* 330:1335–1340, 1994.

34. Leach SD, Toole AL, Stern H, et al: Effect of β-adrenergic blockade on the growth rate of abdominal aortic aneurysms. *Arch Surg* 23:606–609, 1988.
35. Gadowski GB, Pilcher DP, Ricci MA: Abdominal aortic aneurysm expansion rate: Effect of size and beta-adrenergic blockade. *J Vasc Surg* 19: 727–731, 1994.
36. Laupacis A: Propranolol for small abdominal aortic aneurysms. *Chron Dis Can* 15 (suppl 4):S40-S41, 1991.
37. Lederle FA, Parenti CM, Chute EP: Ruptured abdominal aortic aneurysm: The internist as diagnostician. *Am J Med* 96:163–167, 1994.
38. Schilling FJ, Hempel HF, Becker WH, et al: Asymptomatic aortic aneurysms detected on the abdominal roentgenogram. *Circulation* 33(Suppl 3): 209, 1966.
39. Harris PL. Reducing the mortality from abdominal aortic aneurysms: Need for a national screening programme. *Br Med J* 305:697–699, 1992.
40. Oboler SK, LaForce FM: The periodic physical examination in asymptomatic adults. *Ann Intern Med* 110:214–226, 1989.
41. Canadian Task Force on the Periodic Health Examination: Periodic health examination, 1991 update: 5. Screening for abdominal aortic aneurysm. *Can Med Assoc J* 145: 783–789, 1991.
42. Scott RAP, Wilson NM, Ashton HA, et al: Influence of screening on the incidence of ruptured abdominal aortic aneurysm: 5-year results of a randomized controlled study. *Br J Surg* 82:1066–1070, 1995.
43. Lederle FA: Screening for snipers: The burden of proof. *J Clin Epidemiol* 43:101–104, 1990.
44. Lederle FA: Looking for asymptomatic abdominal aortic aneurysms. *J Gen Intern Med* 11:774–775, 1996.
45. St. Leger AS, Spencely M, McCollum CN, et al: Screening for abdominal aortic aneurysm: A computer assisted cost-utility analysis. *Eur J Vasc Endovasc Surg* 11:183–190, 1996.
46. Frame PS, Fryback DG, Patterson C: Screening for abdominal aortic aneurysm in men ages 60 to 80 years: A cost-effectiveness analysis. *Ann Intern Med* 119:411–416, 1993.

Chapter 27

Diagnosis and Management of Peripheral Arterial Disease

Timothy J. Wilt

Peripheral arterial disease (PAD) produces symptomatic disability in greater than 1 million people in the United States each year.[1] In addition to functional impairment and potential for limb loss, the presence of PAD is associated with atherosclerosis in other vascular beds and early mortality.[2-4] The presence of PAD is the strongest age-adjusted predictor of survival in patients recovering from an acute myocardial infarction as well as in individuals undergoing coronary artery bypass surgery.[5-8] Additionally, asymptomatic but hemodynamically significant PAD is present in as many as 15% of individuals. Asymptomatic disease has also been associated with reduced length and quality of life as well as more advanced or complicated coronary heart disease (CHD).[9]

Most patients with PAD do not require invasive therapy. The nonsurgical management of patients with PAD involves a multidisciplinary approach using the combined expertise of a primary care physician, vascular surgeon, radiologist, and vascular internist.[10-12] This review focuses on diagnostic and management approaches in patients with lower extremity vascular disease that are of greatest relevance to the internist.

Epidemiology and Natural Course of Peripheral Arterial Disease

The prevalence of symptomatic PAD ranges from 0.4%–20% depending on the age, gender, and health care characteristics of the popu-

From *Clinical Cardiology in the Elderly. Second Edition,* edited by Elliot Chesler. © 1999, Futura Publishing Company, Armonk, NY.

lation studies.[4] The annual incidence of intermittent claudication is approximately 20 per 1000 in men and women older than 65 years.[13] The incidence rises with age, atherosclerotic risk factors, and the presence of CHD, occurring at about one-fourth of the incidence of CHD. It is estimated that up to 1.3 million elderly persons can be expected to develop disabling claudication symptoms every 2 years during the next 50 years. Consequently, PAD will be an increasing cause of disability.

Approximately one-half of patients with PAD remain symptomatically stable or show some improvement 5 years after onset of symptoms.[14,15] Sixteen percent have worsening of symptoms, 25% have tissue loss or require surgery, and only 4% eventually require an amputation. In contrast to the favorable limb prognosis in patients with mild to moderate claudication, 15% of patients presenting with severe claudication required an amputation within 2.5 years. In patients developing ischemic ulcerations or rest pain, an immediate intervention (surgery, angioplasty, or amputation) was required in almost 20% of cases.[14,16] Cigarette smoking and diabetes accelerate PAD progression and are associated with worsening of symptoms, increased frequency of ischemic rest pain, and amputation.[16-21]

While the risk of limb loss is low, the mortality rate for patients with intermittent claudication is 2 to 3 times that of age- and sex-matched controls and almost three-quarters die from atherosclerotic causes.[3,4] The mean 5-, 10-, and 15-year survival after the diagnosis of PAD is approximately 70%, 50%, and 30%, respectively. Atherosclerosis in other vascular beds further reduces survival. Only 60% of patients with associated symptomatic cerebrovascular or coronary artery disease survive for 5 years. In these patients 60% died from CHD, 24% from cerebral vascular disease and 10% from other vascular disorders such as ruptured aortic aneurysms.[4]

The prevalence of comorbid conditions is considerably higher in patients with PAD than the general population. Estimated prevalence rates include: past or current history of tobacco use (80%), hypertension (20%–40%), hypercholesterolemia (30%), CHD (28%), diabetes (20%), and cerebrovascular disease (10%).[14,22] Thus management of patients with PAD needs to incorporate a knowledge of their overall prognosis as well as the risk and benefits of treatment.

Clinical Presentation and Physical Examination

History

The characteristic symptom of PAD, intermittent claudication, is described as muscle pain, cramping, fatigue, or weakness produced by walking that is relieved within minutes by rest. Claudication means "to limp" and results from inadequate tissue perfusion during exertion.

Symptoms consists of 3 essential features: the pain is always experienced in a functional muscle unit (eg, calf, buttock); it is reproducibly precipitated by exercise; and it is promptly relieved by rest. The pain description and physical examination findings depend on the location and severity of arterial occlusion and have prognostic significance.

Physical Examination

Physical examination can assess the presence, location, and severity of lower extremity vascular disease. Inspection of the affected leg and foot and comparison with the opposite extremity may reveal signs of chronic arterial insufficiency. Limbs should be examined for evidence of hair loss, poor nail growth, dry, scaly atrophic skin, dependent rubor, pallor with leg elevation, and delayed color return and venous filling. Hemodynamically significant atherosclerosis is considered present if extremity pallor is noted after elevation at 60° for 1 minute. Time for color return and venous filling is 10–15 seconds in a normal extremity and greater than 40 seconds in a limb with severe ischemia.[23] Absent or diminished femoral or pedal pulses generally indicate advanced atherosclerosis, but may overestimate the presence of disease. While the dorsalis pedis pulse alone may be absent in as many as 8% of the normal population the posterior tibial pulses should be palpable in patients with normal arterial supply. The lack of a posterior tibial pulse may be the single best clinical predictor of atherosclerotic peripheral vascular disease.[24] If pedal pulses are present at rest, exercising the limb or foot may result in transient loss of these pulses, indicating PAD. Because the prevalence of asymptomatic aortic aneurysms in elderly individuals is almost 2%, palpation of the abdominal aorta should be part of the vascular examination.[26] PAD is not independently associated with the presence of aortic aneurysms.[25-27]

Ischemic rest pain characteristically is worse when individuals are in the supine position due to leg elevation. Pain frequently involves the foot diffusely and distal to the metatarsals. Patients with rest pain may have tissue necrosis, gangrene, or nonhealing ulcers. Ischemic ulcers are usually painful and located on the dorsal or lateral aspect of the foot distally. In contrast, stasis ulcers usually occur without pain and are located on the lower third of the leg and medial malleolus. Neurotrophic ulcers generally form under calluses or pressure points. Chronic ischemic ulcers have a punched out appearance and have little bleeding with manipulation. Ischemic rest pain or ulceration implies a reduction of extremity blood flow below that required for resting tissue metabolism. These patients are at high risk for limb loss and require surgical consultation.

Differential Diagnosis

The differential diagnosis of intermittent claudication includes nonvascular causes such as arthritis of the hips, restless leg syndrome,

Table 1
Differential Diagnosis of Intermittent Claudication

- Arthritis
- Prolapsed intervertebral disk
- Spinal stenosis (pseudoclaudication)
- Peripheral neuropathy
- Restless leg syndrome
- Deep venous thrombosis
- Arterial embolus
- Thromboangiitis obliterans (Buerger's disease)
- Musculoskeletal leg cramps

peripheral neuropathies, and spinal stenosis (Table 1). Their presence can usually be determined by location, duration, and precipitating factors of the pain as well as physical examination and noninvasive vascular testing. For example, in contrast to neuropathic pain, ischemic rest pain is typically relieved by placing the foot in a dependent position. Symptoms of spinal stenosis (pseudoclaudication) are frequently brought on by extension of the lumbar spine. Weight-bearing activities, including standing for long periods and walking, precipitate pain. Relief usually requires sitting for 15–20 minutes with forward flexion at the hips and not merely standing still as with vascular claudication. Nocturnal calf cramps are common in patients with PAD. They are due to muscle spasm, relieved by massage, and are not due to resting tissue ischemia. Symptoms of "cold feet" in the absence of other clinical findings usually do not indicate arterial insufficiency.

Disease Classification

PAD is generally classified anatomically as aortoiliac, femoropopliteal, or tibioperoneal disease, each with distinctive clinical features and prognosis. One-third of patients, however, have more than one area involved. *Aortoiliac disease* occurs in approximately 15% of patients with PAD and they have suffer from claudication in the thigh or buttock due to arterial occlusive disease in the aortoiliac distribution. In males, impotence is common and normal erectile function argues against an ischemic etiology. Claudication in the aortoiliac distribution is typically described as an aching discomfort associated with weakness rather than pain. Aortoiliac disease commonly occurs in patients who are in their fifth and sixth decades of life, smoke or have hypercholesterolemia. Femoral pulses are often diminished but distal pulses may be intact at rest because of development of collateral circulation. Patients with aortoiliac disease usually have segmental lesions and two-thirds of all patients can be managed successfully without operative intervention.[16] Worsening symptoms indicate progressive stenoses or more frequently, distal progression.

Femoropopliteal disease occurs in approximately two-thirds of patients with PAD and is associated with hypertension, diabetes, and especially cigarette use. Patients present with symptoms of exercise-induced cramping pain and weakness in the affected calf. Femoral pulses are usually normal, but popliteal and pedal pulses are generally reduced or not palpable. Because of the extensive nature of this disease, symptomatic progression is more common than in aortoiliac disease. Limb loss occurs in 5% of patients followed for 5 years without surgical intervention. Relief of symptoms is limited by graft failure in up to 50% of patients undergoing surgery, especially in those with poor proximal and distal blood flow or who continue to smoke.[28] Because of coexisting diseases, perioperative mortality is relatively high (up to 10%) and atherosclerosis is often too extensive to be amenable to angioplasty.[29]

Tibioperoneal disease (alone or in combination with superficial femoral and popliteal artery atherosclerosis) occurs predominately in older or diabetic patients. Trophic changes such as skin atrophy, hair loss, and skin ulceration are common. Intervention for claudication symptoms is generally not recommended because the risk of immediate limb loss is low and atherosclerosis is often too distal and extensive for angioplasty or bypass surgery to be effective. Furthermore, because of comorbid conditions, these patients are at increased operative risk and often have a reduced activity and life expectancy.

PAD in patients with diabetes develops at an earlier age, progresses more rapidly, and has a different distribution than in patients without diabetes. The popliteal, tibial, and profunda femoris arteries are more severely and diffusely involved, while the aorta and iliac arteries may remain relatively disease free. The combination of neuropathy and distal atherosclerosis make diabetic patients particularly vulnerable to foot lesions. Pain may be absent or if present, due to a neuropathic rather than an ischemic process. Noninvasive blood pressure measurements are frequently confounded by the presence of calcific medial sclerosis, making vessels virtually incompressible and ankle blood pressure measurements unreliable. Diabetic patients with neuropathy may develop ulcerations on the plantar surface of the foot secondary to undetected pressure sores. Progression of this ulceration due to infection and marginal tissue perfusion may require surgical intervention before tissue ischemia *per se* causes tissue necrosis.

Diagnostic Studies

Questionnaires

Much of what is known about the natural course of PAD is derived from epidemiological studies that used questionnaires to detect patients with symptoms. The sensitivity of the Rose claudication questionnaire in detecting subjects with a disruption to arterial blood flow assessed by noninvasive techniques is less than 20%. However, it is greater than 50% in detecting severe arterial occlusion demonstrated by angiography.[3,21] The questionnaire is highly specific—correctly identifying over 98% of healthy individuals.[17,24,30] When administered on multiple occasions, the reproducibility is 80%–90%.[31] False-positive results are usually due to musculoskeletal and venous disorders while false-negative results are due to sedentary lifestyle, asymptomatic disease, or concurrent illnesses that limit exercise and prevent the onset of symptoms. In a study of more than 18,000 subjects aged 40–64 years, 2% were classified as having probable or possible intermittent claudication by the Rose Questionnaire. A 17-year follow-up of subjects demonstrated a 2-fold increase in cardiovascular and all-cause mortality rates in patients with probable or possible intermittent claudication that was independent of coronary risk factors.[32]

Symptom questionnaires or interviews are limited because patients with asymptomatic disease are also at increased risk for atherosclerotic morbidity and mortality.[33,34] After a detailed interview, one third of presumed healthy asymptomatic volunteers (n = 64) had arteriographically proven occlusions.[3] In hypertensive patients with mild carotid artery plaque 42 of 369 (11%) had evidence of obstructive lower extremity atherosclerosis as determined by noninvasive blood pressure measurements but only 1 was symptomatic.[35] In men with CHD, PAD was evident in 18%, of which only one-third (6%) were symptomatic.[36]

Noninvasive Laboratory Studies

Noninvasive vascular tests for diagnosing the presence, location, and severity of disease as well as for monitoring progression include segmental blood pressure, plethsymography, Doppler flow velocity, and tissue oxygenation measurements. Tests that duplicate or mimic the stress of walking are often used to enhance the sensitivity of these noninvasive measurements and include treadmill exercise testing and postocclusive reactive hyperemia. These tests provide supplementary diagnostic information to the history and physical examination and can assist in therapeutic decisions. Noninvasive testing also provides evidence of physiological obstruction that is not available using angiography.[37] The high prevalence of asymptomatic PAD and the ease and reliability of noninvasive tests have prompted the suggestion that screening for asymptomatic PAD should occur.[17,38]

Segmental Blood Pressure Measurements

Blood pressure recordings over the arm, thigh, calf, and ankles provide a measure of peripheral arterial flow. Blood pressure is recorded with the patient in a supine position. The systolic pressure of the posterior tibial or dorsalis pedis artery (ankle) is compared to the brachial artery pressure. The ratio of the ankle to arm systolic pressure is termed the ankle:brachial index (ABI). The ABI, not the absolute ankle pressure, is most reliable for diagnosing PAD. An ABI of less than 0.9 has a sensitivity of 95% in detecting angiographically positive disease while an ABI of 0.9 or higher is virtually 100% specific in identifying patients without clinical disease.[39–41]

ABI measurements can be obtained in the clinic, require about 5–10 minutes, and have been shown to be more sensitive and reliable than the Rose Claudication Questionnaire. If ABI recordings are normal, further measurements are usually not necessary. Some individuals with symptoms strongly suggestive of intermittent claudication may have a discrepancy between demand and supply only during periods of increased demand. In these patients blood pressure measurements after exercise, postocclusive reactive hyperemia testing, or the use of Doppler velocity determinations may be beneficial.

If abnormal results are obtained, segmental pressure measurements at the thigh, knee, and toes can be used to determine (along with clinical symptoms) the severity of disease and the approximate location of hemodynamically significant obstruction. Table 2 illustrates segmental blood pressure measurements from a vascular laboratory in normal subjects and patients with angiographically confirmed PAD. Patients with ABI indicating PAD and who have functionally limiting disease should be referred for surgical evaluation. If noninvasive management is selected, a repeat study in approximately 6 months could be performed to assess for disease progression. Changes in ABI of ± 0.15 are

Table 2
Ratio of Leg:Arm Arterial Pressure in Patients with Peripheral Arterial Occlusive Disease*

Functional Index	Normal Subjects	Group 1 (localized aortoiliac obstruction)	Group 2 (localized femoropopliteal obstruction)	Group 3 (aortoiliac and femoropopliteal obstruction)
Segmental Blood Pressure**				
Upper thigh/arm	1.34 ± 0.27	0.72 ± 0.25	1.26 ± 0.39	0.97 ± 0.34
Above knee/arm	1.32 ± 0.23	0.70 ± 0.24	0.92 ± 0.39	0.79 ± 0.32
Below knee/arm	1.26 ± 0.24	0.62 ± 0.21	0.73 ± 0.30	0.61 ± 0.28
Above ankle/arm	1.08 ± 0.10	0.57 ± 0.18	0.51 ± 0.28	0.48 ± 0.31

* From Bernstein EF, Fronek A: Current status of noninvasive studies in diagnosis of peripheral arterial disease. *Surg Clin North Am* 62:473–487, 1982.
** Mean ± standard deviation.

considered clinically significant. Patients with diabetes may have vascular calcifications resulting in noncompressible vessels and unreliable ankle blood pressure measurements. These patients should be assessed by complete segmental blood pressure measurements or other noninvasive methods.

ABIs have considerable prognostic value. An ABI less then 0.8 indicates moderate disease and less then 0.6 indicates severe or multilevel involvement. ABI less then 0.4 are often associated with limb-threatening complications including ulceration and gangrene. Jelnes[42] analyzed 257 patients with intermittent claudication and reported that no patient with an initial ABI over 0.5 or an ankle pressure over 70 mm Hg progressed to critical ischemia or required surgery during a 6.5 year follow-up. Additionally, an ABI is a powerful tool for predicting survival in patients with known PAD and should be incorporated in decision making.[43] Patients with ABI 0.3 or less have poorer survival than do patients with ABI 0.31–0.91. The mean survival in these patients was about 4 years.

Segmental blood pressure data can also be analyzed by determining the pressure gradient between any 2 sites in a single extremity or by comparison with the identical site on the contralateral leg. Reductions in pressure from proximal to distal sites of 20 mm Hg or greater (vertical pressure gradient) are considered clinically significant and indicate disease proximal to the pressure drop. Similarly, a 20 mm Hg difference between legs at the same site (horizontal pressure gradient) also indicates hemodynamically significant disease (Figure 1).[37] Repeated measurements produce an average range in ABI of ± 16%, comparable to arm systolic blood pressure measurements.

Segmental blood pressure measurements are not able to determine the length or exact location of arterial lesions or whether there is occlusion or focal stenosis. Angiography or ultrasound techniques must be utilized for further assessment in patients with evidence of PAD who are candidates for interventional therapy. Patients with calcified vessels (in particular patients with diabetes) may have noncompressible arteries resulting in markedly elevated blood pressure recordings that are not reliable. These patients can be assessed with plethsymography.

Plethsymography

Plethsymography records changes in flow volume to toes, fingers, or entire limbs that occur with each pulse beat as blood flows in or out of the digit or extremity.[44] These pulse volume recordings are helpful in the assessment of perfusion of the forefoot and digits, areas not easily measured by the Doppler unit, or in patients with unreliable segmental blood pressure readings. A normal pulse volume recording waveform has a rapid systolic upslope and a downslope that bows toward the baseline. With obstruction, the pulse wave becomes rounded, diminished in amplitude, and the downslope bows away from the baseline

Segmental Pressures

Segmental Pressures

R [115] ARM [117] L   R [152] ARM [152] L

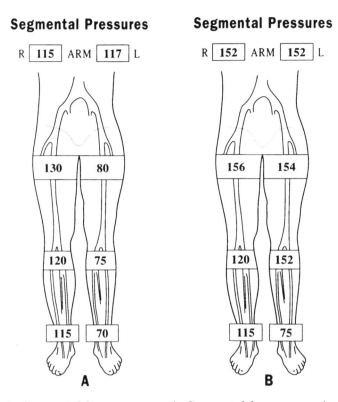

Figure 1: Segmental leg pressures. *A: Segmental leg pressure in a normal right lower extremity (ABI: 115/115 = 1.00) and one with an isolated left iliac artery occlusion (ABI:70/117 = 0.60). Both horizontal and vertical pressure gradients exist at the thigh. B: Segmental leg pressures in a patient with an isolated focal right superficial femoral artery stenoses and a distal left tibial artery occlusion.*

(Figure 2). Photoplethsymography utilizes a light sensor and photoelectric detector to qualitatively assess perfusion in distal extremities. The recorded pulse wave is helpful in providing qualitative recordings in patients suspected of distal or calcified atherosclerosis. A quantitative assessment can be obtained using a mercury strain gauge sensor or plethsymograph to record digital pressures.

Toe pressures typically average about 5–10 mm Hg below those in the arm in healthy subjects. A toe/brachial pressure index less than 0.6 is abnormal, and values less than 0.15 are commonly found in patients with rest pain (toe pressures less than 20 mm Hg).[45] Spuriously high pressures due to arterial calcification seldom occur at toe level. For this reason toe indices are a reliable indicator of the physiological severity of arterial occlusive disease and should be used when there is doubt about the validity of the ankle pressure or when arterial disease

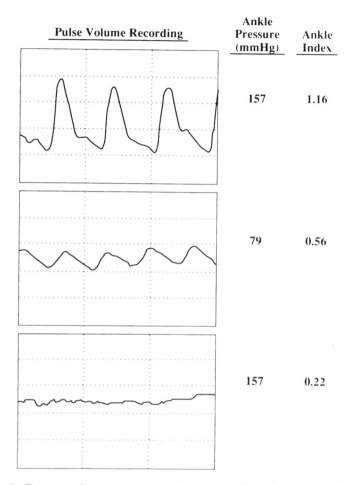

	Pulse Volume Recording	Ankle Pressure (mmHg)	Ankle Index
		157	1.16
		79	0.56
		157	0.22

Figure 2: Pressure data and pulse volume recordings in three patients with arterial disease. **Upper panel:** *Normal perfusion;* **middle panel:** *borderline perfusion;* **lower panel:** *ischemia.*

is confined to the digital arteries (Figure 3).[46] In limbs with ischemic ulcers or gangrene normal ankle pressures may be present indicating atherosclerosis located primarily in pedal or digital arteries. Plethsymographic toe pressures or wave forms can be helpful in these cases to assess wound healing potential.

Transcutaneous Oxygen Tension Measurements

Transcutaneous oxygen tension ($tcPo_2$) measurements can assess tissue viability for wound healing potential, determine the optimal level

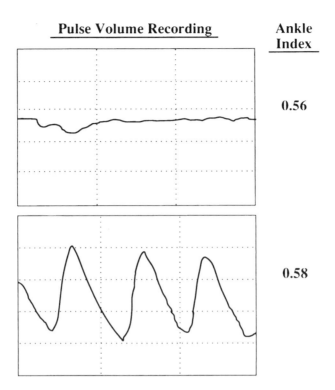

Figure 3: Use of pulse volume recordings to measure digital perfusion. *The patient in the **upper panel** has poor digital perfusion as demonstrated by a low ankle index and markedly diminished digital pulse volume recording. The patient in the **lower panel** has adequate digital perfusion demonstrated by normal pulse volume recordings despite a low ankle index.*

of amputation if necessary, or differentiate ischemic rest pain from neuropathic discomfort.[47] tcPo$_2$ is recorded by small electrodes placed on any area of the body and reflect the level of tissue perfusion. As tissue perfusion becomes marginal, capillary oxygen and tcPo$_2$ levels begin to fall. They are generally not indicated in patients whose only symptom is intermittent claudication because tcPo$_2$ levels are normal at rest. tcPo$_2$ can be unreliable with increased skin thickness (obesity, hyperkeratosis), edema or cellulitis. tcPo$_2$ measurements of greater than 55 mm Hg are normal, levels less than 30 mm Hg suggest arterial ischemia, and tcPo$_2$ levels less than 20 mm Hg generally are associated with nonhealing ulcers.

Doppler Velocity Measurements Duplex and Color Doppler Ultrasound

A Doppler probe placed over the femoral, popliteal, posterior tibial, or dorsalis pedis artery provides an assessment of the arterial velocity profile and reveals the presence, location, and degree of PAD. The signals are not affected by arterial calcifications, and can by evaluated subjectively by interpretation of audible signal. The use of a directionally sensitive Doppler device and graphic recorder permits quantitative measurement of the shape and slope of waveforms. The studies are subject to operator skill and training, and thus, standardization is limited.[39]

Duplex scanning combines conventional B-mode ultrasound imaging with Doppler analysis. This allows the examiner to determine the location and extent of obstructions or stenoses as well as the presence, direction, and velocity of flow in that vessel.[48] Sensitivity and specificity of this method have been reported at 82% and 92%, respectively.[49] Examination time is approximately 1–2 hours and inter-reader reliability is comparable to angiography. Color Doppler ultrasound combines real-time ultrasound imaging with semiquantitative color coding of the Doppler information. The color assignment depends on the velocity and direction of flow.

Exercise Testing

Exercise treadmill testing is rarely needed to make a diagnosis or assess disease severity. Patients with ischemic rest pain, ulcers, or gangrene, and the vast majority of individuals with atherosclerotic induced intermittent claudication have decreased lower extremity blood pressures at rest. Furthermore, intraindividual variation in exercise performance as well as benefits due solely to training limit the use of treadmill testing for assessing a patient's response to therapy.[50] Assessment of walking distance utilizing a standardized treadmill protocol can assist in judging the relative magnitude of the disability produced by arterial obstructions or in differentiating vascular from neurogenic or musculoskeletal induced claudication.[51] Treadmill testing may also provoke claudication symptoms and hemodynamic abnormalities in patients with lesions that are only present during exercise.

A normal response to exercise is a slight increase or no change in the ankle systolic pressure or pulse volume recording compared with the resting value. Patients with symptomatic obstructive arterial disease will seldom be able to walk on a treadmill longer than 5 minutes at 2 mph on a 10% grade. In contrast to neurogenic claudication, an exercise-induced reduction in ankle systolic pressure (usually to <60 mm Hg) occurs in vascular claudication. The magnitude of the ankle pressure drop and the alteration in the pulse volume recording reflects the extent of the anatomic impairment and degree of functional disability.[37,52] In general, the more proximal the disease the more effect it has on the ankle pressure response to exercise.

Postocclusive Reactive Hyperemia Testing

Although less physiological than the treadmill test, postocclusive reactive hyperemia measurements are an objective, quantitative, and quick method to assess PAD. Cardiac monitoring is not required, testing is not affected by patient effort or training, the test can be performed on patients unable to complete a treadmill examination, and each leg is independently evaluated.[39] By increasing the rate of blood flow through stenotic arteries, a drop in the ankle pressure similar to that observed after exercise occurs. A pneumatic cuff, placed around the thigh, is inflated above systolic pressure for 4–5 minutes. After release of the compression, ankle pressures are monitored at 15–30 second intervals for 3–6 minutes. In normal limbs, ankle pressures immediately decrease to about 80% of preocclusion levels, but reach 90% levels within 30 to 60 seconds. In limbs with obstructive arterial disease, the decrease in pressure coincides with that seen after exercise. The magnitude of the pressure drop depends on the anatomic extent of the disease and on the degree of functional impairment. In addition to pressure measurements, the reappearance time of toe pulsation or mean Doppler femoral artery velocity can also be measured. Disadvantages include discomfort, potential hazard for femoropopliteal grafts, and the difficulty in obtaining rapid pressure measurements.

Angiography

Angiography is most useful for determining location and extent of atherosclerosis and is the gold standard by which noninvasive studies are measured.[53] Use of angiography to classify degree of atherosclerosis is invasive and expensive, and limited by interobserver variability.[54] Diabetic patients with compromised renal function are at increased risk for renal failure from the iodinated angiographic contrast material. Complications due to angiography occur in about 1% of all cases with mortality in about 0.05%.[55,56] Angiography should be reserved for patients with functionally disabling PAD as determined by history, physical examination, and noninvasive vascular testing and in whom an invasive procedure is being considered. Percutaneous transluminal angioplasty can be performed at the time of angiography.

Medical Management

The goals for the internist are to detect PAD early and intervene to limit local and systemic atherosclerotic progression. The medical management of intermittent claudication involves 3 complementary modalities: risk factor modification, exercise training or rehabilitation, and pharmacological therapy (Table 3). Optimal management requires an individualized approach based on disease severity and location, functional limitations, and comorbid conditions. Patients with mild to moderate symptoms can usually be reassured about the prognosis for limb viability, although functional impairment and morbidity exist. Pa-

Table 3
Medical Management in Peripheral Arterial Disease

- Risk factor modification
  General Measures (treatment of COPD, CHF, obesity)
  Local measures (nail trimming, shoe selection, foot and skin care.)
  Treatment of diabetes, hypertension, hypercholesterolemia
  Smoking cessation
- Exercise training or rehabilitation
  Walking
  Weight training
- Pharmacological therapy
  Antiplatelet agents
    Aspirin
    Ticlopidine
    Clopidogrel
  Rheologic agents
    Pentoxifylline
  Fibrinolytic agents
    Defibrotide
  β-Blockers
  Calcium channel blockers
  Ginkgo biloba
  Garlic
  Antioxidants
  Chelation
  Ketanserin

tients with severe claudication have a worse prognosis with regard to limb salvage, job productivity, daily activities, and survival.[1,9,17,38]

General Health Care Measures and Risk Factor Modification

Minor local trauma to an ischemic limb such as pressure sores, thermal or chemical injuries, and ensuing infections are inciting yet preventable events in almost half of patients requiring amputation. Patients with a history of smoking, hypertension, diabetes, cerebral, or coronary vascular disease should receive a thorough evaluation for signs or symptoms of PAD, and be instructed in methods to limit disease progression. Detection in these high-risk patients should begin as early as possible and could include screening for asymptomatic flow disturbances. Treatment modalities should offer a wide range of preventive and therapuetic approaches that improve functional status and reduce progression of systemic atherosclerosis.

Initial treatment should be aimed at optimizing the patients' general medical condition. This can often improve the functional status to an acceptable level. The presence and severity of underlying medical problems not only influences the course of the disease but may determine if invasive therapy is feasible and the type of reconstruction possible. Patients whose lifestyle or survival are limited by factors other than claudication are generally not candidates for invasive therapy. Obese patients should receive dietary counseling to lose weight in an attempt to decrease the effort of ambulation. Patients with chronic lung disease or CHF should receive medical therapy to improve their dyspnea and increase tissue oxygenation. Patients with CHF may have improvement in lower extremity perfusion with ulcer healing and relief of claudication or resting ischemia when their cardiac output is improved.

Cigarette Smoking

Smoking is the major modifiable risk factor in patients with PAD.[57] Over 80% of patients with claudication have a history of smoking and they develop symptoms 5–10 years earlier than nonsmokers.[58] Population studies calculate that the risk of developing claudication is up to 9 times higher in smokers compared to nonsmokers and is related to the number of cigarettes smoked.[13,18] Juergens et al[19] demonstrated that 11% of those who continued smoking required limb amputation versus none of those who abstained.[20] The prognosis is worse in diabetics who continue to smoke. Compared to patients who continued to smoke those who discontinued smoking had a 40% improvement in pain-free walking distance 10 months after smoking cessation. Ankle blood pressures also increased significantly in the smoking cessation group.[59] In addition to accelerated progression of disease in native vessels, patients who continue to smoke also have a higher failure rate of angioplasty and arterial bypass grafts.[19,60] A 5-year patency rate of approximately 90% for aortofemoral and 80% for femoropopliteal grafts occurred in patients who either stopped smoking or smoked fewer than 5 cigarettes per day postoperatively. In contrast 30% and 45% of aortofemoral and femoropopliteal grafts occluded in patients continuing to smoke more than 5 cigarettes daily.

The importance of smoking cessation must be emphasized regardless of whether medical or invasive management is undertaken. Nicotine replacement therapy (patches or gum) is effective for reducing smoking rates and has been demonstrated to be safe in subjects with known vascular disease.[61] Sustained-release buproprion (150 mg once or twice a day for 7 weeks) has also been demonstrated to be effective for smoking cessation and was accompanied by reduced weight gain and minimal side effects.[62] Long-term use of other nicotine-containing products such as smokeless tobacco should also be discouraged because nicotine absorbed from the oral mucosa may still accelerate atherosclerosis.

Hypertension

As many as 40% of patients with PAD have hypertension.[14,22] Hypertension increases the extent and severity of atherosclerosis, and when combined with elevated serum cholesterol levels, appears to accelerate arterial wall injury.[63,64] Hypertension is the most important risk factor for both and thrombotic and hemorrhagic strokes and a strong contributor to cardiovascular complications and all-cause mortality.[65] Several randomized trials have demonstrated that treating systolic and diastolic hypertension reduces morbidity and mortality from stroke, coronary heart disease, and renal failure.[66] However, data are not available to determine whether treatment will alter the course of PAD.

Nonpharmacological therapy and lifestyle modification including weight loss, sodium, and alcohol restriction have been recommended as first-line intervention to prevent or treat hypertension.[66,69] Modest weight reduction, of 5–10 pounds can normalize blood pressure in many patients with mild hypertension even before desirable weight is reached.[67] Sodium intake should be limited to 70–100 mEq/d (4–6 g of table salt) and alcohol to 30 g/d (approximately 2 ounces of 100-proof whiskey, 8 ounces of wine, or 24 ounces of beer).[67]

On the basis of outcomes data from randomized controlled trials, pharmacological therapy beginning with diuretics and β-blockers is recommended. The dosing convenience and low cost of these agents can improve patient compliance. Thiazide diuretics have been demonstrated to reduce stroke and cardiovascular morbidity and mortality in several large randomized trials. Many participants in these trials were elderly or had known atherosclerosis. The low cost and demonstrated reduction in mortality in patients with hypertension and CHD make β-blockers a good choice either as monotherapy or in combination with thiazide diuretics. A meta-analysis of randomized controlled trials indicated that β-adrenergic blocker therapy does not worsen intermittent claudication in subjects with PAD.[69]

Angiotensin-converting-enzyme (ACE) inhibitors have also been shown to improve length and quality of life in subjects with vascular disease and hypertension. Patients with claudication frequently smoke cigarettes, have diffuse atherosclerosis, and are more likely to have renal artery stenosis. Therefore, caution should be taken to ensure that ACE inhibitors do not worsen kidney function. Vasodilating agents used for blood pressure control, such as prazosin or methyldopa, have not been found to reduce claudication symptoms.[70] However, reserpine has been shown to reduce vascular related morbidity and mortality.[66] The calcium channel blocker nitrendipine has demonstrated a decrease in the rate of cardiovascular complications (primarily cerebrovascular and coronary heart disease events) in elderly patients with isolated systolic hypertension.[71] Whether nitrendipine improves claudication symptoms is not known.

Hyperlipidemia

Hyperlipidemia is present in almost half of patients with PAD. The Framingham study found that a fasting cholesterol greater than 7 mmol/L (270 mg/dL) was associated with approximately twice the risk of development of claudication than lower levels.[72] Subjects with low high-density lipoprotein (HDL) cholesterol levels despite acceptable low-density lipoprotein (LDL) cholesterol levels are also at increased risk for having PAD. Whether drug treatment to specifically raise low HDL-cholesterol will reduce future vascular morbidity and mortality is currently being studied.[73] Several clinical trials have shown regression of coronary atherosclerosis in hypercholesterolemic patients treated with different cholesterol-lowering medications.[74–76] Additionally, some studies have investigated the effects of cholesterol lowering on PAD. Treatment of hyperlipidemia for 19 months resulted in a two-thirds reduction in atherosclerotic progression in lower extremity arteries.[77] The Lipid Research Clinic Coronary Primary Prevention Trial found a 15% reduction in new intermittent claudication in the cholestyramine group, although this was not statistically significant.[78] The POSCHE study demonstrated a lower rate of intermittent claudication and abnormal ABI in postmyocardial infarction patients treated with intestinal bypass surgery for hypercholesterolemia.[79,80] The statin drugs have been demonstrated to provide a large reduction in cholesterol levels and the rate of stroke, coronary heart disease, and total mortality.[81] Many subjects enrolled in these studies had PAD. Guidelines regarding lipid management are identical for patients with clinically evident atherosclerosis regardless of whether their disease is manifested as lower extremity, coronary, or cerebrovascular.

Diabetes

No controlled trials have been performed to evaluate the effects of diabetic therapy on PAD. However, patients with diabetes and PAD have a worse prognosis and 7-fold higher amputation rate compared to nondiabetic patients.[82,83] This increased risk of amputation may be due to more distal and diffuse atherosclerosis. The results of recent trials in patients with type 1 diabetes indicate the beneficial effect on morbidity and mortality of strict glycemic control.[84] This may result in regression or lack of progression of peripheral microvascular atherosclerotic lesions. Poor distal blood flow combined with sensory neuropathy in diabetic patients contributes to traumatic ulcerations and infections with limited wound healing potential. Patient education and instruction in self-care to prevent ulceration is critical in optimizing limb survival rates. For example, the amputation and ulceration rate was 3 times higher in a no-education group (21 amputations and 8 ulcerations of 177 limbs) compared to a group of diabetic patients who received a 1-hour educational program consisting of 14 simple instructions for foot care (7 amputations and 8 ulcerations of 177 limbs).[85] Diabetic patients should be counseled about the importance of glycemic control, assessed for peripheral neuropathy, instructed in meticulous foot care including wearing comfortable shoes, avoidance of excessively hot water, use of lanolin to prevent skin fissuring, drying between toes to prevent maceration, treatment of lower extremity ulceration, and careful nail trimming. Referral to a podiatrist is indicated for advanced management of calluses and corns and evaluation for orthotic devices.

Exercise Rehabilitation and Training

Exercise rehabilitation is a noninvasive, relatively inexpensive, and effective method for improving claudication pain symptoms. It is an alternative to drug or surgical treatment for intermittent claudication. Pharmacological treatment is expensive and provides minimal improvement. The cost of surgical procedures has increased in recent years, yielding an estimated 1994 national health care cost of $3.3 billion per year.[86] Surgery also carries risks of cardiovascular complications, which for some patients may outweigh the benefits.

Exercise has been demonstrated to provide reproducible increases in pain-free walking distance in patients with intermittent claudication. A meta-analysis of 21 studies demonstrated that exercise training increased the distance to the onset of claudication by 179% (from 126 meters to 351 meters) and the distance to maximal claudication pain by 122% (from 325 meters to 723 meters).[86] These results are superior to pharmacological interventions and comparable to invasive treatments. The beneficial effects appear to result from improved tissue oxygen extraction, muscle function and coordination, and alterations in abnormal hemorheology rather then development of collateral blood supply.[89-90] The optimal program should consist of walking to the point of claudication, followed by rest, then resumption of activity for a total of 30 minutes at least 3 times per week for 6 months.[85,89-92]

Pharmacological therapy

Pharmacological therapy should be utilized in patients who have functionally limiting claudication symptoms despite risk factor modification and exercise rehabilitation, and in whom invasive therapy is not indicated or desired. Pharmacological therapy generally consists of rheologic modifiers, antiplatelet agents, vasodilators, fibrinolytics, and agents affecting the vascular endothelium.

Rheologic Modifiers

Pentoxifylline is the only drug approved for the symptomatic relief of claudication. It is believed to improve blood flow and walking capacity by altering erythrocyte deformability, platelet hyperreactivity, and blood viscosity. Study designs have varied and often use co-interventions such as exercise therapy, smoking cessation, and improved self-care. End points such as treadmill walking distance are highly variable and influenced by subjects motivation, disease duration, training, or placebo effect, and presence or absence of diabetes, age, cigarette smoking, and gender. Overall, pentoxifylline appears to provide modest improvement in the treadmill walking capacity of patients with moderate intermittent claudication. A meta-analysis of 11 placebo controlled randomized trials among patients with moderate intermittent claudication concluded that pentoxifylline increased the distance walked on a treadmill before the onset of calf pain and the maximum distance walked on a treadmill by 29 and 48 meters, respectively.[95] This improvement may not be clinically important and is less than occurs with a supervised exercise program. Side effects such as light-headedness, dyspepsia, and nausea and cost limit its use. A trial of 400 mg 3 times a day with meals for 3 months is reasonable in patients who have not benefited from other modalities.

Antiplatelet Agents

Several studies have assessed the effects of aspirin, ticlopidine, dipyridamole, clopidogrel, or combinations of these drugs in patients PAD. Antiplatelet therapy has been demonstrated to maintain vascular graft of arterial patency. In an overview of 14 randomized studies (most using aspirin), the odds of an occlusion after a peripheral artery procedure was reduced from 25% (control) to 16% (antiplatelet group) benefiting 90 patients per 1000 treated for 19 months.[98] A meta-analysis from 31 randomized trials of antiplatelet therapy involved more than 29,000 patients and noted that aspirin therapy reduced vascular mortality by 15% and nonfatal stroke and myocardial infarction by 30%.[95] Similar benefits were noted in the largest of 2 primary prevention trials in patients without systemic vascular disease taking low-dose aspirin.[98,99] Results from randomized trials of platelet-active agents have shown improvement in angiographic disease progression, claudication, or healing of ischemic ulcers in patients with chronic arterial insufficiency.[100–102] Their effect in improving claudication symptoms is only modest. Because of the safety, low cost, and effectiveness of aspirin in reducing cardiac and cerebrovascular morbidity and mortality it should be prescribed to all patients with PAD. If individuals cannot tolerate aspirin, other agents such as ticlopidine or clopidogrel are effective, although more expensive.[103–104] Ticlopidine has been demonstrated to increase the distance that patients with PAD are able to walk, reduce the rate of death, myocardial infarction, and stroke and need for reconstructive lower extremity arterial surgery.[105–109] It also improves the long-term patency of saphenous-vein bypass grafts.[110]

Anticoagulants have not been shown to improve claudication symptoms.[111] Vasodilators are generally not felt to provide symptomatic relief because they rarely increase blood flow beyond the level produce by maximally tolerated exercise.[89,112] Calcium channel blockers may theoretically benefit patients by decreasing platelet aggregation, vascular thrombosis, and oxygen metabolism.[113,114] In a small randomized placebo-controlled study verapamil increased mean pain-free walking distance by 29% (45–58 meters) and maximal walking distance by 49% (111–150 meters).[115]

Drugs that have been observed to lower fibrinogen levels, decrease arterial vasoconstriction, alter lipids, platelet, white, and red blood cell, and endothelial interactions and thereby alter the course of atherosclerosis have been studied. Defibrotide is an oral fibrinolytic agent that has been demonstrated to provide a net gain in absolute walking distance of approximately 75 meters when compared with placebo.[116] Antioxidant vitamins have not been shown to be effective in either peripheral arterial or other vascular diseases.[117] Omega-3 fatty acids found in fish oil, ketanserin,[118] a serotonin antagonist, the prostaglandin E analogue, iloprost, ethylenediaminetetraacetic acid (EDTA) for chelation therapy,[119] garlic, and *Ginkgo biloba*[120] have also been investigated. They are generally not indicated as they have limited or no clinical effect.

Role of Invasive Therapy

Invasive therapy consists of essentially two modes of treatment: surgical bypass or percutaneous transluminal angioplasty (PTA). Both technologies are evolving rapidly and future results will undoubtedly alter treatment decisions. Neither of the invasive strategies, however, affect the progression of systemic atherosclerosis that increases mortality in these patients. Therefore patients still require management of the coexisting medical problems and risk factors. The initial clinical evaluation should determine the benefits and risks of intervention as outlined above by establishing the degree of disability, the threat to limb viability, the general location and severity of the occlusive lesions, the anesthetic risk, and the patient's prospects for long-term survival. Indications for invasive therapy include symptoms significantly interfering with a person's lifestyle, rest pain (indicating potential tissue ischemia), or ischemic ulcers/gangrene.

Percutaneous Transluminal Angioplasty

The role of invasive therapy in the management of PAD has changed with the availability of angioplasty.[12,29,121–124] Patency rates of PTA are dependent on location and type of lesion with proximal short lesions being ideal.[125] Initial success rates are over 90% for aortic dilation. Follow-up studies for 3–7 years show a continued patency rate of approximately 80%. Both the primary and long-term success rates decrease for more distal lesions. Angioplasty for iliac stenoses has a primary success ranging from 33%–83% with approximately 85% of these remaining patent at 2–4 years. Femoral angioplasty has a primary success rate of about 75% with a follow-up patency of 30%–75%.[29,126] Redilation of failed angioplasty sites is possible.[127] Disease greater than 10 cm in length, arterial occlusion, multiple stenoses, eccentric plaque formation, calcified plaque, poor distal runoff, and limb salvage indications decrease the efficacy of PTA.[128]

Complications of PTA are divided into those related to the arterial puncture such as groin hematoma formation and those associated with the dilation procedure itself. The latter include subintimal guidewire passage, distal embolization, and vessel occlusion. Significant complications requiring operative management, transfusion or permanent renal failure are seen in 1%–8% of cases. A 3%–15% rate is noted for all complications and mortality is less than 0.5%.

A recent review compared angioplasty versus noninvasive management for mild to moderate claudication.[128] At 6 months follow-up, ABI were higher in the angioplasty group. Angioplasty improved walking distance when compared to a group treated with aspirin but not in another trial that used an exercise program in the control group. In patients with mild to moderate symptoms, angioplasty may have short-term benefits that appear to be no better than those achieved with an exercise program.

Angioplasty is generally reserved for patients with moderate to severe symptoms and who have segmental stenosis demonstrated on angiography in the aortoiliac or femoral region. Occasionally, patients who are at high surgical risk may undergo angioplasty in more distal arterial beds in attempts to salvage a limb or receive angioplasty of a proximal lesion with subsequent revascularization of the distal segments.[129] Nonoperative modalities such as laser angioplasty, atherectomy, and percutaneously placed intravascular stents are options that may be used in selected patients at centers with experience in these methods.

Vascular Surgery

Arterial surgical reconstruction is utilized in cases with arterial occlusion, or diffuse, extensive, or multiple in-series lesions. Because these are more common than single, short lesions, PTA can be considered as the sole or initial invasive treatment of occlusive arterial disease in only 10%–40% of patients who are candidates for invasive therapy.[126,128] Surgical series report perioperative complications between 2% and 12% and death rates of 2%–5%. Patency rates vary with surgical center, disease location (proximal better then distal), type of surgical procedure (surgical bypass using native vessels versus synthetic graphs or endarterectomy), and coexisting risk factors (diabetes, cigarette use, etc.). Doubilet[29] has reviewed several clinical series and reports 1- and 5-year patency rates of 98% and 88% for aortoiliac and aortofemoral surgery and 79% and 60% for femoropopliteal surgery.

Comparison of PTA versus Surgery

A randomized trial compared the effectiveness of PTA with surgery in the treatment of severe occlusive disease of the iliac, femoral, or popliteal arteries.[130] Twenty-five patients (20%) having PTA were considered early treatment failures. At 4.5 years, 50 deaths (21% in the surgical group and 18% from the PTA group) and 24 major amputations of legs occurred. Both angioplasty and surgery provided similar improvements in ankle-brachial indices, relief of symptoms, and functional status. A subsequent vascular operation on the study limb was required in 16% of surgical patients and 23% of patients having PTA. Repeat PTA procedures were performed more frequently on patients initially receiving PTA than on those receiving surgery.

When the costs of PTA and reconstructive surgery are compared in a patient with a lesion that could be treated by either method, PTA is about one-fifth the cost of operation.[29,131] A decision and cost-effectiveness analysis concluded that angioplasty is the preferred initial treatment in patients with disabling claudication and a femoropopliteal stenosis or occlusion and in those with chronic critical ischemia and a stenosis. Bypass surgery is the preferred initial treatment in patients with chronic critical ischemia and a femoropopliteal occlusion.[123] The introduction of transluminal angioplasty has generally lowered the threshold for invasive therapy as well as provided an alternative means of treatment in those with threatened limb loss.

Conclusions

PAD is common and results in reduced length and quality of life. Disease in one vascular bed is a strong indicator of diffuse atherosclerosis. The majority of patients are managed without invasive therapy. The role of the internist is to provide a systematic and systemic approach to diagnosis and therapy. Patients should receive a thorough history and physical examination to evaluate the severity of disease as well as detect other comorbid conditions. An individualized approach to control risk factors such as smoking, hypertension, hypercholesterolemia, and diabetes as well as to ensure meticulous foot and lower extremity care is indicated. An exercise program using intermittent walking to near-maximal pain is effective and should be encouraged to enhance functional performance. Pharmacological agents provide only a modest improvement in claudication symptoms. Patients with mild to moderate symptoms resulting in minimal interference with their lifestyle should be managed by their primary physician. Patients who develop worsening symptoms interfering with their daily activities or have signs of impending tissue ischemia should be evaluated by vascular surgeons, radiologists, or interventional intermists for consideration of surgical bypass or angioplasty.

Recommendations for angioplasty or bypass are based on severity and location of disease with angioplasty being most effective for short segmental proximal lesions.

References

1. Peripheral Vascular Disease: Report by NHLI Panel on Peripheral Vascular Disease, Feb. 28–29, 1972.
2. Kannel WB, Skinner JJ, Schwartz M, et al: Intermittent claudication incidence in the Framingham study. *Circulation* 1:875–883, 1970.
3. Widmer LK, Greensher A, Kannel WB: Occlusion of peripheral arteries. A study of 6400 working subjects. *Circulation* 30:836–884, 1964.
4. Dormandy J, Mahir M, Ascady G, et al: Fate of the patient with chronic leg ischemia. *J Cardiovasc Surg* 30:50–57, 1989.
5. Eagle KA, Rihal CS, Foster ED, et al, for the CASS Investigators. Long-term survival in patients with coronary artery disease: importance of peripheral vascular disease. *J Am Coll Cardiol* 23:1091–1095, 1994.
6. Criqui MH, Langer RD, Fronek A, et al: Mortality over a period of 10 years with peripheral arterial disease. *N Engl Med* 326:381–386, 1992.
7. Pardaens J, Lesaffre E, Willems JL, et al: Multivariant survival analysis for the assessment of prognostic factors and risk categories after recovery from acute myocardial infarction: The Belgian situation. *Am J Epidemiol* 122:805–819, 1985.
8. Varnaukas E, the European Coronary Surgery Study Group: Survival, myocardial infarction, and employment status in a prospective randomized study of coronary bypass surgery. *Circulation* 72(suppl V):V-90–V-101, 1985.
9. Wilt TJ, Rubins HB, Collins D, et al: Correlates and Consequences of Diffuse Atherosclerosis in Men with Coronary Heart Disease. *Arch Intern Med* 156:1181–1188, 1996.
10. Radack K and Wyderski RJ: Conservative management of intermittent claudication. *Ann Intern Med* 113:135–146, 1990.
11. Findgarde F, Jelnes R, Bjorkman H, et al: Conservative drug treatment in patients with moderately severe chronic occlusive peripheral arterial disease. *Circulation* 80:1549–1556, 1989.
12. Cooke JP, Dzau VJ: The time has come for vascular medicine. *Ann Intern Med* 112:138–139, 1990.
13. Kannel WB, McGee DL: Update on some epidemiologic features of intermittent claudication: The Framingham Study. *J Am Geriatr Soc* 33:13–18, 1985.
14. McDaniel MD, Cronenwett JL: Basic data related to the natural history of intermittent claudication. *Ann Vasc Surg* 3:273–277, 1989.
15. Peabody CN, Kannel WB, McNamara PM: Intermittent claudication. Surgical significance. *Arch Surg* 109:693–697, 1974.
16. Imparato AM, Kim GE, Davidson T, et al: Intermittent claudication: Its natural course. *Surgery* 78:795–799, 1975.

17. Fowkes FGR: The measurement of atherosclerotic peripheral arterial disease in epidemiologic surveys. *Int J Epidemiol* 17:248–254, 1988.
18. Hughson WG, Mann JI, Garrod A: Intermittent claudication: Prevalence and risk factors. *Br Med J* 1:1379–1381, 1978.
19. Juergens JL, Barker NW, Hines EA Jr: Arteriosclerosis obliterans: Review of 520 cases with special reference to pathogenic and prognostic factors. *Circulation* 21:188–195, 1960.
20. Jonason T, Bergstrom R: Cessation of smoking in patients with intermittent claudication. *Acta Med Scand* 221:253–260, 1987.
21. Myers KA, King RB, Scott DF, et al: The effect of smoking on the late patency of arterial reconstruction in the legs. *Br J Surg* 65:267–271, 1978.
22. Criqui MH, Browner D, Fronek A, et al: Peripheral arterial disease in large vessels is epidemiologically distinct from small vessel disease: An analysis of risk factors. *Am J Epidemiol* 129:1110–1119, 1989.
23. Spittell JA: Diagnosis and management of occlusive peripheral arterial disease. *Curr Probl Cardiol* 1–33, 1990.
24. Criqui MH, Fronek A, Klauber MR, et al: The sensitivity, specificity, and predictive value of traditional clinical evaluation of peripheral arterial disease: Results from noninvasive testing in a defined population. *Circulation* 71:516–522, 1985.
25. Lederie FA, Johnson GR, Wilson SE, et al: Prevalence and associations of Abdominal Aortic Aneurysm Detected through Screening. *Ann Intern Med* 126:441–449, 1997.
26. Lederie FA, Walker JM, Reinke DB. Selective screening for abdominal aortic aneurysms with physical examination and ultrasound. *Arch Intern Med* 148:1753–1756, 1988.
27. Allardice JT, Allwright GJ, Wafula JMC, et al: High prevalence of abdominal aortic aneurysm in men with peripheral vascular disease: Screening by ultrasonography. *Br J Surg* 75:240–242, 1988.
28. Imparato AM, et al: Comparisons of three technique for femoral-popliteal arterial reconstructions. *Ann Surg* 177:375, 1973.
29. Doubilet P, Abrams HL: The cost of underutilization. Percutaneous transluminal angioplasty for peripheral vascular disease. *N Engl J Med* 310:95–102, 1984.
30. Schroll M, Munck O: Estimation of peripheral arteriosclerotic disease by ankle blood pressure measurements in a population study of 60 year old men and women. *J Chron Dis* 34:261–269, 1981.
31. Reunanen A, Takkunen H, Aromaa A: Prevalence of intermittent claudication and its effect on mortality. *Acta Med Scand* 11:249–256, 1982.
32. Smith GD, Shipley MJ, Rose G: Intermittent claudication, heart disease risk factors, and mortality. The Whitehall Study. *Circulation* 82:1925–1931, 1990.
33. Criqui MH, Coughlin SS, Fronek A: Noninvasively diagnosed peripheral arterial disease as a predictor of mortality. *Circulation* 72:768–773, 1985.
34. Rose G, McCartney P, Reid DD: Self administration of a questionnaire on chest pain and intermittent claudication. *Br J Prev Soc Med* 31:42–48, 1977.
35. Wilt TJ, Sprinkle JW, Flack JM, et al: Prevalence and correlates of lower extremity arterial disease in hypertensive patients with carotid atherosclerosis: Baseline results from the Multicenter Isradipine/Diuretic Atherosclerosis Study (MIDAS). *J Vasc Med Biol* 4:95–101, 1993.
36. Wilt TJ, Rubins HB, Robins SJ, et al: Carotid atherosclerosis in men with low levels of HDL cholesterol. *Stroke* 28:1919–1925, 1997.

37. Raines JK, Darling RC, Buth J, et al: Vascular laboratory criteria for the management of peripheral vascular disease of the lower extremities. *Surgery* 79:21–29, 1976.
38. Prineas RJ, Harland WR, Janzon L, et al: Recommendations for use of non-invasive Methods to detect atherosclerotic peripheral arterial disease in population studies. *Circulation* 65:1561A–1566A, 1982.
39. Bernstein EF, Fronek A: Current status of noninvasive tests in the diagnosis of peripheral arterial disease. *Surg Clin North Am* 62:473–487, 1982.
40. Laing S, Greenhalgh RM: The detection and progression of asymptomatic peripheral arterial disease. *Br J Surg* 70:628–630, 1983.
41. Lynch T, Hobson RW, Wright CB, et al: Interpretation of Doppler segmental pressures in peripheral vascular occlusive disease. *Arch Surg* 119:465–467, 1984.
42. Jelnes Gaardsting O, Jensen KH, et al: Fate in intermittent claudication: outcome and risk factors. *Br Med J* 293:1137–1140, 1986.
43. McDermott MM, Feinglass J, Slavensky R, et al: The ankle-brachial index as a predictor of survival inpatients with peripheral vascular disease. *J Gen Intern Med* 9:445–449, 1994.
44. Summer DS: Volume plethysmography in vascular disease: An overview. *In* Bernstein EF (ed): *Noninvasive Diagnostic Techniques in Vascular Disease.* 3rd ed. CV Mosby Co, St. Louis, 1985. pp 97–118.
45. Ramsey DE, Manke DA, Sumner DS: Toe blood pressure-a valuable adjunct to ankle pressure measurement for assessing peripheral arterial disease. *J Cardiovasc Surg* 24:43, 1983.
46. Vollrath KD, Salles-Cunha SX, Vincent D, et al: Noninvasive measurement of toe systolic pressures. *Bruit* 4:27, 1980.
47. Cina C, Katsamouris A, Megerman J, et al: Utility of transcutaneous oxygen tension measurements in peripheral arterial occlusive disease. *J Vasc Surg* 1:362, 1984.
48. Jager KA, Phillips DJ, Martin RL, et al: Noninvasive mapping of lower limb arterial lesions. *Ultrasound Med Biol* 11:515–521, 1985.
49. Kohler TR, Nance DR, Cramer MM, et al: Duplex scanning for diagnosis of aortoiliac and femoropopliteal disease: a prospective study. *Circulation* 76:1074–1080, 1987.
50. Ouriel K, McDonnell AE, Metz CE, et al: A critical evaluation of stress testing in the diagnosis of peripheral vascular disease. *Surgery* 91:686, 1982.
51. Goodreau JJ: Rational approach to the differentiation of vascular and neurogenic claudication. *Surgery* 84:749, 1978.
52. Carter SA: Response of ankle systolic pressure to leg exercise in mild or questionable arterial disease. *N Engl J Med* 287:578, 1972.
53. Thiele BL, Strandness DE: Accuracy of angiographic quantification of peripheral atherosclerosis. *Prog Cardiovasc Dis* 26:223–235, 1983.
54. Bruins SH, Strihbosch L, Greep JM: Inter-observer variability in single plane aortography. *Surgery* 90:497–503, 1981.
55. Hessel SJ, Adams DF, Abrams HL: Complications of angiography. *Radiology* 138:273, 1981.
56. Rose JS: Contrast Media. Complications, and preparation of the patient. In: RB Rutherford, ed. *Vascular Surgery* 2nd ed. Philadelphia, Saunders, 1984, pp 244–252.
57. Kannel WB, Shurtleff D: Cigarettes and the development of intermittent claudication. *Geriatrics* 28:61–68, 1973.

58. Rosen A, DePalma RG, Victor Y: Risk factors in atherosclerosis. *Arch Surg* 107:303–308, 1973.
59. Quick CRG, Cotton LT: The measured effect of stopping smoking on intermittent claudication. *Br J Surg* 69(suppl):524–526, 1982.
60. Ameli FM, Stein M, Provan JL, et al: The effect of postoperative smoking on femoropopliteal bypass graphs. *Ann Vasc Surg* 3:20–25, 1989.
61. Joseph AM, Norman SM, Ferry LH, et al: The safety of transdermal nicotine as an aid to smoking cessation in patients with cardiac disease. *N Engl J Med* 335:1792–1798, 1996.
62. Hurt RD, Sachs DPL, Glover ED, et al: A comparison of sustained-release bupropion and placebo for smoking cessation. *N Engl J Med* 337: 1195–1202, 1997.
63. Robertson WB, Strong JP: Atherosclerosis in persons with hypertension and diabetes mellitus. *Lab Invest* 18:538–551, 1968.
64. Chobanian AV: The influence of hypertension and other hemodynamic factors in atherogenesis. *Prog Cardiovasc Dis* 26:177–196, 1983.
65. Rutan G, Kuller LH, Neaton JD, et al: Mortality associated with diastolic hypertension and isolated systolic hypertension among men screened for the Multiple Risk Factor Intervention Trial. *Circulation* 77:504–514, 1988.
66. The Sixth Report of the Joint National Committee on Prevention, Detection, Evaluation and Treatment of High Blood Pressure. *Arch Intern Med* 157:2413–2446, 1997.
67. National Education Programs Working Group Report on the Management of Patients with Hypertension and High Blood Cholesterol. *Ann Intern Med* 114:224–237, 1991.
68. Stamler R, Stamler J, Grimm R, et al: Nutritional therapy for high blood pressure. *JAMA* 257:1484–1491, 1987.
69. Radack K, Deck C: Beta-adrenergic blocker therapy does not worsen intermittent claudication in subjects with peripheral arterial disease. A meta-analysis of randomized controlled trials. *Arch Intern Med* 151:1769, 1991.
70. Coffman JD: Vasodilator drugs in peripheral vascular disease. *N Engl J Med* 300:713–717, 1979.
71. Staessen JA, Fagard R, Thijs L, et al: Randomised double blind comparison of placebo and active treatment for older patients with isolated systolic hypertension. *Lancet* 350:757–764, 1997.
72. Kannel WB, Skinner JJ, Schwartz MJ, et al: Intermittent claudication. Incidence in the Framingham study. *Circulation* 41:875–883, 1970.
73. Rubins HB, Robins SJ, Iwane MK, et al: Rational and design for the Department of Veterans Affairs Lipoprotein Cholesterol Intervention Trial (HIT) for secondary prevention of caronary artery disease in men with low high-density lipoprotein cholesterol and desirable low-density cholesterol. *Am J Cardiol* 71:45–52, 1993.
74. Blankenhorn DH, Nessim SA, Johnson RL, et al: Beneficial effects of combined colestipolniacin therapy on coronary atherosclerosis and coronary venous bypass grafts. *JAMA* 257:3233–3240, 1987.
75. Brown BG, Lin JT, Schafer SM, et al: Niacin or lavastatin, combined with colestipol, regress coronary atherosclerosis and prevent clinical events in men with elevated apolipoprotein B (abstract). *Circulation* 80:Suppl II: II-266, 1989.
76. Nikkila EA, Viikinkoski P, Valle M, et al: Prevention of progression of coronary atherosclerosis by treatment of hyperlipidaemia: a seven-year prospective study. *BMJ* 289:220–223, 1984.

77. Duffield RGM, Lewis B, Miller NE, et al: Treatment of hyperlipidaemia retards progression of symptomatic femoral atherosclerosis. *Lancet* 2: 639–642, 1983.
78. Lipid Research Clinics Program: The Lipid Research Clinics Coronary Primary Prevention Trial Results. I. Reduction in incidence of coronary heart disease. *JAMA* 251:351–364, 1984.
79. Buchwald H, Varco RL, Matts JP, et al: Effect of partial ileal bypass surgery on mortality and morbidity from coronary heart disease in patients with hypercholesterolemia. *N Engl J Med* 323:946–955, 1990.
80. Buchwald H, Bourdages HR, Campos CT, et al: Impact of cholesterol reduction on peripheral arterial disease in the Program on the Surgical Control of the Hyperlipidemias (POSCH). *Surgery* 120:672–679, 1996.
81. Hebert PR, Gaziano JM, Chan KS, et al: Cholesterol lowering with statin drugs, risk of stroke, and total mortality. An overview of randomize trials. *JAMA* 278:313–321, 1997.
82. Jonason T. Ringvist I: Diabetes mellitus and intermittent claudication: Relation between peripheral vascular complications and location of the occlusive atherosclerosis in the legs. *Acta Med Scand* 218:217–221, 1985.
83. Jonason T, Ringqvist I: Factors of prognostic importance for subsequent rest pain in patients with intermittent claudication. *Acta Med Scand* 218: 27–33, 1985.
84. The Diabetes Control and Complications Trial Research Group: The effect of intensive treatment of diabetes on the development and progression of long-term complications in insulin-dependent diabetes mellitus. *N Engl J Med* 329:977, 1993.
85. Malone JM, Snyder M, Anderson G, et al: Prevention of amputation by diabetic education. *Am J Surg* 158:520–523, 1989.
86. Gardner AW, Poehlman ET: Exercise rehabilitation programs for the treatment of claudication pain. A meta-analysis. *JAMA* 274:975–980, 1995.
87. Ernst EE, Matral A: Intermittent claudication, exercise, and blood rheology. *Circulation* 76:1110–1114, 1987.
88. Schoop W: Mechanism of beneficial action of daily walking training of patients with intermittent claudication. *Scand J Clin Lab Invest* 31 (suppl 128):197–199, 1973.
89. Dahllof AG, Bjorntorp P, Holm J, et al: Metabolic activity of skeletal muscle in patients with peripheral arterial insufficiency. *Eur J Clin Invest* 4:9–15, 1974.
90. Eckroth R, Dahllof AG, Gundevall B, et al: Physical training of patients with intermittent claudication: indications, methods, and results. *Surgery* 84:640–643, 1978.
91. Ernst E: Physical exercise for peripheral vascular disease-a review. *Vasa* 16:227–237, 1987.
92. Skinner JS, Strandness DE: Exercise and Intermittent Claudication. I. Effect of repitition and intensity of exercise. *Circulation* 36:15–22, 1967.
93. Skinner JS, Strandness DE: Exercise and Intermittent Claudication. II. Effect of physical training. *Circulation* 36:23–29, 1967.
94. Larsen OA, Lassen NA: Effect of daily muscular exercise in patients with intermittent claudication. *Lancet* 2:1093–1096, 1966.
95. Hood SC, Moher D, Barber GG: Management of Intermittent claudication with pentoxifylline: Meta-analysis of randomized controlled trials. *Can Med Assoc J* 155:1053–1059, 1996.

96. Antiplatelet Trialists' Collaboration: Collaborative overview of randomised trials of antiplatelet therapy: II: Maintenance of vascular graft or arterial patency by antiplatelet therapy. *Br Med J* 308:159–168, 1994.

97. Antiplatelet Trialists' Collaboration: Secondary prevention of vascular disease by prolonged antiplatelet treatment. *Br Med J* 296:320–323, 1988.

98. Research Study Group: Preliminary report: findings from the aspirin component of the ongoing physicians' health study. *N Engl J Med* 318:262–264, 1988.

99. Peto R, Gray R, Collins R, et al: Randomized trial of prophylactic daily aspirin in British male doctors. *Br Med J* 296:313–316, 1988.

100. Jones NAG, DeHaas H, Zahavi J, et al: A double-blind trial of suloctidil v placebo in intermittent claudication. *Br J Surg* 69:38, 1987.

101. Katsumura T, Mishima Y, Kamiya K, et al: Therapeutic effect of ticlopidine, a new inhibitor of platelet aggregation on chronic arterial occlusive disease, a double-blind study versus placebo. *Angiology* 33:357, 1982.

102. Hess H, Miewtaschik A, Deichsel G: Drug-induced inhibition of platelet function delays progression of peripheral occlusive arterial disease: A prospective double-blind arteriographically controlled trial. *Lancet* 1:416, 1985.

103. Fagher B: Long term effects of ticlopidine on lower limb blood flow, ankle/brachial index and symptoms in peripheral arteriosclerosis. A double-blind study. The STIMS Group in Lund. Swedish Ticlopidine Multicenter Study. *Angiology* 45:777–788, 1994.

104. Gent M: A randomised, blinded, trial of clopidogrel versus aspirin in patients at risk of ischaemic events (CAPRIE) *Lancet* 348:1329–1339, 1996.

105. Arcan JC, Blanchard J, Boissel JP, et al: Multicenter double-blind study of ticlopidine in the treatment of intermittent claudication and the prevention of its complications. *Angiology* 39:802–811, 1988.

106. Boissel JP, Peyrieux JC, Destors JM: Is it possible to reduce the risk of cardiovascular events insubjects suffering from intermittent claudication of the lower limbs? *Thromb Haemost* 62:681–685, 1989.

107. Janzon L, Bergqvist D, Boberg J, et al: Prevention of myocardial infarction and stroke in patients with intermittent claudication: effects of ticlopidine: results from STIMS, the Swedish Ticlopidine Multicentre Study. *J Intern Med* 227:301–228, 1990 [Erratum, *J Intern Med* 228:659, 1990].

108. Bergqvist D, Almgren B, Dickinson JP: Reduction of requirement for leg vascular surgery during long-term treatment of claudicant patients with ticlopidine: results from the Swedish Ticlopidine Multicentre Study (STIMS) *Eur J Vasc Endovasc Surg* 10:69–76, 1995.

109. Blanchard J, Carreras LO, Kindermans M, EMATAP Group: Results of EMATAP: a double-blind placebo-controlled multicentre trial of ticlopidine in patients with peripheral arterial disease. *Nouv Rev Fr Hematol* 35:523–528, 1993.

110. Becquemin J-P, et al: Effect of Ticlopidine on the long-term patency of saphenous-vein bypass grafts in the legs. *N Engl J Med* 337:1726–1731, 1997.

111. Kretcschmer GJ, Wenzl E, Wagner O, et al: Influence of anticoagulant treatment inpreventing graft occlusion following saphenous vein bypass for femoropopliteal occlusive disease. *Br J Surg* 73:689–692, 1986.

112. Clagett GP, Genton E, Salzman EW: Antithrombotic therapy in peripheral vascular disease. *Chest* 95(supp):128S–139S, 1989.

113. Snyder SH, Reynolds IH: Calcium-antagonist drugs: Receptor interactions that clarify therapeutic effects. *N Engl J Med* 313:995, 1985.

114. Weinstein DB, Heider JG: Antiatherogenic properties of calcium antagonists: State of the art. *Am J Med* 86(4A):27–32, 1989.
115. Bagger-JP; Helligsoe-P, Randsbaek-F, et al: Effect of verapamil in intermittent claudication. A randomized, double-blind, placebo-controlled, cross-over study after individual dose-response assessment. *Circulation* 95:411–414, 1997.
116. Ferrari P, Clerici G, Gussoni G, et al: Defibrotide versus placebo in the treatment of intermittent claudication: a met-analysis. *Drug Investigation* 7:157–60, 1994.
117. Jha P, Flather M, Lonn E, et al: The antioxidant vitamins and cardiovascular disease: a critical review of epidemiologic and clinical trial data. *Ann Intern Med* 123:860–872, 1995.
118. Clement DL, Duprez D. Effect of ketanserin in the treatment of patients with intermittent claudication: results from 13 placebo-controlled parallel group studies. *Cardiovasc Pharmacol* 10:S89–S95, 1987.
119. van Rij AM, Solomon C, Packer SG, et al: Chelation therapy for intermittent claudication. A double-blind, randomized, controlled trial. *Circulation* 90:1194–1199, 1994.
120. Blume J, Kieser M, Holscher U: Placebo-controlled double-blind study of the effectiveness of Ginkgo biloba special extract Egb 761 in trained patients with intermittent claudication. *Vasa* 25:265–274, 1996.
121. Zarins CK: The vascular war of 1988. *JAMA* 261:416–417, 1989.
122. Jeans WD, Danton RM, Baird RM, et al: The effects of introducing balloon dilatation into vascular surgical practice. *Br J Radiol* 59:457–459, 1986.
123. Anderson JB, Wolinski AP, Wells IP, et al: The impact of percutaneous transluminal angioplasty on the management of peripheral vascular disease. *Br J Surg* 73:17–19, 1986.
124. McKlean L, Jeans WD, Horrocks M, et al: The place of percutaneous transluminal angioplasty in the treatment of patients having angiography for ischaemic disease of the lower limb. *Clin Radiol* 38:157–160, 1987.
125. Widlus DM, Osterman FA: Evaluation and percutaneous management of atherosclerotic peripheral vascular disease. *JAMA* 261:3148–3154, 1989.
126. Johnston W, Rae M, Jogg-Johnston SA, et al: Five-year results of a prospective study of percutaneous transluminal angioplasty. *Ann Surg* 206: 403–413, 1987.
127. Joly S, Bonan R, Palisaitis D, et al: Treatment of recurrent restenosis with repeat percutaneous transluminal coronary angioplasty. *Am J Cardiol* 61: 906–908, 1988.
128. Fowkes FGR, Gillespie IN. Angioplasty (versus non surgical management) for intermittent claudication. In: Fowkes FGR, Janzon L, Kleijnen J, Leng GC (eds.) Peripheral Vascular Diseases Module of the Cochrane Database of Systematic Reviews, [updated 28 August 1997]. Available in The Cochrane Library [database on disk and CDROM]. The Cochrane Collaboration; Issue 4. Oxford: Update Software; 1997. Updated quarterly.
129. Wilson SE, White GH, Wolf G, et al: Proximal percutaneous balloon angioplasty and distal bypass for multilevel arterial occlusion. *Ann Vasc Surg* 4:351–355, 1990.
130. Wilson SE, Wolf GL, Cross AP: Percutaneous transluminal angioplasty versus operation for peripheral arteriosclerosis. Report of a prospective randomized trial in a selected group of patients. *J Vasc Surg* 9:1–9, 1989.

131. Jeans WD, Danton RM, Baird RN, et al: A comparison of the costs of vascular surgery and balloon dilatation in lower limb ischaemic disease. *Br J Radiol* 59:453–456, 1986.
132. Hunink MGM, Wong JB, Donaldson MC, et al: Revascularization for femoropopliteal disease. A decision and cost-effectiveness analysis. *JAMA* 274:165–171, 1995.

Chapter 28

Preoperative Risk Assessment in the Elderly Patient Undergoing Elective Noncardiac Surgery

Edward O. McFalls

The preoperative assessment of a high-risk patient in need of a major elective operation is a difficult task. Presently, there is enormous controversy regarding the appropriate strategy to diagnose and manage coronary artery disease prior to surgery. Overall, general surgical procedures carry a low risk of perioperative cardiac events, with an incidence of myocardial infarction and/or death of less than 1%.[1] Among elderly patients with peripheral vascular disease, the prevalence of coronary artery disease is high and may exceed 50%. It is not surprising therefore, that there is a high risk of unexpected perioperative morbidity and mortality from cardiac complications. In such patients, a cursory risk assessment based on history and physical examination alone may be suboptimal, justifying additional tests to evaluate left ventricular function and potentially ischemic myocardium.

The objective of this chapter is to identify factors that predict perioperative cardiac events in elderly patients, so that appropriate diagnostic and therapeutic decisions can be made. Internists often express a desire to perform coronary angiography prior to major vascular procedures. In fact, the primary goal of the preoperative cardiac "work-up" is to identify those individuals in need of diagnostic coronary angiography. The decision to perform coronary angiography however is only one aspect of the entire problem and is often much less difficult than decid-

From *Clinical Cardiology in the Elderly. Second Edition,* edited by Elliot Chesler. © 1999, Futura Publishing Company, Armonk, NY.

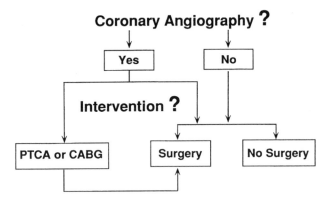

Figure 1: *This figure summarizes the 2 critical decisions in the preoperative work-up and the possible outcomes.*

ing on the optimal management of the patient following coronary angiography (Figure 1).

From a technical point of view, coronary artery revascularization in elderly patients with advanced coronary artery disease can be very complex, with procedural-related complications higher and long-term success lower than in younger patients with less advanced atherosclerosis. Therefore, the second part of management decision following diagnostic coronary angiography may be more uncertain. Unfortunately, there are no randomized trials that have identified those patients who are likely to benefit from prophylactic coronary revascularization prior to elective noncardiac surgery. Until this information becomes available, decisions must be individualized and predicated on the long-term success of the revascularization procedure.[2,3]

Perioperative Cardiac Morbidity in High-Risk Patients

In order to understand the risk-benefit ratio of the preoperative cardiac work-up, one should take into account the expected incidence of cardiac complications in the perioperative period. The latter is dependent upon a number of factors and includes: (1) the nature of the operation; (2) the population at risk; and (3) expertise of the anesthesiologist and surgeon.[4]

Among individuals with a high prevalence of coronary artery disease, cardiac morbidity in the perioperative period is not trivial. Table 1 summarizes the incidence of perioperative cardiac complications in patients undergoing elective noncardiac surgery.

In the above series, perioperative cardiac morbidity is defined as either myocardial infarction or occurrence of one or more of the follow-

Table 1
Incidence of Perioperative Cardiac Complications
in High Risk Patients

Series	Number	Morbidity		Mortality
		MI	Total	Cardiac in Origin
*Cooperman (5)	566	5%	17%	6%
*Eagle (6)	200	6%	15%	3%
*Cutler (7)	130	7%	12%	5%
*Carliner (8)	200	3%	17%	2%
*Pastemack (9)	100	14%	—	2%
*Leppo (10)	100	17%	—	1%
*Arous (11)	135	14%	—	10%
*Baron (12)	457	5%	19%	2%
*McFalls (13)	116	19%	—	2%
+ Von Knorring (14)	214	18%	—	8%
+ Steen (15)	587	6%	—	5%
+ Foster (16)	458	1%	—	1%
# Gerson (17)	100	3%	13%	6%
Pooled Average	—	**9%**	**16%**	**4%**

MI (myocardial infarction); * Peripheral vascular disease; + known coronary artery disease; # elderly (age >65 years).

ing: unstable angina, congestive heart failure, and serious dysrhythmias. Cardiac mortality is defined as death from a primary cardiac event. As shown, perioperative cardiac morbidity occurs in 12%–19% of high-risk patients and death in approximately 1%–10%. This is much higher than might be expected in general medical patients without cardiac disease, where the incidence of perioperative cardiac morbidity is less than 1%.[1,18]

Our experience at the Veterans Medical Center, Minneapolis, Minnesota, is in accord with the above studies.[13] In 116 consecutive patients (male; average age 67 years) undergoing elective vascular operations, there were 22 perioperative myocardial infarctions (19%) including 2 cardiac deaths (2%). Of patients with myocardial infarctions documented by enzyme and elctrocardiographic (ECG) changes, 10 were non-Q wave without subsequent complications. The remaining 10 with nonfatal myocardial infarction had heart block requiring temporary pacing (n = 1), persistent ventricular or supraventricular arrhythmias requiring antiarrhythmic therapy (n = 5) and congestive heart failure requiring diuretics and nitrates (n = 4).

Comparing our experience with other reported series, the number of documented myocardial infarctions is high.[19] This might be explained by the inherent risk in our veteran population who present with advanced atherosclerosis. Likewise, the differences may also reflect the intensity of surveillance in the perioperative period that in our series, involved routine blood sampling for cardiac enzymes every 8 hours for the first 24 hours and daily for the next 3 postoperative days. This differs from other reports where blood is not routinely drawn in all patients for the first 3 postoperative days.[20] When the acquisition of blood for creatine kinase (CK) enzymes and ECGs is dependent on altered clinical status, it could be expected that many subtle cardiac events might be unrecognized.[21] A second consideration in understanding differences between studies is the criteria by which perioperative myocardial infarction is diagnosed. Our study relied on a rise in the specific CK-MB isoenzyme above the upper limits for normal of the laboratory and ECG changes compatible with ischemia. Although these criteria may be too nonspecific in the perioperative period, they are more sensitive than those which depend on evolution of new Q-waves and/or an abnormal technitian pyrophosphate scan.[18]

Despite the variability between studies, we can reasonably assume that the incidence of perioperative myocardial infarctions and morbid events is approximately 20% in high risk patients. Although this may seem prohibitively high, the overall 30-day mortality of these operations is low and in patients without unstable cardiac symptoms is less than 5%. This should be understood when considering prophylactic coronary artery revascularization in high risk patients, particularly when such procedures may carry higher risk than the intended noncardiac surgery.[22,23]

Risk Assessment Based on Clinical Variables

In a well-designed prospective study of over 1000 medical patients undergoing noncardiac surgery, Goldman et al[24] identified a number of clinical factors associated with increased perioperative morbidity and mortality (Table 2). By assigning a numerical score to each variable and adding up the total, one can estimate the relative risk of the operation. This approach is popular among consultants responsible for preoperative risk assessment and has been validated in subsequent prospective studies.[25]

Although the Goldman Criteria are widely accepted, there are certain limitations in its application to the elderly in need of elective vascular surgery. The prevalence of coronary artery disease in Goldman's population was lower than might be expected compared with other high risk groups since less than 7% had angina and only 27% had signs or symptoms of coronary artery disease. This is much lower than the clinical suspicion of coronary artery disease among patients with vascular disease[26] and may explain why angina was not identified as an independent risk factor.

In another prospective study of 455 patients undergoing elective

Table 2
Goldman Criteria
Clinical Variables Associated with Increased
Perioperative Complications

History

- Age >70 years
- Myocardial infarction within 6 months
- Chronically debilitated state

Physical Examination

- Increased jugular venous distention
- S₃ gallop
- Significant aortic stenosis

Electrocardiogram

- Heart rhythm other than normal sinus
- Premature atrial contractions
- Premature ventricular contractions (>5 per minute)

noncardiac surgery, Detsky et al[27] confirmed many of the Goldman Criteria and devised a new set of criteria called the Modified Multifactor Index. In addition to the Goldman Criteria, this study identified angina functional class III and IV by the Canadian Heart Association classification as an exceedingly high-risk factor for perioperative cardiac events.

Risk Assessment Based on Surgical Procedure

The Goldman study was important in showing that the type of surgery influences the incidence of perioperative events. For instance, emergent operations or procedures involving the abdominal or thoracic aorta were associated with the highest risk. Interestingly, nonaortic vascular surgery was not found to be associated with increased cardiac complications, compared with other surgical procedures.

Because the Goldman data were derived from a large group of surgical patients, less than 16% of whom underwent elective vascular surgery, it is probable that the risk for vascular surgery was underestimated. Similar to the Goldman study, Detsky et al[27] showed that the pretest probability of cardiac event was highly dependent upon the type of operation. In contrast however, they found that vascular procedures were associated with at least a 13% incidence of severe cardiac complications. Other studies support these findings.[28]

The reasons for increased perioperative risk among patients undergoing vascular operations are multifactorial. The Cleveland Clinic reported that coronary artery disease, defined by greater than 70% stenosis of at least one major epicardial artery, is present in more than 50% of patients scheduled for elective vascular surgery.[26] This includes nearly 80% of "suspected" and 40% of "unsuspected" individuals. Moreover, fewer than 8% of patients referred for vascular surgery were found to have normal coronary angiograms. Additionally, the risk of vascular surgery is often increased due to prolonged operations, often with wide fluctuations in intraoperative blood pressure and intravascular volume.[29]

Cardiac Risk Assessment Prior to Elective Noncardiac Surgery

One of the most important aspects of the preoperative assessment is to synthesize available clinical variables with judicious utilization of ancillary tests. A simple pneumonic for remembering appropriate items is to seek **help**:

History and physical examination;
Electrocardiogram;
Left ventricular function;
Provocative tests for detecting ischemia.

Initial Screen

The importance of the history, physical examination, and baseline ECG cannot be overemphasized. In addition to the Goldman Criteria and the Modified Multifactorial Index, specific clinical variables in high-risk patients must be identified. Among 566 patients undergoing vascular surgery, 5 clinical variables were shown by Cooperman et al[5] to be independently associated with increased perioperative cardiac complications. These include a history myocardial infarction, cerebrovascular accident, congestive heart failure, arrhythmia, and an abnormal ECG. The incidence of cardiovascular complications was 1.3% among patients with no risk factors but exceeded 23% in patients with all 5 factors. Similarly, in 200 patients undergoing vascular surgery, Eagle et al[6] showed that the presence of Q waves on ECG and a history of ventricular ectopy requiring treatment were independently associated with increased perioperative cardiac risk. Advanced age, diabetes, and a history of angina were additional independent risk factors for perioperative cardiac events. The latter factors have also been associated with a decreased 5-year survival following elective vascular surgery.[30]

We have found similar results in terms of univariate predictors of perioperative cardiac complications.[13] Consistent with prior studies, risk of perioperative myocardial infarction was higher among patients with a history of coronary artery disease (P < .001), including previous myocardial infarction (P < 0.001), angina (P < 0.0001), and an abnormal ECG (P < 0.05). Diabetes mellitus as a risk factor, achieved borderline statistical significance (P = 0.06).

Left Ventricular Function

Patients with left ventricular dysfunction are at increased risk for perioperative cardiac complications. Therefore, the screening history and physical exam are important. Dyspnea on exertion[15] or the presence of either increased jugular venous pressure or a third heart sound[24] independently identify individuals at increased risk. When the initial clinical work-up is inconclusive regarding left ventricular impairment, further studies may be indicated.

Studies of left ventricular function may be a useful adjunct for preoperative risk stratification for patients scheduled for elective operation. In 100 patients referred for elective vascular surgery, radionuclide left ventricular ejection fraction correlated inversely with the incidence of both perioperative myocardial infarction and death.[9] Among 1600 patients in the CASS registry who subsequently underwent major noncardiac surgery, left ventriculograms were retrospectively analyzed for wall motion abnormalities in 5 segments.[16] This showed that the degree of left ventricular dysfunction was a strong independent predictor of perioperative cardiac complications and was more predictive than clinical assessment. In contrast, other studies have not shown ejection fraction to be an independent predictor of perioperative cardiac events in either high-risk vascular patients undergoing abdominal aortic aneurysm repair[31] or in elderly patients undergoing noncardiac surgery.[17]

In our series of 116 patients,[13] 108 received preoperative radionuclide angiography. The ejection fraction of patients with and without complications was 45% ± 3% and 55% ± 2%, respectively (P < 0.005). By multivariate analysis however, ejection fraction was not shown to be an independent risk factor. It therefore remains controversial whether studies of left ventricular function should be performed in all high-risk patients prior to elective operation. Although left ventricular ejection fraction is a univariate predictor of cardiac complications in the perioperative period, it may not be an independent risk factor and therefore its utility in the preoperative evaluation is not clear.

Exercise Performance

Functional class provides important predictive information, in both general medical and high-risk vascular patients. Unfortunately, many patients do not give a history of impaired functional status either because of coexisting pulmonary or peripheral vascular disease, or because their coronary artery disease is asymptomatic. Exercise testing therefore, may provide additional information. Among patients over 65 years of age, inability to perform 2 minutes of exercise on a supine bicycle or to raise heart rate above 99 beats per minute is independently associated with perioperative cardiac complications.[17] Arm ergometry is also useful among elderly patients unable to perform standard exercise treadmill tests. Among 284 patients having elective vascular procedures, the ability to achieve greater than 75% maximum heart rate without evidence of ischemic ECG changes identified a group without cardiac complications. Those patients who did not achieve 75% of their maximum heart rate and developed ischemia, had an incidence of perioperative complications of 19%.[7]

Although exercise electrocardiography may be useful in some patients, interpretation can be difficult, particularly among vascular patients where prevalence of abnormal baseline tracings exceeds 60%.[5] Among 200 patients having preoperative exercise testing prior to noncardiac surgery, the exercise ECG was found to have low sensitivity and specificity for identifying individuals who developed perioperative myocardial infarction, compared to the baseline ECG that was highly predictive of events.[8] Because of poor exercise capacity and poor predictive accuracy of the exercise ECG in high-risk patients, other strategies have been developed for identifying individuals with significant myocardium at risk for ischemia.

In our group of 116 patients undergoing elective vascular surgery, 88 performed exercise treadmill or arm ergometry with thallium-SPECT.[13] An abnormal thallium scan was more frequent in the group with cardiac complications, although there was no difference in either exercise time or double product between groups. The data demonstrate that the predictive accuracy of exercise testing can be enhanced with thallium in high risk patients disabled by peripheral vascular disease.

Ambulatory ECG

Identifying patients with asymptomatic coronary artery disease who have increased cardiac risk for elective surgery can be facilitated by ambulatory ECG. In 176 patients undergoing 24–48 hour Holter monitoring within 9 days of elective vascular surgery, 32 (18%) had preoperative ischemic ST-segment depression. Thirteen (7%) met strict criteria for major postoperative cardiac events, and only 1 patient had a negative preoperative Holter study.[32] The data showed that an abnormal preoperative Holter monitor was 92% sensitive and 88% specific for a perioperative event, suggesting that this may be a useful screening test. Of concern however, is that the predictive value of a positive result was only 38%, meaning that other testing would be needed to further stratify such groups. Clearly, more studies are needed to determine whether its application will prove to be a cost-effective screening test.

Stress Imaging Modalities

Dipyridamole thallium scintigraphy has gained widespread acceptance as a means of identifying patients at increased operative risk, particularly for those unable to exercise. Although stress imaging tests are not cost-effective for all individuals undergoing elective operation,[12] they may provide important information in certain groups at intermediate risk. Dipyridamole infused intravenously in a dose of 0.56 mg/kg over 4 minutes increases coronary blood flow 4–5 times in myocardium perfused by normal coronary arteries.[33] In regions perfused by critically stenosed arteries, the coronary vasculature is already maximally vasodilated so that a drop in coronary perfusion pressure decreases flow distal to the stenosis resulting in subendocardial ischemia. This phenomenon has been termed "coronary steal" because in other regions, myocardial blood flow increases, at the expense of the jeopardized regions.

Among high-risk vascular patients undergoing elective surgery, a reversible thallium defect following infusion of intravenous dipyridamole identifies patients at risk for perioperative cardiac complications.[10,34] In combination with clinical variables, it has been shown to be a cost effective way of identifying high risk patients. For example, among 200 patients with vascular disease followed prospectively, it was found that age over 70 years, Q waves on the ECG, and a history of either angina, diabetes, or ventricular ectopy were independent predictors of perioperative cardiac complications. Dipyridamole thallium was found to be most useful in patients with "intermediate" risk; that is, when only 1 or 2 of the clinical variables were present. Patients with none of the clinical variables were at low risk and needed no further testing while patients with 3 or more variables were high risk with a complication rate of 50%. This group would be best managed by coronary angiography without noninvasive testing.[6]

This previous study proposed a cost-effective approach for deciding which patients need preoperative invasive testing, without need for expensive testing in all surgical candidates. However, concern has been raised over the sensitivity and specificity of dipyridamole thallium tests in an intermediate group of patients. For example, Mangano et al[35] reported that 10 of 20 patients undergoing elective vascular surgery with negative preoperative dipyridamole thallium tests had perioperative ischemia demonstrated by intraoperative transesophageal echocardiogram and 1 patient suffered fatal myocardial infarction. In addition, the specificity of dipyridamole thallium testing for identifying myocardium at risk may also be lower than prior reports, particularly in relation to fixed defects. Other studies suggest that fixed thallium defects identify patients at increased risk for developing subsequent cardiac complications.[36]

Our experience is in agreement with the concept that partially reversible thallium defects after exercise or dipyriamole identifies viable myocardium at risk for ischemia. Among 88 patients who had exercise thallium tests prior to elective vascular surgery, 46 had abnormal scans including 20 reversible, 11 persistent, and 15 mixed defects.[13] The presence of a nonreversible thallium defect was an independent predictor of perioperative myocardial infarction, with an odds ratio of 2.48 (95% confidence interval of 1.03–5.95). The only other independent risk factor was angina, with an odds ratio of 6.81 (95% confidence interval of 0.97–47.80).

With the advent of stress ECHO, high-risk individuals can also be identified by visualizing altered regional myocardial function during infusion of high dose dobutamine with atropine. Among individuals in whom satisfactory images can be obtained, stress ECHO is comparable to nuclear-imaging tests in diagnosing significant coronary artery disease. In patients undergoing elective vascular operations, stress induced wall motion abnormalities provide important information about the extent of myocardium at risk and predict both early and late cardiac events following surgery.[37] Whether the test is more accurate than other modalities depends on the image quality and the technical expertise of the ECHO laboratory. The advantages over nuclear studies are less expense and the ability to assess valvular and global left ventricular function; disadvantages are that adequate imaging may be technically difficult in a significant percentage of patients.

Prophylactic Coronary Artery Revascularization

In many large series of patients having elective vascular surgery, coronary artery disease has been reported to be the leading cause of post operative mortality, both at 30 days and at 5 years.[30] Because patients who have had coronary artery bypass surgery have a lower incidence of perioperative complications, it has been suggested that prophylactic coronary artery revascularization may be indicated in all patients undergoing elective vascular surgery.[26,32,38] These results must be interpreted with caution because the studies were not randomized and therefore are subject to selection bias. For example, data from the Cleveland Clinic have shown that although 80% of patients in need of vascular surgery have symptomatic coronary artery disease, less than half are amenable to coronary artery revascularization.[26]

For a better understanding of the long-term prognosis in elderly patients undergoing elective vascular surgery, vital status was determined for all patients in our original series for a median of 4 postoperative years.[39] Although the 30-day mortality was low (3%), the mortality

Table 3
Univariate Predictors of Total Post-Operative Mortality
at 1 and 4 Years

	1 Year Mortality	4 Year Mortality
Prior Coronary Artery Disease	NS	NS
Abnormal EKG	$P < 0.05$	NS
≥ Moderate Sized Thallium Defects¶	$P < 0.05$	NS
LV Ejection Fraction ≤40%*	$P < 0.01$	NS
Perioperative Myocardial Infarction	$P < 0.01$	$P = 0.06$
non-AAA Surgery	NS	$P < 0.01$
Diabetes Mellitus	NS	$P < 0.05$

NS (Nonsignificant by Chi Square Analysis); ¶ Thallium defects are defined as persistent or reversible and were graded as small, moderate or large by an independent observer.
* LV Ejection Fraction was arbitrarily categorized into above and below 40% to allow for Chi Square Analysis. (Reproduced with permission from McFalls et al.[39]).

at 4 years was 39%. Of the 45 patients who died within 4 years after surgery, the major causes of death were cardiac (4%), cancer (18%), and cerebrovascular (13%). Univariate predictors of 1- and 4-year mortality are shown in Table 3. In addition, life table analyses are shown for individuals with and without a perioperative myocardial infarction and for the type of surgery (Figure 2). By logistic regression, the independent predictors of 4-year mortality were vascular surgery involving infrainguinal procedures and diabetes mellitus with perioperative myocardial infarction showing marginal significance ($P = 0.06$).[40] The data reemphasize that long-term survival is more predicated by advanced atherosclerotic disease, particularly among patients who require surgery for distal limb salvage Although the data show that the major cause of death in these patients is cardiac, we cannot necessarily assume that the long term prognosis could have been improved with preoperative coronary artery revascularization.

Presently, there are no data to show that coronary artery revascularization prior to elective vascular operations improves long-term survival. Patients with peripheral vascular disease in the CASS Trial who were randomly assigned to coronary artery bypass surgery did show improved survival.[41] However, these patients were not elderly individuals with severe comorbid illnesses and advanced peripheral vascular disease. Among Cleveland Clinic patients with coronary artery disease needing elective vascular surgery, the perioperative mortality from prophylactic coronary artery bypass surgery was at least 5%, which is 2- to 3-fold higher than that of the CASS study.[42] Similarly, other centers have reported that the risk of prophylactic coronary artery bypass surgery in elderly patients with advanced vascular disease is fraught with complications.[22,23] This emphasizes that even with selection, high-risk

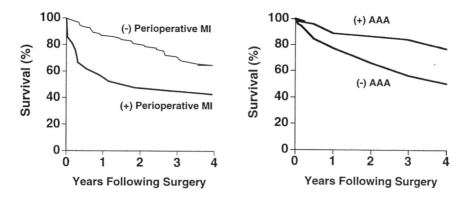

Figure 2: *These life table analyses show the long-term survival for 93 patients without and 22 patients with a perioperative myocardial infarction (**left**) as well as the long-term survival of 44 patients undergoing abdominal aortic aneurysm (AAA) surgery compared with 71 patients undergoing infrainguinal surgery (**right**). Differences in survival curves were statistically significant at 4 years for both variables (P < 0.05). Reproduced with permission from McFalls E, Ward H, Santilli S, et al: The influence of perioperative myocardial infarction on long term prognosis following elective vascular surgery. Chest 113:681–686, 1998.*

vascular patients are technically difficult surgical candidates with a high incidence of perioperative morbidity and mortality.

There are some small nonrandomized series which have suggested that an aggressive preoperative strategy is beneficial. A Mayo Clinic report of 50 patients with severe coronary disease who had PTCA within 9 days of noncardiac operation showed that the incidence of perioperative myocardial infarction and death was 6% and 2%, respectively. Although this would appear to be an acceptably low incidence among high risk patients, the risk-benefit ratio of prophylactic coronary artery revascularization may not have been so favorable. The original patient cohort consisted of 55 patients, 5 of whom had failed PTCA and required urgent coronary artery bypass surgery; also, 3 patients who had successful PTCA suffered perioperative myocardial infarction.[43]

To clarify this problem of preoperative management of patients with coexistent coronary artery and vascular diseases, the VA Cooperative Studies Program has funded a feasibility pilot study to test whether prophylactic coronary artery revascularization prior to elective vascular surgery improves long term survival. The coronary artery revascularization prophylaxis (CARP) trial will hopefully provide important information about which subsets of patients should be subjected to expensive and risky strategies to diagnose and manage coronary artery disease. Until information from that trial is available, it is clear that the actual decision to proceed with aggressive coronary artery revascularization procedures needs to weigh the long- term benefit of the pro-phylactic procedure as well as the immediate short-term risks.[2,3]

Tentative Therapeutic Strategy

Until the results from a cooperative study become available, the optimal management of a patient with coronary artery disease in need of major noncardiac surgery will have to be individualized. At this point however, we recommend a number of considerations for the preoperative risk assessment. As shown from Figure 3, the decision to proceed with coronary angiography is made by synthesizing all relevant univariate and multivariate clinical risk factors. Because coronary artery disease accounts for the majority of cardiac complications perioperatively, the patient should be evaluated initially with a history, physical examination and baseline ECG.

Based on the findings of many trials, it is advisable to withhold or delay elective procedures among patients who have had myocardial infarction within the preceding 3 months. Among patients less than 70 years of age and without: a history of recent myocardial infarction, angina, arrhythmia, or diabetes, signs of congestive heart failure (presence of a third heart sound or elevated jugular venous pressure), or Q

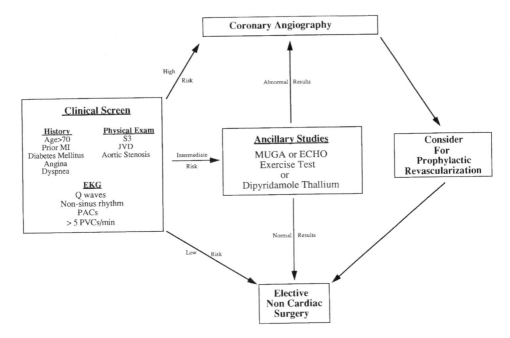

Figure 3: *This figure demonstrates a generalized strategy for the preoperative work-up of the high-risk patient scheduled for elective noncardiac surgery.*

waves on the ECG, the incidence of cardiac complications can be expected to be low and further studies are not required. In the presence of most of these variables, the risk is high and a decision to proceed with coronary angiography is reasonable. In the intermediate group, where risk assessment is not clear from clinical variables, ancillary tests are advisable to assess (1) degree of myocardial impairment and/or (2) degree of myocardium at risk for ischemia. The most appropriate tests would be a combination of ECHO or radionuclide angiography and stress tests with or without imaging modalities.

Once a decision to perform coronary angiography has been made, the possibility of prophylactic revascularization arises. With 2- or 3-vesslel coronary artery disease and mild left ventricular dysfunction, it is reasonable to proceed with coronary artery revascularization in otherwise good candidates. When the risk-benefit ratio for prophylactic revascularization is excessive (such as poor target vessels, left ventricular dysfunction and significant other illnesses), it may be advisable to reassess the need for elective noncardiac surgery. When the patient is not amenable to coronary artery revascularization but needs an elective procedure, several precautions should be taken. These include pre and perioperative hemodynamic monitoring for optimizing intravascular volume and arterial blood pressure, adding β-blockers[43] and in some situations, simplifying the surgical procedure.[29]

Cardiac Risks Other Than Coronary Artery Disease

Valvular Heart Disease

Both the Goldman Criteria and the Modified Multifactorial Index identify significant aortic stenosis as a major cause of perioperative morbidity and mortality. Many elderly patients have coexistent medical diseases that would preclude aortic valve replacement. Although there are no data on effectiveness, percutaneous aortic valvuloplasty might serve as a temporary solution but would only be considered when the situation is urgent. In other instances, it might be reasonable to proceed with elective noncardiac surgery, accepting the risks without a definitive prophylactic procedure. In 48 elderly patients with severe aortic stenosis, elective vascular surgery was performed with a favorable surgical outcome with aggressive pre and postoperative hemodynamic monitoring.[44]

Patients with critical mitral stenosis are at increased risk for perioperative pulmonary edema, particularly during episodes of rapid supraventricular tachycardia. In addition, the added risk of cardiac thromboembolic disease would contraindicate any elective surgical procedures in this group. The presence of mitral regurgitation on the other hand, has not been shown to be a significant risk factor in the absence of congestive heart failure. Goldman et al[24] showed that a systolic murmur not consistent with aortic stenosis was not associated with increased risk.

Hypertrophic Cardiomyopathy

In the early postoperative period, volume depletion, tachycardia and increased systemic catecholamines may critically aggravate dynamic outflow tract obstruction. Shulman et al[45] reported 35 patients with symptomatic hypertrophic cardiomyopathy who underwent 56 surgical procedures (4 with spinal anesthesia); all survived without complications with the exception of 1 patient who had myocardial infarction and congestive heart failure. The authors concluded that surgery can be performed safely, but spinal anesthesia and associated coronary artery disease increase perioperative risk.

Conclusion

Coronary artery disease accounts for the majority of complications after elective noncardiac surgery and its prevalence among elderly patients with peripheral vascular disease is of great concern. The history, physical examination and baseline ECG allow the clinician to identify low-, intermediate-, and high-risk groups. Further stratification should be directed among the intermediate-risk patient, using a variety of noninvasive tests. Coronary angiography needs to be considered in high-risk individuals and the decision to undertake subsequent prophylactic revascularization should be made on clinical grounds. There is a definite need for controlled, multicentered trials to define which patients are likely to benefit from an invasive approach.

References

1. Tarhan S, Moffitt E, Taylor W, et al: Myocardial infarction after general anesthesia. *JAMA* 220:1451–1454, 1972.
2. Gersh B, Rihal C, Rooke T, et al: Evaluation and management of patients with both peripheral vascular and coronary artery disease. *J Am Coll Cardiol* 18:203–214, 1991.
3. Fleisher L, Eagle K: Screening for cardiac disease in patients having noncardiac surgery. *Ann Intern Med* 124:767–772, 1996.
4. Mangano D: Perioperative cardiac morbidity. *Anesthesiology* 72:153–184, 1990.
5. Cooperman M, Pflug B, Martin EJ, et al: Cardiovascular risk factors in patients with peripheral vascular disease. *Surgery* 84:505–509, 1978.
6. Eagle K, Coley C, Newell J, et al: Combining clinical and thallium data optimizes preoperative assessment of cardiac risk before major vascular surgery. *Ann Intern Med* 110:859–866, 1989.

7. Cutler B, Wheeler H, Paraskos J, et al: Applicability and interpretation of electrocardiographic stress testing in patients with peripheral vascular disease. *Am J Surg* 141:501–506, 1981.
8. Carliner N, Fisher M, Plotnick G, et al: Routine preoperative exercise testing in patients undergoing major noncardiac surgery. *Am J Cardiol* 56: 51–58, 1985.
9. Pasternack P, Imparato A, Riles T, et al: The value of the radionuclide angiogram in the prediction of perioperative myocardial infarction in patients undergoing lower extremity revascularization procedures. *Circulation* 72(Suppl 2):II13-II17, 1985.
10. Leppo J, Plaja J, Gionet M, et al: Noninvasive evaluation of cardiac risk before elective vascular surgery. *J Am Coll Cardiol* 9:269–276, 1987.
11. Arous E, Baum P, Cutler B: The ischemic exercise test in patients with peripheral vascular disease. *Arch Surg* 119:780–783, 1984.
12. Baron J, Mundler O, Bertrand M, et al: Dipyridamole-thallium scintigraphy and gated radionuclide angiography to assess cardiac risk before abdominal aortic surgery. *N Engl J Med* 330:663–669, 1994.
13. McFalls E, Doliszny K, Grund F, et al: Angina and persistent exercise thallium defects: Independent risk factors in elective vascular surgery. *J Am Coll Cardiol* 21:1347–1352, 1993.
14. Von Knorring J: Postoperative myocardial infarction: A prospective study in a risk group of surgical patients. *Surgery* 90:55–60, 1981.
15. Steen P, Tinker J, Tarhan S. Myocardial reinfarction after anesthesia and surgery. *JAMA* 239:2566–2570, 1978.
16. Foster E, Davis K, Carpenter J, et al: Risk of noncardiac operation in patients with defined coronary disease: The Coronary Artery Surgery Study (CASS) Registry experience. *Ann Thorac Surg* 41:42–49, 1986.
17. Gerson M, Hurst J, Hertzberg V, et al: Cardiac prognosis in noncardiac geriatric surgery. *Ann Intern Med* 103:832–837, 1985.
18. Ashton C, Petersen N, Wray N, et al: The incidence of perioperative myocardial infarction in men undergoing noncardiac surgery. *Ann Intern Med* 118: 504–510, 1993.
19. Mangano D, Goldman L: Preoperative assesssment of patients with known or suspected coronary disease. *N Engl J Med* 333:1750–1756, 1995.
20. Taylor L Jr, Yeager R, Moneta G, et al: The incidence of perioperative myocardial infarction in general vascular surgery. *J Vasc Surg* 15:52–61, 1991.
21. Charlson M, MacKenzie C, Alex K, et al: Surveillance for postoperative myocardial infarction after noncardiac operations. *Surg Gynecol Obstet* 167:407–414, 1988.
22. Birkmeyer J, O'Connor G, Quinton H, et al, for the Northern New England Cardiovascular Disease Study Group: The effect of peripheral vascular disease on in-hospital mortality rates with coronary artery bypass surgery. *J Vasc Surg* 21:445–452, 1995.
23. Mesh C, Cmolik B, Van Heekeren D, et al: Coronary byass in vascular patients: A relatively high-risk procedure. *Ann Vasc Surg* 11:612–619, 1997.
24. Goldman L, Caldera D, Nussbaum S, et al: Multifactorial index of cardiac risk in noncardiac surgical procedures. *N Engl J Med* 297:845–850, 1977.
25. Zeldin R: Assessing cardiac risk in patients who undergo noncardiac surgical procedures. *Can J Surg* 27:402–404, 1984.

26. Hertzer N, Beven E, Young J, et al: Coronary artery disease in peripheral vascular patients: A classification of 1000 coronary angiograms and results of surgical management. *Ann Surg* 199:223–233, 1984.
27. Detsky A, Abrams H, Forbath N,et al: Cardiac assessment for patients undergoing noncardiac surgery: A multifactorial clinical risk index. *Arch Intern Med* 146:2131–2134, 1986.
28. Jeffrey C, Kunsman J, Cullen D, et al: A prospective evaluation of cardiac risk index. *Anesthesiology* 58:462–464, 1983.
29. Rao T, Jacobs K, El-Etr A: Reinfarction following anesthesia in patients with myocardial infarction. *Anesthesiology* 59:499–505, 1983.
30. Jamieson W, Janusz M, Miyagishima R, et al: Influence of ischemic heart disease on early and late mortality after surgery for peripheral occlusive vascular disease. *Circulation* 66:92–97, 1982.
31. Kazmers A, Cerqueira M, Zierler R: The role of preoperative radionuclide ejection fraction in direct abdominal aortic aneurysm repair. *J Vasc Surg* 8:128–136, 1988.
32. Ruby S, Whittemore A, Couch N, et al. Coronary artery disease in patients requiring abdominal aortic aneurysm repair. *Ann Surg* 201:758–764, 1985.
33. Araujo L, Lammertsma A, Rhodes C, et al: Noninvasive myocardial blood flow measurements using 0–15 labeled water and positron emission tomography. *Circulation* 83:875–885, 1991.
34. Boucher C, Brewster D, Darling R, et al: Determination of cardiac risk by dipyridamole-thallium imaging before peripheral vascular surgery. *N Engl J Med* 312:389–394, 1985.
35. Mangano D, London M, Tubau J, et al: Dipyridamole thallium-201 scintigraphy as a preoperative screening test: A reexamination of its predictive potential. *Circulation* 84:493–502, 1991.
36. McEnroe C, O'Donnell TJ, Yeager A, et al: Comparison of ejection fraction and Goldman risk factor analysis to dipyridamole-thallium 201 studies in the evaluation of cardiac morbidity after aortic aneurysm surgery. *J Vasc Surg* 11:497–504, 1990.
37. Poldermans D, Arnese M, Fioretti P, et al: Sustained prognostic value of dobutamine stress echocardiography for late cardiac events after major noncardiac vascular surgery. *Circulation* 95:53–58, 1997.
38. Crawford E, Morris GJ, Howell J, et al: Operative risk in patients with previous coronary artery bypass. *Ann Thorac Surg* 26:215–220, 1978.
39. McFalls E, Ward H, Santilli S, et al: The influence of perioperative myocardial infarction on long term prognosis following elective vascular surgery. *Chest* 113:681–686, 1998.
40. Krupski W, Layug E, Reilly L, et al, and The Study of Perioperative Ischemia (SPI) Research Group. Comparison of cardiac morbidity between aortic and infrainguinal operations. *J Vasc Surg* 15:354–365, 1992.
41. Rihal C, Eagle K, Mickel M, et al: Surgical therapy for coronary artery disease among patients with combined coronary artery and peripheral vascular disease. *Circulation* 91:46–53, 1995.
42. Hertzer N, Young J, Bevern E, et al: Late results of coronary bypass in patients with peripheral vascular disease. *Cleve Clin J Med* 54:15–23, 1987.
43. Huber K, Evans M, Bresnahan J, et al. Outcome of noncardiac operations in patients with severe coronary artery disease successfully treated preoperatively with coronary angioplasty. *Mayo Clin Proc* 67:15–21, 1992.

44. Mangano D, Layug E, Wallace A, et al: Effect of atenolol on mortality and cardiovascular morbidity after noncardiac surgery. *N Engl J Med* 335: 1713–1720, 1996.
45. O'Keefe J, Shub C, Rettke S: Risk of noncardiac surgical procedures in patients with aortic stenosis. *Mayo Clin Proc* 64:400–405, 1989.
46. Shulman S, Amren D, Bisno A, et al: Prevention of bacterial endocarditis: A statement for health professionals by the Committee on Rheumatic Fever and Infective Endocarditis of the Council on Cardiovascular Disease in the Young. *Circulation* 70:1123A–1127, 1984.

Part 6

ETHICS

Chapter 29

Attaining and Maintaining Autonomy

Henry D. McIntosh

Since the most ancient of times, humans have sought to function independently of others and, in their personal lives, to **attain and maintain their autonomy.** Such a goal continues to be actively sought by members of contemporary societies, not just during the prime of life, but during the twilight years as well. These efforts have fostered an increasing interest in establishing advance directives, such as living wills and in the designation of a durable power of attorney for health. Some have even favored adopting the practice(s) of assisted suicide and/ or euthanasia.

But surprising as it may seem, few members of the medical profession have attempted to contribute to the evolution of the social attitudes, practices, and/or laws that will significantly influence the final years of many of their patients. As a result, it is uncertain what influence, if any, members of the profession will have on future discussion(s), customs, and laws regarding the final care of members of our aging society.

When confronted by such uncertainties regarding the future, it has been my habit to follow the advice of Oliver Wendell Holmes, the renowned American jurist of the first third of this century. He said,

"When I want to understand what is happening today, or try to decide what will happen tomorrow, I look back."

A Review of History

In looking back we learned that since ancient times and until the decade following World War II, despite the desire to maintain auton-

From *Clinical Cardiology in the Elderly. Second Edition,* edited by Elliot Chesler. © 1999, Futura Publishing Company, Armonk, NY.

omy, society has, without questions, granted physicians, many special privileges. The public wanted to accept that medical decision-making and other patient-related actions by physicians were guided by the principle of beneficence. This implied that every effort of the physician was to promote the well-being of the patient. This belief by most of society led to the widespread promotion and acceptance of the philosophy of medical paternalism: the physician was considered the devoted father and the patient was considered the accepting, dependent child. The public wanted to believe that only the physician possessed the requisite knowledge and judgement to make decisions regarding the appropriate course of action for a patient. The physician, like a loving, caring father, was able to transfer to the patient the image of "truly caring." These philosophical principles—beneficence and paternalism—served for century after century as guideposts for the ideal practice of medicine. They are at the core of the Hippocratic tradition[1,2] that dates back to the 5th century B.C.[3]

The Doctor

When I was a medical student in the late 1940s after World War II at the University of Pennsylvania, my mentors frequently reminded me that Francis Peabody taught that "The secret of the care of the patient is in caring for the patient."[4] When I graduated from medical school, the Wyeth Pharmaceutical Company gave each member of the class a reproduction of "The Doctor" (Figure 1). We were told, and it was so stated in the University of Pennsylvania School of Medicine Yearbook,[5] that "The Doctor" was painted in 1891 by Sir Luke Fildes on the order of Queen Victoria of England. According to that report, the physician represented at the bedside in the painting was Sir James Clark. Allegedly, when Queen Victoria was at her summer home in Scotland, the only child of her favorite personal servant became ill. The Queen was concerned by the gravity of the child's appearance and summoned her personal physician, Dr. Clark, from London. Dr. Clark arrived promptly by special train and immediately went to the child. He too was concerned about the appearance of the child and sat at the bedside to observe and comfort the child and allay the anxiety of the parents. We were told that the Queen was so impressed by the compassion and dedication of Dr. Clark that she commanded Sir Luke Fildes to preserve the scene for posterity. As we received the M.D. degree, we were given a reproduction of the painting with a brief history and were told that it "represented what medicine was all about."

But was the physician immortalized in the widely viewed painting of "The Doctor" really Queen Victoria's personal physician, Dr. James Clark? Possibly not. Sylvan Lee Weinberg, in his American College of Cardiology President's Page, "Remembering Keats in Rome,"[6] reported that Dr. James Clark attended the renowned poet, John Keats, until his death in Rome in 1821. Then, in 1826, Dr. Clark moved his practice

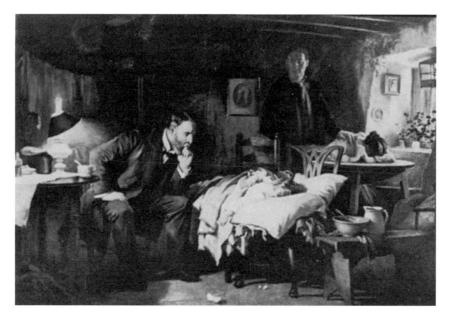

Figure 1: *A copy, done with oil (1993) by Joseph Tomanek, of a painting by Sir Luke Fildes (1891) of "The Doctor" (see text). Reproduced with permission of Wyeth-Ayerst Laboratories, Philadelphia, PA.*

from Rome to London and became the physician to Queen Victoria. She died in 1901, 10 years after "The Doctor" was painted. So Dr. Clark could have attended the "only child of the favorite servant" of the Queen in Balmoral Castle prior to 1891. But Dr. Weinberg's probing research of the practice of Dr. Clark led to a detailed ichnographical report by Albert Rinsler[7] of the origin of the painting, "The Doctor." No reference is made in that report of Dr. Clark. To the contrary, Albert Rinsler reported that the death of the artist's, Sir Luke Fildes, first-born son on Christmas morning in 1877 probably did have a significant influence on the evolution of "The Doctor" 3 years later. He quoted the artist's son, L.V. Fildes, as reporting in the biography of his father that "The character and bearing of their doctor, Dr. Gustavus Charles Philip Murry, throughout the time of their anxiety, made a deep impression on the parents. Apparently Dr. Murry became a symbol of professional devotion which would one day inspire the painting of "The Doctor." Rinsler reported how Henry Tate, a most generous philanthropist, particularly for British art, after seeing preliminary sketches by Luke Fildes of a doctor at the bedside, commissioned him for 3000 pounds to produce the work. The painting has hung in the Tate Gallery in London since that day.

It would appear that the "facts" about the characters and other details in the painting that were given to medical students and reported by this author on numerous occasions, have possibly been incorrect.[1,2,8] But does the name of the doctor used to project the "image of caring" make a difference? I think not. Does "The Doctor" immortalized by Fildes, regardless of the name of the physician, still not portray, as they told us at graduation, "what medicine is all about"? Furthermore, is it not remarkable that there are widely circulated reports of the radiation of the "spirit of love and compassion and of beneficence" from the manner and appearance of at least 2 physicians perceived years ago by the families of the ill? Are patients and their families likely to get the same visual message from their doctor today? Are medical students taught how to deliver that message? Unfortunately, this author fears that the answer to those last two questions is, "No!"

The Evolution of Clinical Investigation

We are indebted to Dr. D.J. Rothman, in his very readable historical review, entitled *Stranger at the Bedside,*[9] for reporting that before World War II, the medical research enterprise was typically a small-scale, intimate, cottage industry. Medical researchers were few in number. They frequently worked alone. Their experiments were usually carried out on themselves, their families, and/or their immediate neighbors. The research questions, for which answers were sought, were usually therapeutic in nature. The experimental subject usually benefitted directly, if the experiments were successful; if not successful, little harm was done.[9,18,19]

Now when the world went to war for the second time, the potential and importance of medical research was recognized. In the summer of 1942, 6 months after the United States had joined the Allied Forces, President Franklin Delano Roosevelt created the Office of Scientific Research and Development (OSRD) to oversee the work of 2 parallel committees. One committee was devoted to weapons research and the other to medical research (Committee on Medical Research [CMR]). Over the course of World War II, the CMR recommended to OSRD some 600 research proposals for funding. The OSRD, in turn, contracted with investigators in some 135 university hospitals and research institutions to carry out the research. Most of the research dealt with the treatment of illnesses or physical afflictions common to combat and/or military life such as dysentery, wound infection, venereal disease, sleep deprivation, exposure to extremes of temperatures, etc. Many of these studies involved the use of humans as experimental subjects. Answers were the most important, if not the only, goal. How the answers were obtained seemed to be immaterial. The country was at war and if good came from the research at the expense of a few, how different was that from what was taking place at the front against the common enemy where soldiers were being killed for the common good?[9,30–32]

The Nazi Practices

Such a philosophy had been adopted by the Nazis. In 1942, Hitler proclaimed that "as a matter of principle, if it is in the interest of the state, human experiments were to be permitted." It was, according to Hitler, "unacceptable for someone in a concentration camp or prison to be untouched by the war, while German soldiers had to suffer the unbearable."[9,61]

The War Ends

In 1945, the war finally ended. The nation had learned that battles could be won, not only against the German and Japanese War Machines, but also against death due to organisms and even cancer. In the fall of 1945, Vannevar Bush, the director of the OSRD, emphasized the accomplishments of the research community in a report entitled "Science, The Endless Frontier." He first listed the achievements of medical research during the 200 years preceding World War II. He then cited victories over smallpox, typhoid, tetanus, yellow fever, and other infectious diseases. He mentioned the introduction of sulfa drugs and even penicillin. He then listed the spectacular discoveries of medical research during World War II. He concluded that "Medicine is on the verge of its most heroic explorations—it would be foolhardy to close off the Frontiers of Science by ending federal support."[9,51–54]

Dr. Bush's message was supported by many in public office. Senator Joseph Ransdell from Louisiana stated: "We have found the cause of a number of epidemic diseases and have practically conquered them. May we not expect the same kind of success against the so-called degenerative diseases if we work hard enough?"[9,51–54]

The New York Times, in 1945, published: "It is sad to realize that, had it not been for the war, penicillin might not have been placed in the hands of physicians. We need something more than the natural curiosity of the research scientist to speed discovery that means so much to mankind."[9,51–54]

Establishing the National Institutes of Health

The whole nation was enthusiastic about continuing a strong medical research program and support of the organization of the postwar National Institutes of Health (NIH) was widespread. In 1945, the NIH had a budget of $700,000. As a result of the enthusiastic support of the public, the budget for the NIH was $36 million by 1955. Little did anyone realize, when the war ended, that in 1965 the budget would be $436 million and, in 1970, $1.5 billion. The National Heart Institute was founded in 1948, and ushered in the golden era of clinical investigation in cardiology.[9,51-54]

After the war ended, the wartime research scientists, who had predominantly been faculty members of medical schools, returned to their campuses and applied for NIH grant support and continued their research, with "hardly a dropped beat." When a researcher applied for another grant or a renewal of an existing grant, the major question asked of the researcher was not: "How many questions have you answered?" but rather, "How many papers have you published?" (H.D. McIntosh, personal observations).

Clinical Investigation in the Medical Schools

Medical students were attracted by the excitement of the research laboratories and soon were following in the footsteps of their mentors. They soon appreciated the importance of obtaining answers. But they also realized the importance of the length of the bibliography. In the postwar years, the mentality of "publish or perish" took a firm hold on the American scientific community. It was accepted that without a long list of publications, there were no grants. Without grants, there was no promotion. Without a promotion, there was no financial security. The mentor taught his scientists-in-training these lessons that had been learned during the urgency of wartime research. It was a case of "like father, like son." But unfortunately, little attention was directed to teaching the doctors-to-be to radiate the image of truly "caring for the patient" as seen by Sir Luke Fildes in Dr. James Clark and/or Dr. Gustavus Charles Philip Murry (H.D. McIntosh, personal observation).[1]

Now, during the postwar scientific expansion, as had been the practice during the wartime effort, all types of research were done on hospitalized patients, frequently with little relation to the disease process for which the patient was hospitalized. Young patients, hospitalized for a nonbleeding and occasionally even a bleeding peptic ulcer, were ideal subjects for cardiac catheterization and studies of the hemodynamic effects of new drugs. The patient or, really, the "experimental subject," was given only the most cursory explanation as to why the study was being carried out. The Doctrine of Informed Consent had yet to be established (H.D. McIntosh, personal observations). Few considered that the patient had Autonomy. The philosophy of medical paternalism was still operative.

The Evolution of the Nuremberg Code

Surprising as it may seem, these attitudes and practices persisted, despite the conduct at that time of the Nuremberg War Trials of the

Nazi physicians and others responsible for the glaring atrocities at Hadamar and other death mills. Not only was attention at the trial being directed to the assault on Jews, Poles, and other people, but special attention was also directed, during those trials, to the widespread practice(s) of human experimentation that had been conducted by the Nazis.

A code containing 10 Moral Principles for Conducting Human Research evolved. The opening provision of this Nuremberg Code declared: "The voluntary consent of the human subject is absolutely essential. This means that the person involved should have legal capacity to give consent." Moreover, the Code insisted that the research subject "should be so situated as to be able to exercise free power of choice" and "should have sufficient knowledge and comprehension of the elements of the subject matter involved to make an understanding and enlightened decision."

But these pronouncements from Nuremberg had little immediate effect on the American academic medical community. Many investigators had developed a large research effort during the war—a program that generated much new knowledge—but possibly even more important, a program that generated money. Research grants paid for new, expensive scientific equipment. Research grants also paid for construction of research space, and for salaries for scientists, technicians, and other support staff (H.D. McIntosh, personal observations).

Rothman, in the previously quoted publication entitled "Strangers At The Bedside,"[9,51–54] reported that the Nuremberg War Trials were mentioned in fewer than a dozen articles in *The New York Times* during 1945–1946. The announcement of the guilty verdict in August 1947, was on the front page of *The New York Times,* but the story of the execution of the 7 defendants in 1948 was on the back page of that same newspaper. Four of those tried were university-trained and university-appointed researchers who had first-rate medical credentials (L. Jaworski, U.S. Military Prosecutor at the Nuremberg International War Crimes Tribunal, personal communication).

Now the medical profession did not give the Nuremberg Trials, or the 10 Moral Principles that the Nuremberg Code defined, as much attention as did *The New York Times* (H.D. McIntosh, personal observations). The average research scientist accepted that "madness, not medicine, was implicated at Nuremberg." Furthermore, "science was pure—it was politics that was corrupting."[9,51–54]

But the decrees from Nuremberg were responsible for eventually introducing a new element into medical decision making. The Nuremberg Code outlawed medical paternalism and introduced, as the guideline for the patient-doctor relationship, the Principle of Autonomy—the right of the individual to exercise control of the course of his or her life. It is of interest that this was a right that the individual, since antiquity, had sought in all other relationships save with their physician.

Some were concerned that their institutions conform to the dictums of the Nuremberg Code. They established research committees. In 1960, Louis Welt circulated a questionnaire to 80 university departments of medicine inquiring about the practice guidelines in human experimentation. Only 8 of those 80 university departments of medicine had a procedural documentation, and only 24 had, or favored having, a committee to review problems in human experimentation. Dr. Welt concluded: "A committee cannot take responsibility. This must be in the hands of the individual investigator."[10]

By 1965, the NIH had funded between 1500 and 2000 research projects that, by title, indicated that the research would be done on humans. But the NIH had no requirements to be certain that the directives of the Nuremberg Code, published 20 years before, were being followed.[9,51–56] They accepted the conclusions of Dr. Welt.

Henry K. Beecher "Blows the Whistle"

But one physician found this total ignoring of the Nuremberg Code troublesome. That physician was Henry K. Beecher, the Door Professor of Research Anesthesiology, Harvard Service of the Massachusetts General Hospital in Boston. Beecher was impressed with the principles of the Nuremberg Code and believed that the directives of that Code not only applied to the work of physicians involved in politically directed activities but in all activities involving patients. But he saw report after report of research done in respected university laboratories and published in respected peer reviewed journals that openly violated the Nuremberg Code.

Beecher, therefore, on June 16, 1966, published in *The New England Journal of Medicine (NEJM)* a 6-page article entitled "Ethics and Clinical Research."[11] That article included abstracts of 22 studies of human subjects in the most prestigious institutions in the country and published in the most respected medical journals. Thirteen of the 22 studies were carried out in university medical centers and 3 had been carried out at the Clinical Center of the NIH. Six of the articles had been published in the *NEJM,* 5 in the *Journal of Clinical Investigation,* 2 in the *Journal of the American Medical Association (JAMA),* and 2 in *Circulation.* One of the cited articles was published in 1948, 13 were published between 1950–1959, and the remaining 8 were published between 1960–1965.

It is noteworthy that Dr. Beecher had first submitted his manuscript to *JAMA.* When originally submitted in 1965, it contained citations to 50 published studies with which he found serious criticism(s). *JAMA* rejected the manuscript, so Beecher reworked it for publication in the *NEJM.* To encourage publication, he shortened the manuscript and reduced the number of citations from 50 to 22.

Beecher's opening sentence in the article stated: "Human experimentation since World War II has created some difficult problems with increasing employment of patients as experimental subjects when it must be apparent that they would not have been available if they were truly aware of the uses that would be made of them." Beecher further stated: "An experiment is ethical or not at its inception. It does not become ethical post hoc; ends do not justify means." Beecher concluded the article by stating: "The ethical approach to experimentation in man has several components: two are more important than the others. The first being informed consent—the second is the more reliable safeguard provided by the presence of an intelligent, informed, conscientious, compassionate, responsible investigator."[11]

This article by Dr. Beecher was widely discussed in the lay press, but it caused little discussion and no significant changes in the activities in the "house of medicine." However, the publication did get the attention of the administration of the NIH and the Food and Drug Administration (FDA). On August 30, 1966, 44 days after the publication of Beecher's article, the FDA published a statement on policy concerning consent for use of investigational new drugs in humans. The following year, the NIH added a new paragraph to the Clinical Center Manual. It stated: "While there is general agreement that informed consent must be obtained, there is also the reservation that it is not possible to convey all of the information to the subject or patient upon which he can make an intelligent decision. There is a strong feeling that the protection of the subject is best achieved by group consideration and peer judgement."[9,85-93]

The Evolution of the Doctrine of Informed Consent

Walter Mondale, United States Senator from Minnesota, was concerned about Beecher's report and, in February 1968, introduced legislation to establish a Commission on Health and Society. This commission had little effect on the conduct of medical research. Finally, in 1973, Senator Edward Kennedy stated: "The question is whether or not we can tolerate a system where the individual physician is the sole determinant of the safety of an experimental procedure. After all, it is the patient who must live with the consequences of the decision." Shortly after that, 7 years after the article by Beecher, and 25 years after the Nuremberg Code was established, Senator Kennedy introduced legislation to establish the National Commission for the Protection of Human Subjects. Soon thereafter, the Doctrine of Informed Consent was established. Thus, history reveals that the Doctrine of Informed Consent was not generated by physicians/scientists in the halls of the "house of medicine." The Doctrine was established (with credit for the phrase to David J. Rothman) by "Strangers at the Bedside"—lawyers, public officials, the clergy, and ethicists.[9,85-93]

As I reflect on the revelations by Beecher and try to recall my reaction(s) at the time (1966), I don't recall a reaction. I had been a professor of medicine at Duke University for 4 years; that year, I had been named chief of the cardiovascular division of the Department of

Medicine. The Division had a very active research program using many human subjects. I do not recall reading the article by Beecher or a description thereof. Nor do I recall any discussion about the subject at scientific meetings. Furthermore, I do not recall having engaged in conversations or read about the deliberations of the National Commission for The Protection of Human Subjects, which had been established by legislation introduced by Senator Edward Kennedy (H.D. McIntosh, personal observations).

In the initial paragraphs of this document, comments were made about the lack of current interest by the medical profession in guiding of the evolution of opinions regarding Advance Directives, Durable Power of Attorney for Health, Assisted Suicide and Euthanasia. Is it not an example of history repeating itself? Would Oliver Wendell Holmes have been surprised?

The Evolution of the Living Will

The principle of autonomy embraces the right of the individual to exercise control of the course of his or her own life. Never is that right more important as when death approaches. By the mechanism of advance directives, a competent individual may decide, after thoughtful consideration, what he or she might wish to have done when death becomes inevitable. To fill this logical need, the concept of a living will evolved as the first recognized advance directive for matters of health. The term "living will" was introduced for the first time in 1967, the year after Beecher's article.[12] It was intended to serve as a testament of an individual, signed when in sound mind, regarding the use of life-sustaining medical interventions. In 1976, California became the first state to legalize such a document. It was titled The California National Death Act. As of December 1990, 41 states had enacted a living will statute. According to Basta,[13] all states now have one form or another of advance directives regarding health legislation. But there are no uniform guideline(s) that define what living wills should cover and how they should operate. All states do require an individual to be competent when signing such a document. Some states require that even if a valid living will had been signed, it would not become operative until the individual was "qualified." To become "qualified," 2 physicians must examine the patient, 1 of whom must be the attending physician and must certify in writing that the patient is suffering from a terminal illness. In such states, only under these circumstances can the living will become operative. Some states require that a person cannot sign a binding living will until he or she is suffering from a terminal illness. Other states require that a living will be reaffirmed at specific intervals. Furthermore, states vary as to whether or not life-sustaining procedures include nutrition and/or hydration. In some states, nutrition and hydration are considered therapy. They may be administered as needed. Thus, a physician must be aware of the statutes operative in the state in which he/she practices.[14]

Dr. Basta has become a vocal advocate of shifting from "terminal illness to medical planning in the last chapter of life." He states that "there is a pressing need to develop rational guidelines for end of life medical interventions." Furthermore, he emphasizes that "appropriate legislation is necessary to establish the framework to carry out agreed upon recommendations." But he emphasized that "the weighty issues must not be relinquished to medical ethicists, health care alliances, or the courts. It is the domain of physicians and the public at large." But will we and our colleagues accept the challenge and act?

The Contribution of Karen Ann Quinlan

The complexities of the problems embraced by the living will were emphasized in 1990 by the Nancy Cruzan case. But new ground that had made the introduction of the living will possible and desirable had been previously broken by the Karen Ann Quinlan case in New Jersey in 1976.[9,221–229,14,15] On the night of April 15, 1975, Karen Ann Quinlan, a 22-year-old woman, was brought to a New Jersey emergency department in a coma. The etiology of the coma was never explained. She was placed on a respirator. After several months of hoping against hope, her parents asked the physician to take her off the respirator. The Quinlans were practicing Catholics and had sought guidance from their church before requesting that the respirator be removed. They had been told that the respirator was "extraordinary care" and that returning Karen to her "natural state," that is, taking her off the respirator even if she would die, was a morally correct action. The physician first agreed to remove the respirator. He and the officials at the hospital prepared a document relieving the hospital and the staff and the physician of legal liability. But during the night, attitudes changed. The physician informed the family that taking Karen off the respirator might kill her, and he declined to commit the act.

The Quinlans asked a lower court in New Jersey to order that the physician and the hospital remove the respirator, but the court refused. The Quinlans sought help from the Supreme Court of New Jersey, which agreed to hear the case in June 1976. The court finally agreed that the family did, indeed, have the right to order the respirator to be removed. This was the first time that a court had given orders regarding therapy that did not support the orders of the physician. This was, indeed, a landmark case that involved not just the patient's right to die but also the concept of a living will. But it involved something far more specific and fundamental. It defined, "Who ruled at the bedside!"[9,221–229] The Quinlan case was a contest between physicians and patients and families and legal advisors. Until that case, the physician was presumed to represent and be the spokesperson for the patient. With the Quinlan case, the court and the lawyers gave the order and the respirator was removed. As is well known, despite the predictions by the physicians of imminent death, Karen Ann Quinlan survived off the respirator for 9 more years.

It is of more than passing interest that the United States Supreme Court, 3 years earlier, had reduced the supremacy of the physician in the *Roe v Wade* decision regarding abortion.[9,221–229] That decision claimed that the constitutionally protected right to privacy overlaid the physician-patient relationship. On the basis of that earlier decision, the New Jersey Supreme Court declared: "Presumably, the Right to Privacy is broad enough to encompass a patient's decision to decline medical treatment under such circumstances, in much the same way that it is broad enough to encompass a woman's decision to terminate pregnancy under certain conditions.[9,225] But the Court stated that the patient's right to privacy was not absolute. For example, in an abortion, the right to privacy carried little weight in the third trimester of pregnancy. The court had to decide the balance between the State's interest in preserving life and the right of the physician to exercise his or her best professional judgement. The Court declared: "We think that the State's interest, *contra* withdrawal of the respirator, weakens and the individual's Right To Privacy grows as the degree of bodily invasion increases and the prognosis dims."[9,225] Ultimately, there comes a point at which the individual's right overcomes the State's interest to preserve life. Furthermore, the Court indicated that it had the authority to challenge prevailing medical standards. The Court declared that the social values and medical values might well diverge and, when that occurred, medical practice "must, in the ultimate, be responsive to the concepts of medicine but also to the common moral judgement of the community at large."[9,225] If that occurred, it was claimed that the Court was best situated to define and implement community standards. When the New Jersey Supreme Court adjourned in 1976, the "house of medicine" had been changed forever.[9,221–229]

The Contribution of Nany Cruzan

As indicated, the events surrounding the terminal years of Nancy Cruzan also had a significant effect on the practice of medicine.[16,17] In 1983, Nancy Cruzan, a woman in her twenties, lost control of her car. The vehicle overturned, and Miss Cruzan was found lying face down in a ditch, without detectible respiratory or cardiac function. It was later estimated that she had been deprived of oxygen for about 12 to 14 minutes. Paramedics were able to restore respiratory function and she was taken to a hospital and received maximal acute care. She remained in a coma for 3 weeks but then progressed to a conscious state and was able to ingest nutrients. Later, a gastrostomy tube was implanted. Finally, a persistent vegetative state was diagnosed.

After it became apparent that Nancy had little chance of advancing from a vegetative state, her parents asked the hospital authorities in

Missouri to terminate nutrition and hydration by the gastrostomy tube. Miss Cruzan had made no advance directive as to what she wished to be done under such circumstances. She had, however, made statements to a friend and roommate that she "wouldn't want to live as a vegetable."

The hospital refused to honor the parents' request without court approval. The trial court approved the termination, but that decision was contested, and the case was taken to the state's supreme court. The Supreme Court of the State of Missouri rejected the termination, stating that "No person can assume that choice (i.e., the choice to terminate nutrition and hydration) for an incompetent person without the formalities required by Missouri's Living Will Statute."[17] The Court rejected the roommate's statement as unreliable.

The parents appealed the decision to the U.S. Supreme Court. The Supreme Court accepted Missouri's decree, and stated that individual states do have the right to demand, if life-sustaining treatment is to be withdrawn from an incompetent person, that the person must have, while competent, previously established by clear and convincing evidence that he or she would not want to be kept alive by artificial means. Thus, because Miss Cruzan had no advance directive, she had to continue to receive parenteral hydration and nutrition despite continuing to exist in a vegetative state.

Despite the lack of support of the Supreme Court, the parents persisted. They identified new and more persuasive witnesses. They took the case back to the original trial court in Missouri. After hearing testimony from the new witnesses, the judge ruled that there was now clear and convincing evidence that Miss Cruzan would not want to continue to live in a vegetative state. The gastrostomy tube that had kept the patient alive for 7 years was removed and, 12 days later, on December 26, 1990, Miss Cruzan died.

It is of more than passing interest that on December 26, 1990, when Nancy Cruzan died in the Missouri Rehabilitative Center, Mount Vernon, Missouri, rather than there being only a single security guard, as was the custom, there were 35 armed guards patrolling the premises to keep euthanasia opponents who were camped outside, from breaking into Miss Cruzan's room. The police arrested 19 individuals who had stormed the center in an attempt to find Miss Cruzan to forcefully resume the feedings.

It should be noted that, if Nancy Cruzan had a living will, it would not have altered her care in Missouri or in many other states. Many states, including Missouri, consider that life-sustaining treatment serves only to postpone the moment of death. Implicitly, treatments intended to restore function are considered to be technological interventions, not simply food and water. Furthermore, the U.S. Supreme Court established that each state could establish its own standards allowing a substitute decision maker to exercise decision making for an incompetent person. Finally, it is usually considered that living wills are intended for members of the older segment of our society. Nancy Cruzan was in her twenties when she needed it.[16]

It is of more than passing interest that the decision of the U.S. Supreme Court in the Cruzan case was split, 5:4. Supreme Court Justice Brennan, in dissenting, stated eloquently: "Too few people execute Living Wills or equivalent forms of Directives for such an evidentiary rule to ensure adequately that the wishes of an incompetent person will be honored. When a person tells family or close friends, however, that she does not want her life sustained artificially, she is expressing her wishes in the only terms familiar to her. To require more is unrealistic for all practical purposes. It precludes the right of the patient to forego life-sustaining treatment." (Cruzan, U.S. Supreme Court, June 1990.)

The Evolution of the Durable Power of Attorney

Now the concept of advance directives, of which a living will is a recently established example, has been for centuries firmly established in the legal system. The most familiar form is the last will and testament. Such a directive serves, upon death, as an instructional device to designate, for example, how property is to be distributed. It may serve to donate organs or support a specific organization. The last will and testament may also designate a surrogate as an executor. In that capacity, the executor would act in the individual's behalf, but not in matters of health.

Because of limitations of existing living wills, in 1989 California broadened the authority of advance directives and established a durable power of attorney.[18] Such a directive expressly authorizes the appointment of proxies for making health care decisions and specifies how individuals may identify a person to make decisions about their health care if they are no longer competent to decide for themselves.

Now the authority of a durable power of attorney is different from a traditional power of attorney. A power of attorney becomes invalid when the principal, that is, the individual being represented, becomes incompetent. A durable power of attorney, however, remains valid after the principal becomes incompetent. Therefore, the principal can personally choose those who will have authority over his or her affairs by this procedure. But the durable power of attorney must be executed while the principal is still competent.

The surrogate's actions, that is, the person acting for the principal, should be guided by the principle of substituted judgement. The surrogate will hopefully make the decisions that the patient would have made had he or she been able to do so. The durable power of attorney for health care confers on the surrogate great power over the well-being of another person. It therefore engenders the potential for abuse. The decision of the surrogate cannot command the ethical force of contemporaneous decision making by the informed, competent patient. Therefore, if the surrogate's decision(s) appear to the physician to be unreasonable or contrary to the patient's best interests, the physician must seek advice of a hospital ethics committee, or even the courts, before following instructions.[16,19]

As previously stated, all states now have one form or another advance directive legislation; over 30 states have proxy statutes.[13] Establishment of such a vehicle is generally inexpensive and does not require court involvement.

Do Not Resuscitate Order

The most widely publicized and simplest to establish advance directive is the do not resuscitate (DNR) order. But a decision to initiate or forego life-prolonging procedures such as cardiopulmonary resuscitation, can present profound medical and ethical dilemmas for the physician, the nurse, the patient, the family, and society at large. Physicians are trained, from the outset, always to act in favor of sustaining life. But this objective can conflict with another fundamental objective of medicine: the relief of suffering. These dilemma were intensified by the evolution of increasingly sophisticated technology and its potential use in an aging population[20–22] adding further difficulties to easily defining a course of action are economic factors.

But it has been well established that the public has not been encouraged by physicians and other health care providers to establish such directives regarding their preferences for treatment as death becomes imminent.[13–15,23–27] So it should not be surprising that in the absence of a leadership role by the "house of medicine" to encourage the patient to establish advance directives, some other force would.

The Patient's Self-Determination Act

The Cruzan case served as the stimulus to popularize the concept of advance directives. Senator John Danforth, from Missouri, was acutely aware of the burdens that situations similar to Nancy Cruzan's placed on all parties—the families, physicians, nurses, and other health care professionals, the health care facilities, and the courts. He assumed that agonizing situations of this sort could be avoided if patients like Nancy Cruzan had known about, and taken advantage of, laws allowing people to exercise advance directives while still competent. Despite the policies, few took proper advantage of what could be done. Therefore, in October 1989, Senator Danforth and Senator Daniel Moynihan from New York, introduced in the U.S. Congress the Right of Self-determination Act.[23]

As a result of this effort, the Patients' Self-determination Act (PSDA) was enacted in 1991. Since then, if an individual in the United States is admitted to a hospital or a nursing home that is reimbursed by Medicare or Medicaid, or if that individual receives care from any federally reimbursed health care maintenance organization, hospice, or other type of health care company, that facility must provide the patient with written legal rights concerning advance directives. In addition, the patient must be informed of the health care organization's policies insuring the implementation of such rights. Furthermore, the health care provider must note in the medical record of the patient if he/she had made an advance directive.[23,24]

The stated purpose of the legislation was to assist the individual to attain and maintain autonomy. Unfortunately, these legally mandated exchanges frequently take place hurriedly in the emergency department or admitting office of the health care facility when the patient may be physically and/or emotionally unstable; furthermore, the health care provider may be represented by a harassed, overworked admission clerk (H.D. McIntosh, personal observation).

It is, indeed, unfortunate that although by tradition physicians were considered to perform their activities for patients with beneficence and were encouraged to practice medical paternalism, physicians have shown no interest, in an organized manner, to insure that their patients attain and maintain their autonomy through a legally recognized advance directive. Thus, Senators Danforth and Moynihan, and others in the federal government, bypassed physicians and granted the responsibility of attaining and maintaining autonomy to third party deliverers of health care.

As previously stated, the Act mandated that health care professionals discuss with all hospitalized or nursing home patients who receive Medicare or Medicaid reimbursements, the importance and types of advance directives. But despite this Federal Directive and several educational campaigns, such as the Study to Understand Prognosis and Preferences for Outcomes and Risks of Treatments (SUPPORT), funded by the Robert Wood Johnson Foundation in the amount of $28 million, many patients and families are still ambivalent about what to do when serious illness and death becomes a real possibility. Only about 15% of persons in the United States had, in 1996, executed such documents.[27] Unfortunately, physicians rarely initiate discussions with their patients about even the most widely used advance directive: the DNR order.[4,18,19,27]

Physician–assisted Suicide and Euthanasia

Patients are frequently confused about having to make life and death decisions far in advance. How can one be sure how much pain one would tolerate to participate in some event that was really important?

It is not surprising that much widespread ambivalence has fueled intense national debate over legalizing the practice of physician-assisted suicide or active euthanasia. On November 8, 1994, Oregon became the first state to legalize physician-assisted suicide. Previous efforts, in Washington State in 1991 and California in 1992, to legalize euthanasia had failed. The Oregon Death with Dignity Act was passed by the slim margin of 51.3% to 48.7%.[28] But subsequent legal challenges kept the law from going into effect. The U.S. Supreme Court recently heard the case and ruled that states in fact have the right to outlaw physician-assisted suicide.

The court further held that there is no fundamental right to assistance in committing suicide and that legally, distinguishing between refusing life-saving medical treatment and requesting assistance in suicide, comports with fundamental legal principles of causation and intent. Chief Justice Rehnquist stated that the right to commit suicide with another's assistance is not one of the "fundamental rights and liberties deeply rooted in the national history and tradition."[29] The Supreme Court also invalidated the earlier decision by the Ninth Circuit Court of Appeals, which had concluded that a competent adult ". . . has a strong liberty interest in choosing a dignified and humane death . . . including not just refusal of treatment but also 'hastening one's own death'".[29]

In an attempt to settle the issue once and for all, Oregon's legislators offered the voters another chance at the polls. The citizens responded with the largest voter turnout in years and voted $3:2$ in support of physicians being able to assist a patient die. The law allows physicians to give lethal doses of drugs, but not lethal injections, to patients who have 6 months or less to live, as determined by at least 2 physicians, provided the patient is of sound mind and makes a written request to die. But as of this publication, the law has not been implemented. The Drug Enforcement Agency (DEA) has warned that the measure violates federal narcotics laws and doctors risk losing their licenses by writing prescriptions to assist patients commit suicide.[28]

Even proponents of the Oregon law are concerned that the practice of assisted suicide could gradually be expanded from physician-assisted suicide to active euthanasia, both nonvoluntary (when the patient is unable to request or consent) or involuntary (when the patient is competent and does not request to consent). This development is usually referred to as the "slippery slope" and if and when that occurs, our patients will clearly have lost their hard fought for autonomy.[29]

Complacency of Physicians

But the medical profession must appreciate the feelings of the public. While this document was being prepared, the December 30, 1997, local paper described a 71-year-old lady, living only 40 miles away, traveling from Eureka Springs, Florida, to Detroit, Michigan, "to end her life with the help of physician Jack Kevorkian." The patient allegedly had "cancer in the left breast which had spread to her lungs." The paper reported her friend of 40 years stating that, "I guess she just got tired of being sick" . . . "Kevorkian and a medical associate, George Reding, delivered Langford's body, slumped over in a wheelchair to the Oakland County Medical Examiners' Office about 7:10 PM Saturday".[30]

Unfortunately, no physician group was heard in the halls of Congress during the hearings devoted to developing the PSDA. However, at the same time elsewhere in the halls of Congress, legislation regarding reimbursement for the interpretation of electrocardiograms was being discussed. More than 2 dozen medical organizations had representatives speaking out for physicians to receive reimbursement for the interpretation of ECGs (A.A. Hutter, Jr, personal communication).

If the "house of medicine" was and is interested in continuing to be thought of as practicing with beneficence and deserving to be considered paternalistic, which of the 2 hearing would have, or should have had, the largest medical representation? One cannot help wondering which hearing Sir James Clark,[5] the physician of Queen Victoria, or Dr. Gustavus Charles Philip Murry,[7] or Dr. Francis Peabody[4] would have attended.

Is it not time for the members of the "house of medicine" assume the responsibility for discussing, at the time of each complete physical evaluation of a patient or evaluation of a new major symptom complex in the physician's office, whether that patient has established an advance directive, ideally, a durable Power of attorney? If the patient has established such a directive, should not the physician then review the decisions embraced by the directive with the patient to be sure that the patient has considered what will be necessary to maintain his or her autonomy and be certain that, if changes in attitude have occurred since the last discussion, they are incorporated into the existing directive? If the patient does not have an appropriate advance directive, should not the physician assist the patient in attaining one? Then, should not the physician give the patient a wallet-sized card that contains information regarding the advance directives that could be presented in the future to the "harassed, overworked admitting clerk" representing the health care provider, who was attempting to fulfill the requirements of PSDA of 1991? At that time, should not the patient of the beneficent, paternalistic physician, showing the card to the health care worker, be able to say "You may relax, I've done it!'"?

But the lack of interest in formulation of policies to assist the patient to attain and maintain autonomy should not be surprising. Unfortunately, organized medicine is rarely, if ever, *anticipatory;* rather, organized medicine is almost always *reactionary.* Should not the "house of medicine" have been able to predict that advance directives would become a universally adopted document and, anticipating that to be the case, should not the "house of medicine" have taken the lead in developing the process? If the answer is "yes," why should not we, as physicians, develop, even if a bit late, guidelines for The End of Life

Medical Interventions proposed by Dr. Basta[13] and the "I've Done It" card? If we don't, it may soon be too late to prevent having to "read more unpleasant history!"

References

1. McIntosh HD: The maturation of a cardiologist with reflections on the "Passing Sands of Time." *Ann Emerg Med* 15:1101–1110, 1986.
2. McIntosh HD: From academia to private practice, or the maturation of a physician. *Int J Cardiol* 5:260–268, 1984.
3. Council on Ethical and Judicial Affairs, American Medical Association, Code of Medical Ethics, 1997.
4. Peabody FW: *Doctor and Patient: Papers on the Relationship of the Physician to Men and Institutions.* New York, NY, Macmillan & Co, 1930.
5. Tomanek J: *The Doctor.* Philadelphia, PA, Scope, Philadelphia Campus Publishing, 1950, p 115.
6. Weinberg SL: President's Page. Remembering Keats in Rome. *J Am Coll Cardiol* 22:943–945, 1993.
7. Rinsler A: "The Doctor." *J Med Biography* 1:165–170, 1993.
8. McIntosh HD: Attaining and maintaining autonomy. In: E. Chesler, ed. *Clinical Cardiology in the Elderly.* Armonk, NY, Futura Publishing Co, Inc, 1994, pp. 547–563.
9. Rothman DJ: *Strangers at the Bedside. A History of How Law and Bioethics Transformed Medical Decision Making.* New York, NY, Basic Books, 1991.
10. Welt LG: Reflection on the problems of human experimentation. *Conn Med* 25:75–78, 1961.
11. Beecher HK: Ethics and clinical research. *N Engl J Med* 274:1354–1369, 1966.
12. Lazaroff AE, Orr WF: Living wills and other advance directives. *Clin Geriatr Med* 2:521–534, 1986.
13. Basta L, Tauth J: *High Technology Near End of Life: Setting Limits. J Am Coll Cardiol* 28:1623–1630, 1996.
14. Doudera AE: Developing issues in medical decision-making: The durable power or attorney and institutional ethics committees. *Prim Care* 13:315–325, 1986.
15. Caralis PV: Withdrawal and withholding of life-supporting food and fluids. One state's struggle. *J Fla Med Assoc* 77:821–828, 1990.
16. Saultz J: Routine discussion of advance health care directives: Are we ready? An affirmative view. *J Fam Pract* 31:653–655, 1990.
17. Rodriguez GS: An opposing view. *J Fam Pract* 31:656–659, 1990.
18. Steinbrook R, Lo B: Decision making for incompetent patient by designating proxy—California's new law. *N Engl J Med* 310:1598–1601, 1984.
19. Gillon R: Living wills, powers of attorney and medical practice. *J Med Ethics* 14:59–60, 1988.
20. Fox M, Lipton HL: The decision to perform cardiopulmonary resuscitation. *N Engl J Med* 309:607–608, 1983.
21. President's Commission for the Study of Ethical Problems in Medicine and Biomedical and Behavior Research. Deciding to forego life-sustaining treatment: A report on the ethical, medical and legal issues in treatment decisions. Washington, DC: Government Printing Office. 1983:15.

22. Lo B: Unanswered questions about DNR orders. *JAMA* 265:1874–1875, 1991.
23. Capron AM: The Patient Self-determination Act: New responsibilities for health care providers. *J Am Health Policy* January/February: 140–143, 1992.
24. Charnow JA: Law spurs upfront talk with patients about advance directives. *ACP Observer* December 1991, p 4.
25. Cohen CB: 1990 and beyond: The genie out of the bottle. *Hastings Cent Rep* September/October: 33–35, 1990.
26. Gamble ER, McDonald PJ, Lichstein PR: Knowledge, attitudes, and behavior of elderly persons regarding living wills. *Arch Intern Med* 151:277–280, 1991.
27. Feinberg AW: The care of dying patients. *Ann Intern Med* 126:164–165, 1997.
28. Wilson JF: Oregon voters reaffirm physician assisted-suicide law. *ACP Observer* 12:3, 1997.
29. Churchill LR, King NMP: Physician-assisted suicide, euthanasia, or withdrawal of treatment. *Br Med J* 315:137–138, 1997.
30. Sloan J: Woman's use of Kevorkian surprises neighbors. *The Tampa Tribune* December 30:1, 1997.

Chapter 30

Cardiopulmonary Resuscitation in the Elderly

Philip J. Podrid

Each year 350,000 to 500,000 Americans experience sudden cardiac death, the leading cause of mortality in the United States.[1] Sudden death is one of the principal complications of heart disease, particularly coronary artery disease (CAD) with or without myocardial infarction (MI) and cardiomyopathy. Because the incidence of heart disease, particularly CAD, increases with age and is a frequent problem in the elderly, a substantial number of those experiencing sudden cardiac death are older patients, above age 65 years. In addition to the presence of structural heart disease, which is often diffuse and severe in the older patient, other chronic medical problems are often present that can also have an independent impact on survival. These cardiac and noncardiac factors have a particularly important impact on the short- and long-term survival of patients after a cardiac arrest and hence they need to be considered in regard to resuscitation. Since the incidence of sudden cardiac death is high among the elderly, it is important to review the outcome of resuscitation in this group for estimating the cost/benefit of this procedure, thus permitting establishment of guidelines for not performing cardiopulmonary resuscitation (CPR).

Sudden Cardiac Death: Mechanism and Defibrillation

It has been well established that the mechanism of sudden cardiac death in the vast majority of patients is a ventricular tachyarrhythmia,

From *Clinical Cardiology in the Elderly. Second Edition,* edited by Elliot Chesler. © 1999, Futura Publishing Company, Armonk, NY.

principally ventricular fibrillation.[2] This arrhythmia is the result of chaotic electrical activity originating within the ventricular myocardium. A necessary precondition for this disorder of electrical impulse conduction is an abnormal substrate which includes diffuse myocardial disease or the presence of localized areas of tissue necrosis and patchy fibrosis. These conditions disrupt the normal electrical system of the heart, ie, the His Purkinje system that often survives despite the underlying disease.[3,4] As a result of areas of delayed conduction and altered repolarization or recovery, the ventricular myocardium is electrically unstable and capable of developing multiple microreentrant circuits, necessary for the establishment of continuous reentry, the usual mechanism for serious ventricular tachyarrhythmias. Under the appropriate conditions, multiple reentrant circuits become simultaneously activated, resulting in localized areas of continuous electrical activity.[5] The multiple wavelets of activation produce small areas of independently contracting myocardium resulting in the inability of the ventricle to contract uniformly, With the absence of any effective contraction there is no cardiac output. Since there is a total absence of blood flow and tissue perfusion and no supply of glucose or oxygen, ischemia occurs and, if prolonged, cellular and tissue damage occur. After approximately four minutes, cellular damage becomes irreversible and ultimately death of tissue ensues.[6] The brain is perhaps the organ most vulnerable to the effect of acute hypoxia. Unless there is prompt restoration of organized electrical activity and effective cardiac pumping action leading to an increase in cardiac output with the resumption of tissue perfusion and sufficient supply of oxygen, the outcome is death of the individual.

Once ventricular fibrillation is established, it is invariably persistent unless interrupted by another, usually external, source of electrical current that produces simultaneous global depolarization of all myocardial tissue, therefore terminating reentry.[7] During ventricular fibrillation, multiple reentrant circuits are active and with defibrillation, they become simultaneously depolarized and inactivated, unable to continue generating reentry, permitting resumption of sinus node activity and restoration of its role as dominant pacemaker. In the presence of a normal sinus impulse, ventricular activation is organized and orderly, resulting in effective myocardial contraction.

The technique of delivering a high-energy, nonsynchronized shock to the heart is known as direct current external defibrillation.[8] During the performance of CPR, 2 paddle electrodes are placed on the chest, one to the right of the sternum and the other at the apex of the heart. In this way, the 2 paddles are separated from each other by an adequate distance. An electric shock of 200 to 400 W seconds (Joules) is delivered via these electrodes, thereby causing the entire heart to become depolarized simultaneously.

Defibrillation renders all myocardial tissue and, hence, reentrant circuits refractory in a homogeneous fashion. Ventricular fibrillation ceases since the appropriate conditions necessary for its precipitation are no longer present. Although defibrillation is highly effective for terminating ventricular fibrillation and reestablishing sinus rhythm, the ability to successfully defibrillate the heart decreases as the duration of the arrhythmia increases.[9] It has been observed in both an animal model and in clinical practice that with the onset of ventricular fibrillation, the electrical activity is manifest as fibrillatory waves on the surface electrocardiogram (ECG) that are rapid in rate, very irregular in morphology and interval and are coarse, ie, of high amplitude, indicating the presence of chaotic electrical activity involving the entire myocardium. As the duration of fibrillation continues and there is death of myocardial tissue, these fibrillatory waves become progressively reduced in amplitude or finer, eventually resulting in the absence of all electrical activity, represented as a flat line on the ECG, or asystole.[10] Since successful defibrillation requires the presence of some electrical activity, asystole cannot be reverted with defibrillation and there is generally little, if any, chance for survival once asystole occurs. This has been confirmed in a number of clinical studies that have reported virtually no survival when the initial rhythm documented on the ECG is asystole, while 20% to 50% of patients with out-of-hospital ventricular fibrillation survive to be admitted to a hospital.[11]

Outcome of Cardiopulmonary Resuscitation and Defibrillation

Although ventricular fibrillation can often be terminated with the use of a defibrillator, in-hospital mortality is high and the percentage of patients surviving the hospitalization and ultimately being discharged is still low (Table 1).[11] Interestingly, the majority of hospital deaths in patients successfully resuscitated from a ventricular tachyarrhythmia result from either irreversible brain damage or pulmonary and infectious complications due to the prolonged intubation and respiratory support often necessary in these patients. In the experience of Myerburg and coworkers[12] 30% of the in-hospital deaths were caused by a low output state and cardiogenic shock, 38% were a direct result of anoxic encephalopathy, and in 21% had an infection due to a prolonged period of respirator dependency. Only 10% of the deaths were the result of recurrent ventricular tachyrhythmia.

One of the earliest reports of survival after resuscitation from out-of-hospital ventricular fibrillation comes from the Seattle Heart Watch Program, which reported on 146 patients, average age 60 years, who were successfully resuscitated from out-of hospital sudden death and subsequently discharged from the hospital.[13] These patients represented 16% of a total of 886 patients who had received out-of-hospital CPR. The authors reported that the outcome of CPR was related to the status of the patient at the time emergency medical technicians (EMTs) arrived and the etiology of the initial rhythm on the ECG. The survival

Table 1
Outcome of Cardiopulmonary Resuscitation

Study	Group	No.	Success CPR (%)	Discharged
Liberthson 15	Outpatient	301	99 (33)	42 (14)
Thompson 16	Outpatient	316	199 (63)	88 (28)
Fusgen 29	Outpatient	335	335 (100)	23 (7)
Taffet 24	Inpatient/Outpatient	399	160 (40)	24 (6)
Bedell 25	Inpatient	294	129 (44)	41 (14)
Bayer 28	Inpatient/Outpatient (Elderly)	95	37 (39)	16 (17)
Murphy 31	Inpatient/Outpatient (Elderly)	503	110 (22)	19 (4)
Wuerz 32	Outpatient	563		
	<65	212	34 (16)	11 (5)
	>65	320	58 (18)	13 (4)
Bonnin 33	Outpatient	986		
	<70	619	160 (26)	73 (12)
	>70	367	81 (22)	24 (7)
Myerburg 11	Outpatient	352	200 (57)	67 (19)
Ritter 17	Outpatient	2142	407 (19)	171 (8)
Greene 22	Outpatient	447	268 (60)	89 (20)
Varon 51	Inpatient (elderly)	89	18 (20)	8 (9)
O'Keefe 52	Outpatient	274	82 (30)	25 (9)
	<70	99		19 (19)
	>70	175		6 (3)
Juchems 53	Outpatient	898		
	<70	495		71 (14)
	>70	403		44 (11)
	Inpatient	572		
	<70	245		70 (28)
	>70	327		46 (140)
Overall		8475	2194 (31)*	979 (12)
Schneider 14	Metaanalysis inpatient	19,955		2994 (15)
	<70			(16.2)
	>70			(12.4)

* 2194/7003 (does not include Juchems study for which there is no data about successful CPR)

rate was 15% among the 821 patients who were in ventricular fibrillation when EMTs arrived, compared with a 37% survival rate among 65 patients who were initially conscious and in sinus rhythm but who developed ventricular fibrillation after the arrival of EMTs. This difference in outcome was likely related to the promptness with which CPR was instituted and defibrillation performed, limiting the duration of ventricular fibrillation among whom its onset is observed.

It is important to recognize that this survival rate of 16% represented the best that could be achieved at the time, since the Seattle Heart Watch Program was a community-based CPR program with a well- organized and efficient emergency medical system that responded quickly to a call allowing for the initiation of CPR within 4 to 5 minutes after the onset of ventricular fibrillation. Unfortunately, the results of CPR for out-of-hospital sudden death have not improved substantially over the years. For example, Schneider and coworkers[14] reported a meta-analysis of 98 reports involving in-hospital CPR performed on 19,955 patients. Overall, 15% of patients survived to be discharged and this was constant over the 30-year period. In this review, age was a factor in the outcome and the success rate was lower in those over 70 years of age, ie. 12.4% versus 16.2% for those less than 70 years of age.

In the study from Seattle, electrocardiographic evidence of acute MI was observed in only 24 patients (17%), although lactate dehydrogenase isoenzyme patterns indicated some myocardial necrosis in 57% of the patients. In many of these cases, it is unclear whether the myocardial damage was actually a result of the ventricular fibrillation and myocardial hypoxia, rather than the cause. Although the frequency of an acute MI was low, in the Seattle experience, the presence of an acute infarction was more frequently documented in patients who developed ventricular fibrillation after the arrival of EMTs while the incidence was very low in those who were in ventricular fibrillation on the arrival of emergency personnel.

During an average follow-up of 418 days, a significant number of the 146 patients who were discharged from the hospital had a recurrent episode of ventricular fibrillation and the mortality rate at 1 year was 26% and at the end of two years it was 38%. However, among the patients with ventricular fibrillation precipitated by an acute MI, the 1- and 2-year mortality was 14% and 25%, respectively, compared with a 30% and 47%, respectively, among those without an acute MI. Therefore, when ventricular fibrillation is provoked by a definable and often transient event, such as an MI, outcome is better and arrhythmia is less likely to recur during follow-up. In contrast, the prognosis is worse when ventricular fibrillation is primary and unassociated with any definable precipitating cause.

Another report by Liberthson and coworkers[15] involved 301 patients, average age 63 years, who were in ventricular fibrillation on arrival of EMTs. Although initial defibrillation was successful in 199 patients (66%), 98 patients died at the scene or in the ambulance before admission to the hospital, an additional 59 patients died in the hospital, while only 42 patients (14%) were discharged. In this study, 57% of those hospitalized experienced recurrent arrhythmia (ventricular tachycardia [VT] or ventricular fibrillation), which generally occurred within the first 24 hours after admission. Congestive heart failure (CHF) was present in 63% of the patients, cardiogenic shock in 25%, and pulmonary complications developed in 42%. Of the 42 patients who survived to be discharged from the hospital, 28% had mild and 12%

had severe neurological deficits. Interestingly, the average age of those discharged from the hospital was 8 years less than those who were initially resuscitated but who died in the hospital, suggesting that age was a factor influencing ultimate outcome. Of prognostic importance was the first rhythm documented by EMTs after resuscitation and defibrillation which may reflect the amount of myocardial damage. Patients who had sinus tachycardia or atrial fibrillation had a better outcome than those with sinus bradycardia or a junctional or idioventricular rhythm. This is likely related to the duration of the ventricular fibrillation before defibrillation is performed.

It is apparent that one of the important factors related to survival is the time delay between the onset of cardiac arrest, the initiation of CPR, and the administration of definitive therapy (ie, defibrillation), since the duration of hypoxia is an important factor determining extent and reversibility of damage to the brain and other organs. As indicated, the longer the interval between the onset of the arrhythmia and restoration of a stable rhythm, cardiac function, and sufficient blood flow to the brain, the lower the survival rate. There is a greater chance for long-term survival if CPR is bystander-initiated, which shortens the duration of ventricular fibrillation compared to the delay that occurs when waiting for the arrival of emergency personnel.

In the Seattle Heart Watch Program, Thompson and coworkers[16] reviewed data on 316 patients, average age 63, initially resuscitated at the scene from out-of-hospital sudden cardiac death. There were 117 patients (37%) who died prior to hospitalization (at the scene in the ambulance, or in the emergency room) and 106 (34%) who died in hospital despite successful resuscitation. The average age of those patients who were successfully resuscitated at the scene and admitted to the hospital was 58 years, less than that of the entire group, suggesting that age was a factor in the ability to resuscitate the patient from ventricular fibrillation, and was associated with a better initial survival. Of the 199 patients resuscitated and admitted to the hospital, only 90 patients (28% of the entire group of 316) were ultimately discharged home. Survival was related to the duration of ventricular fibrillation prior to CPR, ie, whether CPR was bystander-initiated or EMT-initiated. Earlier CPR was initiated by a bystander in 109 patients and 73 (67%) were successfully resuscitated and admitted to the hospital. Ultimately, 47 of these patients (43% of the total group, 64% of those successfully resuscitated) were discharged from the hospital. Delayed resuscitation by EMTs was performed in 207 patients and 126 (61%) were initially resuscitated and admitted to the hospital (P = not significant compared to the group with bystander-initiated CPR). However, only 46 of these patients (22% of the total group and 37% of those initially resuscitated) were discharged from the hospital ($P < 0.001$ compared to those with bystander-initiated CPR). While the duration of ventricular fibrillation and an earlier time for initiating CPR was not associated with the ability to resuscitate a patient, it did have a favorable impact on hospital outcome and ultimate survival. This is largely the result of less time for cerebral hypoxia, ischemia of other organs and, hence, less tissue damage.

An association between delay in instituting CPR and performing defibrillation and outcome has been reported by others. Ritter and co-workers[17] retrospectively analyzed the outcome of 2142 patients who experienced a cardiac arrest. When CPR was initiated by a bystander, 22.9% of patients survived to be admitted to the hospital and 11.9% of these patients were ultimately discharged. In contrast, when CPR was not initiated by a bystander, resuscitation was successful in 14 % who were then admitted to the hospital, but only 4.7% were discharged (P < 0.001). Guzy and coworkers[18] also reported a lower survival rate when CPR was not initiated by bystanders (5%) compared to a 22% survival rate when CPR was bystander-initiated (P < 0.001).

The better outcome from effective bystander-initiated CPR is due to the more rapid restoration of some cerebral blood flow and perfusion to other vital organs resulting in maintenance of oxygenation. This reduces the amount of neurological damage prior to delivering definitive therapy, ie, defibrillation, and reestablishment of hemodynamic stability and normal tissue perfusion. However, even when CPR is initiated early and defibrillation is performed promptly, the overall survival of patients resuscitated from out-of-hospital sudden death is still low. This is likely due to other factors that have an impact on the severity and extent of the brain damage resulting from cessation of blood flow for even a brief period. Of major importance is the presence of underlying cerebrovascular disease such as that associated with hypertension; carotid artery atherosclerosis; or previous cerebrovascular accident resulting from any cause such as thrombosis, embolism, or ruptured aneurysm. In patients with these underlying abnormalities, the presence of even a brief period of cerebral ischemia might result in severe irreversible brain damage.

Another factor associated with poor outcome is the severity of heart disease and presence of CHF. In these situations, the absence of myocardial perfusion, even if brief, may result in further myocardial damage and dysfunction aggravating the underlying abnormalities. In these cases, the restoration of electrical activity, even if prompt, may not result in adequate mechanical function and a low output state and cardiogenic shock may occur. Additionally, there is a risk of recurrent ventricular fibrillation even when antiarrhythmic drug therapy is administered in these patients who usually have very advanced and severe heart disease. Even if successfully resuscitated, these patients also have an increased mortality as a result of progressive CHF.

The presence of underlying chronic diseases involving other organ systems is an additional factor that has an impact on survival after cardiac arrest. If there is preexisting hepatic or renal insufficiency, progressive deterioration of organ function may result from ventricular fibrillation and the absence of cardiac output. Ultimately, hepatic or renal failure may cause severe metabolic and electrolyte disorders that have significant impact on cardiac function, can result in a recurrence of arrhythmia, and can affect survival. These factors have a substantial effect on the ultimate outcome of patients initially resuscitated from cardiac arrest and admitted to the hospital, and may contribute to the high in-hospital mortality.

Age and Relationship to the Outcome of Cardiopulmonary Resuscitation

Although the long-term survival is poor in most studies reporting the outcome of patients resuscitated from out-of-hospital or in- hospital sudden death, the majority of these studies involve patients of all ages. While most of these studies do not specifically analyze the outcome based on age, there is a suggestion that age is a factor. Dickey and coworkers[19] reported on 190 patients who underwent CPR and were discharged from the hospital. In this trial, survival at 1, 2, 5, 10, and 20 years after hospitalization was 76%, 60%, 41%, 27%, and 12%, respectively. Factors related to long-term survival were ventricular fibrillation as the presenting arrhythmia, ventricular fibrillation associated with an MI, the duration of the arrest before resuscitation, the presence of hypotension after the arrest, use of digoxin, need for diuretics (indicating the presence of left ventricular [LV] dysfunction and CHF), and age greater than 60 years.

In a review of 710 patients who had a cardiac arrest, Marwick and coworkers[20] reported on a cohort of 193 patients (27%) who were successfully resuscitated from out-of-hospital sudden death. Variables associated with successful CPR and in-hospital survival were the nature of the rhythm at the time of the arrest, a delay in instituting CPR, and age. Factors related to long-term survival were the need for intubation during hospitalization, the time delay in administering CPR, and age. Tortolani et al[21] reported similar results in a cohort of 407 patients who experienced an in-hospital cardiac arrest. After 24 hours, 153 patients (38%) were alive, but ultimately only 69 patients (45% of initial survivors and 17% of total population) were discharged from the hospital. Independent predictors of hospital survival were the location of arrest (ie, general medical ward versus intensive care unit or emergency room), CPR duration of less than 15 minutes, a nonasystolic arrest not the result of a cardiac cause, and the need for less than one intravenous medication during the hospitalization. In addition to these factors, other independent predictors of long-term survival were the need for intubation after CPR and the patient's age.

The Seattle Heart Watch Program reported the outcome of 447 patients with out-of- hospital sudden death who underwent CPR [22]. There were 269 (60%) patients who were initially resuscitated, but only 114 patients (26%) were discharged from the hospital. Predictors of overall mortality were poor LV function and a low ejection fraction, presence of extensive heart disease, primary ventricular fibrillation not associated with an MI, frequent ventricular premature beats on ambulatory monitoring, inducibility during an electrophysiological study, exercise-induced angina or hypotension, and age. George and coworkers[23] performed a multivariate analysis of patients undergoing CPR and reported that independent predictors of overall mortality were postarrest hypotension, azotemia, and age greater than 65 years. Similar results were reported by Taffet and coworkers[24] in a retrospective analysis of 399 patients. CPR was initially successful in 48 of cardiac arrests that were witnessed and in only 30 of those not witnessed. When analyzed according to age, 31% of CPR attempts were successful in those patients over the age of 70 years, but none of these patients survived hospitalization. Among patients younger than 70 years of age, CPR was successful in 43 percent, although only 10% of these patients survived the hospitalization and were discharged. Predictors of poor outcome were the presence of sepsis after CPR, a diagnosis of cancer, the number of medications being administered, a cardiac arrest that was unwitnessed, and age.

Therefore, successful resuscitation and long-term survival of a patient resuscitated from out-of- hospital sudden death is related to a number of factors, but the most important are age, the duration of ventricular fibrillation, the nature and extent of underlying heart disease, and the presence and severity of other chronic disease states such as hypertension, diabetes, renal or liver disease, and central nervous system (CNS) abnormalities (Table 2). While the presence of chronic disease is a concern in any patient, it is particularly important in the elderly who often have more advanced cardiac and cerebrovascular disease and a higher incidence of other chronic diseases.

While the poor outcome of patients with out-of-hospital cardiac arrest is associated with delay in defibrillation, similar results and low survival rates have also been reported among hospitalized patients who

---

Table 2
Predictors of Outcome from
Cardiopulmonary Resuscitation

Age
Initial rhythm (VT, VF, asystole)
Absence of vital signs
Duration of arrest prior to CPR
Duration of CPR
Need for intubation
Poor LV function
Presence of multiple chronic diseases
Hypotension after CPR
Anemia prior to CPR
Sepsis post-CPR
Debilitated state prior to arrest

have a witnessed cardiac arrest and undergo CPR. Bedell and coworkers[25] prospectively analyzed data on 294 consecutive patients, average age 70 years, who had ventricular fibrillation and were resuscitated during hospitalization in a university teaching hospital. CPR was performed in the intensive care unit or emergency room in 61% of the patients and was performed in a general ward in 25%. Despite prompt CPR, 166 (56%) patients died while 144 (49%) initially survived after early CPR attempts. However, of the 144 patients successfully resuscitated, 31 died within 24 hours (11% of the total group, 22% of the initial survivors) and ultimately 56 patients (19% of the total group and 39% of the initial survivors) died in the hospital. Overall, only 41 patients (14% of the total group or 28% of those initially resuscitated) were discharged from the hospital. The median duration of hospitalization was 6 days (range 1 to 61 days) for those who died in the hospital and was 26 days (range 8 to 61 days) for those who were discharged. At 6 months, 8 of these 41 patients had died, while 33 were still alive, yielding an overall survival at 6 months of 11%. Interestingly, in this study, the etiology of the arrest was a ventricular tachyarrhythmia in only 33% of patients, while 27% had respiratory arrest, 18% had asystole as the first rhythm documented, 16% had electromechanical dissociation, and in 4% complete heart block was the presumed cause. Unlike the population of patients with out-of hospital cardiac arrest, the delay before initiating CPR was short and, in 89% 5 minutes after the arrest. The duration of CPR was less than 15 minutes in 16% of patients, over 15 minutes in 82%, and over 30 minutes in 61%. Using a logistic regression multivariate analysis, factors present before the arrest that predicted mortality after CPR were hypotension, pneumonia, renal failure, cancer, and a homebound lifestyle prior to hospitalization. Significant factors associated with failure to resuscitate the patient during the arrest included an arrest duration longer than 15 minutes, need for intubation, hypotension, pneumonia, and homebound lifestyle prior to hospitalization. Conditions present after CPR that predicted in-hospital mortality included coma, need for pressors, and duration of CPR longer than 15 minutes. Notable was the fact that there was no survival among patients who had sepsis during hospitalization or who presented initially with an acute stroke associated with a neurological deficit. In this study, age itself was not a predictor of outcome, but important factors associated with prognosis were the presence and extent of underlying heart disease and the presence of other systemic diseases, both of which increase with age.

Although the majority of studies have reported that advanced age is a predictor of poor outcome, several have reported that age is not an important factor. Linn and Yurt[26] retrospectively reviewed the records of 292 patients successfully resuscitated and hospitalized after a cardiac arrest and compared the outcome of those older than 60 years to those younger than age 60 years. Survival rates were identical in both groups. When the authors compared the patients who survived with the non survivors, they reported that age did not influence outcome.

Gordon and Hurowitz[27] also reported that age itself was not an important predictor of survival after CPR. In their study, the most important prognostic factors were impaired physical and mental states as well as the presence of underlying chronic illnesses.

Several studies have specifically examined the outcome of elderly patients resuscitated from out-of-hospital sudden death. Bayer and coworkers[28] reported the outcome of 95 patients aged 65 to 90 (mean age 77). Resuscitation was successful in 37 patients (39%), but 21 (22%) died in the hospital. Only 14 patients (15%) were alive at three months, a survival rate similar to that reported in younger patients. In this study, there was no relation between survival and the age of the patient. Of note was the presence of a significant degree of mental, physical, and emotional disability among the survivors and a substantial impairment in the ability to readjust to routine home situations or social life. However, none of these patients expressed regret over being resuscitated. Fusgen and Summa[29] reviewed the records of 657 resuscitations performed in 335 patients, 239 of whom were more than 60 years of age. In the group of patients age younger than 60 years, 17% were discharged from the hospital and 14% were alive at 6 months, while only 5% of those older than age 60 years were discharged from the hospital and only 3% were alive at 6 months. While advanced age itself affected the survival rate, the more important factor was the presence of chronic illness. However, age is an important concern since the elderly are more likely to have multiple chronic diseases. Among the survivors the prevalence of neurological impairment or need for placement in an extended care facility was similar in those younger or older than 60. After a follow-up of 35 months, 49% of patients discharged from the hospital died. Hospital mortality and discharge from the hospital were related to age, although long-term outcome of survivors after discharge from the hospital was not associated with age. In this study, an important finding was the patient's attitude towards resuscitation. Although patients older than age 60 years had acceptable lifestyles after CPR, most did not wish to be resuscitated again.

Tresch and coworkers[30] reported on 214 consecutive patients, 112 of whom were over 70 years of age and 102 of whom were younger than 70 years of age. As expected, a prior history of heart failure was more common in the elderly (42% vs. 18% for younger patients), while younger patients were more likely to have an acute MI precipitating the cardiac arrest (33% vs. 16%). The etiology of the arrest was ventricular fibrillation in 83% of the younger patients compared to 71% of the elderly. Electromechanical dissociation was 5 times more common in the elderly. Hospital deaths were more frequent in the elderly (71% vs. 53%), although length of hospitalization and stay in an intensive care unit were equivalent. Overall survival was higher in the younger patients (47% vs. 28%, $P < 0.005$) and the difference was more striking when younger patients were compared to those over age 80 years who had a survival rate of 18%.

A large study reporting the outcome of CPR in the elderly is that of Murphy and coworkers[31] who prospectively followed 503 consecutive patients over age 70 years who sustained a cardiac arrest and in whom CPR was initiated. CPR was initially effective in 22% who were admitted to the hospital, but only 19 patients (3.8%) survived the hospitalization and were discharged. In this study, there was a relationship between the location of the cardiac arrest and outcome (ie, home versus hospital). Among 244 patients having an out-of-hospital cardiac arrest, 8.2% were initially resuscitated, and only two patients (0.8%) were discharged from the hospital. Of 259 patients who had an in-hospital cardiac arrest, 82 (32%) were successfully resuscitated initially, but only 17 patients (6.5%) were discharged from the hospital. Also of importance is the fact that there were no survivors among the 88 patients who had an unwitnessed out-of-hospital arrest, while there was a 1.7% survival (2 patients) among the 120 witnessed out-of-hospital arrests. In the group of patients who sustained a cardiac arrest in the hospital, survival was 7.4% when witnessed (15 of 204 patients) and 3.6% (one out of 28 patients) when not witnessed.

Among the group with an out-of-hospital cardiac arrest, an important prognostic factor was the absence of detectable vital signs at the time of the arrest. This was associated with no survival, while survival was 7.4% when vital signs were detected during the arrest. For the in-hospital patients, survival was 2.7% and 11.1%, respectively, when vital signs were absent or present.

Among the hospitalized patients other factors associated with poor outcome and no survival were hematocrit less than 35%, the presence of 2 or more diseases before the arrest, the use of a greater number of medications (6.4 vs, 4.9 for survivors, $P < 0.05$), and the initial rhythm. When VT or ventricular fibrillation were observed, there was a 20.8% survival compared to a 2.6% survival when the initial ECG showed any other rhythm, particularly electromechanical dissociation, asystole, or a junctional rhythm. Lastly when the duration of CPR was greater than five minutes, survival was 2.6% compared with 22.5% when CPR lasted less than 5 minutes.

Among the 19 patients who survived and were discharged from the hospital, 9 (1.8% of total patient population) had little or no neurological impairment, while the remaining 10 patients had moderate or severe deficits, 5 of whom were discharged to a rehabilitation hospital. Overall among the elderly who experienced a primary cardiac arrest only 1.8% were able to return home and could resume their normal lifestyle. This is a substantially lower success rate than that reported for a younger population of patients.

Another large study of rural advanced life support was reported by Wuerz and coworkers.[32] This study involved 563 patients, 320 of whom (60%) were over 65 years of age. CPR was successful in 18% of those over 65 and in 16% less than 65. The rates of survival to hospital discharge were 4% and 5%, respectively. The results from CPR in an urban setting are similar. Bonnin and coworkers[33] reported on 989 patients, 367 of whom were elderly. CPR was successful in 22% of the elderly patients, but only 7% survived to be discharged from the hospital. Survival was better in those patients with ventricular tachycardia or fibrillation (14%).

Applebaum and coworkers[34] reported on the long-term outcome of 705 patients over 65 years of age who had CPR initiated in a nursing home. There were 117 permanent residents of the nursing home and 580 nonresidents who were there for management of an acute problem. Only 2 (1.7%) of the permanent residents were successfully resuscitated and, while 11% of the nonresidents survived. This study suggested that poor survival among the elderly in nursing homes is related to the presence of underlying chronic diseases and a state of debilitation. requiring constant medical care. Several other studies have also reported that survival among elderly patients in a long term facility is very poor and there is no survival among those with an unwitnessed cardiac arrest.[35,36] It has been recommended that CPR in a nursing home be initiated only in those with a witnessed cardiac arrest and be continued only if ventricular tachycardia or ventricular fibrillation are initially documented.[37]

Role of Do Not Resuscitate Orders

The poor results of CPR and the low survival rates suggest that a hospital policy for do not resuscitate (DNR) orders should be established and the issue of DNR status discussed with all patients admitted to the hospital. This is especially important for the elderly, who represent the largest proportion of hospitalized patients and who often have multiple acute and chronic diseases as well as underlying neurological or CNS abnormalities that contribute to their poor survival after CPR. Additionally, the elderly who are resuscitated are likely to have a prolonged hospital course after CPR resulting from multiple complications that require costly intensive hospital care prior to death.

When the elderly patient has an out-of-hospital cardiac arrest, the presence of asystole or electromechanical dissociation on the initial ECG tracing and the absence of measurable vital signs on physical examination are associated with 100% mortality regardless of whether or not a medical history is known at the time CPR is begun. Under these circumstances, CPR should probably not even be initiated. If initially begun, it should be terminated after 5 minutes if not effective, as the chances of successful resuscitation are very small and the percentage of survival is extremely low. When the patient is in the hospital and has a witnessed cardiac arrest, these factors are also important, especially if the patient is known to have multiple chronic diseases (Table 3).

An important medical and economic issue is the need for DNR orders when an elderly patient is admitted to the hospital for therapy of an acute or chronic disorder. When the elderly patient has multiple underlying chronic ailments, is anemic, and has a superimposed acute disease process, it is appropriate and necessary that such orders be

---

Table 3
Considerations for No Cardiopulmonary
Resuscitation or for Discontinued
Cardiopulmonary Resuscitation

Absence of any vital signs
Asystole or electromechanical dissociation on initial ECG
CPR lasting for >5 minutes
Multiple chronic diseases
Sepsis
Cerebrovascular accident and severe neurological deficit
Cancer or Alzheimer's disease

---

discussed with the patient and the data about long-term outcome after cardiac arrest be presented. If the patient is mentally impaired or has a severe neurological deficit precluding sufficient understanding, this should be discussed with the family so that the proper decision about CPR or DNR orders may be made. This should be rediscussed during the hospitalization if there are changes in the patient's clinical status that would affect the outcome of CPR.

Patient and Family Views About CPR

In the Murphy study,[31] 90% of patients did not discuss resuscitation with the health-care providers. While resuscitation was discussed with 10% of patients, a decision was made in only 2.8% of patients that resuscitation was to be attempted. Miller and coworkers[38] surveyed 248 elderly patients and reported that they overestimated the survival rate from a cardiac arrest by 300%. However, these patients felt that DNR orders were appropriate when cancer or Alzheimer's disease were present. Another study also reported that elderly patients and their families overestimated the effectiveness of CPR largely because their only source of information was television drama.[39] However, 86% of patients were willing to consult with a physician about their own CPR and 64% of patients ultimately followed this advice. Another study of 287 patients 60 years of age or older reported that 41% preferred CPR before obtaining any information about the effectiveness of CPR while only 22% overall and 6% of those over 86 opted for CPR after learning about the probability of survival.[40] When the patient was asked about CPR if they had a chronic illness which would limit their life expectancy, 11% opted for CPR before learning about the probability of survival while only 5% wanted CPR after discussing the probable outcome. It has been reported that quantitative information about the outcome of CPR has more of an impact on decision making that does descriptive information.[41]

Torian and coworkers[42] reported that the elderly who agreed to have DNR orders placed in the chart were generally more functionally dependent and more frequently had acute and chronic illnesses. Unfortunately, these patients were less likely to participate in decision making about this issue; rather, the decision was made by family members or other surrogates in most cases. These authors reported that in most instances, patients and families considered the severity of the illness and the presence of other chronic diseases in making a decision about DNR.

Another study reported that most patients and families prefer measures that provide comfort, but life-sustaining measures are nevertheless frequently used.[43] Other studies have indicated that an important consideration is the quality of life.[44] Nevertheless, patient's attitudes cannot be predicted reliably and surrogate decision making is inadequate. Since the majority of patients make decisions based on prognostic information as well as personal health and social circumstances, most welcome a discussion about resuscitation and prefer that this be initiated by their physicians.[45] Schonwitter and coworkers[46] also reported that the elderly overestimated their chances for survival, but this was based on a lack of information, as only 17% of the patients in this study had previously discussed CPR with a physician. Shmerlling and coworkers[47] interviewed 75 elderly patients and only 7% had an understanding of what CPR involved and about the prognosis after CPR. However, 78% of patients wanted to discuss this with health care providers, 70% felt it should be discussed at the time of hospitalization and 84% wanted CPR or DNR orders to be part of the hospital record.

Economic Implications

The need to establish DNR orders has an important economic impact. Kvale and D'Elia[48] reviewed the records of 86 patients over the age of 75 who underwent CPR. Resuscitation was successful in 41%, 23% regained consciousness, and 7% were alive at 1 year. The cost for CPR itself was $100,000 (in 1987) and one-half of this cost was allocated to the patients who remained unconscious before ultimately dying. Another factor is the length of hospitalization after successful CPR. As indicated, a substantial number of patients are in intensive care units and, before death, they often live days or weeks, requiring intensive, sophisticated, and costly care during this time. It is not unusual for the hospital costs to be in excess of $100,000 per patient, which is an enormous economic burden on the health care delivery system, especially when the patient does not survive. For the very few who do survive, continued care in a rehabilitation center, chronic care hospital, or nursing home is often required. The cost for such care will continue to escalate since the elderly represent a growing percentage of the population and they are the majority of patients who require hospitalization.

The use of DNR orders has an important impact on health care.

Quill and Bennett[49] reviewed the use of DNR orders in those over 79 years of age. Prior to institution of a policy permitting CPR or DNR orders, only 21% of charts had such orders, compared to 76% after the policy was adopted. When CPR was ordered, it was performed in 92% of cases after the policy was initiated, compared to only 29% before the policy. Importantly, the overall survival of patients over 79 years of age was 34%, likely to be the result of better patient selection. Unfortunately, in only 25% of cases was a decision about CPR or DNR orders made by patients themselves after being provided with necessary information.

In view of these conclusions, the need for decision making in this regard is a medical and economic reality.[50-53] For each patient admitted to the hospital, particularly the elderly, consideration must be given to the likely short- or long-term outcome of a cardiac arrest should it occur, and the possible impact this will have on lifestyle. While age is an important concern, other factors to consider are underlying medical problems and the social background of the patient. DNR orders are an important consideration for those patients likely to have a cardiac arrest but unlikely to survive. This may also be a concern for those unlikely to resume a normal or reasonable lifestyle even if they survive and are discharged from the hospital. For those patients without DNR orders, a decision about initiating CPR should be also based on these concerns. For the patient who has a cardiac arrest, there are objective factors that should be considered before instituting CPR even if there are no DNR orders, including the initial rhythm on the ECG, the absence of vital signs, and a history of chronic diseases. Such decision making will reduce the economic burden placed on society and will eliminate many of the emotional and ethical concerns faced by patients and families.

References

1. Lown B: Sudden cardiac death: The major challenge confronting contemporary cardiology. *Am J Cardiol* 43:313, 1979.
2. Cobb LA, Baum RS, Alverez H, et al: Resuscitation from out of hospital ventricular fibrillation. *Circulation* 51:111, 1975.
3. Bharati S, Lev M: The pathology of sudden death. In: Josephson ME, ed. *Sudden Cardiac Death,* Cardiovascular Clinics, FA Davis, Philadelphia 1985, p 1.
4. Friedman PL, Stewart JR, Fenoglio JJ, et al: Survival of subendocardial Purkinje fibers after extensive myocardial infarction in dogs. *Circ Res* 33:597, 1973.
5. El Sherif N, Sherlag JB, Lazzara R, et al: Re-entrant arrhythmias in the late myocardial infarction period. II. Patterns of initiation and termination of re-entry. *Circulation* 55:702, 1971.
6. Myerburg RJ, Castellanos A: Cardiac arrest and sudden cardiac death. In: Braunwald E, ed. *Heart Disease. A Textbook of Cardiovascular Medicine.* Philadelphia, WB Saunders Co, 1988, p 742.

7. Lown B, Neuman J, Amarasingham R, et al: Comparison of alternating current with direct current electroshock across the closed chest. *Am J Cardiol* 10:223, 1962.
8. DeSilva RA, Graboys TB, Podrid PJ, et al: Cardioversion and defibrillation. *Am Heart J* 100:881, 1980.
9. Weaver WD, Cobb LA, Hallstrom AP, et al: Factors influencing survival after out-of-hospital cardiac arrest. *J Am Coll Cardiol* 7:752, 1986.
10. Pratt CP, Francis MJ, Luck JC, et al: Analysis of ambulatory electrocardiogram in 15 patients during spontaneous ventricular fibrillation with special reference to preceding arrhythmic events. *J Am Coll Cardiol* 7:789, 1985.
11. Myerburg RJ, Conde CA, Sung RJ: Clinical electrophysiologic and hemodynamic profile of patients resuscitated from in-hospital cardiac arrest. *Am J Med* 68:568, 1980.
12. Myerburg RJ, Zaman L, Luceri RM, et al: Clinical characteristic of sudden death. Implications for survival. In: Josephson ME, ed. *Sudden Cardiac Death*. Cardiovascular Clinics, FA Davis, Philadelphia 1985, p 107.
13. Baum RS Alvarez H, Cobb LA: Survival after resuscitation from out-of hospital ventricular fibrillation. *Circulation* 50:1231, 1974.
14. Schneider AP, Nelson DJ, Brown DD: In-hospital cardiopulmonary resuscitation: A 30 year review. *J Am Board Fam Pract* 6:191, 1993.
15. Liberthson RR, Nagel EL, Hirschman JC, et al: Pre-hospital ventricular fibrillation. *N Engl J Med* 291:317, 1979.
16. Thompson RG, Hallstrom AP, Cobb LA: Bystander initiated cardiopulmonary resuscitation in the management of ventricular fibrillation. *Ann Intern Med* 90:737, 1979.
17. Ritter G, Wolfe RA, Goldstein S, et al: The effect of bystander CPR on survival of out-of-hospital cardiac arrest victims. *Am Heart J* 110:932, 1985.
18. Guzy PM, Pearce ML, Greenfield S: The survival benefit of bystander cardiopulmonary resuscitation in a paramedic served metropolitan area. *Am J Public Health* 73:766, 1983.
19. Dickey W, MacKenzie G, Adgey AA: Long-term survival after resuscitation from ventricular fibrillation occurring before hospital admission. *Q J Med* 80:729, 1991.
20. Marwick TH, Case CC, Siskind V, et al: Prediction of survival from resuscitation: A prognostic index derived from multivariate logistic model analysis. *Resuscitation* 22:129, 1991.
21. Tortolani AJ, Resucci DA, Rosati RJ, et al: In-hospital cardiopulmonary: Patient arrest and resuscitation factors associated with survival. *Resuscitation* 20:115, 1990.
22. Greene HL: Sudden arrhythmic cardiac death mechanism, resuscitation and classification: The Seattle perspective. *Am J Cardiol* 65:4B, 1990.
23. George AL, Folk BP, Criceluis PL, et al: Pre arrest morbidity and other correlates of survival after in-patient cardiopulmonary arrest. *Am J Med* 87:28, 1989.
24. Taffet GE, Teasdale TA, Luchi RJ: In-hospital cardiopulmonary resuscitation. *JAMA* 260:2069, 1998.
25. Bedell SE, Delbanco TL, Cook EF, et al: Survival after cardiopulmonary resuscitation in the hospital. *N Engl J Med* 309:569, 1983.
26. Linn BJ, Yurt RW. Cardiac arrest among geriatric patients. *Br Med J* 2: 25, 1970.

27. Gordon M, Hurowitz Z: Cardiopulmonary resuscitation of the elderly. *J Am Geriatr Soc* 32:930, 1984.
28. Bayer AJ, Ang HC, Pathy MSJ: Cardiac arrests in a geriatric unit. *Age Ageing* 14:271, 1985.
29. Fusgen I, Summa JD: How much sense is there in an attempt to resuscitate an aged person. *Gerontology* 24:37, 1978.
30. Tresch DD, Thakur RK, Hoffman RG, et al: Should the elderly be resuscitated following out-of-hospital cardiac arrest. *Am J Med* 86:145, 1989.
31. Murphy DJ, Murray AM, Robinson BE, et al: Outcomes of cardiopulmonary resuscitation in the elderly. *Ann Intern Med* 111:199, 1989.
32. Wuerz RL, Holliman CJ, Meador SA, et al: Effect of age on prehospital cardiac resuscitation outcome. *Am J Emerg Med* 13;389, 1995.
33. Bonnin MJ, Pepe PE, Clark PS: Survival in the elderly after out of hospital cardiac arrest. *Crit Care Med* 21:1645, 1993.
34. Applebaum GE, King JE, Finucane TE: The outcome of CPR initiated in nursing homes. *J Am Geriatr Soc* 38:197, 1990.
35. Awoke S, Mouton CP, Parrott M: Outcomes of skilled cardiopulmonary resuscitation in a long-term-care facility: Futile therapy? *J Am Geriatr Soc* 40:593, 1992.
36. Gordon M, Cheung M: Poor outcomes of on-site CPR in a mulit-level geriatric facility: Three and a half years experience at the Baycrest Centre for Geriatric Care. *J Am Geriatr Soc* 41:163, 1993.
37. Tresch DD, Neahring JM, Duthie EH, et al: Outcomes of cardiopulmonary resuscitation in nursing homes: Can we predict who will benefit? *Am J Med* 95:123, 1993.
38. Miller DL, Jahnigem DW, Gorbien MJ, et al: Cardiopulmonary resuscitation. How useful? Attitudes and knowledge of an elderly population. *Arch Intern Med* 152:578, 1992.
39. Mead GE, Tumbull CJ: Cardiopulmonary resuscitation in the elderly: Patients' and relatives' views. *J Med Ethics* 21:39, 1995.
40. Murphy DJ, Burrows D, Santilli S, et al: The influence of the probability of survival on patients' preference regarding cardiopulmonary resucitation. *N Engl J Med* 330:545, 1994.
41. Schonwitter RS, Walker RM, Kamer DR, et al: Resuscitation decision making in the elderly: The value of outcome data. *J Gen Intern Med* 9:57, 1994.
42. Torian LV, Davidson EJ, Fillit AM, et al: Decisions for and against resuscitation in an acute geriatric medicine unit serving the frail elderly. *Arch Intern Med* 152:561, 1992.
43. Lynn J, Teno JM, Phillips RS, et al: Preceptions by family members of the dying eperience of older and seriously ill patients. SUPPORT Investigators. Study to Understand Prognoses and Preferences for Outcome and Risks of Treatments. *Ann Intern Med* 126:97, 1997.
44. Bruce-Jones PN: Resuscitation decisions in the elderly: A discussion of current thinking. *J Med Ethics* 22:286, 1996.
45. Bruce-Jones P, Roberts H, Bowker L, et al: Resuscitating the elderly: What do patients want? *J Med Ethics* 22:154, 1996.
46. Schonwitter RS, Teasdale RA, Taffet G, et al: Educating the elderly: Cardiopulmonary resuscitation decisions before and after intervention. *J Am Geriatr Soc* 152:372, 1991.
47. Shmerlling RH, Bedell SE, Lilenfeld A, et al: Discussing cardiopulmonary resuscitation: A study of elderly outpatients. *J Gen Intern Med* 3:317, 1988.
48. Kvale JN, D'Elia G: Resuscitation of the elderly. *Fam Pract Res J* 7:78, 1987.

49. Quill TE, Bennett NM: The effects of a hospital policy and state legislation on resuscitation orders for geriatric patients. *Arch Intern Med* 152:569, 1992.
50. Podrid PJ: Resuscitation in the elderly: A blessing or a curse? *Ann Intern Med* 111:193, 1989.
51. Varon J, Fromm RE: In-hospital resuscitation among the elderly: Substantial survival to hospital discharge. *Am J Emerg Med* 14:130, 1996.
52. O'Keefe S, Redahan C, Keanem P, et al: Age and other determinants of survival after in-hospital cardiopulmonary resuscitation. *Q J Med* 81:1005, 1991.
53. Jurgems R, Wahlig G, Frese W: Influence of age on the survival rate of out-of-hospital and in-hospital resuscitation. *Resuscitation* 26:23, 1993.

Chapter 31

Socioeconomic Circumstances and the Elderly

Leighton E. Cluff

The organization, delivery and financing of health care for Americans, including care for cardiovascular disorders, is increasingly determined by private and public insurers. Physicians and hospitals are responsible for most health care in the United States, but where, when and how this care is provided is less and less determined by the physician and hospital. "Managed care" organizations and Health Maintenance Organizations (HMOs) now enroll most people in systems of care whose development has been fostered by efforts to control unacceptable expense. Initially, constraints on health care were directed at the care of patients in hospitals, but there is a growing effort to control home care that has become equally expensive. Nursing home care is largely subsidized by state-federal Medicaid programs, and states especially, have been forced to restrain this expenditure.

During all of this, the elderly population continues to grow, and those over age 75 years are the greatest consumers of health-care services. Added to this is the acceleration in development of new medical technology, more and more of which can be used at home and in the nursing home, thus changing the way medical care is provided. A major national study, moreover, shows that physicians pay little if any attention to "living wills" or the expressed wishes of patients and families in the use of life extending technology for terminally ill persons.[1,2] These are a few of the socioeconomic circumstances that will continue to shape health care into the future.

From *Clinical Cardiology in the Elderly. Second Edition,* edited by Elliot Chesler. © 1999, Futura Publishing Company, Armonk, NY.

Payment for Health Care

Americans older than 65 years constitute about 13% of the total population, and it is anticipated that this figure will rise to 20% by the year 2030.[3,4] This is not unique to the United States; in several developed and developing countries, age-adjusted mortality rates show the greatest decline among people older than 80 years. Chronic illnesses account for three quarters of all health care expenditures in the United States of which cardiovascular conditions are responsible for a significant proportion.[3,5] Almost all elderly persons have Medicare as their first means of financing their medical care. There is evidence that poor, uneducated, and minority people, especially African American, even with Medicare and Medicaid, may be less likely than others to receive treatment and procedures for cardiovascular disease. Thus, the social context in which cardiovascular care is provided further compounds the fragmentation, uneven distribution, and provision of medical services. Physicians have probably paid too little attention to the availability, allocation and provision of services to people in need who face different socioeconomic circumstances. The elderly consume about 40% of the nation's health-care expenditure, provided by public tax-supported funds yet a large percentage of children do not have any health insurance. In the future we will have to choose whether we should spend more of our resources to help those at the end, as compared to those at the beginning of their lives.

Intensive Care at the End of Life

Performance of expensive cardiovascular procedures in patients 80 years of age or older, with short life expectancy, should be a concern for cardiovascular physicians and surgeons. Additionally, excessive use of life sustaining technology in intensive care units for patients who are likely to die soon confronts medicine with an enormous challenge to reexamine its purpose, value system, and ethical standards.[1,2] These practices may result in financial disaster for the patient and family when insurance is inadequate and providers do not accept insurance payments only. The question to be addressed is whether procedures or technologies applied in diagnosis and treatment improve the quality of life for the patient, whether it is in the best interest for society, or whether they meet only a special interest of a physician. Our attention should be directed to criteria governing admission of terminally, or severely ill, old persons to an intensive care unit, where the intensity of care often seems uncontrollable. While age alone is not a risk factor, associated conditions such as pneumonia, adult respiratory distress syndrome, myocardial infarction, and unsuccessful cardiopulmonary resuscitation certainly are. Furthermore, it must not be overlooked that some diagnostic and therapeutic procedures, themselves may be responsible for adverse effects, even death. Unfortunately, too many patients are sent to hospitals dying, only to be subjected to excessive interventions. It is not surprising that patients admitted to hospital from nursing homes have a much higher mortality rate than those admitted from home.[3] Admission of dying patients to hospitals from nursing homes may not justify the expense and requires greater moral and ethical, as well as medical judgment. Most physically ill but mentally well and many mentally impaired elderly persons who remain in nursing homes for long periods of time experience great decline in the quality of their lives. The availability of care by physicians in nursing homes is often poor and many residents are sent to the hospital for their terminal event. Physicians need to examine the probability of patients spending the remaining days of their lives in a nursing home before they embark on an aggressive course of medical care. If a patient's quality of life is not likely to be improved following medical care, they should reexamine their course of action.

Coordination of Health Care

Elderly persons account for about 50% of all days of hospital care and their average stay is longer than for those who are younger.[3] Hospital expenses account for the largest share of their health cost, but increasing use of home care services is now the most rapidly growing segment of health care.[6] Yet, at the same time, it is estimated that 1 in 3 persons older than 65 years of age will spend some time in a nursing home. Those with long-term care insurance are few, and those with financial resources are obliged to pay out-of-pocket for nursing home and home care services. Many eventually spend down their funds, or legally divest themselves of their assets to qualify for Medicaid. Medicaid is the single largest insurer of nursing home care, and this expenditure impacts on state resources to such an extent that Medicaid becomes an intolerable burden on state budgets.

Among the elderly, women outnumber men by 3 to 2, a disparity that is even greater over age 85 years. About two-thirds of women age 65 or older are widows, living with relatives or alone, whereas two-thirds of men age 65 or older are married and only 18% live with relatives.[3] This says much about the social support for older men as compared to women. Men are more likely to have a wife, who often is younger. For this reason, men with cardiovascular or other health problems, are more likely to be cared for at home when they are ill. There is abundant evidence that a good support system is important to convalescence, recovery, and prevention of some diseases and their complications. Visiting nurses, home care, and other professional services cannot compensate for the lack of natural or informal support at home. An aging population of very old women and the prevalence of cardiovascular disease will pose additional problems for the providers of healthcare. Many believe that case management is the way for the future in controlling rising health-care costs and improving the quality of care. It is widely recognized that patients are frequently dependent on many different physicians for their care. Elderly patients are particularly vulnerable to the adverse consequence of fragmented care whereby they may receive multiple expensive, potentially dangerous medications. Coordination of their care by a case manager would improve the quality of care and decrease the cost.

Hospice Care

The hospice is the only organized institution designed to provide supportive care but its focus had been on palliative care for terminally-ill cancer patients.[7] Conceivably, the hospice could become a more important mechanism to provide the supportive and caring function for many severely ill patients with cardiovascular disease. Cardiac patients generally are not included or considered as candidates for Hospice care, largely because hospices have not expanded their role and financing mechanisms to provide care for more people who are severely ill. Hospices, also, remain very much dependent on volunteer services by members of the community. It is my view that neither government, personal finances, or other social benefits will ever be able to afford the cost of professional services for those who are seriously, as well as those who are terminally ill.

"Managed care" has become the instrument to organize the financing, delivery, and organization of medical care, whose major purpose is to control the price of health care.[8] During the past few years, managed care systems, including for-profit and not-for-profit organizations, have captured a large proportion of the population. It is estimated that about 70% or more of insured people are enrolled in one or other Managed Care Program or Health Maintenance Organization.[3] National health-care costs have risen at a slower rate, proportionate with the growth of managed care systems. In 1980, the rate of increase in health care costs was 11.6%; in 1985 8.3%, in 1990 8.0%, and in 1995 4.5%.[3] However, in 1998, it is anticipated that this rate will rise again, attributable, to an aging population, costly technology, and growing public demand for highly specialized services. There are also increasing concerns regarding the quality and adequacy of care in many of these programs. Congress and the current administration are beginning to place demands on services provided by managed care plans that, in and of themselves, may further increase costs. I believe that the organization, delivery and financing of health care will remain in a state of change for several years, before citizens, politicians and private insurers come to some agreement as to what should be provided.

Certainly, the magnificent advances in medical technology have prolonged the useful life of many individuals with cardiovascular diseases but this romance of medicine and industry with technology has also created major social, ethical and medical dilemmas. Medicine can no longer stand aloof and assume an attitude that its only task is to prevent death and preserve "meaningless" life at any price. Inevitably, balancing individual rights, socioeconomic benefits, and societal rights and responsibilities creates conflicts. Physicians caring for geriatric patients must recognize their central role in resolving such conflicts. The United States and the rest of the industrialized world face a problem never faced by nations before—a time when life expectancy and an aging population is becoming dominant. Medicine and society are in this together, and together they must strive to deal with the changes in demography, population and socioeconomic disparities with a view to the future, and not only to the solution of today's problems.

References

1. Isaacs JL, Knickman , eds: *To Improve Health and Health Care 1997. The Robert Wood Johnson Foundation Anthology.* San Francisco, Joseey-Bass Publishers, 1997.
2. Hoffman JC, et al: Patient preferences for communication with physicians about end-of-life decisions (SUPPORT). *Ann Nit Ed* 1:127(1):1–12, 1997.
3. *Statistical Abstract of the United States, 1996*, 116th Ed., U.S. Department of Commerce, Bureau of the Census, Washington, DC.
4. *U.S. Population Estimates by Age, Sex, and Hispanic Origin, 1989*, U.S. Bureau of the Census, Current Population Reports, Series P-25, No 1057, Washington, DC, 1990.
5. Nelson EC, et al: A longitudinal study of hosptalization rates for patients with chronic diseases. *Health Services Res* 32(Feb):774–749, 1998.
6. Arras JD, ed: *Bringing the Hospital Home: Ethical and Social Implications of High Tech Home Care.* Baltimore, John Hopkins University Press, 1995. 7. Sheehan DC, Forman WB, eds. *Hospice and Paliative Care.* Massachusetts, Jones and Bartlett Publishers, 1996.
7. Sheehan DC, Forman WB, eds. *Hospice and Paliative Care.* Massachusetts, Jones and Bartlett Publishers, 1996.
8. Johnson H, Broder Sd: *The System. The American Way of Politics at the Breaking Point.* Boston-New York, Little Brown and Co, 1996.

Chapter 32

Reflections on Bioethics in the Elderly Cardiac

Howard B. Burchell

So even while avoiding philosophic systems, I like philosophers and greatly enjoy their converse. Philosophy embodies the eternal aspiration of human reason toward knowledge of the unknown...therefore philosophers always live in controversial questions and in lofty regions.

Claude Bernard[1]

A chapter on ethics in a cardiological text is not a usual finding; indeed, neither is it found in numerous volumes on the practice of medicine. With some educational background in the humanities, and trained in medicine by teachers, presumed exemplars of professional behavior, it has been generally assumed that physicians would do the right thing for their patients. People have traditionally ranked them high on the scales of moral behavior, although there have always been the salutary effects of a few detractors and satirists. In recent decades the criticisms of the profession from the increasing population of bioethicists, in the parlance of the business world, a "growth industry," have been more scholarly, but no less acerbic. However, the new bioethical group has not escaped critical assessment; a rather caustic one is that of Ruth Shalit (*New Republic,* April 29, 1997).

About 200 years ago, Thomas Percival began discourses on a code of professional behavior, and these were published under the title of Medical Ethics. Chauncey Leake[2] has analyzed the impact of this book on English medicine in a new edition in 1975. Leake's historical commentary is instructive, emphasizing that Percival was detailing largely etiquette, not ethics; how to conduct oneself in relation to the hospital, colleagues, the community and the law courts.

From *Clinical Cardiology in the Elderly. Second Edition,* edited by Elliot Chesler. © 1999, Futura Publishing Company, Armonk, NY.

Times certainly have changed, as exemplified in the title of Paul Starr's book, *Social Transformation of American Medicine.*[3] One of the challenges thrown up to debate was whether a physician, largely compensated by a third-party payer, rather than directly from the patient, could have sensitivity and responsiveness to the complete needs of the sick and troubled. In some instances physicians have become prey to aggressive marketing practices of corporations, proposing a new technological gadget to increase the physician's income. Hospitals may spend considerable sums of "physician bonding" activities to recruit and retain physicians who sometimes become prone to "self-referral" through partnership in facilities where they treat their patients. Thus, properly, there is the increased attention paid to "conflict of interest" problems in recent years. Because reimbursement for their services is now so replete with rules and paperwork, it could become a "game," an attempt to beat the system through bypassing the rules even though this could actually be to the detriment of the patient's welfare.[4]

The tremendous advances in technology have aroused concerns that the physician has become an automaton, an historic analysis epitomized in the title of Reiser's book, *Medicine and the Reign of Technology.*[5] Many medical leaders are aware of the problems engendered by this technological age, as examples, Thomas,[6] Kjellstrand,[7] and Chinard.[8] There has been concern too that technology might attract the narrow-minded to medical schools with the premedical courses being "dehumanizing."[9]

Another exposition of the revolutionary change in the physician's relationship to the patient; particularly terminally, has been written by the historian David Rothman under the provocative title of *Strangers at the Bedside.*[10] Therein, he outlines the train of events in the past half century whereby he asserts that the physician has been replaced by the ethicist and lawyer as the primary decision maker, in the patient's care, particularly in a terminal illness.

Physicians have undoubtedly taken much for granted regarding the acquisition of skills in the identification and solving of ethical problems, while focusing their goals in medical school on the mastering of medical technology and the understanding of the mechanisms of physical disease. However, despite their college degree, medical students have been foremost in requesting more education in ethics, which is laudable, not only for their recognition of its importance, but also perhaps for an awareness of the increasing legal regulations that engulf us.

Historically, this attitude is in striking contrast with the statement made by the president of the first meeting of the elite Association of American Physicians: "We, all of us, know why we are assembled here today. It is because we want an association in which there is no medical politics and no medical ethics—(we) want a society in which we can learn something." How strange and seemingly paradoxical that Osler, a penultimate ethicist, should say 30 years later, that Delafield had "struck the right note" and quoted the above sentences.[11] Both these physicians had their basic training and extended experience in pathology! Maurice Fishbein, long-time editor of the *Journal of the American Medical Association* and potent force in American medical politics, is reputed to have said regarding the history of ethics, "unnecessary and of no significance."[12] I do not believe he could have meant it; and to be noted is that he was referring to the *ancient* history of ethics not the current problems.

In the arena of bioethics, the clinician may sometimes feel "put down" by the apparent self-confidence and specialized jargon of the professional ethicist, moral philosopher, law judges, or clergy. However, it is pertinent to recall that decisions reached by judges are often based on data supplied by those physicians and nurses who had closely observed the patient first hand, and their prognosis had been ventured on the basis of knowledge of human pathophysiology and their long experience. But, physicians should recognize that they also may be susceptible to subconscious self-deception, and could have prematurely made a diagnosis or come to a conclusion and fabricated some supporting facts. Students and physicians of all ages have probably found refuge in the first of Hippocrates 411 aphorisms: "Life is short, the art long, experience deceptive and judgment difficult." I like the challenge of Richards' translation of the last two lines *viz.* "and the trial precarious and the crisis grievous."[13] Arguing from the British scene, Thompson[14] has written a rather scathing indictment of both physicians and philosophers in their conduct and discourses on the complexities in the training of students in medical ethics. This underscores the plethora of opinion currently being published in this field.

Our library shelves are burgeoning with new texts and journals pertaining to medical ethics and geriatric medicine, designed to inform both undergraduates and postgraduates. Ethical instruction have valid claims to time in the undergraduate curriculum[15-18] and this is further illustrated by a whole issue of the journal of *Academic Medicine* recently being given to the topic (December, 1989).

It is noteworthy that the American College of Cardiology asked the bioethicist physician, Engelhardt, to give the convocation lecture in 1991, which he entitled "Medical Ethics for the 21st Century."[19] He predicted a continuing expansion of technology and of complicated services; and emphasized the central role "that physicians can play in helping the public understand how to come to terms with the finitude of life, medical capacities, economic resources and moral authority."

Can ethics be taught in didactic courses? Definitely yes! Certainly, many problems can be illustrated, classified, opinions aired and logic criticized. Acquaintance with different terminologies will be expanded, and physicians will be less bewildered by philosophical terms. My view, concordant with that of many others, is that ethics in medicine is to be derived mainly from individual cases. Despite repetitive stereotyped situations, there are, however, unique features to be discovered in each one.

Another method of interesting students in ethics is by courses in literature, discussions of classic books and plays, and of selected current novels. In the solution of moral problems, the novelist has often directed decisions perhaps with, perhaps without, recourse to the law courts. As a single example I mention the story by Mary Webb—"Precious Bane," wherein an elderly ailing woman is coaxed into a euthanasia mood by her cruel son, and death follows his administration of a digitalis tea. Her physician is suspicious, but decides against a coroner's investigation. Not only can ethics be taught from the classics, but from current novels, which medical students may have authored. One review in support of this viewpoint is that by Radwany and Adelson[20] and, an exposition on literary medical eponyms by Rodin and Key[21] is instructive and entertaining.

The revered scholar in thanatology Kubler-Ross[22] has given no specific opinions pertinent to the care of the cardiac patients. In general, I have not recognized her five stages in attitude (denial, anger, bargaining, depression and acceptance in sequence) to dying in the elderly patient with heart disease. It has seemed that a cardiac illness has been more acceptable to the afflicted than that of cancer.

Textbooks on ethics generally present cases for discussion from which guidelines for management can be derived. This successful format in teaching, is akin to that of the clinical pathological conference or legal case presentation in law school. Sometimes there may be deficiencies in the ethical conclusions, when for example, a patient may have had varying evaluations and prognoses by different experts, and, when a course of action has been advocated and implemented, details of the follow-up may have been skimpy. It may be difficult to decide by the limited reported subsequent events whether the management plan had been optimal or not. Such drawbacks to the evaluation of the result do not pertain in the majority of the illustrative case reports included in a recommended book *Medical Ethics and Elderly People* edited by R. John Elford,[23] and *Ethical Problems in Geriatric Medicine* by Cassel et al.[24]

While the term "elderly" has often referred to those subjects over 65, it is the increasing population of older octogenarians and nonagenarians that is particularly projected to increase in the next decade. The elderly population itself is aging, that is, the proportion of people over 80, in the over-70 age groups is increasing. This "old-old" group will have many with heart disease as well as general debility. The prevalence of coronary heart disease in the women (in their 70s + ,) will have become equal, (they will have "caught-up") to that of men in this old age group.

The Living Will

Two tenets, basic to a physician's actions, to which he or she pledges allegiance, are the recognition of the sanctity of life and the right of the individual to determine his or her destiny (autonomy). Having acclaimed these ruling concepts, I submit that many times "absolutes are in the dark" and we struggle with gray areas and seeming exceptions, a stance that identifies me as a pragmatist or casuist. In the very elderly in particular, autonomy may be illusionary, and the patient willingly dependent on the physician's and family's guidance in any decision making. I rather like Jay Katz's assertion, who frequently goads the profession for its complacency in ethical controversies, when he bluntly implies that in the present climate of physician-patient decision-making the "informed consent" procedure may have become a charade.[25] The definition of this phrase is a perennial challenge and myths abound.[26] However, in a claim for autonomy, a new problem has arisen, the relatives or a surrogate insisting on therapy that the physicians believe to be overtly futile but the courts forbid its cessation.[27]

The aged person often becomes fragile in structure and brittle in intellect. Often an early grievance is loss of their independence, and the good physician will be sensitive to this change in status and respect their desire for autonomy, no matter how illusionary. First name usage will be deferred and any challenge to the patient's memory of events or orientation, delicately approached. If this be just good manners, so be it, but surely such is encompassed in ethics.

If the alert physician suspects the beginning of Alzheimer's disease, it will require all the skill and tact that he possesses as to when and how this information is imparted to the patient and the relatives. The astute physician will also recognize depression, which will be a common occurrence among his elderly, particularly male, cardiac patients, and assess the need for consultation. He will be cognizant of the fact that his psychiatric associates have been outspoken in declaring depression to be grossly underdiagnosed and inadequately treated. When a patient appears confused or depressed, obviously his medications require review; even if rare, digitalis for example, can cause depression.

In respect to definitions, it should be now accepted that perfused visceral organs do not constitute "a life" and the diagnosis of "brain death" is legally recognized in most countries. The criteria for the diagnosis of "brain-dead" have been carefully spelled out.[28] but there continue to be disputations, frequently seemingly semantic, from the ethicists.[29] There will always be mystery, wonder, and perplexity about exactly when a life ends and this is clearly portrayed in the opinions of the United States Supreme Court justices in the recent, now famous, case of Nancy Cruzan.[30,31] However, great difficulties arise in the completely incompetent patient, labeled as being in the vegetative state, requiring varied respiratory, alimentary, cardiac or renal technologic support. Perhaps some glimmer, suggesting cerebral function, as from a seeming recognition of a family member, deters the label of death. In the United States, the authority to discontinue supportive therapy has been delegated by the Supreme Court to the individual states and the final judgment stems from the best determination of what the patient would have wished to be done ("that there be clear and convincing evidence") as gathered from relatives and close acquaintances, and ideally from a living will, if one has been made.

Beginning in 1992, patients receiving medical care financed by the government in the United States are required by law to be informed of their rights, and availability of instructions on the living will, and of the durable power of attorney[32] and this is reason for concern.[33] Courts in the United States are now unanimous in allowing the terminally ill patient who is alert and declared competent, to have his or her wish to stop supportive therapy. Regardless of the proper emphasis on the autonomy of the patient as the determining factor in decisions by legal and philosophic leaders, I have observed that many elderly are quite passive and desire a maternalistic or paternalistic voice to guide their care.

When there has been controversy regarding cessation of therapy in the incompetent subject, there appears to have been some gender discrimination in the courts, more credence seems to have been given to the male's reported verbal wishes than that of the female's. This conclusion stemmed from a result of an analysis by Miles and August[34] wherein the judgements of courts allowed termination of supportive therapy in a larger percentage of men than of women. In at least one instance, the judge's commentary was disparaging to the woman's capacity to express her convictions and to be more fickle in changing her mind. As a general rule, the written word has carried a greater weight and given more serious credence than the spoken one. It is not expected that uniformity in the courts will be attained and there are lingering concerns that, toward the end, patients might change their minds and their autonomy not be respected.

It is to be hoped that elderly patients with known heart disease, or those at high risk for it, will utilize the method of the living will and name a designated health care proxy, to emphasize their wishes regarding resuscitative and supportive management, and most of the 50 states have given legal recognition for the document. The potential problems arising from disobeying stated wishes of a subject in a living will, by relatives or bystanders, will require additional time and experience for its solution.

In a prospective study, Emmanuel and associates[35] found that patients wished to discuss advance directives for life-sustaining care, that this did not provoke undue anxiety, and a perceived barrier was lack of physician initiative. Similarly, in a small sample of rural residents, Gamble et al[36] found that "many elderly want to share planning for terminal illness, but had never demanded or been given the opportunity." There is apathy or lack of concern, particularly among younger people (including many physicians) about drawing up a living will, perhaps based on denial or rationalization that fatal illness will befall people other than themselves; an attitude similar to that, I have seen in many fighter pilots facing combat. I have been astonished by the number of our colleagues who have not prepared living wills, as learned from conversations and observing a hand count in a recent meeting.

The Do–Not–Resuscitate Order

One of the thorniest clinical riddles in recent decades relates to the writing of the positive order "do not resuscitate" (DNR) on the patient's chart, clearly forbidding resuscitation procedures in case of cardiac arrest. Nurses, understandably, have desired to have the directive as a written order rather than a vague vocal order. It is manifestly less agonizing for most physicians to write such an order for a patient with end-stage metastatic cancer than for a senescent patient with chronic, but stable heart disease. Amazing improvements in cardiac function sometimes do occur unexpectedly. There should be no hesitation in the minds of physicians in writing a DNR order for some patients in severe intractable cardiac failure in whom the suffering and prognosis may be equal to that of many cancers . . . perhaps the profession should be thinking of hospices for such cardiovascular cases. The DNR issue does have to be faced and the relatives may be the first to raise the question despite their possible feelings of guilt in doing so. Here again, the usefulness of prior communication with the patient and of a living will is self-evident. That the physician needs to fully document his actions and the patient's responses on the chart requires repeated emphasis. Also, he must be cognizant of local laws, in some areas the physician may be legally bound to discuss such an order with a competent patient.

Old adages have force from logic and tradition, *viz.* Clough's irreverent doggerel, "Thou shalt not kill, but need not strive officiously to keep alive", or Thomas Fuller's "good physician" quoted by Osler,[37] "When he can keep life no longer in, he makes a fair and easy passage for it to go out." Osler gives this quotation in a letter to the editor of *The Spectator* protesting against a paper with pictures therein, depicting the act of dying as one of horror and torment. He identifies himself "as a student for many years of the art and the act of dying" and opines "no death need be physically painful" and that "there were no circumstances contradicting the practice" advocated by "Fuller's physician."

Although the argument continues,[38] I cannot accept a fundamental moral difference between the withholding and the withdrawing of any life-sustaining therapy in a patient in a terminal illness. This position is supported by the American Thoracic Society[39] and the Council on Ethics and judicial affairs of the American Medical Association. I emphasize that, in my opinion, the easing of the death event is distinct from euthanasia or assisted suicide.

One of the most emotionally traumatic scenarios in medicine arises when family, nurses and physicians disagree about resuscitation plans for a patient, with a resulting paralysis of that action that may seem so rational to the physician. It is often more difficult to refrain from initiation of resuscitative efforts, than to discontinue them after a trial period.

While the successes in resuscitation from cardiac arrest and the quality of life in those saved, is approximately equal in the junior elderly, age 65 to 75, to that of young subjects, the data for those over 80, though better within the hospital, present a dismal picture,[40-43] and this is discussed by Podrid in another chapter. The advice and cooperation of the listed "health care proxy" is invaluable under these circumstances. How the physician behaves when the "person-hood" he or she knew as his or her patient, has disappeared, with only a somatic shell remaining, will reflect his personal philosophy. The physician may well benefit from listening to the reasoning of the professional ethicist but not necessarily be completely servile to him or her. Representatives from any profession may have developed strong convictions, dispelling humility and leading to autocratic paternalism or maternalism.

Ethics of Surgery in the Elderly
'Cardiac'

Details of the surgical treatment in the aged are given in other chapters. I am in complete agreement with the frequent assertion that "age is never a contraindication to surgery." Yes, but age, particularly near its upper limit, has brought deterioration in many organ systems, and this may be a valid contraindication. Equally important in the decision process, that takes into account the increased risk of operation, should be a consideration that the betterment in the quality of life in survivors may be disappointing. There is an old adage, "the surgeon should not hurry the hand of God." Courage is not enough, on the part of the surgeon or patient. While the principle of autonomy mandates that the patient make the decision; in practice, the doctor dominates. Overtly, surgery as a "way out" of a perilous terminal state cannot be condoned.

It is germane to emphasize that the results of aortic valve surgery in the elderly have generally been excellent. This is true also for coronary bypass surgery and angioplasty in well-selected cases. Usually, patients in their 60s can be expected to be good risks equivalent to those in younger decades, those in their 80s and 90s give more concern. As general examples, I would be aggressive in the recommendation for surgery for a proximal aortic dissection, with extensive distal involvement, or for a rupture of the ventricular septum with acute myocardial infarction, in persons of 65, but much less likely to be so in one of 85. Heart disease is a risk factor for noncardiac surgery and the markers for that risk have been elaborated upon in another chapter.

The physician's "ethics" require an intimate knowledge of the institution's capabilities and that he or she present them fairly to the patient and the relatives. Decisions to refer patients to another institution are often difficult. The physician's quasi-acceptance of an alternate or "complemental care" wished for by a patient and/or relatives is quasi-ethical. The moral responsibility in obtaining consent for a surgical procedure is better met by the sincerity of the process than simply obtaining a signature on a piece of paper. In countries other than the United States, "autonomy" and "informed consent" seem to be not prominent in the desideratum of practice: it has been argued in a case appealed to the House of Lords, that Britain cannot afford "the American informed consent rule" with its National Health Service.[44] The English psychiatrist Jones[45] also states that there are differences between the legal concept of consent in the United Kingdom and the United States; English law recognizing only "real consent." If true, this generates a seeming paradox; the English physician plays the dominant role, while in the United States the onus is more on the patient to make his or her decision.

Euthanasia

Euthanasia is defined in 2 ways: easing a patient's death or actively causing death in an ill or crippled subject. A century ago, physicians acted in concert with the first definition, for instance Munk whose book in 1897 was entitled *Euthanasia of Medical Treatment in Aid of an Easy Death* endorsing the value of love, opium, and brandy. The recommendations therein were endorsed by Osler. Euthanasia has in large part earned its bad name from an identification with what has been called social Darwinism, the survival of the socially most fit, often inviting a political decision to cull out from a population the designated unfit: "lives not worth the living." The outstanding, never-to-be-forgotten example, the Holocaust, occurred in Germany under Hitler, with a planned systematic extermination of Jews and Gypsies, initiated by the killing of imbeciles. This was frank genocide, a devilish variety of active involuntary homicide, engendered by a racial hygiene cult, masquerading as under the name of euthanasia.

Although there have been objections to the classification of euthanasia into the "active" and "passive," there is pragmatic value in it (as well as a potential entrance to an abyss of uncertainties). The contrast is between a positive killing procedure contrasted with withholding somatic supportive therapy. In reality, for the physician, an aid to the dying process is not truly euthanasia. For the incompetent patient, the guidelines have been given. For the elderly competent subject, weary of life and wishing relief from physical and mental discomfort, physicians sometimes have acceded to the patient's wish for help in such escape. Despite strong arguments advanced in support of such collaboration, and of its occurrence (the most publicized being in the Netherlands), many physicians, myself included, would be uncomfortable playing a co-conspirator role in a homicidal event, (labeled so even in the Netherlands where the practice seems tolerated).[46,47] The medical profession of the world may best regard The Netherlands' practice as exploratory, willing to wait later analyses before emulating it. Another act called "assisted suicide," whereby for example, physicians may hasten the end is by prescribing more sedative than immediately needed. Sometimes they may even have included an opinion of the probably lethal dosage. I believe the physician could become morally supportive of such an act, but should not participate in the act directly, a course of action deemed ethical by the ethicist-chaplain, Ernle Young.[48] In a recent confession, one doctor[49] mentioned to his patient a way of obtaining informational material from the Hemlock Society (an organization espousing the propriety of suicide, when the burdens and discomforts are assessed as intolerable and this judgment having been arrived at in a methodical careful way).

This doctor, Quill, has been a cautious witness before the US Supreme Court in support of the principle of a physician legally helping a patient to commit suicide. Quill recently has recorded his views and experience in a full length text (1997). The brash proponent and implementor of the procedure, Kevorkian, has become notorious. Some medical editors have suggested a hero status for him, but not in my book. Kevorkian continues to be an aggressive activist in his cause particularly via the lay press.

The meaning of the term assisted suicide may appear clear, but ambiguity and complexity are quickly revealed in any discussion. Indeed, a strict grammarian might deny its existence; a dreamy sociologist might assert all suicides are assisted and an ambivalent philosopher might claim that Socrates' death was not truly a suicide, because of the coercion and the choice that faced him. The aversion to physician assisted suicide relates to the traditional belief that the physician's role is to heal, relieve suffering but not to kill. Arguments favoring the act have focused mainly on the assertion that the patient had a constitutional right, the "liberty" to have it, for help in self-destruction. The Supreme Court justices, in what I would regard as "common sense" opinions denied such a "right," or the constitutionality of any law enacted by a state legalizing such a procedure. However, they seemed unanimous in their support of palliation therapy in end stage therapy. Since the June 1997 decision of the US Supreme Court, innumerable articles have appeared in the lay press, professional journals, and brochures of varied groups with the objective of clarifying its legal and social significance. One article that I think may be particularly helpful in the legal interrelations to the physician is that by Annas entitled "The Bell Tolls for a Constitutional Right to Physician Assisted Suicide."[48a*]

Euthanasia and suicide have long troubled the profound thinkers of the world. Contemporary differing opinions were expressed at a recent international colloquy, entitled "Dying Well," and reports of the meeting appeared in a special issue of the *Hastings Center Report* (March-April 1992) the Dutch and German practices were analyzed. The director of the Hastings Center, Daniel Callahan, argued strongly

---

* *U.S. Law Week,* June 24, 1997.

against the physician assisting suicide, reflected in the choice of his title "When Self-Determination Runs Amok." Society, not physicians, will eventually determine the practice. There will be increasing acrimony in debates with legal arguments to be expected in this area, with patients preparing advanced directives regarding their desires. Numerous surveys have indicated that a large number of patients have felt deserted by their physicians in their terminal days. Perhaps Bernard Shaw was prescient when entering the opinion in his preface to the *Doctor's Dilemma:* "The theory that every individual alive is of infinite value is *legislatively* impracticable." One should proceed on the principle that invalids, meaning persons who cannot keep themselves alive by their own activities, cannot beyond reason, expect to be kept alive by the activity of others. I wish that some segments of the world's cultures were more tolerant of the suicidal act in the elderly and would not be ashamed or regard it as a stain on the family escutcheon. Over the ages, suicide may have been regarded as either a cowardly or a heroic act, depending on the circumstances. The giving of one's life for child or friend has been generally praised, and the act of Sidney Carter in Dickens' *A Tale of Two Cities,* is a fictional example.

Currently, the law courts seem unpredictable regarding labeling of acts terminating a life labeled as euthanasia. A modest proponent Fletcher[50] asserts that a solution to the suicide-euthanasia problem might reside in decriminalized euthanasia. "If I were myself to formulate a solution of the suicide-euthanasia problem in succinct terms, I would say that just as we have decriminalized suicide we ought to decriminalize euthanasia" I believe each case requires individual attention. As a guiding principle I am empathetic with Fletcher's view, but strongly disagree with his recommendations. One must remember that while the quality of life is largely intrinsic, dependent on the patient's health, the extrinsic factor of how society and a family treat the problem overtly affects the quality of life.

The phrase "dying with dignity" might be emblazoned on a banner under which most, if not all, of us would gather. Our journals are inundated with articles with this title. As a cause of the brain-dead, or the vegetative state, a sudden, unexpected cardiac arrest has been a frequent initiating event. This known hazard underlies the expressed wish of some elderly persons not to have resuscitation from a "natural death" of cardiac origin.

In the maintenance of life, a cardiac pacemaker may play an essential role. In rare instances, when a temporary one has been used, but the quality of what life remains is pathetic, turning it off is clearly indicated. This is an unusual problem compared to the numbers of patients where respiratory support, special alimentation or renal dialysis may require a decision for their cessation.

The Postmortem

In the last few decades, there has been a marked decrease in the number of postmortems performed, particularly in the elderly. This has been in large part explained by the number and accuracy of diagnostic tests now available to the physician, which have established the presence of a fatal disease. Autopsies on elderly bodies do sometimes reveal clinically undiagnosed disease, some of which, if known, would have altered therapy.[51] If there is a sudden, unattended, unexpected death, the patient's physician is expected to notify the coroner (or medical examiner) who can sign the death certificate. If the physician has known the patient well, and is confident of the diagnosis of heart disease, he, or she, may well be justified in signing the certificate, without (regrettably) seeking consent for a postmortem. The physician may be placed in a quandary, just how to list the cause of death when, for example, a supposed routine postmortem examination on a victim of heart failure, included drug screening that revealed suggestive fatal quantities of digoxin. Some physicians have confided to me that their fear of medico-legal actions, had influenced their decision not routinely aggressively to request a postmortem examination, for fear that the examination might reveal conditions not suspected during life. However in my experience, the testimony of the pathologist based on postmortem findings generally has been supportive of the physician's decisions and satisfying to the deceaseds' relatives. A potential ethical dilemma does exist that could have unfortunate consequences on teaching: Osler's dictum still has validity "As is our pathology, so is our practice."[52]

Clinical Trials

In popular parlance, randomized clinical trials are "the current rage," and their ethical content may not always have had the depth of study reviewing panels should have demanded. There is always the obvious question how well investigators may have complied with the "informed consent" requirement, particularly in quasi-competent subjects, perhaps, for instance, in a nursing home population. In one small sampling of a myocardial infarction trial,[53] about half of the subjects later could not recall the details of their consent forms. Interestingly, patients over the age of 75 years had been excluded from that study. In many trials of therapeutic regimens projected to last over some years, the very elderly have been arbitrarily excluded, presumably because of concern over noncompliance, the frequency of confounding items, and the steepness of the normal mortality curve in this age group. Many of the elderly may also have anxiety and suspicions, if not a little paranoia, about being the subject of an "experiment," or being "guinea pigs." Despite these drawbacks, the elderly are deserving of being participants in therapeutic trials when management dilemmas are present.[54]

In general, I am content that most large publicized trials have had adequate surveillance by ethicists. But constant vigilance in asking questions is a virtue. An ethical problem, not infrequently encountered, in a proper "blinded" randomized trial, is when to declare a statistical difference between treated and placebo groups and stop the trial[55]; to carry on could be considered unethical despite the strong wish to obtain data, that would be convincing to the rankest skeptic. When differences are marginal and confounding factors present, statistical analyses are difficult and the old bogey of "clinical significance," contrasted with "statistical significance" often arises and its credence respected. "Informed" consent, autonomy of the patient, and a collective professional equipoise regarding different arms of the treatment protocol form the basis for an ethical trial.

Although he makes the answer sound easy, Claude Bernard's dictum over a century ago, is pertinent[56]: "For we must not deceive ourselves, morals do not forbid making experiments on one's neighbors or on oneself, in everyday life men do nothing but experiment upon one another. Christian morals forbid only one thing, doing ill to one's neighbor. So among experiments to be tried on man, those that can do only harm are forbidden, those that are innocent are permissible, those that can do good, obligatory." Overtly, Bernard's manifesto is the epitome of socialistic paternalism. Another frequently encountered quotation from his work is "The principle of medical and surgical morality consists in never performing on man an experiment that might be harmful to him to any extent even though the result might be highly advantageous to science, that is the health of others." Clinical investigators cannot expect the luxury of assuming a subject's consent in their investigations particularly when the subject will not be directly benefited. They will, perforce, be knowledgeable of the Nuremberg and Helsinki codes of conduct and in the United States, of the guidelines regarding the use of human volunteers, from the National Institutes of Health.

Rationing of Health Measures

The principle of rationing has a very long history, exemplified in recent centuries, by the rule in a shipwreck, women and children "first" for the available lifeboats, or the custom in famine, the priority given to children for any food in the country. When the need surpasses supply there is the necessity of selection of those to be given the therapeutic item. In a catastrophic event with many casualties, triage must be practiced, so that the greatest benefits to the greatest number may be achieved. When rapid technological advances occur, the number of life-saving devices may be greatly exceeded by the number of suitable candidates, for example the story of the respirator (the iron lung) for respiratory paralysis in victims of poliomyelitis. Dialysis for end-stage renal failure is an even greater problem, with the actual escalating costs to the public health system becoming a prominent factor. A recent entrant to this technology requirement is that of the implantable antiarrhythmic devices. These problems have been historically ably outlined by Rothman in his book. *Beginnings Count* (1997).

Physicians may often opt to close their eyes to the reality of needed rationing of some items of medical care. An understandable attitude is: "we can show you what we can do; others in the society can supply the money *or* declare its unavailability." However, there are limits that the citizen MD would recognize, for example, in the transplantation of organs and renal dialysis. There are not enough donor organs, nor will there be in the future, and a societal discrimination against the very elderly, creates no ethical problem for me. It is doubtful whether such medical consensus could ever be attained and a rigid policy would be inimical to the treasured doctor-patient relationship.[57] Very intensive studies have been carried out on the quality of life in patients undergoing renal dialysis and the sometimes decision underlying the stopping of the dialysis, is often made by the patient. One occasionally encounters elderly nursing home occupants, who very passively continue on dialysis despite what seems a poor quality of life and it seems that maybe no one has the courage, or think it ethical to stop it. The definition of what rationing entails that has had much publicity and debate is that established in the State of Oregon in the Oregon list of Health Services.[58]

When there is discrimination against the elderly, there would be a gender difference in the numbers of men and women excluded from a possible therapy, as there are more women older than 75 years of age than men. Such an event has been regarded as a gender discrimination[59] and, although secondary to the age discrimination, planners should be aware that such a result might engender, unjustly, charges of unfairness.

The physician has a dual role, not only to care for, and support the autonomy (self determination) of, his patients but also to society by influencing the rational allocation of society's finite resources. The latter is an issue that may not be readily solved by government edict or private enterprise. When, and how to limit or stop treatment, deciding on the most cost-effective investigation or treatment and avoiding the use of inappropriate high technology, are complex issues that span the whole field of geriatric medicine and will be agonized over because they have a profound effect on the nation's resources. In this regard, the development of the implantable defibrillator, for which many elderly patients will be candidates, has the potential of bankrupting the fiscal medical system. In this task of apportioning resources, the clinically experienced, benevolent physician should be better oriented than government agencies, professional ethicists, and philosophers to guide the decisions that will benefit his particular patient and society as a whole. Regrettably, many of us in the profession have not had the interest or capability to enter this turbulent revolutionary field. Carleton Chapman[60] from his background of a career in clinical investigation and medical education has also analyzed the changing position of the physician relative to the law and the ethicist. He acridly opines that "two millennia of mistaken emphasis (by the medical profession) is surely enough. "Medicine at long last (may) be approaching ethical maturity if one defines maturity in terms of placing the patient before the brotherhood or guild." I laud his scholarship and respect his opinion, but believe he overstates his case.

Ethical dilemmas will remain. Should a physician ever support an educational movement based on a justice principle, wherein the aging population was encouraged to reject the notion that they have rights to unlimited dollars and to equal access to scarce technology?[61] I submit that morally, the primary care physician, might well be a passive supporter for such a view, but should not be an activist in any movement to establish it; his duty is to his patient.

Some patients with a Judeo-Christian background may have found solace in psalmists' song that "the days of our years are three score years and ten."[62] Many biologists now think this might be projected to 4 score years and 10 as an ideal. The admonition in the psalm: "So teach us to number our days that we may apply our hearts unto wisdom" remains. When a physician has struggled with a hard decision regarding a patient's care, it has been alluded to as "playing God." While this has underscored the gravity of the act, it has become a trite remark and I think inappropriate, a judgment to which I believe Young[48] would agree.

A concluding plea to my fellow physicians; one needs to listen to the counsel of the legal profession, to be exposed to the convictions of the professional ethicists, to be guided by the ideals of religious leaders, and to conform, if possible, to the wishes of relatives, but not to take a back seat in the judgment process. Overtly, the autonomy of the patient should dominate the final process in the decision, however, there are worrisome illusions in any acceptance of this, in reality. The challenge has been thrown out, "philosophers do not belong at the bedside"[63]; in such a pedagogic debate, I would choose the opposition; that they should see the patient and the relatives, sharing the burden and perplexities. Compliance with the law is primal; however, its interpretation and application are open to appeal. In the United States, when our courts have disagreed among themselves, and the Supreme Court justices are divided on critical issues, the study of dissenting opinions is worthwhile, and we can temporarily accept our differences or when so motivated, work for changes.

Practicing physicians may be overwhelmed by the mass of philosophic theory, but regain their confidence when, eschewing self referral traps, returns to the care of the patient. As counselor to the patient, sometimes family friend, and not always a stranger at the bedside, the physician may justly claim to be the best director of the patient's management, but never again in quite the same traditional authoritarian way.

Acknowledgment

The author is deeply appreciative of the encouragement and suggestions of the editor of this volume, Elliot Chesler, in the writing of this chapter. The endeavor has turned out to be my vision of the optimal care of the patient and the advancement of scientific medicine and not, it is realized any penetrating analysis of bioethical teaching. Overtly too, it was impossible to mention all the worthy contributors to the subject.

References

1. Bernard C; Greene HM, trans.: *An Introduction to the Study of Experimental Medicine 1865.* Henry Schuman, 1949, p 221.
2. Leake C: *Percival's Medical Ethics.* New York, NY, Krieger Publishing Co., 1975.
3. Starr P: *Social Transformation of American Medicine.* New York, NY, Basic Books, 1949.
4. Morreim EH: Gaming the system. Dodging the rules, ruling the dodgers. *Arch Intern Med* 151:443–447, 1991.
5. Reiser SJ: *Medicine and the Reign of Technology.* New York, Cambridge University Press, 1978.
6. Thomas L: *The Technology of Medicine—The Lives of a Cell Notes of a Biology Watcher* New York, Bantam Books, 1974, pp 35–42.
7. Kjellstrand CM: *Giving Life—Giving Death. Ethical Problems of High Technology Medicine.* Stockholm, 1988, Thesis.
8. Chinard FP: Ethics and technology. *J Med Soc New Jersey* 82:119–123, 1985.
9. Coombs RH, Aulson MJ: Is Pre-medical education dehumanizing? A literature review. *J Med Humanities* 11:13–22, 1990.
10. Rothman D: *Strangers at the Bedside. A History of How Law and Bioethics Transformed Medical Decision Making.* New York, NY, Basic Books, 1991.
11. Osler W: *Quoted from Cushing—Life of Sir William Osler.* London, Oxford University Press, 1940, p 269.
12. Leake C: Preface. In: Percival's Medical Ethics. New York, NY, Krieger Publishing Co., 1975.
13. Richards D: The first aphorism of Hippocrates. In: *Medical Priesthoods and Other Essays.* Private Printing, 1970, p 23.
14. Thompson IE: The implications of medical ethics *J Med Ethics* 2:74–82, 1976.
15. Rosen B, Caplan A: *Ethics in the Undergraduate Curriculum. The Teaching of Ethics.* Hastings-on-Hudson, NY, Hastings Institute, 1980.
16. Pellegrino ED, et al: Relevance and utility of Courses in medical ethics. *JAMA* 253:49–53, 1985.
17. Dartmouth Conference Report: Basic Curricular Goals in Medical Ethics. *New Engl J Med* 312:253–356, 1983.
18. American Geriatrics Society: Curriculum guidelines on the care of the elderly for internal medicine residency training programs. *Am J Med* 91: 449–452, 1991.
19. Englehardt HT: Medical ethics for the 21st century. *J Am Coll Cardiol* 257:303–307, 1991.
20. Radwany SM, Adelson BH: The use of literary classics in teaching medical ethics to physicians. *JAMA* 257:1629–1631, 1987.
21. Rodin AE, Key JD: Humanizing medicine through literary medical eponyms. *Houston Med* 6:181–185, 1990.

22. Kubler-Ross E: *One Death and Dying.* London, Tavistock, 1970.
23. Elford JR, ed. *Medical Ethics and the Elderly People.* Edinburgh Churchill Livingstone, 1987.
24. Cassel CK: Ethical problems in geriatric medicine. In: Cassel CK, Riesenberg DE, Sorenson LB, Walsh JR, eds. *Geriatric Medicine.* Springer Verlag. (2nd Ed.) 1990, pp 14–90.
25. Katz J: *Judges, Physicians and Patients in the Silent World of Physician and Patient.* New York, NY, The Free Press, 1984.
26. Meisel A, Kuezewski M: Legal and ethical myths about informed consent. *Arch Intern Med* 156:2551–2556, 1996.
27. Miles SH: Informed demand for non-beneficial medical treatment. (Editorial Comment: Angell M). *N Engl J Med* 325:512–515, 1991.
28. Guidelines for the determination of death. *JAMA* 246:2184, 1981.
29. Veatch RM: Defining death anew. Technical and ethical problems. In: Weir RF, (ed). *Ethical Issues in Death and Dying.* New York, NY Columbia University Press, (1986).
30. Annas GJ: Sounding board: Nancy Cruzan and the right to die. *N Engl J Med* 323:670–672, 1990.
31. Lo B, Steinbrook R: Beyond the Cruzan case: The US Supreme Court and Medical Practice. *Ann Intern Med* 114:895–901, 1991.
32. Annas GJ: The health care proxy and the living will. *N Engl J Med* 324: 210–213, 1991.
33. Multi-disciplinary group (Special Report): Sources of concern about the Patient Self-determination Act. *N Engl J Med* 325:1666–1671, 1991.
34. Miles SH, August A: Courts, gender and "the right to die" law. *Med Health Care* 18:85–93, 1991.
35. Emmanuel LL. Advance directions for patient care—A case for greater use. *N Engl J Med* 324:889–895, 1991.
36. Gamble ER, McDonald PJ, Lichstein PR: Knowledge, attitudes, and behavior of elderly persons regarding living wills. *Arch Intern Med* 151:277–280, 1991.
37. Osler W. Letter to the Editor of *The Spectator* (Nov 4 1911) Reproduced in Cushing H. *The Life of Sir William Osler.* London, Oxford University Press, London, 1940. (Thomas Fuller - The Holy State and the Profane State. Tegg London, 1841).
38. Dagi TF: Letting and making death happen—Is there a difference? The problem of moral linkage. *J Med Humanities* 11:81–82, 1990.
39. American Thoracic Society Bioethics Task Force: *Position paper: Withholding and withdrawing life sustaining therapy. Ann Intern Med* 115:478–483, 1991.
40. Gulati RS, Bhan GL, Horan MA: Cardiopulmonary resuscitation in old people. *Lancet* II:267–269, 1983.
41. Murphy DS, Murray AM, Robinson BF, et al: Outcomes of cardiopulmonary resuscitation in the elderly. *Ann Intern Med* 111:199–205, 1989.
42. Longstreth WT, Cobb LA, Fahrenbruch CE, et al. Does age affect outcomes of out-of-hospital cardiopulmonary resuscitation. *JAMA* 264:2109–2110, 1990.
43. Tresch DD: CPR in the elderly: When should it be performed? *Geriatrics* 46:47–59, 1991.
44. Schwartz R, Srubb A: Why Britain can't afford informed consent. *Hastings Cent Rep* 15:19–25, 1985.
45. Jones RW: Problems in senile dementia. In ER Elforo, (ed). *Medical ethics and Elderly People.* Edinburg, Churchill Livingstone, 1987, pp 49–67.

46. de Wachter NAM: Active euthanasia in The Netherlands. *JAMA* 262:3316, 1989.
47. Battin MP: Seven caveats concerning the discussion of euthanasia in Holland. *Perspect Biol Med* 34:73–77, 1990.
48. Young EWD: Alpha and omega. Ethics at the frontiers of life and death Chapter 10, Assisted Suicide. The Portable Stanford, Stanford Alumni Association, Stanford, CA. 1988.
48a. Annas, GJ: The bell tolls for a constitutional right to physician-assisted suicide. *N Engl J Med* 337:1098, 1997.
49. Quill TE: Death and dignity. A case of individualized decision making. *New Engl J Med* 324:691–694, 1991.
50. Fletcher J: The courts and euthanasia. Law medicine and public health. *Law Med Health Care* 15:223–2350, 1987/1988.
51. Butler RN: Autopsy: the final peer review. *Geriatrics* 46:11–12, 1991.
52. Osler W: Treatment of disease. *B Med Jnl (Toronto)* 42:896–913, 1909.
53. Okene IS: The Consent Process in the thrombolysis in Myocardial Infarction. TIMI (Phase 1) Trial. *Clin Res* 39:13–17, 1991.
54. Sacks GA, Cassel CK. Biomedical research. Involving older human subjects. *Law Health Care* 18(3):234–243, 1990.
55. Browner WS: Ethics, statistics and technology assessment. The use of a stopping rule and an independent policy and data monitoring board in a cohort study of perioperative cardiac morbidity. *Clin Res* 39:7–11, 1991.
56. Bernard C, Greene HM, trans.: *Introduction to the Study of Experimental Medicine.* (1865). Henry Schuman, 1949, p 102.
57. Hunt RW: A critique of using age to ration health care. *J Med Ethics* 19: 19–23, 1993.
58. Fox DM: The ups and downs of Oregon's rationing plan. *Health Affairs* 12: 66–70, 1993.
59. Jecker NS: Age-based rationing and women. *JAMA* 266:3012–3015, 1991.
60. Chapman CB: *Physicians, Laws and Ethics.* New York, NY, New York University Press, 1984, p 147.
61. Hartwig J: Is there a duty to die. *Hastings Cent Rep* 27:34–42, March April 1997.
62. Knight JA: Ethics in the Caring for the Elderly. *J South Med Assoc* 87: 909–917, 1944.
63. Sullivan P: Philosophers have no place at bedside, physician-lawyer maintains. *Can Med Assoc J* 140:1195–1196, 1989.

Index